Autoimmune Diseases: A Pathophysiological Approach

Autoimmune Diseases: A Pathophysiological Approach

Edited by Dallas Lynch

hayle medical
New York

Hayle Medical,
750 Third Avenue, 9th Floor,
New York, NY 10017, USA

Visit us on the World Wide Web at:
www.haylemedical.com

ISBN: 978-1-63241-587-5

Printed in China.

Cataloging-in-Publication Data

Autoimmune diseases : a pathophysiological approach / edited by Dallas Lynch.
p. cm.
Includes bibliographical references and index.
ISBN 978-1-63241-587-5
1. Autoimmune diseases. 2. Physiology, Pathological. 3. Immunologic diseases. I. Lynch, Dallas.
RC600 .A98 2019
616.978--dc23

Table of Contents

Preface

This book has been a concerted effort by a group of academicians, researchers and scientists, who have contributed their research works for the realization of the book. This book has materialized in the wake of emerging advancements and innovations in this field. Therefore, the need of the hour was to compile all the required researches and disseminate the knowledge to a broad spectrum of people comprising of students, researchers and specialists of the field.

Autoimmune disease is the clinical condition that arises due to an abnormal immune response to a body part. There are around 80 different kinds of autoimmune diseases. Certain common autoimmune diseases are diabetes mellitus type 1, psoriasis, rheumatoid arthritis, multiple sclerosis, etc. The diagnosis of an autoimmune disease can be difficult to determine and depends on the type of the condition or its severity. Autoimmune diseases may have certain pathological effects such as damage or destruction of tissues and altered organ function or organ growth. They may evolve into chronic, debilitating and even life-threatening conditions in some cases. The treatment of an autoimmune disease generally targets the symptoms rather than the disease itself as the causative factor is still not defined. Immunosuppressants, nonsteroidal anti-inflammatory drugs (NSAIDs) and intravenous immunoglobulin are commonly used for treatment. This book explores all the important aspects of autoimmune diseases in modern day healthcare. It strives to provide a fair idea about the diagnosis and treatment of autoimmune diseases and to help develop a better understanding of the latest advances in this area. This book will serve as a reference to a broad spectrum of readers.

At the end of the preface, I would like to thank the authors for their brilliant chapters and the publisher for guiding us all-through the making of the book till its final stage. Also, I would like to thank my family for providing the support and encouragement throughout my academic career and research projects.

Editor

1

Autoimmunity and the Gut

Andrew W. Campbell

The Wellness Center, 23144 Emerson Way, Land O Lakes, FL 34639, USA

Correspondence should be addressed to Andrew W. Campbell; immunedoctor@gmail.com

Academic Editor: Aristo Vojdani

Autoimmune diseases have increased dramatically worldwide since World War II. This is coincidental with the increased production and use of chemicals both in industrial countries and agriculture, as well as the ease of travel from region to region and continent to continent, making the transfer of a pathogen or pathogens from one part of the world to another much easier than ever before. In this review, triggers of autoimmunity are examined, principally environmental. The number of possible environmental triggers is vast and includes chemicals, bacteria, viruses, and molds. Examples of these triggers are given and include the mechanism of action and method by which they bring about autoimmunity.

1. Introduction

Autoimmune diseases have registered an alarming increase worldwide since the end of the Second World War. This pandemic includes more than 80 autoimmune disorders and increases in both the incidence and prevalence of autoimmune disorders such as Crohn's disease, rheumatoid arthritis, multiple sclerosis, and type I diabetes [1, 2]. In the United States, it is far more commonly found in women and is one of the top 10 leading causes of death in female children and women of all age groups. The National Institutes of Health (NIH) estimates that 23.5 million Americans have an autoimmune disease. In contrast, cancer affects 13 million Americans. Symptoms involve many medical specialties and can affect all body organs (http://www.aarda.org/autoimmune-information-statistics/).

Genetic predisposition, environmental factors (including infections), and gut dysbiosis play major roles in the development of autoimmune diseases (Figure 1). Autoimmunity develops over time, and preclinical autoimmunity precedes clinical disease by many years and can be detected in the peripheral blood in the form of circulating autoantibodies [3]. Initially, symptoms of autoimmune disorders are vague and include fatigue, low-grade fever, muscle and joint aches, and malaise. They usually progress and become debilitating with significant morbidity. Patients are often seen by physicians only after their disease process has become symptomatic, clouding the understanding of the early events leading to disease. The clinician familiar with triggers for autoimmunity can order the right combination of laboratory analyses necessary to elucidate the type and stage of the patient's autoimmune reaction. This in some cases may help the clinician initiate preventive therapies aimed at removing the offending triggers and thereby reverse the progression of the autoimmune disorder with the possibility of eliminating the autoimmune disease.

2. Genetics

There are genetic variants that predispose humans to multiple autoimmune diseases and, secondly, multiple genes predispose humans to each disease. The major histocompatibility complex (MHC) is central in mediating inflammatory responses to pathogens. The unique coding or noncoding genetic variations of HLA alleles determine the antigenic responses to self- or non-self-antigens [4]. One of the most common genetic associations with autoimmune disorders is the protein tyrosine phosphatase gene PTPN22 expressed in lymphocytes. The tryptophan allele within PTPN22 has been found in patients with many autoimmune disorders, including type 1 diabetes mellitus, rheumatoid arthritis (RA),

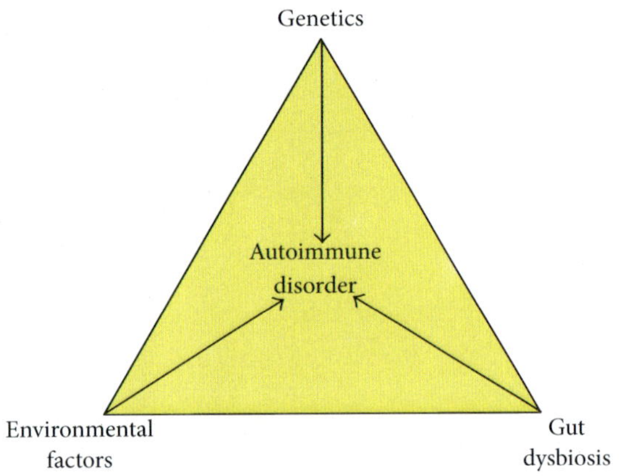

FIGURE 1: The triangle of autoimmune triggers. Gut dysbiosis and genetic and environmental factors play major roles in the development of autoimmune diseases.

systemic lupus erythematosus (SLE), and autoimmune thyroiditis [5, 6]. Cytokines and cytokine receptors are also associated with autoimmune disorders, as can be seen in IL-12/IL-23 pathway in inflammatory bowel disease (IBD), ankylosing spondylitis, and psoriasis [6]. Tumor necrosis factor (TNF) has been linked with autoimmune disorders, notably the TNF-inducible protein A20, which has been associated with RA, psoriasis, and SLE [7]. The importance of CD40 in the maintenance of effector T cell populations in autoimmune diseases has been described in recent studies. Patients with type 1 diabetes (T1D) have increased $CD4^{lo}CD40^{+}$ T cells in peripheral blood compared with T2D patients or healthy controls [8]. A polymorphism of CD40 that enhances CD40 signaling is common in patients of Mexican and South American descent; these two groups are known to have increased severity of SLE [9]. In celiac disease (CD), 95% of patients possess the HLA DQ gene; in RA, the HLA variants are DR genes.

There is familial clustering in some autoimmune diseases, suggesting common genetic, developmental, and environmental factors. This has been demonstrated in twin studies with higher disease concordance in monozygotic twins as compared to dizygotic twins. A large population-based survey revealed patients with multiple sclerosis (MS) or rheumatoid arthritis (RA) were more likely to have other autoimmune diseases [10, 11]. However, this concordance rate is only 10–40% for most autoimmune diseases, indicating environmental factors as playing a major role [12].

3. Environmental Factors

There are a host of environmental factors that trigger autoimmune disorders, including chemical toxicants, heavy metals, viruses, bacteria, emotional stress, and drugs. For example, adjuvants, such as aluminum hydroxide used in vaccines and medical silicones used in breast implants, can cause an autoimmune disorder known as Shoenfeld's syndrome [13]. A recent study published in the journal Apoptosis demonstrates that hepatitis B vaccine causes liver cell destruction in Hepal-6 cells. This cell death is attributed to the use of the adjuvant aluminum hydroxide, increasingly identified as a contributing cause of autoimmune disease in immunized patients [14]. Studies show that hepatitis C is almost indistinguishable from autoimmune hepatitis based on biochemical and clinical features. Autoantibodies detected in patients with autoimmune hepatitis are also frequently found in patients with hepatitis C, and both groups of patients suffer from the same immune-mediated symptoms and diseases with chronic hepatitis C [15]. Indeed, 40–70% of patients suffering from hepatitis C also develop at least one extrahepatic inflammatory disorders, including arthritis, vasculitis, and sicca syndrome [16].

Women with silicone breast implants frequently fulfill the diagnostic criteria for autoimmune syndrome induced by adjuvants, known as autoimmune syndrome induced by adjuvants (ASIA). Although the exact mechanism is not known, medical silicones in breast implants are associated with systemic lupus erythematosus, rheumatoid arthritis, vasculitis, and progressive systemic sclerosis [17, 18].

Smoking is a known risk for RA and recent studies have demonstrated that cigarette smoking may induce citrullination of proteins in pulmonary alveolar cells. This is an important finding because antibodies to citrullinated peptides are highly specific for RA as are the HLA associations that are related to the development of these autoantibodies [19, 20].

Infectious agents, including bacteria, viruses, fungi, and parasites, are also known to trigger autoimmune disorders through several mechanisms: molecular mimicry, epitope spreading, standard activation, viral persistence, polyclonal activation, dysregulation of immune homeostasis, and autoinflammatory activation of innate immunity. It is important to note that an infection may not necessarily be the inducer but rather the total burden of infections from childhood on that trigger autoimmunity [21]. Moreover, an infection can amplify an autoimmune disease by either exacerbating an ongoing disorder, including a relapse, or by leading to chronic progressive disease [22].

An example of infectious agents associated with autoimmune disorders is the link between dysregulation of Epstein-Barr virus (EBV) with the occurrence of systemic autoimmune diseases (SADS), a group of connective tissue diseases, including systemic lupus erythematosus (SLE), rheumatoid arthritis (RA), Sjogren's syndrome (SS), and mixed connective tissue disease (MCTD), with overlapping symptoms and antibody development. EBV is an omnipresent infectious virus, affecting approximately 95% of the world's population [23]. It is a DNA virus of the herpes family transmitted in saliva and initially infects epithelial cells in the oro- and nasopharynx. Afterwards, EBV enters the underlying tissues and infects B-cells [24]. In childhood, EBV causes a mild asymptomatic infection; in adolescents, it causes infectious mononucleosis (IM) in 30–70% of cases, and up to 20% of B-cells are infected with EBV [25]. After the first lytic infection, EBV persists in resting memory B-cells for the rest of the patient's life and can switch between an active lytic cycle and a latent state from which it occasionally reactivates, making it a continuous challenge to the patient's immune system [26].

Patients with SLE have an elevated viral load in the peripheral blood mononuclear cells (PBMCs) compared to healthy controls, anywhere from 10 to 40 times higher. The viral load is coupled with disease activity and unrelated to any immunosuppressive medication. A study found an elevated EBV DNA in the serum in 42% of patients compared with 3% of healthy controls [27–29]. Lastly, elevated levels of IgA antibodies to early antigen diffuse (EA/D) were found in 58% of SLE patients versus healthy controls and unrelated to immunosuppressive medication, demonstrating that the antibodies were not due to reactivation of EBV due to a suppressed immune system from medications [30].

In patients with RA, EBV DNA/RNA has been found in PBMCs in saliva, synovial fluid, and synovial membranes, as well as a 10-fold higher frequency of EBC-infected B-cells than in healthy controls [31–33]. This demonstrates widespread lytic EBV infection in RA patients that is also localized in the joints, signifying EBV-infected cells in the synovial inflammation that is characteristic of RA patients [34].

EBV infection has also been demonstrated in SS patients, with EBV-directed antibodies and increased viral load [35, 36]. Patients with SS also have a higher risk for EBV-associated lymphomas [37]. Elevated levels of antibodies to EBNA, VCA, and EA have been found in the serum of SS patients [38, 39]. One study showed IgG antibodies to EA/D in 36% of SS patients compared to 4.5% of healthy controls; these antibodies were not associated with immunosuppressive medication [40].

In conclusion, EBV infection is an example of one of the causal environmental factors in autoimmune disorders. As discussed above, EBV infection can lead to SADS as it can persist in the patient as a latent infection that can occasionally reactivate and cause flares as seen in chronic SADS and other autoimmune disorders.

4. Mucosal Immunity

The diet of humans has changed dramatically since the Second World War, especially in industrialized countries and in urban areas. For thousands of generations, humans ate food shortly after harvesting and when it was in season. Meat was occasionally consumed and much of it was caught in the wild. In the past 50 or so years, our foods have undergone a considerable transformation. We have developed new strains of grains, especially in wheat, rice, soy, and corn. In the United States, we use more genetically modified crops than the rest of the world combined. We use chemicals such as pesticides, fungicides, and insecticides for other crops such as fruits and vegetables; we inject dairy cows with hormones passing them on into dairy products; antibiotics, heavy metals, such as arsenic, and hormones are used in concentrated animal feeding operations (CAFO's) which include cattle, hogs, turkey, and chicken; we have chemical ingredients in our foods such as artificial preservatives, colorings, and flavorings; we use artificial sweeteners abundantly, especially in soft drinks; we consume more than twice the amount of salt that we should, leading to cardiovascular disorders and contributing to immune reactions leading to autoimmune disorders [41–44]. Our abundant use of plasticizers such as bisphenol A in food and beverage containers contributes to this overreaching environmental exposure to xenobiotics as well. The widespread use of antibiotics, antacids, proton pump inhibitors, histamine 2 blockers, and other drugs, many of which are available over the counter, adds to what we consume.

Parallel to these dietary changes, there has been a considerable increase in autoimmune diseases such as type 1 diabetes, Crohn's disease, and multiple sclerosis (MS), especially in developed industrialized countries, suggesting a link between diet and autoimmune problems. For example, it has been established that ingestion of gluten leads to gluten enteropathies and vitamin D deficiency has been epidemiologically correlated with a higher risk for autoimmune diseases [45]. Indeed, type 1 diabetes and MS are also linked to low vitamin D levels as are other autoimmune diseases [46].

There are a large number of bacteria in the oral cavity, approximately 10^{12}, which include the tongue, teeth, and periodontal tissues. In contrast, the stomach has only 10^3-10^4 bacteria and there are 10^8-10^9 in the terminal ileum. The greatest number of bacteria is in the large intestine. The majority of these bacteria, approximately 70%, cannot be cultivated by current laboratory microbiological methods [47]. The gut, with a surface area of approximately 200 square meters, is where we come into greatest contact with the outside world and it follows that the gut also has the largest collection of immune cells, consisting of 70% of all lymphoid tissues in the body [48, 49]. It serves to prevent the outgrowth of pathogenic organisms. Recent studies have discussed the human microbiome and its composition in the healthy gut [50, 51]. We carry approximately $1 \times 10^{(13)}$ microorganisms in our gut, more than 10 times the total number of cells in our bodies [52]. The two predominant bacterial phylotypes are *Bacteroidetes* and *Firmicutes* [53]. Interestingly, the number of genes of our intestinal microbiota is 150 times greater than the number of genes in the human genome (Figure 2) [54]. Diet can substantially effect the microbiota. For example, in a diet that is high in fat and protein, *Bacteroides spp.* enterotype predominate, whereas in a diet that is high in carbohydrates, *Prevotella spp.* enterotypes predominate [55].

Mucins are highly glycosylated macromolecules, forming the first barrier between the contents of the gut and epithelial cells. This barrier provides protection for the epithelial cells from direct contact with commensal bacteria and their elements (Figure 3). Changes in either the composition or amount of mucus may lead to inflammatory responses [56]. Secretory IgA is one of the main humoral defense mechanisms ensuring the proper functioning of the mucosal surface barrier. It prevents the adherence of bacteria to mucosal surfaces and the penetration of antigens into the internal environment of the host by specific and nonspecific mechanisms [57, 58]. However, in persons with selective IgA deficiency, the mucosal barrier is deficient and more permeable to immunogens and allergens. Dendritic cells are the main cells that present antigens to the adaptive arm of the mucosal immune system [59]. A mucosal immune

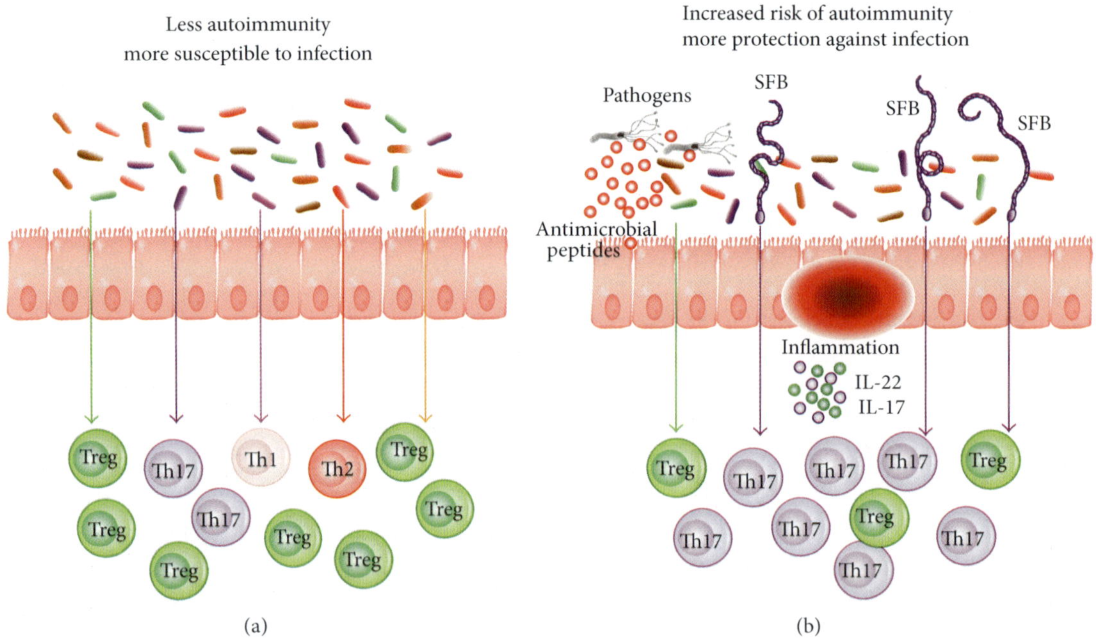

Figure 2: The composition of the intestinal microbiota is involved in the regulation of immune homeostasis. (a) Signals from different components of the microbiota (different colored arrows) regulate different branches of mucosal T cell response (corresponding color immune cells) in the lamina propria. (b) Changes in the composition of commensal bacteria, for example, the introduction of segmented filamentous bacteria (SFB), effect a change in the immune homeostasis, in this case, increasing the signals mediating induction of Th17 cells (purple arrows). This changes the immunological fitness of the individual. In the case of SFB, the increased production of Th17 cell effector cytokines, for example, IL-17 and IL-22, and the consecutive increase in antimicrobial peptide production from epithelial cells (red circles) increase the ability of the host to fight off intestinal infections. However, this increase in proinflammatory cytokines may also render the host more susceptible to chronic autoimmune inflammation. In this way, differences in the composition of the commensal bacteria in the gut may account for differences in individual response in the face of similar environmental challenges. (Adapted from: Ivanov I, Littman D. Segmented filamentous bacteria take the stage. Mucosal Immunology, 3(3):209-12, 2010.).

response, either one of tolerance or stimulation, depends on the partaking of different populations of dendritic cells responsible for the activation of regulatory T-cells subpopulations [60]. Activation of regulatory T-cells that inhibit the immune response and induce mucosal tolerance is dependent on the production of IL-10 and transforming growth factor-beta [61]. The maturation of dendritic cells is dependent on inducement by pathogenic organisms organisms and this then brings about the activation of effector T cells crucial for clearing infections and the prevention of subsequent infections with the same or related bacteria.

The epithelial cells of the gut have secretory, digestive, and absorptive functions and have receptors to facilitate their participation in immunological processes. The signaling pathways of these cells are highly regulated by pathways and molecules to provide a negative feedback system to avert uncontrolled inflammatory responses [62, 63]. Epithelial cells are the first point of contact for gut bacteria [64]. The epithelial layer of the gut is a major barrier between the host and the environment and is composed of a single layer of interconnected epithelial cells. This layer is reinforced by tight junctions in the paracellular spaces between the epithelial cells. These tight junctions of the epithelial layer of the gut act as a highly regulated entry that open and close depending on signals, such as cytokines and bacterial components from the lumen, lamina propria, and epithelium. Tight junctions are essential to the intestinal diffusion mechanisms [65]. The epithelial cells also make contact with the immune system of the gut and line the lamina propria of the small and large intestines and Peyer's patches which are organized lymphoid tissues. The Peyer's patches are critical for the direct antigen sampling from the gut and are where immune responses are induced and regulated. This is essential for gut health as too little or no bacterial exposure, as in germ-free conditions, can impair immune response, whereas excessive contact with bacteria may cause an increase in proinflammatory immune response. IgA and IgM derived from T-cell dependent and T-cell independent activation of B-cells and their differentiation into immunoglobulin secreting plasma cells are fundamental for the regulation of antigen penetration across the gut [66]. Immune regulation assists the gut to support microbiota and to ensure that effector immune responses are activated as a response to invading pathogens. Studies have shown the importance of Tregs in maintaining tolerance to the microbiota in the gut [67].

5. The Gut Microbiota

The gut microbiota can be influenced by several factors: the motility of the gastrointestinal tract (GIT); the intake of

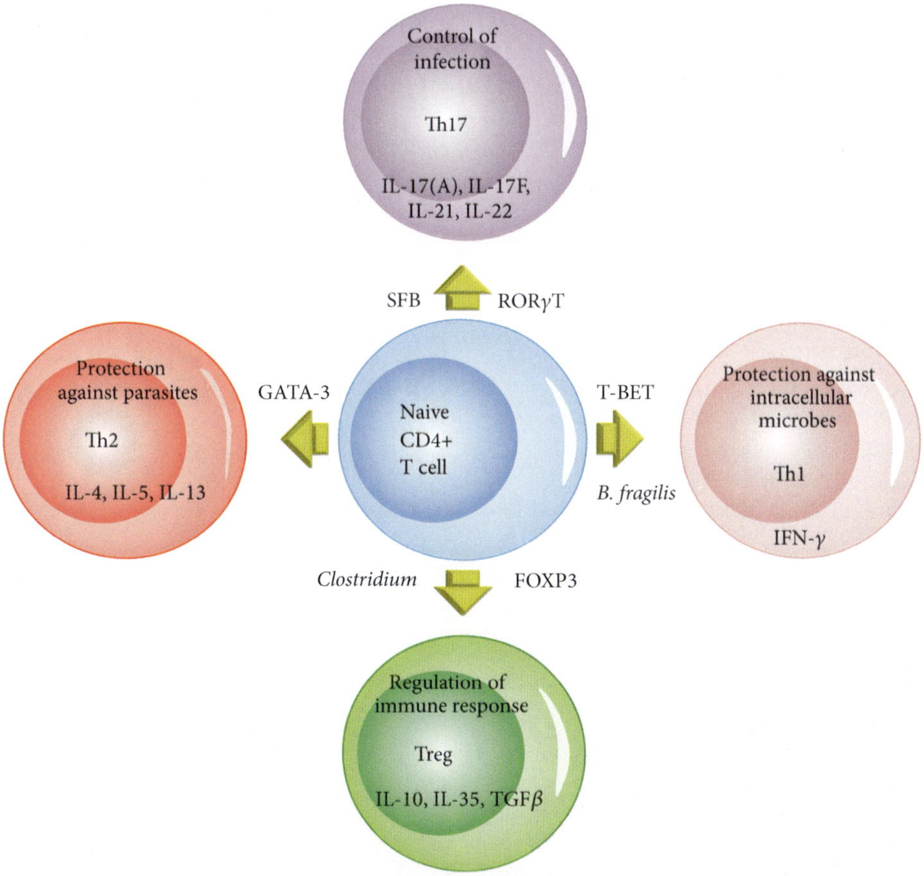

FIGURE 3: Commensal bacteria induce CD4+ T cell differentiation. Naïve CD4+ T cells can differentiate into four major cell types: Th1, Th2, Tregs, and Th17. The differentiation of each lineage requires the induction of a transcription factor that is unique to each lineage. Once differentiated, each lineage secretes a special set of cytokines. Th1 cells play an important role in eliminating intracellular pathogens while Th2 function to control parasitic infection. The primary role of Th17 is to control infection, while that of Tregs is to regulate immune response. The type of bacteria species that has been shown to induce a particular T cell differentiation pathway is also shown. (Adapted from Wu H, Wu E. The role of gut microbiota in immune homeostasis and autoimmunity. Gut Microbes 3 : 1, 4-14, 2012.).

pharmaceutical medications, including antacids, antibiotics, and nonsteroidal anti-inflammatory drugs; smoking; the use of alcohol; the GIT transit time; mucosal blood flow; and renal clearance [68, 69]. These factors can lead to the uptake of antigens from the lumen, which play an important role in the pathogenesis of gastrointestinal disorders (Figure 6). The disproportionate uptake of these antigens, coupled with the suppression of immune responsiveness or the failure in immunological tolerance, can lead to immunological reactions both within the gut and in other organs and follow one of two pathways: physiologic transport and pathological transport. Physiologic transport consists of ligand-receptor uptake, antibody uptake, and lastly microfold or M cell transport. Pathological transport is either antigen-specific or -nonspecific. Antigen specific transport via the transcellular of paracellular pathways has the ability to bring about a specific disease.

Examples include celiac disease (CD), gliadin, and allergic gastroenteropathies with casein and beta-lactoglobulin. The antigen nonspecific transport occurs when the tight junction becomes more permeable due to environmental factors which activate inflammatory cascade via transcellular or paracellular pathways [70, 71]. Vojdani in his recent study concluded that "increased antigen uptake in the intestine precedes the onset of many immunologically mediated gastrointestinal diseases" [72]. CD is frequently associated with other autoimmune disorders, in particular type 1 diabetes (T1D) and thyroiditis. This suggests that CD shares some common pathogenic mechanisms with other autoimmune diseases [73]. Genetic studies in patients with CD and T1D have shown gut mucosal barrier dysfunction [74–76]. In CD, we now know that disease-specific autoantibodies are directed against the enzyme transglutaminase 2 (TG2) brought about by gluten-reactive T cells within the celiac lesions, giving rise to glutamic acid (deaminated glutamine) [77–79].

One of the easiest ways to affect human health is through nutrition and diet. This, in turn, is influenced to a significant degree by the gut microbiota. Going from a low fat, plant polysaccharide rich diet to a high fat, high sugar Western diet changed the microbiota in one day in GF mice. There were more members of the Firmicute classes Erysipelotrichi and Bacilli (Enterococcus) and less Bacteroidetes associated with the Western diet. Another notable finding was that there was a significant increase in adiposity in humanized mice fed the Western diet as compared to those fed the low fat plant polysaccharide diet. These are important findings as they demonstrate that the gut microbiome can change over a very short period of time [80].

Recent studies have shown that the colonization of the small intestine in mice with a single commensal microbe, segmented filamentous bacterium (SFB), induced Th17 cells in the lamina propria. SFB are spore-forming Gram-positive bacteria related to the genus *Clostridium* and are found in many species as well as in humans. They are associated with reduced colonization and growth of pathogenic bacteria in the ileum where they are most abundant and adhere tightly to the epithelium. This colonization with SFB resulted in augmented resistance to *Citrobacter rodentium*, an intestinal pathogen, and with increased expression of genes linked with inflammation and antimicrobial defenses [81]. TGF-β differentiate Th17 and Treg cells and are defined by the expression of lineage-specific transcription factors RORγt and Foxp3 [82–86]. Th17 cells are essential mediators of autoimmune diseases, as they have potent inflammatory effects; they have important roles in protection from bacterial and fungal infections, especially at mucosal surfaces, and secrete IL-17, IL-17F, and IL-22. The increased production of Th17 cell effector cytokines, for example, IL-17 and IL-22, and the consecutive increase in antimicrobial peptide production from epithelial cells augment the ability of the host to fight off intestinal infections. At the same time, however, this increase in proinflammatory cytokines may render the host more susceptible to chronic autoimmune inflammation [87].

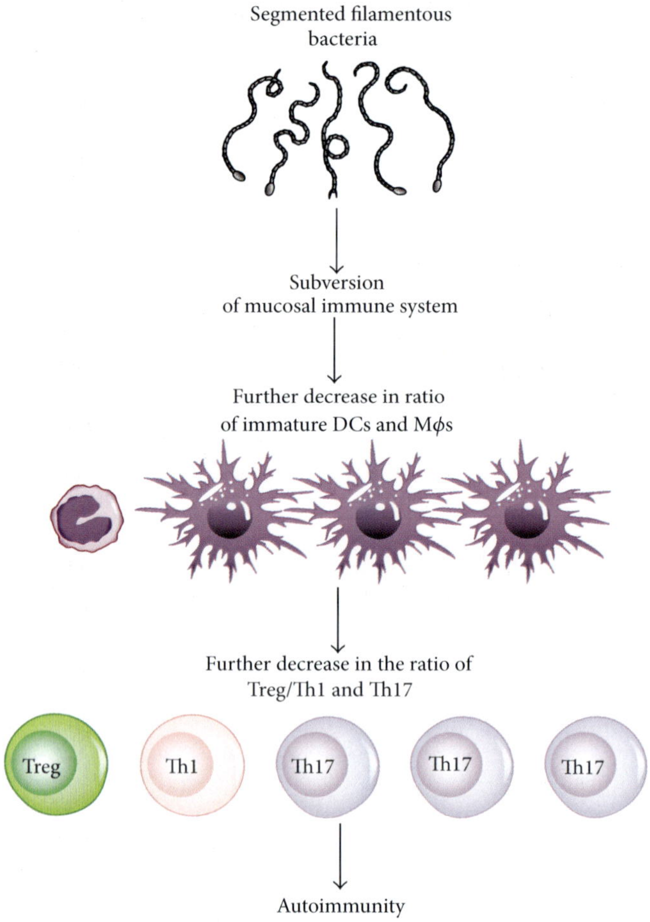

FIGURE 4: How segmented filamentous bacteria (SFB) can change the ratio between Th17 and Tregs, leading to autoimmunity.

6. The Gut and Rheumatic Disease

Rheumatoid arthritis (RA) is one of the most prevalent systemic autoimmune diseases targeting principally the joints. RA leads to joint deformity, disability, and increased mortality without treatment. It is a multifactorial and complex disease caused by genetic and environmental factors with increased production of self-reactive antibodies and proinflammatory T lymphocytes [88]. In RA there is a prolonged period of autoimmunity with circulating autoantibodies such as rheumatoid factor and anticitrullinated peptide antibodies. This preclinical state may last many years without any clinical signs or symptoms of inflammatory arthritis. However, there is an increase in antibody titers and epitope spreading with elevation in circulating proinflammatory cytokines before the onset of clinical disease. In these situations, environmental factors may be the triggering event for systemic joint inflammation. Microbes from the periodontal tissue, the airways, and the gut microbiota have been implicated [89, 90].

RA has pathogenic disease-specific autoimmunity to citrullinated proteins. Citrullination, a modification of arginine catalized by peptidylarginine deiminase enzymes, has the ability to change the structure, antigenicity, and function of proteins. Porphyromonas gingivalis, a major pathogenic bacterium related to gingivitis, is linked to RA in epidemiological studies and is the only bacterium that expresses endogenous citrullinated proteins [91].

The gut microbiota composition can be changed by antibiotics. Studies have shown that antibiotic use reduced Bacteroides and Bifidobacterium and led to the growth of Campylobacter, Streptococcus, Leuconostoc, or yeasts like *Candida Albicans* in the gut [92].

An alteration causing an imbalance in the gut microbiota can change T-cell responses and modulate systemic inflammation. Germ-free mice lack Th17 cells; when the gastrointestinal tract of these mice is colonized with segmented filamentous bacteria (SFB), Th17 cells are induced to accumulate in the lamina propria [81] (Figure 4). Mice raised in germ-free environments are persistently healthy. By introducing specific gut bacterial species, joint inflammation ensues. Treatment with antibiotics in these mice will prevent and negate a rheumatoid arthritis-like phenotype. When the gut of arthritis-prone K/BxN mice gut is colonized with SFB, the inflammatory disease is potentiated by Th17 cells [82]. An imbalance in gut microbiota with predominance of SFB may result in the reduction of functions of Treg cells and a predisposition to autoimmunity. This may affect systemic inflammatory processes and may partially be why there is reduced Treg function in patients with RA. This demonstrates that T cells whose functions are under the control of the gut commensal microbiota can also be the effectors of pathogenesis in autoimmune disorders [83].

A recent study showed that 75% of patients with new onset RA (NORA) carried *Prevotella copri* in their intestinal microbiota. Furthermore, 37.5% of psoriatic arthritis patients also had *Prevotella copri* in their gut compared to 21.4% of healthy controls [93]. This again demonstrates the effects of the environment from the gut microbiota aspect on autoimmune disorders.

Patients with juvenile idiopathic arthritis have been shown to have increased intestinal permeability along with gastrointestinal symptoms, suggesting a role for intestinal changes in the pathogenesis of rheumatic diseases [94]. Arthritis is frequently found in patients with IBD, again suggesting the participation of the gut in immune-mediated rheumatic disorders [95]. IBD is an autoimmune disorder affecting the GI tract in two main forms: Crohn's disease and ulcerative colitis. The phyla of gut microbiota in patients with IBD greatly differ when compared with normal patients [96]. Studies have shown that antibiotics treatment benefits patients as well as animal models of IBD, indicating that bacteria play an important role in the pathogenesis [97]. A recent study has identified the specific microbiota in the dysbiosis of IBD patients. These patients have an overgrowth of proteobacteria and a reduction in Firmicutes and Bacteroides species [98].

Reactive arthritis and autoimmune reactions in joints may be triggered by infections with intestinal microbial pathogens, including Salmonella, Shigella and Yersinia [99]. Antibodies against antigens of certain species of gut bacteria, for example, Proteus, suggest that these bacteria and rheumatoid arthritis have a pathogenic relationship [100]. This parallels the findings in patients with ankylosing spondylitis having increased titers of anti-Klebsiella antibodies suggesting again a bacterial triggering factor [101].

7. The Gut and Neuroautoimmunity

The gut-brain axis acts as a bidirectional communication between the brain and the gut (Figure 5). The brain modulates gastrointestinal function and the gastrointestinal system is monitored by the brain via neural, immunological, and endocrine mechanisms. The development and function of the enteric nervous system are influenced by the intestinal microbiota [102]. The gastrointestinal system is directly controlled by the enteric nervous systems, the "second brain". This system consists of more neurons than the spinal cord, mainly in the myenteric and submucosal plexuses. Neuropeptides are able to increase the permeability of tight junctions to macromolecules and thereby modify the function of the mucosal barrier [103, 104].

In adults, chronic stress affects the composition of the gut microbiota with increase of *Bacteroides* spp. and *Clostridium* spp. Coupled with this are increasing levels of IL-6 indicating immune activation [105]. Chronic stress also makes the gut leaky, increasing circulating levels of LPS. Findings of altered

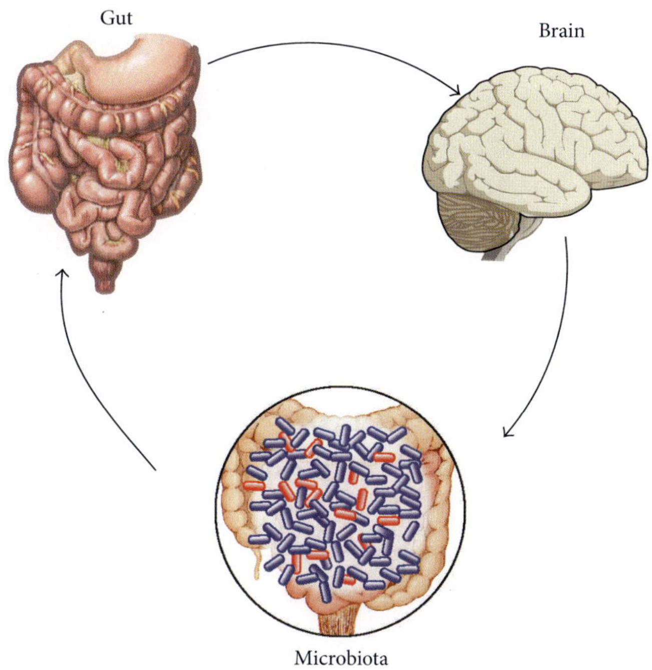

FIGURE 5: The interconnection of the gut, brain, and microbiota.

intestinal permeability (leaky gut) may play a pathogenic role in patients with depression and their first-degree relatives [106, 107].

Multiple sclerosis (MS) is one of the most frequent and severe demyelinating neurological diseases, mainly affecting young people, eventually leading to their becoming disabled. Increased intestinal permeability in these patients and in their relatives has been reported. MS has also been related to infections with bacteria and viruses [108]. Experimental autoimmune encephalomyelitis (EAE) is the animal model widely used for MS. A study in germ-free mice showed attenuated induction of EAE by myelin oligodendrocyte glycoprotein (MOG) peptide in complete Freund's adjuvant [109]. Another study with mice genetically predisposed to develop EAE showed that when they were housed in germ-free or pathogen-free conditions, they were protected from developing EAE. Once they reached adulthood and had normal gut colonization, the protection was lost [110].

There are increasing numbers of studies demonstrating the importance of the permeability of the gastrointestinal tract to large molecules and how this is linked to the development of various neurodegenerative disorders, including Parkinson's disease (PD). Lewy bodies, the pathological hallmark of Parkinson's disease, were found in intestinal biopsies of patients with PD [108–110].

8. The Other Side of the Same Coin

The gut microbiome can also help the host. There are commensal gut bacteria that can ameliorate disease. For example, in immunocompromised mice, *B. fragilis* can lessen the colitis induced by Helicobacter hepaticus via its production of PSA,

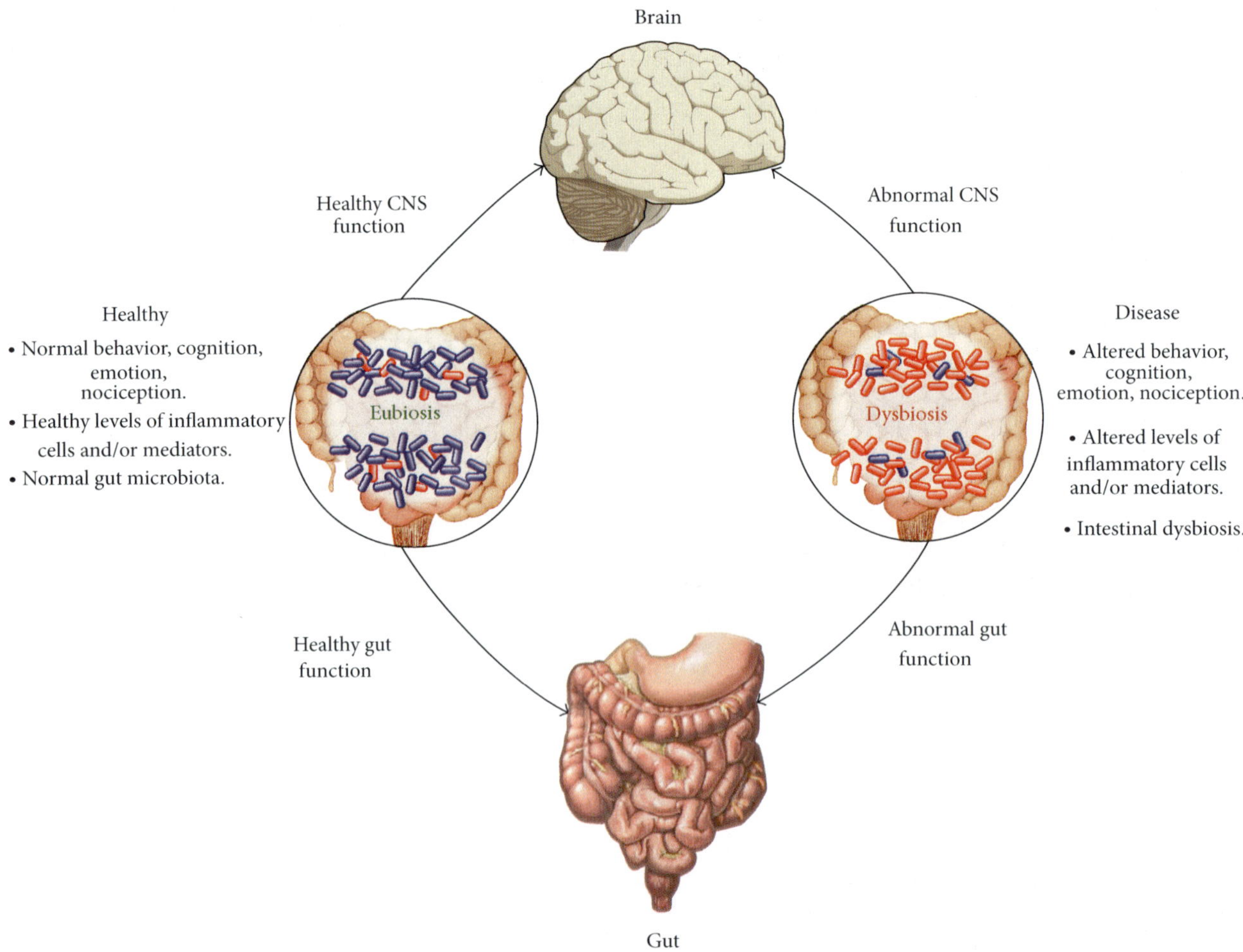

FIGURE 6: Impact of the gut microbiota on the gut-brain axis in health and disease. It is now generally accepted that a stable gut microbiota is essential for normal gut physiology and contributes to appropriate signaling along the gut-brain axis and, thereby, to the healthy status of the individual (a). On the other hand (b), intestinal dysbiosis can adversely influence gut physiology, leading to inappropriate gut-brain axis signaling and associated consequences for CNS functions and resulting in disease states. Conversely, stress at the level of the CNS can affect gut function and lead to perturbations of the microbiota. (Adapted from: Cryan J, Dinan T. Mind-altering microorganisms: the impact of the gut microbiota on brain and behavior. Nat Rev Neurosci., 13(10):701-12, 2012.).

which stimulates the anti-inflammatory IL-10 production from CD4+ T cells and the downregulating of proinflammatory IL-10 production in the colonic tissues. This, in turn, suppresses disease [111]. In another example, short-chain fatty acids (SCFAs) produced by the gut microbiota interact with G-protein-coupled receptors expressed on immune cells and reduce inflammation in the dextran sulfate sodium (DSS-)induced colitis model [112].

9. When Did It All Start?

Bacterial colonization during and shortly after birth plays a major role in the formation of gut microbiota. Factors affecting the communities in this microbiota include premature birth, Caesarean section versus vaginal birth, breast milk versus commercial formula, and many more. For example, premature infants were colonized principally by *C. difficile*. Infants born vaginally were colonized mostly by bacterial communities similar to their mother's vaginal microbiota, including *Lactobacillus*, *Prevotella*, or *Sneathia* spp, whereas Caesarean section born infants were colonized by bacteria found on the skin surface, including *Staphylococcus*, *Corynebacterium*, and *Propionibacterium* species. Formula fed infants had colonization predominantly by *Staphylococci*, *E. coli*, *C. difficile*, *Bacteroides*, *Atopobium*, and *Lactobacilli* [113–117]. Infants delivered via Caesarean section have an increased risk of developing asthma, allergies, and autoimmune disease in later childhood [118, 119]. These are clear demonstrations of the importance of the gut microbiota starting at birth and affecting the patient years later.

10. Conclusion

Factors such as genetics, the environment, infections, and the gut microbiota all play a role in the mediation of autoimmune disorders. There have been tremendous recent advances in our understanding of the interplay of these factors. It is clear that the gut microbiota has a profound and long-term effect starting at birth on the host immune system. It is also evident that it plays a significant role in autoimmune diseases both inside and outside the gut. There are still questions that remain to be answered: does the immune system shape the gut microbiota or vice-versa? This complex and dynamic symbiosis needs further elucidation and may help in determining the outcome of autoimmune diseases in patients. The clinician can assist the patient by being aware of the triggers of autoimmune disorders and monitoring immune and autoimmune markers in the peripheral blood, thereby being able to take preventive measures to hopefully avert the progression towards an autoimmune disease.

Conflict of Interests

The author declares that there is no conflict of interests regarding the publication of this paper.

References

[1] J.-F. Bach, "The effect of infections on susceptibility to autoimmune and allergic diseases," *The New England Journal of Medicine*, vol. 347, no. 12, pp. 911–920, 2002.

[2] G. A. W. Rook and L. R. Brunet, "Microbes, immunoregulation, and the gut," *Gut*, vol. 54, no. 3, pp. 317–320, 2005.

[3] A. Vojdani, "Antibodies as predictors of complex autoimmune diseases and cancer," *International Journal of Immunopathology and Pharmacology*, vol. 21, no. 3, pp. 553–566, 2008.

[4] L. A. Zenewicz, C. Abraham, R. A. Flavell, and J. H. Cho, "Unraveling the genetics of autoimmunity," *Cell*, vol. 140, no. 6, pp. 791–797, 2010.

[5] J. C. Barrett, D. G. Clayton, P. Concannon et al., "Genome-wide association study and meta-analysis find that over 40 loci affect risk of type 1 diabetes," *Nature Genetics*, vol. 41, no. 6, pp. 703–707, 2009.

[6] L. A. Criswell, K. A. Pfeiffer, R. F. Lum et al., "Analysis of families in the multiple autoimmune disease genetics consortium (MADGC) collection: the PTPN22 620W allele associates with multiple autoimmune phenotypes," *American Journal of Human Genetics*, vol. 76, no. 4, pp. 561–571, 2005.

[7] R. P. Nair, K. C. Duffin, C. Helms et al., "Genome-wide scan reveals association of psoriasis with IL-23 and NF-κB pathways," *Nature Genetics*, vol. 41, no. 2, pp. 199–204, 2009.

[8] D. M. Waid, R. J. Wagner, A. Putnam et al., "A unique T cell subset described as $CD4^{lo}CD40^{+}$ T cells (TCD40) in human type 1 diabetes," *Clinical Immunology*, vol. 124, no. 2, pp. 138–148, 2007.

[9] A. L. Peters, R. M. Plenge, R. R. Graham et al., "A novel polymorphism of the human CD40 receptor with enhanced function," *Blood*, vol. 112, no. 5, pp. 1863–1871, 2008.

[10] J.-P. Lin, J. M. Cash, S. Z. Doyle et al., "Familial clustering of rheumatoid arthritis with other autoimmune diseases," *Human Genetics*, vol. 103, no. 4, pp. 475–482, 1998.

[11] S. A. Broadley, J. Deans, S. J. Sawcer, D. Clayton, and D. A. S. Compston, "Autoimmune disease in first-degree relatives of patients with multiple sclerosis. A UK survey," *Brain*, vol. 123, no. 6, pp. 1102–1111, 2000.

[12] M. Salvetti, G. Ristori, R. Bomprezzi, P. Pozzilli, and R. D. G. Leslie, "Twins: mirrors of the immune system," *Immunology Today*, vol. 21, no. 7, pp. 342–347, 2000.

[13] O. Vera-Lastra, G. Medina, M. D. P. Cruz-Dominguez et al., "Human adjuvant disease induced by foreign substances: a new model of ASIA (Shoenfeld's syndrome)," *Lupus*, vol. 21, no. 2, pp. 128–135, 2012.

[14] H. Hamza, J. Cao, X. Li, C. Li, M. Zhu, and S. Zhao, "Hepatitis B vaccine induces apoptotic death in Hepa1-6 cells," *Apoptosis*, vol. 17, pp. 516–527, 2012.

[15] C. P. Strassburg, A. Vogel, and M. P. Manns, "Autoimmunity and hepatitis C," *Autoimmunity Reviews*, vol. 2, no. 6, pp. 322–331, 2003.

[16] C. Palazzi, D. Buskila, S. D'Angelo, E. D'Amico, and I. Olivieri, "Autoantibodies in patients with chronic hepatitis C virus infection: pitfalls for the diagnosis of rheumatic diseases," *Autoimmunity Reviews*, vol. 11, no. 9, pp. 659–663, 2012.

[17] J. W. Cohen-Tervaert and R. M. Kappel, "Siliconeimplantincompatibilitysyndrome (SIIS): afrequentcauseofASIA(Shoenfeld'ssyndrome)," *Immunologic Research*, vol. 56, pp. 293–298, 2013.

[18] N. Agmon-Levin, G. R. V. Hughes, and Y. Shoenfeld, "The spectrum of ASIA: autoimmune (Auto-inflammatory) Syndrome induced by Adjuvants," *Lupus*, vol. 21, no. 2, pp. 118–120, 2012.

[19] L. Klareskog, P. Stolt, K. Lundberg et al., "A new model for an etiology of rheumatoid arthritis: smoking may trigger HLA-DR (shared epitope)-restricted immune reactions to autoantigens modified by citrullination," *Arthritis and Rheumatism*, vol. 54, no. 1, pp. 38–46, 2006.

[20] G. A. Schellekens, H. Visser, and B. A. de Jong, "The diagnostic properties of rheumatoid arthritis antibodies recognizing a cyclic citrullinated peptide," *Arthritis & Rheumatology*, vol. 43, no. 1, pp. 155–163, 2000.

[21] S. Kivity, N. Agmon-Levin, M. Blank, and Y. Shoenfeld, "Infections and autoimmunity: friends or foes?" *Trends in Immunology*, vol. 30, no. 8, pp. 409–414, 2009.

[22] T. F. Davies, "Infection and autoimmune thyroid disease," *Journal of Clinical Endocrinology and Metabolism*, vol. 93, no. 3, pp. 674–676, 2008.

[23] J. A. James, B. R. Neas, K. L. Moser et al., "Systemic lupus erythematosus in adults is associated with previous Epstein-Barr virus exposure.," *Arthritis and Rheumatism*, vol. 44, pp. 1122–1126, 2001.

[24] H. H. Niller, H. Wolf, and J. Minarovits, "Regulation and dysregulation of Epstein-Barr virus latency: implications for the development of autoimmune diseases," *Autoimmunity*, vol. 41, no. 4, pp. 298–328, 2008.

[25] P. Tattevin, Y. Le Tulzo, S. Minjolle et al., "Increasing incidence of severe Epstein-Barr virus-related infectious mononucleosis: surveillance study," *Journal of Clinical Microbiology*, vol. 44, no. 5, pp. 1873–1874, 2006.

[26] D. A. Thorley-Lawson, "Epstein-Barr virus: exploiting the immune system," *Nature Reviews Immunology*, vol. 1, no. 1, pp. 75–82, 2001.

[27] U. Y. Moon, S. J. Park, S. T. Oh et al., "Patients with systemic lupus erythematosus have abnormally elevated Epstein-Barr virus load in blood," *Arthritis Research & Therapy*, vol. 6, no. 4, pp. R295–R302, 2004.

[28] I. Kang, T. Quan, H. Nolasco et al., "Defective control of latent Epstein-Barr virus infection in systemic lupus erythematosus," *Journal of Immunology*, vol. 172, no. 2, pp. 1287–1294, 2004.

[29] J. J.-Y. Lu, D.-Y. Chen, C.-W. Hsieh, J.-L. Lan, F.-J. Lin, and S.-H. Lin, "Association of Epstein- Barr virus infection with systemic lupus erythematosus in Taiwan," *Lupus*, vol. 16, no. 3, pp. 168–175, 2007.

[30] A. Draborg, J. Jorgensen, H. Muller et al., "Epstein-Barr virus early antigen diffuse (EBV-EA/D)-directed immunoglobulin A antibodies in systemic lupus erythematosus patients," *Scandinavian Journal of Rheumatology*, vol. 41, pp. 280–289, 2012.

[31] S. Blaschke, G. Schwarz, D. Moneke, L. Binder, G. Müller, and M. Reuss-Borst, "Epstein-Barr virus infection in peripheral blood mononuclear cells, synovial fluid cells, and synovial membranes of patients with rheumatoid arthritis," *Journal of Rheumatology*, vol. 27, no. 4, pp. 866–873, 2000.

[32] T. Takeda, Y. Mizugaki, L. Matsubara, S. Imai, T. Koike, and K. Takada, "Lytic Epstein-Barr virus infection in the synovial tissue of patients with rheumatoid arthritis," *Arthritis and Rheumatism*, vol. 43, pp. 1218–1225, 2000.

[33] N. Balandraud, J. B. Meynard, I. Auger et al., "Epstein-Barr virus load in the peripheral blood of patients with rheumatoid arthritis: accurate quantification using real-time polymerase chain reaction," *Arthritis and Rheumatism*, vol. 48, no. 5, pp. 1223–1228, 2003.

[34] C. Croia, B. Serafini, M. Bombardieri et al., "Epstein-Barr virus persistence and infection of autoreactive plasma cells in synovial lymphoid structures in rheumatoid arthritis," *Annals of Rheumatic Diseases*, vol. 72, no. 9, pp. 1559–1568, 2012.

[35] X. Mariette, J. Gozlan, D. Clerc, M. Bisson, and F. Morinet, "Detection of Epstein-Barr virus DNA by in situ hybridization and polymerase chain reaction in salivary gland biopsy specimens from patients with Sjogren's syndrome," *American Journal of Medicine*, vol. 90, no. 3, pp. 286–294, 1991.

[36] S. C. Pflugfelder, C. A. Crouse, D. Monroy, M. Yen, M. Rowe, and S. S. Atherton, "Epstein-Barr virus and the lacrimal gland pathology of Sjogren's syndrome," *American Journal of Pathology*, vol. 143, no. 1, pp. 49–64, 1993.

[37] M. Voulgarelis and H. M. Moutsopoulos, "Mucosa-associated lymphoid tissue in lymphoma in Sjogren's syndrome: risks, management, and prognosis," *Rheumatic Disease Clinics of North America*, vol. 34, no. 4, pp. 921–933, 2008.

[38] N. Inoue, S. Harada, N. Miyasaka, A. Oya, and K. Yanagi, "Analysis of antibody titers to Epstein-Barr virus nuclear antigens in sera of patients with Sjogren's syndrome and with rheumatoid arthritis," *Journal of Infectious Diseases*, vol. 164, no. 1, pp. 22–28, 1991.

[39] I. Toda, M. Ono, H. Fujishima, and K. Tsubota, "Sjogren's syndrome (SS) and Epstein-Barr virus (EBV) reactivation," *Ocular Immunology and Inflammation*, vol. 2, no. 2, pp. 101–109, 1994.

[40] S. G. Pasoto, R. R. Natalino, H. P. Chakkour et al., "EBV reactivation serological profile in primary Sjogren's syndrome: an underlying trigger of active articular involvement?" *Rheumatology International*, vol. 33, pp. 1149–1157, 2013.

[41] A. Vojdani, "A potential link between environmental triggers and autoimmunity," *Autoimmune Diseases*, vol. 2013, Article ID 437231, 18 pages, 2013.

[42] A. Campbell, "Pesticides: our children in jeopardy," *Alternative Therapies in Health and Medicine*, vol. 19, no. 1, pp. 8–10, 2013.

[43] A. Campbell, "Neurotoxicity: better living through chemistry," *Advances in Mind-Body Medicine*, vol. 26, no. 2, pp. 6–7, 2012.

[44] A. Campbell, "Organic vs conventional," *Alternative Therapies in Health and Medicine*, vol. 18, no. 6, pp. 8–9, 2012.

[45] N. Agmon-Levin, E. Theodor, R. Segal, and Y. Shoenfeld, "Vitamin D in systemic and organ-specific autoimmune diseases," *Clinical Reviews in Allergy & Immunology*, vol. 45, no. 2, pp. 256–266, 2013.

[46] C. F. Pelajo, J. M. Lopez-Benitez, and L. C. Miller, "Vitamin D and autoimmune rheumatologic disorders," *Autoimmunity Reviews*, vol. 9, no. 7, pp. 507–510, 2010.

[47] F. Bäckhed, R. E. Ley, J. L. Sonnenburg, D. A. Peterson, and J. I. Gordon, "Host-bacterial mutualism in the human intestine," *Science*, vol. 307, no. 5717, pp. 1915–1920, 2005.

[48] S. Salminen, C. Bouley, M.-C. Boutron-Ruault et al., "Functional food science and gastrointestinal physiology and function," *British Journal of Nutrition*, vol. 80, supplement 1, pp. S147–S171, 1998.

[49] M. L. Forchielli and W. A. Walker, "The role of gut-associated lymphoid tissues and mucosal defence," *British Journal of Nutrition*, vol. 93, supplement 1, pp. S41–S48, 2005.

[50] M. Arumugam, J. Raes, E. Pelletier et al., "Enterotypes of the human gut microbiome," *Nature*, vol. 473, no. 7346, pp. 174–180, 2011.

[51] Human Microbiome Project Consortium, "Structure, function and diversity of the health human microbiome," *Nature*, vol. 486, pp. 207–214, 2012.

[52] S. R. Gill, M. Pop, R. T. DeBoy et al., "Metagenomic analysis of the human distal gut microbiome," *Science*, vol. 312, no. 5778, pp. 1355–1359, 2006.

[53] P. Eckburg, E. Bik, C. Bernstein et al., "Diversity of the human intestinal microbial flora," *Science*, vol. 308, pp. 1635–1638, 2005.

[54] J. Qin, R. Li, J. Raes et al., "A human gut microbial gene catalogue established by metagenomic sequencing," *Nature*, vol. 464, no. 7285, pp. 59–65, 2010.

[55] S. Wu and J. Hui, "Treat your bug right," *Frontiers in Physiology*, vol. 2, article 9, 2011.

[56] S. K. Linden, P. Sutton, N. G. Karlsson, V. Korolik, and M. A. McGuckin, "Mucins in the mucosal barrier to infection," *Mucosal Immunology*, vol. 1, no. 3, pp. 183–197, 2008.

[57] J. Mestecky, M. W. Russell, and C. O. Elson, "Intestinal IgA: novel views on its function in the defence of the largest mucosal surface," *Gut*, vol. 44, no. 1, pp. 2–5, 1999.

[58] P. Brandtzaeg, "Update on mucosal immunoglobulin A in gastrointestinal disease," *Current Opinion in Gastroenterology*, vol. 26, no. 6, pp. 554–563, 2010.

[59] M. Rescigno and A. di Sabatino, "Dendritic cells in intestinal homeostasis and disease," *Journal of Clinical Investigation*, vol. 119, no. 9, pp. 2441–2450, 2009.

[60] J. L. Coombes and F. Powrie, "Dendritic cells in intestinal immune regulation," *Nature Reviews Immunology*, vol. 8, no. 6, pp. 435–446, 2008.

[61] M. J. Barnes and F. Powrie, "Regulatory T cells reinforce intestinal homeostasis," *Immunity*, vol. 31, no. 3, pp. 401–411, 2009.

[62] H. Tlaskalova-Hogenova, R. Stepankova, T. Hudcovic, L. Tuckova et al., "Commensal bacteria (normal microflora), mucosal immunity and chronic inflammatory and autoimmune diseases," *Immunology Letters*, vol. 93, pp. 97–108, 2004.

[63] K. Kobayashi, N. Inohara, L. D. Hernandez et al., "RICK/Rip2/CARDIAK mediates signalling for receptors of the innate and adaptive immune systems," *Nature*, vol. 416, no. 6877, pp. 194–199, 2002.

[64] J. R. Turner, "Intestinal mucosal barrier function in health and disease," *Nature Reviews Immunology*, vol. 9, no. 11, pp. 799–809, 2009.

[65] A. Fasano, "Physiological, pathological, and therapeutic implications of zonulin-mediated intestinal barrier modulation: living life on the edge of the wall," *American Journal of Pathology*, vol. 173, no. 5, pp. 1243–1252, 2008.

[66] P. Brandtzaeg, "Homeostatic impact of indigenous microbiota and secretory immunity," *Beneficial microbes*, vol. 1, no. 3, pp. 211–227, 2010.

[67] F. Powrie, "Immune regulation in the intestine: a balancing act between effector and regulatory T cell responses," *Annals of the New York Academy of Sciences*, vol. 1029, pp. 132–141, 2004.

[68] I. Bjarnason, G. Zanelli, and T. Smith, "Nonsteroidal antiinflammatory drug-induced intestinal inflammation in humans," *Gastroenterology*, vol. 93, no. 3, pp. 480–489, 1987.

[69] I. Bjarnason, K. Ward, and T. J. Peters, "The leaky gut of alcoholism: possible route of entry for toxic compounds," *The Lancet*, vol. 1, no. 8370, pp. 179–182, 1984.

[70] O. L. Frick, D. F. German, and J. Mills, "Development of allergy in children. I. Association with virus infections," *Journal of Allergy and Clinical Immunology*, vol. 63, no. 4, pp. 228–241, 1979.

[71] R. P. Ford, I. S. Menzies, A. D. Phillips, J. A. Walker-Smith, and M. W. Turner, "Intestinal sugar permeability: relationship to diarrhoeal disease and small bowel morphology," *Journal of Pediatric Gastroenterology and Nutrition*, vol. 4, no. 4, pp. 568–574, 1985.

[72] A. Vojdani, "For the assessment of intestinal permeability, size matters," *Alternative Therapies in Health and Medicine*, vol. 19, no. 1, pp. 12–24, 2013.

[73] A. Fasano, "Zonulin and its regulation of intestinal barrier function: the biological door to inflammation, autoimmunity, and cancer," *Physiological Reviews*, vol. 91, no. 1, pp. 151–175, 2011.

[74] P. Kucera, D. Novakova, M. Behanova, J. Novak, H. Tlaskalova-Hogenova, and M. Andel, "Gliadin, endomysial and thyroid antibodies in patients with latent autoimmune diabetes of adults (LADA)," *Clinical & Experimental Immunology*, vol. 133, pp. 139–143, 2003.

[75] A. Fasano and T. Shea-Donohue, "Mechanisms of disease: the role of intestinal barrier function in the pathogenesis of gastrointestinal autoimmune diseases," *Nature Clinical Practice Gastroenterology and Hepatology*, vol. 2, no. 9, pp. 416–422, 2005.

[76] M. C. Wapenaar, A. J. Monsuur, A. A. van Bodegraven et al., "Associations with tight junction genes PARD3 and MAGI2 in Dutch patients point to a common barrier defect for coeliac disease and ulcerative colitis," *Gut*, vol. 57, no. 4, pp. 463–467, 2008.

[77] J. Visser, J. Rozing, A. Sapone, K. Lammers, and A. Fasano, "Tight junctions, intestinal permeability, and autoimmunity: celiac disease and type 1 diabetes," *Diabetes/Metabolism Research and Reviews*, vol. 24, pp. 59–63, 2008.

[78] L. M. Sollid, "Coeliac disease: dissecting a complex inflammatory disorder," *Nature Reviews Immunology*, vol. 2, no. 9, pp. 647–655, 2002.

[79] W. Dieterich, T. Ehnis, M. Bauer et al., "Identification of tissue transglutaminase as the autoantigen of celiac disease," *Nature Medicine*, vol. 3, no. 7, pp. 797–801, 1997.

[80] P. J. Turnbaugh, V. K. Ridaura, J. J. Faith, F. E. Rey, R. Knight, and J. I. Gordon, "The effect of diet on the human gut microbiome: a metagenomic analysis in humanized gnotobiotic mice," *Science Translational Medicine*, vol. 1, no. 6, ra14 pages, 2009.

[81] I. I. Ivanov, K. Atarashi, N. Manel et al., "Induction of intestinal Th17 cells by segmented filamentous bacteria," *Cell*, vol. 139, no. 3, pp. 485–498, 2009.

[82] H.-J. Wu, I. I. Ivanov, J. Darce et al., "Gut-residing segmented filamentous bacteria drive autoimmune arthritis via T helper 17 cells," *Immunity*, vol. 32, no. 6, pp. 815–827, 2010.

[83] S. J. Aujla, P. J. Dubin, and J. K. Kolls, "Th17 cells and mucosal host defense," *Seminars in Immunology*, vol. 19, no. 6, pp. 377–382, 2007.

[84] E. Bettelli, M. Oukka, and V. K. Kuchroo, "TH-17 cells in the circle of immunity and autoimmunity," *Nature Immunology*, vol. 8, no. 4, pp. 345–350, 2007.

[85] J. D. Fontenot, M. A. Gavin, and A. Y. Rudensky, "Foxp3 programs the development and function of $CD4^+CD25^+$ regulatory T cells," *Nature Immunology*, vol. 4, no. 4, pp. 330–336, 2003.

[86] I. I. Ivanov, B. S. McKenzie, L. Zhou et al., "The orphan nuclear receptor RORgammat directs the differentiation program of proinflammatory IL-17^+ T helper cells," *Cell*, vol. 126, no. 6, pp. 1121–1133, 2006.

[87] P. Mangan, L. Harrington, D. O'Quinn et al., "Transforming growth factor- beta induces development of the T(H)17 lineage," *Nature*, vol. 441, pp. 231–234, 2006.

[88] I. B. McInnes and G. Schett, "The pathogenesis of rheumatoid arthritis," *The New England Journal of Medicine*, vol. 365, no. 23, pp. 2205–2219, 2011.

[89] K. D. Deane, J. M. Norris, and V. M. Holers, "Preclinical rheumatoid arthritis: identification, evaluation, and future directions for investigation," *Rheumatic Disease Clinics of North America*, vol. 36, no. 2, pp. 213–241, 2010.

[90] J. U. Scher, C. Ubeda, M. Equinda et al., "Periodontal disease and the oral microbiota in new-onset rheumatoid arthritis," *Arthritis & Rheumatology*, vol. 64, no. 10, pp. 3083–3094, 2012.

[91] N. Wegner, K. Lundberg, A. Kinloch et al., "Autoimmunity to specific citrullinated proteins gives the first clues to the etiology of rheumatoid arthritis," *Immunological Reviews*, vol. 233, no. 1, pp. 34–54, 2010.

[92] D. A. Hill, C. Hoffmann, M. C. Abt et al., "Metagenomic analyses reveal antibiotic-induced temporal and spatial changes in intestinal microbiota with associated alterations in immune cell homeostasis," *Mucosal Immunology*, vol. 3, no. 2, pp. 148–158, 2010.

[93] J. Scher, A. Sczernak, R. Longman et al., "Expansion of intestinal Prevotella copri correlates with enhanced susceptibility to arthritis," *ELife*, vol. 2, Article ID e01202, 2013.

[94] P. Weber, T. Brune, G. Ganser, and K.-P. Zimmer, "Gastrointestinal symptoms and permeability in patients with juvenile idiopathic arthritis," *Clinical and Experimental Rheumatology*, vol. 21, no. 5, pp. 657–662, 2003.

[95] T. S. Rodríguez-Reyna, C. Martínez-Reyes, and J. K. Yamamoto-Furusho, "Rheumatic manifestations of inflammatory bowel disease," *World Journal of Gastroenterology*, vol. 15, no. 44, pp. 5517–5524, 2009.

[96] C. Manichanh, L. Rigottier-Gois, E. Bonnaud et al., "Reduced diversity of faecal microbiota in Crohn's disease revealed by a metagenomic approach," *Gut*, vol. 55, no. 2, pp. 205–211, 2006.

[97] K. J. Khan, T. A. Ullman, A. C. Ford et al., "Antibiotic therapy in inflammatory bowel disease: a systematic review and meta-analysis," *American Journal of Gastroenterology*, vol. 106, no. 4, pp. 661–673, 2011.

[98] H. Sokol, P. Seksik, L. Rigottier-Gois et al., "Specificities of the fecal microbiota in inflammatory bowel disease," *Inflammatory Bowel Diseases*, vol. 12, no. 2, pp. 106–111, 2006.

[99] P. Toivanen, "Normal intestinal microbiota in the aetiopathogenesis of rheumatoid arthritis," *Annals of the Rheumatic Diseases*, vol. 62, no. 9, pp. 807–811, 2003.

[100] A. Ebringer, T. Rashid, and C. Wilson, "Rheumatoid arthritis, proteus, anti-CCP antibodies and Karl Popper," *Autoimmunity Reviews*, vol. 9, no. 4, pp. 216–223, 2010.

[101] T. Rashid and A. Ebringer, "Ankylosing spondylitis is linked to Klebsiella—the evidence," *Clinical Rheumatology*, vol. 26, no. 6, pp. 858–864, 2007.

[102] J. Bienenstock and S. Collins, "99th Dahlem conference on infection, inflammation and chronic inflammatory disorders: psycho- neuroimmunology and the intestinal microbiota: clinical observations and basic mechanisms," *Clinical and Experimental Immunology*, vol. 160, no. 1, pp. 85–91, 2010.

[103] S. M. Collins and P. Bercik, "The relationship between intestinal microbiota and the central nervous system in normal gastrointestinal function and disease," *Gastroenterology*, vol. 136, no. 6, pp. 2003–2014, 2009.

[104] M. D. Gershon, "The enteric nervous system: a second brain," *Hospital Practice*, vol. 34, no. 7, pp. 31–42, 1999.

[105] M. T. Bailey, S. E. Dowd, J. D. Galley, A. R. Hufnagle, R. G. Allen, and M. Lyte, "Exposure to a social stressor alters the structure of the intestinal microbiota: implications for stressor-induced immunomodulation," *Brain, Behavior, and Immunity*, vol. 25, no. 3, pp. 397–407, 2011.

[106] J. D. Söderholm and M. H. Perdue, "Stress and the gastrointestinal tract II. Stress and intestinal barrier function," *American Journal of Physiology: Gastrointestinal and Liver Physiology*, vol. 280, no. 1, pp. G7–G13, 2001.

[107] M. Maes, M. Kubera, and J.-C. Leunis, "The gut-brain barrier in major depression: intestinal mucosal dysfunction with an increased translocation of LPS from gram negative enterobacteria (leaky gut) plays a role in the inflammatory pathophysiology of depression," *Neuro Endocrinology Letters*, vol. 29, no. 1, pp. 117–124, 2008.

[108] B. Yacyshyn, J. Meddings, D. Sadowski, and M. B. Bowen-Yacyshyn, "Multiple sclerosis patients have peripheral blood $CD45RO^+$ B cells and increased intestinal permeability," *Digestive Diseases and Sciences*, vol. 41, no. 12, pp. 2493–2498, 1996.

[109] Y. K. Lee, J. S. Menezes, Y. Umesaki, and S. K. Mazmanian, "Proinflammatory T-cell responses to gut microbiota promote experimental autoimmune encephalomyelitis," *Proceedings of the National Academy of Sciences of the United States of America*, vol. 108, no. 1, pp. 4615–4622, 2011.

[110] K. Berer, M. Mues, M. Koutrolos et al., "Commensal microbiota and myelin autoantigen cooperate to trigger autoimmune demyelination," *Nature*, vol. 479, no. 7374, pp. 538–541, 2011.

[111] H. Tlaskalova-Hogenova, L. Tuckova, R. Lodinova-Zadnikova et al., "Mucosal immunity: its role in defense and allergy," *International Archives of Allergy and Immunology*, vol. 128, pp. 77–89, 2002.

[112] C. B. Forsyth, K. M. Shannon, J. H. Kordower et al., "Increased intestinal permeability correlates with sigmoid mucosa alpha-synuclein staining and endotoxin exposure markers in early Parkinson's disease," *PLoS ONE*, vol. 6, no. 12, Article ID e28032, 2011.

[113] A. Fasano, "Zonulin and its regulation of intestinal barrier function: thebiological door to inflammation, autoimmunity, and cancer," *Physiological Reviews*, vol. 91, no. 1, pp. 151–175, 2011.

[114] S. K. Mazmanian, J. L. Round, and D. L. Kasper, "A microbial symbiosis factor prevents intestinal inflammatory disease," *Nature*, vol. 453, pp. 620–625, 2008.

[115] K. M. Maslowski, A. T. Vieira, A. Ng et al., "Regulation of inflammatory responses by gut microbiota and chemoattractant receptor GPR43," *Nature*, vol. 461, no. 7268, pp. 1282–1286, 2009.

[116] M. G. Dominguez-Bello, E. K. Costello, M. Contreras et al., "Delivery mode shapes the acquisition and structure of the initial microbiota across multiple body habitats in newborns," *Proceedings of the National Academy of Sciences of the United States of America*, vol. 107, no. 26, pp. 11971–11975, 2010.

[117] E. Bezirtzoglou, A. Tsiotsias, and G. W. Welling, "Microbiota profile in feces of breast- and formula-fed newborns by using fluorescence in situ hybridization (FISH)," *Anaerobe*, vol. 17, no. 6, pp. 478–482, 2011.

[118] J. Penders, C. Vink, C. Driessen, N. London, C. Thijs, and E. E. Stobberingh, "Quantification of *Bifidobacterium* spp., *Escherichia coli* and *Clostridium difficile* in faecal samples of breast-fed and formula-fed infants by real-time PCR," *FEMS Microbiology Letters*, vol. 243, no. 1, pp. 141–147, 2005.

[119] P. L. Stark and A. Lee, "The microbial ecology of the large bowel of breast-fed and formula-fed infants during the first year of life," *Journal of Medical Microbiology*, vol. 15, no. 2, pp. 189–203, 1982.

2

A Potential Link between Environmental Triggers and Autoimmunity

Aristo Vojdani

Immunosciences Lab., Inc., 822 S. Robertson Boulevard, Suite 312, Los Angeles, CA 90035, USA

Correspondence should be addressed to Aristo Vojdani; drari@msn.com

Academic Editor: K. Michael Pollard

Autoimmune diseases have registered an alarming rise worldwide in recent years. Accumulated evidence indicates that the immune system's ability to distinguish self from nonself is negatively impacted by genetic factors and environmental triggers. Genetics is certainly a factor, but since it normally takes a very long time for the human genetic pattern to change enough to register on a worldwide scale, increasingly the attention of studies has been focused on the environmental factors of a rapidly changing and evolving civilization. New technology, new industries, new inventions, new chemicals and drugs, and new foods and diets are constantly and rapidly being introduced in this fast-paced ever-changing world. Toxicants, infections, epitope spreading, dysfunctions of immune homeostasis, and dietary components can all have an impact on the body's delicate immune recognition system. Although the precise etiology and pathogenesis of many autoimmune diseases are still unknown, it would appear from the collated studies that there are common mechanisms in the immunopathogenesis of multiple autoimmune reactivities. Of particular interest is the citrullination of host proteins and their conversion to autoantigens by the aforementioned environmental triggers. The identification of these specific triggers of autoimmune reactivity is essential then for the development of new therapies for autoimmune diseases.

1. Introduction

The immune system walks a fine line to distinguish self from nonself in preserving the integrity of the host [1]. Interference with this fine line can result in overactivity to self-antigens, leading to autoimmunity. During the past 20 years a significant increase has been observed in the incidence of autoimmune disease worldwide. The etiology and pathogenesis of many autoimmune diseases remain unknown. It does appear that a close interplay between environmental triggers and genetic factors is responsible for the loss of immunological tolerance and autoimmunities [2, 3] (Figure 1). Therefore, in relation to the role of heritability in autoimmunity, genome-wide association studies reported that genetics only accounted for a minority of autoimmunity cases, and in many cases disease discordance exists in monozygotic twins [4]. For this reason, research and publications dedicated to environmental factors in autoimmunity have grown by an average of 7% every year since 1997 [2]. This includes toxic chemicals, infections, and dietary components. Indeed, detection of reactive antibodies to various citrullinated peptides and proteins in autoimmune disease is the best indication for gene-environment interactions [5].

2. Dysregulation of Immune Homeostasis

The full collaboration of both the innate and adaptive arms of the immune system plays a crucial role in the promotion or inhibition of autoimmune disease. Generally, to clear infections the innate immune cells can upregulate costimulatory molecules and produce a mixture of pro- and anti-inflammatory cytokines such as interleukin-1-beta (IL-1β), IL-12, transforming growth factor-beta (TGF-β), IL-23, tumor necrosis factor-alpha (TNF-α), and IL-6 that regulate the adaptive arm of the immune system. However,

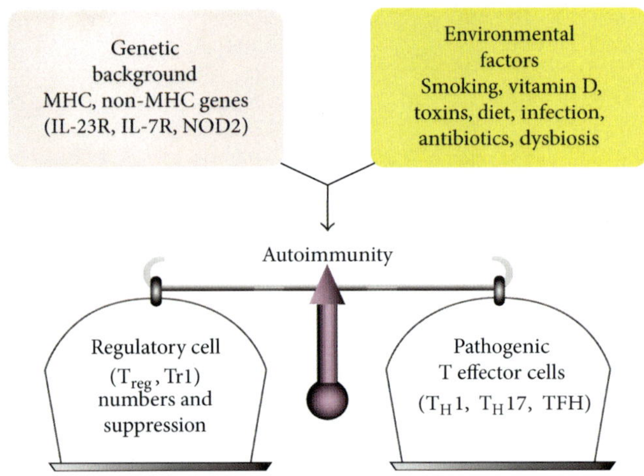

FIGURE 1: The balance of immunity. A combination of host genetic factors and exposure to environmental triggers promote the development of autoimmune disease. A balance must be maintained between the regulatory T cells and the pathogenic T effector cells.

a dysregulated immune response to environmental triggers, such as pathogens, microbiota, or toxins, can initiate a chronic inflammatory response through activation of T-helper-1 (Th1), Th17, and TNF-α and the production of IL-17, IL-22, interferon-gamma (IFN-γ), and IL-21, resulting in inflammation, antibody production and tissue injury [6].

Therefore, a dysregulated adaptive immune system is at the core of the pathogenesis of autoimmune and other immune-mediated diseases. Hyperactivation of innate immune response affects the adaptive immune response as well as development effector T and B cells. Paired with defects in the regulatory T cells, this results in the breakdown of immune homeostasis and the development of autoimmunity [7].

To induce an autoimmune response in the lymph nodes, effector T cells first have to acquire a defined cytokine fingerprint and then must migrate to the appropriate target organs where they initiate tissue inflammation. The effector cells that participate in the induction of autoimmunities are IFN-γ-producing Th1 cells, IL-17- and IL-22-producing Th17 cells, and IL-21-producing follicular Th cells or TFH cells. It has been shown that overactivation or expansion of these newly discovered TFH cells causes antibody production and the development of lupus-like disease in an animal model [8]. In fact, high concentrations of circulating T cells that resemble TFH cells have been detected in a subgroup of patients with lupus. This increased frequency of TFH cells correlated with both disease severity and end-organ damage [9]. Unfortunately, a decrease in frequency and function of FOXP3$^+$T$_{REG}$ cell is often seen in autoimmune diseases. This decrease seems to be associated with the inflammatory environment that contributes to the dysregulation of T$_{REG}$ cells [7].

In the environment of immune homeostasis, the actions of autoreactive Th1, Th17, and TFH cells are countered by FOXP3$^+$ regulatory T cells that produce TGF-β and IL-10. But in an inflammatory milieu the deletion of different transcription factors results in the generation of T$_{REG}$ cells that are unable to suppress the autoreactive T cells (Figure 2).

Thus, tight control of autoreactive T cells, in particular TFH cells, by T$_{REG}$ cells is necessary to suppress the development of autoimmune lupus-like disease.

In order to induce long-lasting remission of immune-mediated diseases, two important factors have to be in place: controlling the inflammatory environment and boosting the frequency and function of FOXP3$^+$ regulatory T cells.

3. Toxicants and Autoimmunity

A number of experimental studies and clinical reports have shown that autoimmune reactivity and/or autoimmune diseases are induced in humans and chronic exposure to various chemicals in animal models. These were summarized by Bigazzi in 1997 [10]. Furthermore, very recently, this role of environmental chemicals, in particular, the induction of autoimmunities by toxicants, was summarized by Pollard et al. [11] in his paper, "Toxicology of autoimmune diseases." The mechanism of toxicant-induced autoimmunity is described by either toxicant induction of aberrant cell death making the hidden cellular material available to anti-gen presenting cells [12, 13] or by immune reactions to xenobiotics through covalent binding of chemicals or haptens to human tissue proteins and formation of neoantigens [14] (Figure 3). This is due to the fact that reactive organic compounds most often bind covalently; that is, their electrophilic properties enable them to react with protein nucleophilic groups such as thiol, amino, and hydroxyl groups. Examples of such reactive, haptenic compounds that frequently lead to sensitization after dermal contact or inhalation are toluene diisocyanate, trimellitic anhydride, phthalic anhydride, benzoquinone, formaldehyde, ethylene oxide, dinitrochlorobenzene, picryl chloride, penicillins, and D-penicillinamine. Sensitizing metal ions react somewhat differently in that they oxidize proteins or

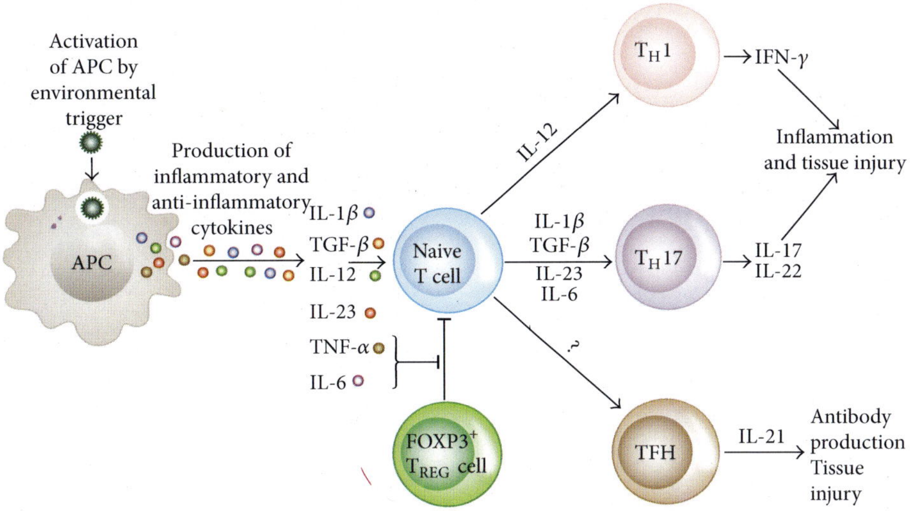

FIGURE 2: Differentiation of naïve T cells into pathogenic effector T cells. APCs can be activated by numerous factors, resulting in the release of cytokines that promote the differentiation of naïve T cells into various subsets of pathogenic effector T cells that drive inflammation, tissue injury, and autoantibody production. Segmented filamentous bacteria (SFB) can also promote the development of Th17 cells and autoimmune responses *in vivo*. Proinflammatory cytokines derived from both innate and adaptive immune cells attenuate T_{REG} cell-mediated suppression of effector T cells.

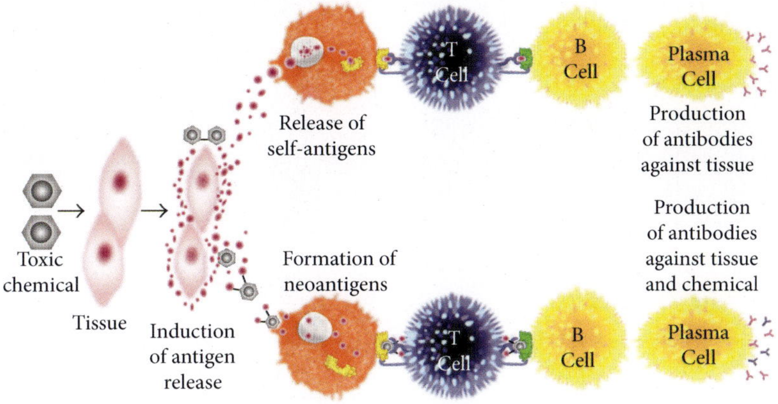

FIGURE 3: Putative mechanism of chemical-induced autoimmunity.

form stable protein-metal chelate complexes by undergoing multipoint binding with several amino acid side-chains [12]. For example, in regard to nail polish and its association with primary biliary cirrhosis (PBC), halogenated compounds could bind to mitochondrial proteins, changing their immunogenicity and inducing antimitochondrial antibodies [10, 15, 16].

In contrast to haptenic compounds, most xenobiotics eliciting adverse immune reaction are unable to bind to proteins when entering the body; however, they can do so after conversion to reactive metabolites. These xenobiotics can be considered as prohaptens, which, after metabolization, manage to bind to human tissue proteins and induce antibody production against both the haptenic chemicals as well as tissue proteins.

Another mechanism is the activation of toll-like receptors by xenobiotics. This predisposes individuals to toxicant-induced inflammatory cytokine production, which exacerbates autoimmune diseases [17].

These and other mechanisms of action were explored in relation to exposure to organic solvents as a risk factor for autoimmune disease in a very extensive systemic review of literature and meta-analysis [18]. After reviewing a total of 103 articles and the inclusion of 33 in the meta-analysis, it was concluded that (1) exposure to organic solvents was associated with systemic sclerosis, primary systemic vasculitis, and multiple sclerosis (MS) and (2) individuals who carry genetic factors for autoimmunities should avoid any exposure to organic solvents in order to avoid increasing their risk for autoimmune diseases.

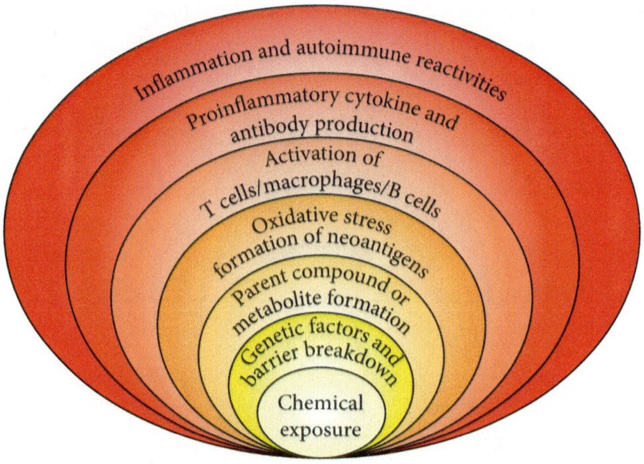

FIGURE 4: Potential molecular mechanisms implicated in chemical-induced autoimmune reactivities.

In addition to the above mechanisms of actions (as shown in Figures 3 and 4), these autoimmune responses and diseases can be induced by solvents and other environmental chemicals through a variety of effects at the biochemical and cellular levels.

(i) Chemicals are capable of altering cellular proliferation, Th1, Th2, Th3, Th17, apoptosis, and tissue-specific function.

(ii) Chemicals are capable of inducing protein or lipid adducts which activate Th17 cells and induce the production of IL-17 and IL-21.

(iii) Chemicals can activate HSP90 and induce production of anti-HSP90 autoantibodies.

(iv) Chemicals are capable of inducing DNA-hypermethylation and change in cellular functions.

(v) Chemicals can increase ROS production and the induction of DNA-fragmentation.

(vi) Chemicals may compete with thyroid hormones or interfere with iodine transportation and induce oxidative stress that leads to an inflammatory response to the thyroid gland.

(vii) Chemicals not only stimulate the release of reactive oxygen species but also stimulate the synthesis of nitric oxide by nitric oxide synthase [18].

Finally, modification of DNA methylation is an additional mechanism by which environmental triggers induce changes in gene expression. For example, environmental pollutants, cigarette smoke and alcohol consumption have been advocated for autoimmunity incidence due to their links with the induction of DNA methylation [10, 19].

Overall, the precise mechanisms responsible for the development of environmentally induced autoimmune disorders are unknown. Additionally, mechanisms involved in the initiation of a disease process might differ from mechanisms responsible for exacerbation of the established illness. Therefore, one or more of these mechanisms either individually or jointly can have strong effects on the development of autoimmune reactivity, which may then be followed by autoimmune disease (Figure 4).

4. Induction of Autoimmunities by Infection

Although some infections can protect individuals from specific autoimmune diseases, infectious agents play a pivotal role in the induction of autoimmune disorders. The question of how infectious agents contribute to autoimmunity has continued to be of interest to clinical and basic researchers and immunologists in general [20].

An autoimmune disease can be induced or triggered by infectious agents, which can also determine its clinical manifestations. Most infectious agents, such as viruses, bacteria, fungi, and parasites, can induce autoimmunity via different mechanisms. In many cases, it is not a single infection but rather the "burden of infections" from childhood that is responsible for the induction of autoimmunity [20].

Almost every autoimmune disease is linked to one or more infectious agent. During the past 50 years molecular techniques have been utilized to explore the interaction between infections and autoimmunities [20–23]. One of the classical examples of this relationship is rheumatic fever, which presents several weeks after infection with beta hemolytic streptococcus. Molecular resemblance between the bacterial M5 protein and human α-myosin results in a breakdown of immunological tolerance and antibody production against α-myosin in genetically susceptible individuals [21, 24]. In the case of antiphospholipid syndrome (APS), anticardiolipin and anti-β_2-glycoprotein I pathogenic (β_2GPI) antibodies are detected. Although there is molecular mimicry between β_2GPI and infections, such as cytomegalovirus, *Haemophilus influenza, Neisseria gonorrhoeae*, rubella, toxoplasma, and tetanus toxoid, and IgM antibodies against them have been detected, the direct connection between these infections and APS has not been established [24]. Another example of associating infection with autoimmune disease is type 1 diabetes. Type 1 diabetes is an autoimmune disease resulting from the destruction of β-islet cells by autoreactive

T cells and the concomitant release of various islet cell antigens [21, 25]. The appearance of antibodies against glutamic acid decarboxylase 65 (GAD-65) and tyrosine phosphatase precedes the onset of the disease by 5–10 years [26, 27]. Several lines of evidence link infections with type 1 diabetes.

(1) A search on PubMed using the keywords "association of viruses with type 1 diabetes" produces close to 1,400 manuscripts.

(2) Enteroviruses such as coxsackie B4 virus and rotavirus, the most common cause of childhood gastroenteritis, not only share homology with GAD-65, but can cause the precipitation of type 1 diabetes when introduced. Higher levels of anti-coxsackievirus and rotavirus antibodies are detected in sera from patients with recent onset of type 1 diabetes [28, 29].

(3) Using PCR technology, coxsackie B4 virus was detected in islet cells of 65% of patients versus only 6% of controls [30].

(4) Inoculation of the virus to genetically susceptible strains of mice resulted in insulitis and diabetes, fulfilling Koch's postulates [21, 31, 32].

(5) Both DNA and RNA viruses are capable of initiating antiviral responses that cross-react with insulin, GAD-65, and other islet cell antigens [21, 33, 34].

Altering the balance of gut microbiota toward either a tolerogenic or nontolerogenic state using antibiotics or probiotics may influence the development of type 1 diabetes [35, 36]. Therefore, just as with their viral counterparts, there is sufficient indirect evidence that gut and other microbial agents, for example, *Mycobacterium avium*, are potential triggers for type 1 diabetes [37].

This multifaceted interaction between genetics, immune dysregulation, various infections, and autoimmune diseases such as rheumatoid arthritis (RA) and thyroid disease reveals many possibilities for pathogenic relationships between different species of infectious agents and autoimmunity [20, 38, 39]. These infectious agents and their association with RA and thyroid autoimmunity are shown in Tables 1 and 2.

4.1. Mechanisms Responsible for the Induction of Autoimmunity by Infection. Autoimmunity can be induced by infectious agents through the following mechanisms: molecular mimicry, epitope spreading, standard activation, viral persistence, polyclonal activation, dysregulation of immune homeostasis, and autoinflammatory activation of innate immunity [20]. In some cases, even if infections are not directly responsible for the induction of autoimmunities, they can often target the site of autoimmune inflammation and amplify the autoimmune disease [68]. In this case, infections can have one of three effects: first, it can exacerbate ongoing disease, leading to greater severity and duration; second, it can induce a relapse; and, third, it can lead to chronic progressive disease.

4.1.1. Molecular Mimicry. In the most likely mechanism by which infection induces autoimmunity, foreign antigens very often may bear sufficient structural similarity to self-antigens.

Table 1: Infectious agents associated with rheumatoid arthritis.

Infection	Reference
Porphyromonas gingivalis	Farquharson et al. 2012 [40]
Segmented filamentous bacteria	Wu et al. 2010 [41]
Yersinia enterocolitica	Gaston and Lillicrap 2003 [42]
Salmonella typhi	McColl et al. 2000 [43]
Shigella flexneri	Hannu et al. 2005 [44]
Proteus mirabilis	Ebringer and Rashid 2006 [45]
Campylobacter jejuni	Pope et al. 2007 [46]
Klebsiella pneumoniae	Domínguez-López et al. 2000 [47]
Clostridium difficile	Cope et al. 1992 [48]
Staphylococcus aureus	Liu et al. 2001 [49]
Streptococcus pyogenes	Faé et al. 2006 [50]
Candida albicans	Hermann et al. 1991 [51]
Leptospira pomona	Sutliff et al. 1953 [52]
Chlamydia	Carter et al. 2010 [53]
Mycoplasma arthritidis	Cole and Ward 1979 [54]
Mycobacterium tuberculosis	Kim et al. 2006 [55]
Borrelia burgdorferi	Imai et al. 2013 [56]
Parvovirus	Kerr et al. 1995 [57]
Epstein-Barr virus	Pratesi et al. 2006 [58]

Table 2: Infectious agents associated with thyroid autoimmunity.

Infection	Reference
Yersinia enterocolitica	Bech et al. 1978 [59]
Epstein-Barr virus	Shimon et al. 2003 [60]
Parvovirus	Mori et al. 2007 [61]
Hepatitis C	Fernandez-Soto et al. 1998 [62]
Mumps	Parmar et al. 2001 [63]
Rubella	Ziring et al. 1977 [64]
Coxsackievirus	Brouqui et al. 1991 [65]
HTLV-1	Kawai et al. 1992 [66]
Human herpes virus types 6 and 7	Leite et al. 2008 [67]

This is called antigenic mimicry or molecular mimicry. Immune response to microbial antigens could result in activation of T cells that are cross-reactive with self-antigens. This is due to the fact that a single T cell can respond to various peptides with similar charge distribution and overall shape [20, 69]. Examples of bacterial or viral antigens, their cross-reactivity with various tissue antigens, and potential ensuing autoimmune diseases are shown in Table 3.

Mechanisms of infection-induced autoimmunity through molecular mimicry are shown in Figure 5.

Initiation of immune response to the foreign antigens such as coxsackievirus that share identical amino acid residues with self-proteins such as GAD-65 may generate a cross-reactive antibody response that incorrectly recognizes the self-protein as a foreign antigen. When the self-antigen is

TABLE 3: Examples of bacterial and viral antigens that can cross-react with self-antigens with potentially resultant diseases.

Pathogen antigen	Cross-reactive self-antigen	Autoimmune disease
Herpes simplex virus	Corneal antigen	Stromal keratitis
Campylobacter jejuni	Ganglioside in peripheral nerve	Guillain-Barré syndrome
Coxsackievirus	Glutamic acid decarboxylase	Type 1 diabetes
Theiler's murine encephalomyelitis virus	Proteolipid protein	Multiple sclerosis
Yersinia enterocolitica	Thyrotropin receptor	Thyroid autoimmunity
Borrelia burgdorferi	Leukocyte function associated antigen	Lyme arthritis
Salmonella typhi and *Yersinia enterocolitica*	HLA-B27	Reactive arthritis
HHV-6, EBV, Rubeolla, influenza virus, and HPV	Myelin basic protein	Multiple sclerosis
Streptococcal M protein	Myosin and other heart valve proteins	Rheumatic fever
Trypanosoma cruzi	Cardiac myosis	Chagas heart disease

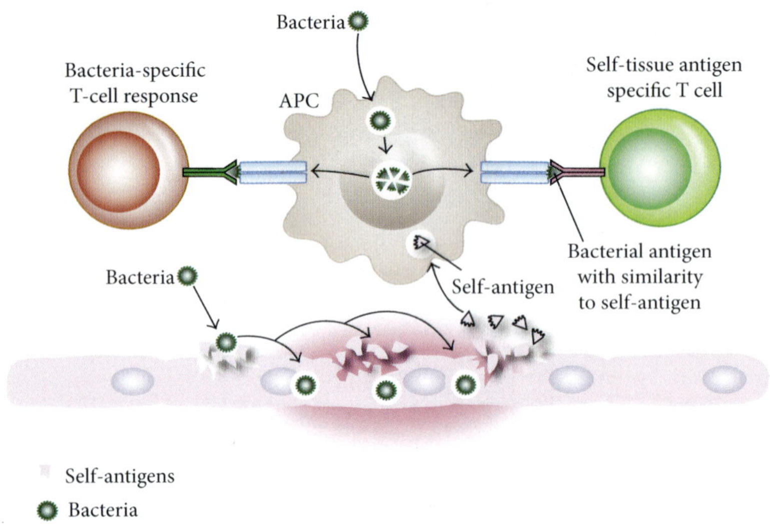

FIGURE 5: Mechanisms of infection-induced autoimmunity through molecular mimicry. Bacterial induction of self-tissue antigen release and simultaneous presentation of bacterial and self-tissue antigens to T cells; activated T cells can produce antibodies against both bacterial and self-tissue antigens.

a cell surface molecule such as GAD-65, the antibody- and cell-mediated immune response can lead to tissue damage [69].

Given the vast numbers of microbial proteins and their cross-reaction with human proteins, immune response against microbial antigens will not always result in autoimmunity. However, such an initial immune response could result in epitope spreading or exposure of other regions of the same self-protein and production of more antibodies [69]. The criteria for the mechanism of autoimmunity induction were reviewed and summarized by Kivity et al. 2009 [20]. In the classical examples of autoimmunities induced by infections summarized in Table 3, all these criteria are present.

4.1.2. Epitope Spreading. Epitope spreading is a phenomenon in which the immune system expands its response beyond the original epitope recognized by T or B cells to induce the release of non-cross-reactive epitopes that are recognized by the immune system later [70]. Epitope spreading can result from a change in protein structure. One such example is protein citrullination, the changing of an amino acid from arginine to citrulline. This can result not only in immune reaction against the original protein or its citrullinated form, but also against other citrullinated proteins.

Epitope spreading is demonstrated in rheumatic fever, in which a chronic autoimmune response against streptococcal M protein and heart valve tissue can result in immune response against collagen or laminin. This immune response against collagen or laminin is no longer specific to the bacterial M protein or its cross-reactive tissue protein. In pemphigus, blistering of the mouth precedes blistering of the skin, and blisters in the mouth are associated with the presence of antibodies against desmoglein-3 protein, which is specific to the mouth epithelial cell antigens. It is only later on when T cells attack skin desmoglein-1 that autoantibodies are produced against skin-specific antigens, and skin blistering develops [71]. In a mouse model of encephalomyelitis, Theiler's murine encephalomyelitis virus T-cell response to myelin develops first against dominant myelin proteolipid (PLP) peptide 139–151. As the disease progresses, response to the different and less dominant epitope PLP peptide 178–191 emerges. This mechanism of

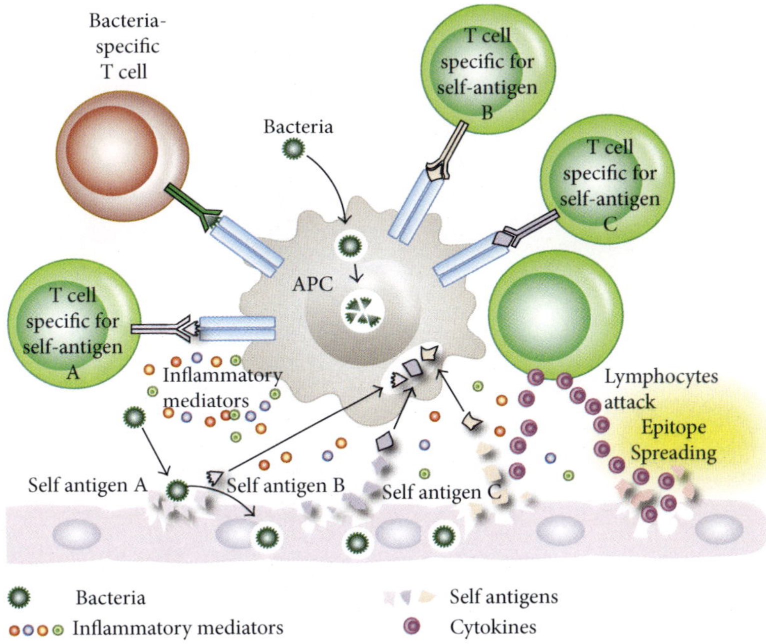

FIGURE 6: Bacterial infection induces release of tissue antigen and presentation of bacterial and self-tissue antigens resulting in the induction of autoreactive T cells. T cells and inflammatory mediators cause the release of more self-antigens which differ from the original antigens. T-cell responses can then spread to involve T cells specific to other self-antigens. This T-cell response against different epitopes results in antibody production against multiple tissue antigens.

infection-induced autoimmunity through epitope spreading is shown in Figure 6.

4.1.3. Bystander Activation and Stimulation of Pattern Recognition Receptors. Bystander activation occurs when viral antigens stimulate toll-like receptors and other pattern recognition receptors become activated in the inflammatory environment [72]. This activation of receptors on an antigen-presenting cell (APC) causes the release of proinflammatory cytokines which can induce tissue damage and the release of hidden antigens (Figure 7). The release of tissue antigens can activate autoreactive T cells that initially were not involved in the immune reactivity against the original infection [20]. Additionally, virally infected APCs and the concomitantly released mediators are able to activate autoreactive Th1 or Th17 cells in a bystander manner. Upon recognition of virally infected tissue cells, viral-specific T cells then release cytotoxic granules such as granzymes and cytokines such as TNF-α, IL-17, lymphotoxin, and nitric oxide. This inflammatory environment can lead to the bystander killing of uninfected neighboring cells. Microbial superantigens can induce a broader form of bystander activation by cross-linking MHC class II molecules to TCRs on APCs and T-cell activation (Figure 8). T cells that are stimulated in this manner may contain a subset recognizing specific tissue antigen [73]. Examples of superantigens are staphylococcal antigens, mycoplasma antigens, enteric-microbiota LPS, EBV, retrovirus, and many heat shock proteins. Some of these superantigens do not cause autoimmune disease but are involved in the exacerbation of EAE, arthritis, IBD, and other disorders [1].

4.1.4. Persistent Infection and Polyclonal Activation of B Cells. In many autoimmune diseases, such as lupus, RA, type 1 diabetes, and MS, B-cell functions are closely correlated with disease activity. Antibodies produced by B-cell-derived plasma cells contribute significantly to disease pathogenesis [69]. In these and other disorders, prolonged infectivity with a virus such as EBV, viral proteins, or viral genomes can lead to autoimmunity by the constant activation and proliferation of B cells.

After a long period of polyclonal B-cell activation, sometimes monospecific clones can emerge, accompanied by very high levels of antibody production and the formation of circulating immune complexes. Finally, this mixture of polyclonal antibodies and immune complexes may cause the autoimmune disease [74], as shown in Figure 9.

5. Dietary Components and Autoimmunities

It is undeniable that the diet of the industrialized and urbanized parts of the world today is vastly different from what it was even two or three decades ago, with a whole new range of novel food experiences that come from new food component sources, new breeds of food plants and food animals, genetic modifications, chemical ingredients, flavors, and preservatives. Over recent decades, a significant increase in the incidence of autoimmune diseases such as diabetes and MS in industrialized countries has led to the postulation that diet is a potential environmental risk factor

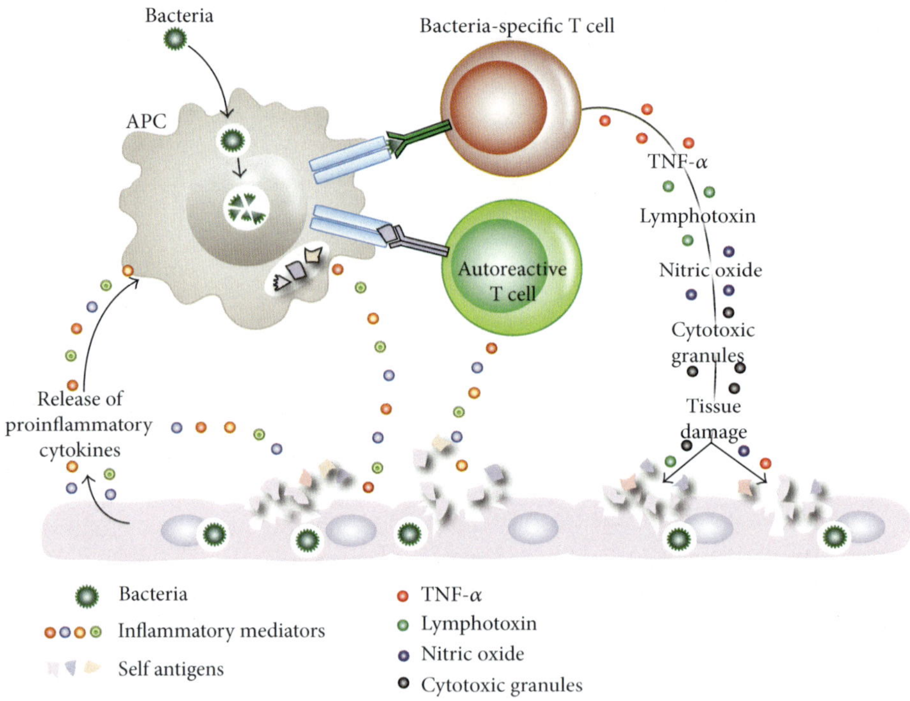

FIGURE 7: Microbial infection stimulates toll-like receptors (TLRs) and other pattern recognition receptors on antigen-presenting cells (APCs), leading to the production of proinflammatory mediators, which in turn can lead to tissue damage. The release of both tissue antigens and bacterial antigens results in bacterial-specific T cells and autoreactive T cells in the process called bystander activation, which contributes to autoimmunity.

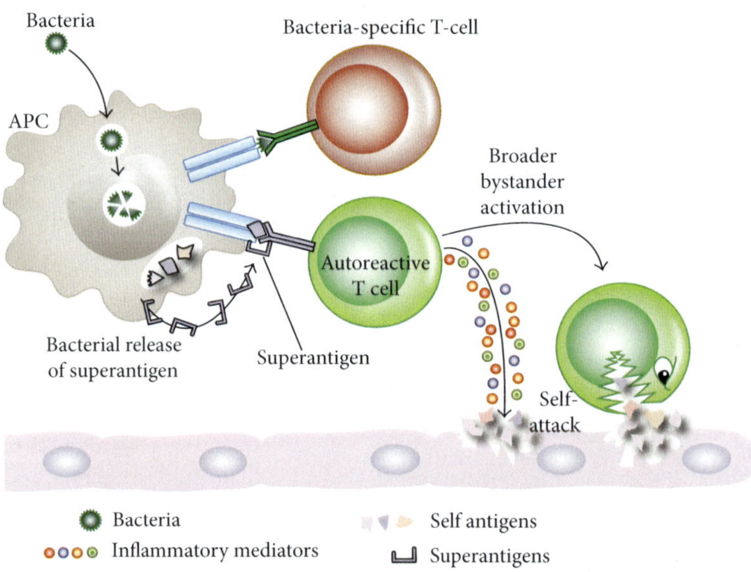

FIGURE 8: Superantigens and autoimmunity. Infection can lead to the release of superantigens, which can cross-link between MHCII and TCR, causing broader bystander activation, some of which may be specific for self-antigens, leading to attack on self-tissues.

for such disorders. The link between gluten ingestion and gluten sensitive enteropathies is already well established and accepted [3]. High levels of dietary sodium are associated with raised blood pressure and adverse cardiovascular health [75] and have been shown to affect the immune system [76]. Low levels of vitamin D have been linked with MS, systemic lupus erythematosus (SLE), RA, and other autoimmune disorders [3]. Lactose intolerance is no laughing matter for those afflicted with it or other milk-related disorders. The pleasures of a modern diet unfortunately come with caveats and unexpected catches that urgently need investigation.

5.1. Sodium Chloride in Diet and Autoimmune Diseases. For the past five decades various studies have been conducted on

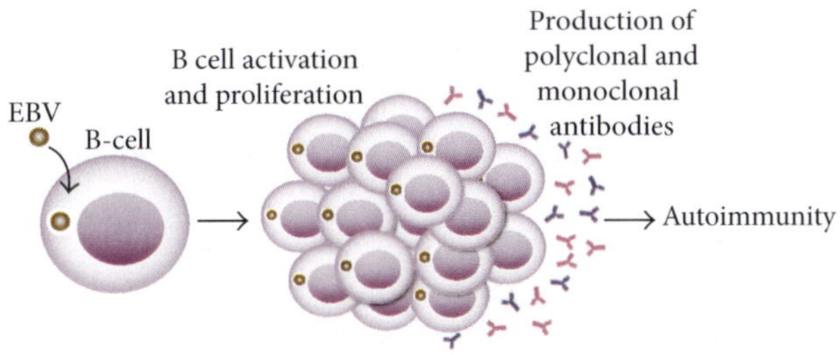

FIGURE 9: Infections, B cells, and autoimmunity. Prolonged infection with a virus, such as EBV, can lead to constant activation and proliferation of B cells, resulting in the production of monoclonal and polyclonal antibodies as well as immune complexes, causing autoimmune disease.

the comparative sodium intake levels in different countries [75, 76]. Animal experiments, epidemiological studies, and clinical trials have provided convincing evidence for the detrimental effect of sodium intake on blood pressure (BP), coronary heart disease, and stroke, as well as noncardiovascular diseases [77–81]. These comparative studies have shown that generally the simpler and less modernized a society and culture are, the lower the sodium intake is, with a concomitant lessening of the associated disorders. Understandably, the high salt content of the modern Asian diet is known worldwide, particularly the use of soy sauce as a seasoning [75, 82]. Indeed, in comparison to home-made meals, the salt content of fast foods can be many times higher [75]. The concentration of Na^+ in plasma similar to standard culture medium is about 149 mM. The consumption of high-salt processed foods may increase this concentration to a higher level and result in a change in physiological conditions. It has been theorized that the consumption of processed foods containing high amounts of salt may in part be responsible for the increasing incidence of autoimmune diseases. In a recent study it was demonstrated that an excess uptake of salt can affect the innate immune system, in particular, macrophage function [83]. However, until very recently little was known about increased NaCl intake, its direct effect on the T-helper cell populations, and the connection of all this to autoimmune diseases. Upon stimulation of the T-cell receptor and the cytokine environment, the naïve $CD4^+$ T cell can differentiate into functionally distinct effector cell subsets. This differentiation is also driven by key transcriptional regulators such as T-bet for Th1, GATA binding protein-3 for Th2, FOXP3 for Th3, retinoid acid receptor-related orphan receptor gamma t (RORγt) for Th17, and transcriptional regulator B-cell lymphoma 6 (BCL6) for T-follicular-helper (TFH) cells [84].

Among these $CD4^+$ T-cell subsets, the IL-23-dependent IL-17-producing $CD4^+$ helper T cells play a pivotal role in autoimmune disease [85]. Adding salt to the wound of complex autoimmune diseases, it has been shown that sodium chloride can drive autoimmune disease by the activation or induction of pathogenic Th17 cells [86]. These elegant experiments were conducted in a culture medium containing an additional 10–40 mM concentration of salt, mimicking animals fed a high-salt diet. Increased NaCl concentrations markedly induced the conversion of naïve $CD4^+$ T cells to $CD4^+$ T cells expressing IL-17A (Figure 10). This effect was dose dependent, and the optimum IL-17A induction was achieved by increasing the concentration of NaCl by 40 mM. Moreover, the authors demonstrated that a high-salt diet could accelerate neuropathology in a mouse model of multiple sclerosis through cellular signaling pathways involving transcription factor NFAT5, the protein kinase enzyme P38, and salt-sensing kinase SGK1. In comparison with the controls, mice on the high-salt diet not only displayed a much higher number of infiltrating $CD3^+$ and $MAC3^+$ cells but also almost doubled the number of $CD4^+$ T cells expressing IL-17A or pathogenic Th17 cells [86, 87]. This effect of the high-salt diet was specific for Th17 conditions, since the high salt levels did not significantly alter cell death, lymphocyte proliferation, or enhancement of Th1 or Th2 differentiations. The mechanism by which a high-salt diet enhances the differentiation of naïve $CD4^+$ cells to pathogenic Th17 cells is shown in Figure 11.

Extracellular NaCl concentration through the activation of IL-23 receptor and its binding by IL-23 influences the activity of SGK1 and NFAT5 which drives the expression of transcription factor RORγt, IL-23R, IL-17A, and IL-17F resulting in the phenotype switch from naïve $CD4^+$ T cells to pathogenic Th17 cells in MS, psoriasis, and other autoimmune disorders (Figure 12). The data presented in these manuscripts [86, 87] clearly indicate that high intake of sodium potentiates pathogenic Th17 cell generation in *in vitro* and *in vivo* systems in an SGK1-dependent manner and, therefore, has the potential of increasing the risk of promoting autoimmune diseases. Moreover, the elevated *in vivo* Th17 resulting from a high-salt diet raises the important question of whether or not increased salt in westernized diets and in processed foods contributes to an increased generation of pathogenic Th17 cells and towards an unprecedented increase in autoimmune diseases [87].

Thus, as indicated, dietary salt is just one of many dietary components that can influence T-helper cell differentiation and the development of autoimmune disease. The effect of other dietary nutrients, for example, vitamins, and other diverse environmental factors on metabolism and microbiota should also be investigated [88].

When this information is taken together with the strong and consistent evidence that implicates high salt intake with high BP and other cardiovascular disorders, it is alarming to note as laid out in all these studies that most adult populations have daily salt intakes well over the recommended US daily

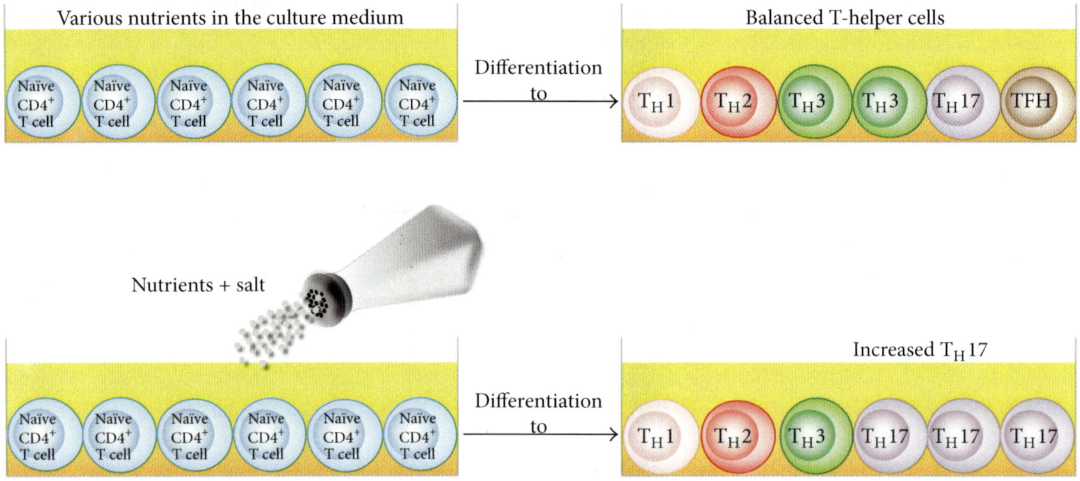

FIGURE 10: Salt affects the differentiation of naïve $CD4^+$ cells. Increased concentrations of salt resulted in the differentiation of naïve $CD4^+$ T cells into a greater number of T_H17 cells.

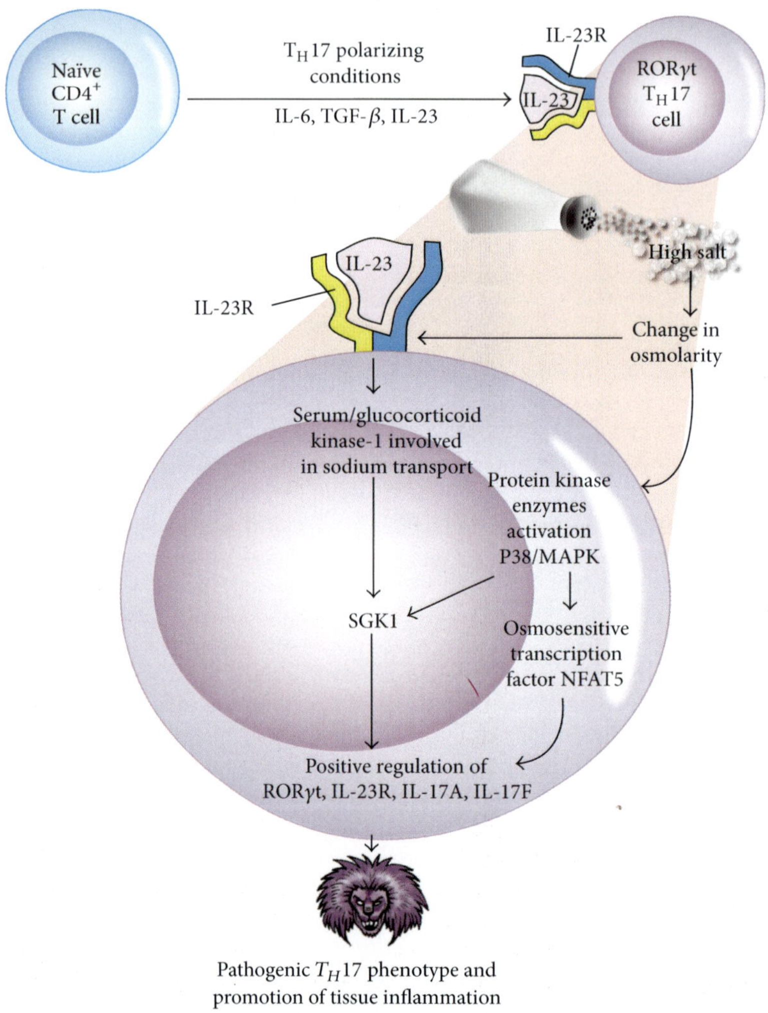

FIGURE 11: Mechanism by which a high-salt diet enhances the differentiation of naïve $CD4^+$ cells to pathogenic T_H17 cells that may exacerbate experimental autoimmune encephalitis. High salt concentration, change in osmolarity, the influence of IL-23 and IL-23 receptor signaling, and the activation of various enzymes drive the expression of T_H17-associated cytokines and the formation of pathogenic T_H17 phenotype.

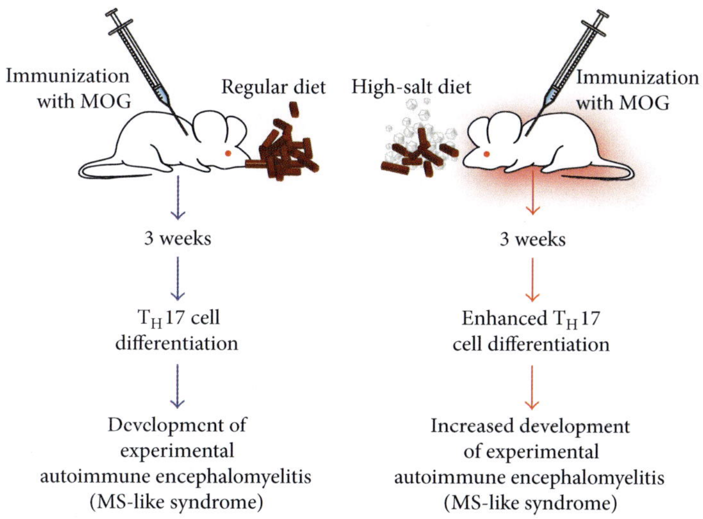

Figure 12: High-salt diet increases risk of autoimmune disease. In two groups of mice, both of which were immunized with MOG to induce EAE, the mice that had been given a high-salt diet (HSD) showed enhanced differentiation of naïve T cells into pathogenic T_H17 cells and a subsequent increased, more profligate development of EAE.

level of 1.5 g/day for middle-aged and older adults [89]. On the face of it a voluntary decrease in salt consumption seems to be an easy policy to implement, but good sense and good health face the formidable opposing forces of flavor, habit, and culture.

5.2. The Role of Milk and Wheat Components in Autoimmune Diseases. In relation to dietary proteins it has been well established that different proteins and peptides in milk and wheat are involved in autoimmune diseases [90–93]. Milk contains more than 400 different proteins, most of which have over 150 amino acids (AA). AA that mimic collagen may induce RA, while those that mimic neural cell antigens may induce multiple sclerosis or other neuroimmune disorders.

For example, a study reports that, as a consequence of immunological cross-reactivity or molecular mimicry between the extracellular IV-like domain of the milk protein butyrophilin and myelin oligodendrocyte glycoprotein (MOG), butyrophilin can modulate the encephalitogenic T-cell response to MOG in experimental autoimmune encephalitis [92]. Epidemiological and ecological investigations suggest that early infant nutrition, particularly drinking cow's milk, may induce autoimmunity, leading to type 1 diabetes. This autoimmune reactivity is due to cross-reactivity of cow's milk, particularly its albumin component, with islet cell antigen-1 and beta cell surface protein. These studies suggest that dysregulation of oral tolerance triggers a cellular and humoral immune response against various components of milk proteins, and cross-reaction with B-cell molecules may result in autoimmunity [94–97]. In association with various autoimmune disorders, wheat proteins and, more specifically, gluten, have received significant attention [98–100]. Indeed, it has been demonstrated that a wheat-based diet induces not only Th1-type cytokine bias in the gut but also increased T-cell reactivity to gluten, with a higher frequency of diabetes [99–101]. In addition to diabetes, it has been shown that celiac disease (CD) is associated with various extraintestinal autoimmune disorders that involve the thyroid, joints, heart, skin, pancreas, bone, liver, reproductive organs, and the nervous system [102–112].

Although the exact mechanisms for the induction of these autoimmunities are not definitely known, there is a growing body of evidence indicating that these diseases may result from molecular mimicry between gliadin or transglutaminase and various tissue antigens, including nervous system proteins [33–35, 68]. Interestingly, the celiac peptide VVKVGGSSSLGW shares more than 30% homology with the trangslutaminase peptide 476–487 (RIRVGQSMNMGS) [113]. Therefore, antibodies generated against transglutaminase in the intestine can bind to extraintestinal tissues such as those of the liver, pancreas, lymph nodes, muscle, heart, and brain [114–117]. Very recently, we used both affinity-purified and, monoclonal antibodies against α-gliadin 33-mer peptide to examine the cross-reaction between gliadin with different food and tissue antigens [91]. We observed significant immune reactivity when these antibodies were applied to cow's milk, milk chocolate, milk butyrophilin, whey protein, casein, yeast, oats, corn, millet, instant coffee, and rice. With regard to the reaction of α-gliadin antibody with various tested tissue antigens, the most significant binding occurred with asialoganglioside, hepatocyte, glutamic acid decarboxylase 65, adrenal 21-hydroxylase, and various neural antigens [92].

These studies collectively indicate that circulating antibodies present in patients with nonceliac gluten sensitivity (NCGS) and CD interact with different food antigens and transglutaminases in various tissues, which may induce the formation of antigen-antibody aggregates that can trigger the activation of the inflammatory cascade.

While most studies about the implications of cross-reactivity with various autoimmunities are limited to milk

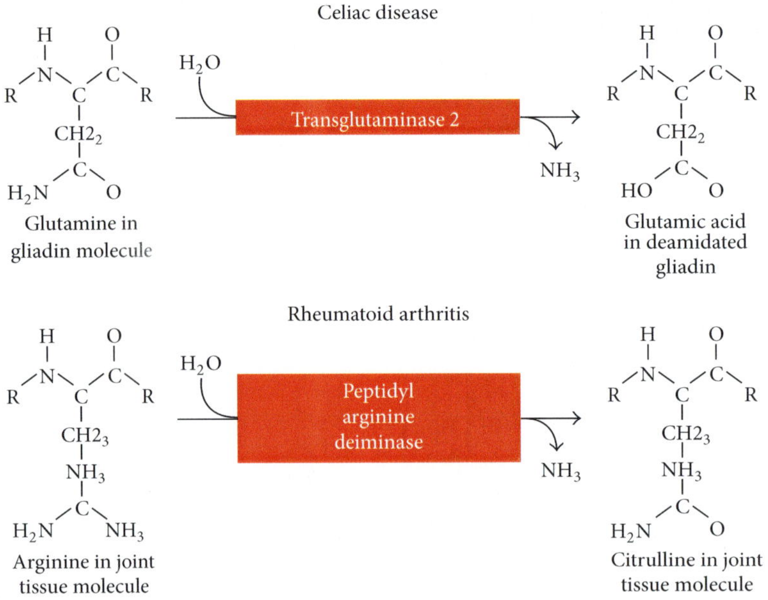

FIGURE 13: The central role of catalytic enzymes in celiac disease and rheumatoid arthritis. Key enzymes that catalyze the modification of glutamine to glutamic acid or arginine to citrulline as new epitopes have a central role in CD and RA.

and wheat, a thorough investigation and understanding of the immunologic cross-reactivity of other food proteins and peptides are essential for advancing our knowledge about the involvement of these dietary components in the development of many autoimmune disorders. Finally, the identification of triggers of autoimmunity can be used in the development of new therapies for autoimmune diseases.

6. Using Gluten Sensitivity, Celiac Disease, and Oral Pathogens to Understand Autoimmunities

There is a lot that clinicians can learn about autoimmune diseases from looking at gluten sensitivity and celiac disease. Some of the features of CD HLA-DQ2/DQ8 association, target organ (villi) T-cell infiltration, and disease-specific autoantibodies produced against modified antigens such as deamidated gliadin and deamidated gliadin-transglutaminase complex [99, 116] are paralleled in chronic joint disorder [94, 118]. These observations suggest that it might be feasible to use CD to identify disease-relevant epitopes in RA and other autoimmune disorders, such as type 1 diabetes and multiple sclerosis [100]. For example, the key enzymes that catalyze the modification of glutamine to glutamic acid or arginine to citrulline as new epitopes have a central role in CD and RA (Figure 13).

It is interesting to note that this process of arginine deamination and the formation of citrullinated proteins and peptides in the joint or other tissues could be potentiated by oral pathogens such as *Porphyromonas gingivalis* [40, 119–124] (Figure 14). That is why RA can also cause inflammation in other organs, including the skin, lungs, heart, and peripheral nerves, often with serious consequences.

This is only one observation suggesting that environmental triggers can change self-tissue antigens to become disease-associated T-cell epitope, resulting in antibody production against the citrulline-containing new epitope. Therefore, if CD as an autoimmune disorder is driven by transglutaminase-2 and deamidated gliadin, then we may state that RA is caused by environmental factors, such as *P. gingivalis* or EBV. These environmental factors, by causing the formation of various citrullinated self-epitopes such as collagen type II, fibrin, vimentin, keratin, α-enolase, and filaggrin, are involved in the induction of RA [119–125]. Experience with CD has taught scientists that genes, environmental factors, and target tissue antigens are all important issues for consideration in understanding the molecular structure of epitopes recognized by T cells and B cells within the inflamed target organ [100, 124].

6.1. Mechanism Involved in the Induction of Autoimmunity by Oral Pathogen. A similar mechanism applies to the autopathogenic correlation of periodontitis induced by *P. gingivalis* and RA [40, 119, 124]. It is possible that both diseases share a common aetiopathogenic background [124]. This mechanism includes the posttranslation modification or citrullination of bacterial proteins and self-antigens simultaneously, generating neoepitope structure. This can result in a breakdown in self-tolerance and antibody production against citrullinated bacterial antigens as well as citrullinated host proteins [125]. One such antigen is α-enolase, which features significant homology between human and bacterial α-enolase. Therefore, antibodies produced against citrullinated bacterial α-enolase will react with human α-enolase, and antibodies produced against human citrullinated α-enolase will react strongly against bacterial α-enolase. For this

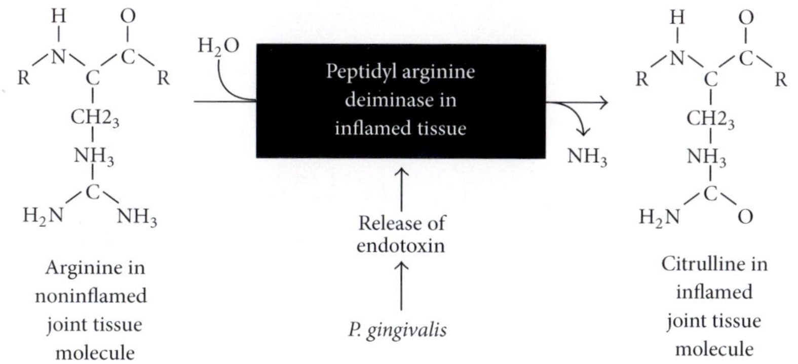

FIGURE 14: Potentiation by oral pathogens. Oral pathogens such as *P. gingivalis* can potentiate the deamination of arginine or formation of citrullinated proteins and peptides in joint and other tissues.

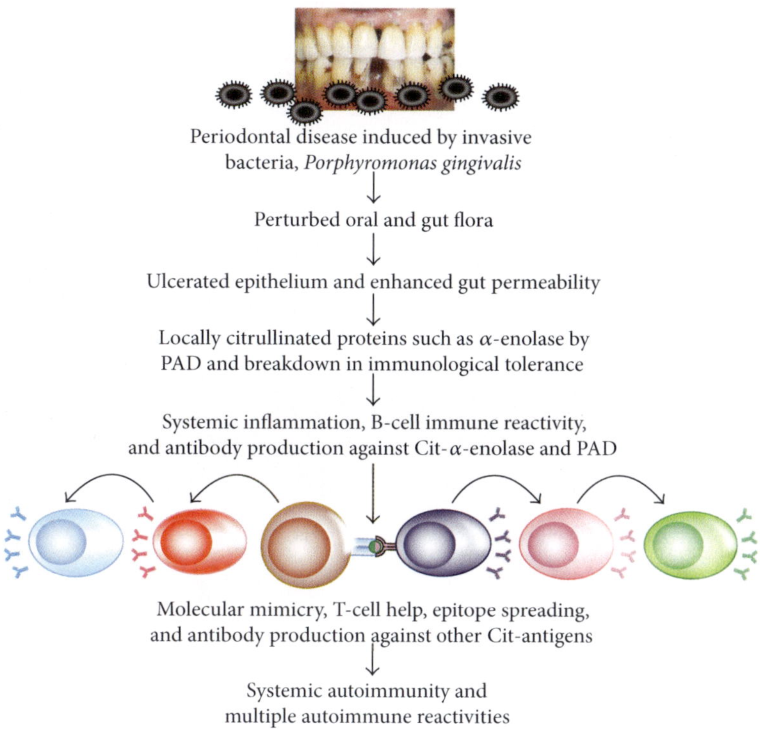

FIGURE 15: Proposed model for the pathogenesis of multiple autoimmune reactivities by infection. Bacterial generation of autoantigens, local inflammation generating autoantigens by PAD, antibody production against one autoantigen, epitope spreading, antibody production against multiple antigens, systemic inflammation, and multiple autoimmune reactivities.

reason, elevated levels of α-enolase antibodies are detected in the synovium of 60% of patients with RA [122]. Indeed, immunological mapping using a library of cyclic citrullinated α-enolase peptides led to the identification of a B-cell-dominant epitope comprising amino acids 5–21 of α-enolase (KIHAREIFDSRGNPTVE) where arginine-9 and arginine-15 are citrullinated, with an 82% sequence similarity with that of *P. gingivalis* [126, 127]. Immunization with citrullinated human and *P. gingivalis* α-enolase and citrullinated fibrinogen causes similar pathology in humanized DR4 transgenic mice. This mechanism may be the common denominator between autoimmunity and cardiovascular disease. These findings suggest that, by mimicking the molecular structure of host-citrullinated proteins, *P. gingivalis* peptidylarginine deiminase-citrullinated bacterial α-enolase could trigger a loss of tolerance to structurally similar host proteins, resulting in expression of anti-citrullinated protein antibodies and the development of RA [128, 129].

These antibodies can be detected up to 10 years before the clinical onset of RA and the production of IgM antibodies against IgG (called rheumatoid factor) in the majority of patients.

In the joint, the specificity of anti-citrullinated peptide is enhanced through epitope spreading to other citrullinated autoantigens such as fibrinogen, collagen, filaggrin, and vimentin (see Figure 15).

7. Conclusion

Putting all this information together, it appears that there are common mechanisms in the immunopathogenesis of multiple autoimmune reactivities. In genetically susceptible individuals, environmental triggers such as xenobiotics and *P. gingivalis* can, respectively, induce the formation of neoantigens, or be capable of inducing the citrullination of host proteins and converting them to autoantigens. These modified proteins can be recognized by the immune system, triggering antibody production and the inflammatory process involved in the clinical manifestations of autoimmune diseases.

To optimize the chances of therapeutic success it is essential to identify the environmental triggers first and then attempt to remove them from the patient's environment (e.g., toxic chemicals and food associated with autoimmunities). In the case of infections, this also helps to guide the clinical use of various medications which are now often used for prophylaxis. Therefore, careful monitoring for the presence of infections in the patient's blood or tissue will be desirable for monitoring the effects of the drug therapy [40, 119–124].

Manipulation of environment triggers and the host immune system during the clinical and in particular preclinical stages of autoimmune disease will offer significant insight and guide early intervention for many autoimmune disorders that, according to the American Autoimmune Related Disease Association, Inc. (http://www.aarda.org/), affects approximately 10% of the world's population [130], while others put it as high as 20%. Finally, identification of triggers of autoimmunities could be used in the development of new therapies for autoimmune diseases.

Conflict of Interests

Aristo Vojdani, PhD, MSc, CLS is the owner, CEO and technical director of Immunosciences Lab., Inc., a clinical reference testing laboratory in Los Angeles, CA, USA.

References

[1] C. Munz, J. D. Lunemann, M. T. Getts et al., "Antiviral immune responses: triggers of or triggered by autoimmunity?" *Nature Reviews Immunology*, vol. 9, pp. 246–228, 2009.

[2] C. Selmi, Q. Lu, and M. C. Humble, "Heritability versus the role of environment in autoimmunity," *Journal of Autoimmunity*, vol. 39, no. 4, pp. 249–252, 2012.

[3] F. W. Miller, K. M. Pollard, C. G. Parks et al., "Criteria for environmentally associated autoimmune disease," *Journal of Autoimmunity*, vol. 39, no. 4, pp. 253–258, 2012.

[4] D. P. Bogdanos, D. S. Smyk, E. I. Rigopoulou et al., "Twin studies in autoimmune disease: genetics, gender and environment," *Journal of Autoimmunity*, vol. 38, no. 2-3, pp. J156–J169, 2012.

[5] H. Mahdi, B. A. Fisher, H. Källberg et al., "Specific interaction between genotype, smoking and autoimmunity to citrullinated α-enolase in the etiology of rheumatoid arthritis," *Nature Genetics*, vol. 41, no. 12, pp. 1319–1324, 2009.

[6] V. K. Kuchroo, P. S. Ohashi, R. B. Sartor, and C. G. Vinuesa, "Dysregulation of immune homeostasis in autoimmune diseases," *Nature Medicine*, vol. 18, no. 1, pp. 42–47, 2012.

[7] J. Bayry, S. Sibéril, F. Triebel, D. F. Tough, and S. V. Kaveri, "Rescuing $CD4^{+}CD25^{+}$ regulatory T-cell functions in rheumatoid arthritis by cytokine-targeted monoclonal antibody therapy," *Drug Discovery Today*, vol. 12, no. 13-14, pp. 548–552, 2007.

[8] M. A. Linterman, R. J. Rigby, R. K. Wong et al., "Follicular helper T cells are required for systemic autoimmunity," *Journal of Experimental Medicine*, vol. 206, no. 3, pp. 561–576, 2009.

[9] N. Simpson, P. A. Gatenby, A. Wilson et al., "Expansion of circulating T cells resembling follicular helper T cells is a fixed phenotype that identifies a subset of severe systemic lupus erythematosus," *Arthritis and Rheumatism*, vol. 62, no. 1, pp. 234–244, 2010.

[10] P. E. Bigazzi, "Autoimmunity caused by xenobiotics," *Toxicology*, vol. 119, no. 1, pp. 1–21, 1997.

[11] K. M. Pollard, P. Hultman, and D. H. Kono, "Toxicology of autoimmune diseases," *Chemical Research in Toxicology*, vol. 23, no. 3, pp. 455–466, 2010.

[12] K. M. Pollard, "Gender differences in autoimmunity associated with exposure to environmental factors," *Journal of Autoimmunity*, vol. 38, no. 2-3, pp. J177–J186, 2012.

[13] D. Germolec, D. H. Kono, J. C. Pfau et al., "Animal models used to examine the role of the environment in the deveopment of autoimmune disease: findings from an NIEHS expert panel workshop," *Journal of Autoimmunity*, vol. 39, no. 4, pp. 285–293, 2012.

[14] P. Griem, M. Wulferink, B. Sachs, J. B. González, and E. Gleichmann, "Allergic and autoimmune reactions to xenobiotics: how do they arise?" *Immunology Today*, vol. 19, no. 3, pp. 133–141, 1998.

[15] M. E. Gershwin, C. Selmi, H. J. Worman et al., "Risk factors and comorbidities in primary biliary cirrhosis: a controlled interview-based study of 1032 patients," *Hepatology*, vol. 42, no. 5, pp. 1194–1202, 2005.

[16] R. Rieger and M. E. Gershwin, "The X and why of xenobiotics in primary biliary cirrhosis," *Journal of Autoimmunity*, vol. 28, no. 2-3, pp. 76–84, 2007.

[17] C. Selmi, "Mechanisms of environmental influences on human autoimmunity: a National Institute of Environmental Health Sciences expert panel workshop," *Journal of Autoimmunity*, vol. 39, no. 4, pp. 272–284, 2012.

[18] C. Barragan-Martinez, C. A. Speck-Hernandez, G. Montoya-Ortiz et al., "Organic solvents as risk factor for autoimmune diseases: a systemic review and meta-analysis," *PLOS ONE*, vol. 7, no. 12, Article ID e51506, 2012.

[19] A. Baccarelli, R. O. Wright, V. Bollati et al., "Rapid DNA methylation changes after exposure to traffic particles," *American Journal of Respiratory and Critical Care Medicine*, vol. 179, no. 7, pp. 572–578, 2009.

[20] S. Kivity, N. Agmon-Levin, M. Blank, and Y. Shoenfeld, "Infections and autoimmunity—friends or foes?" *Trends in Immunology*, vol. 30, no. 8, pp. 409–414, 2009.

[21] M. B. A. Oldstone, M. Nerenberg, P. Southern, J. Price, and H. Lewicki, "Virus infection triggers insulin-dependent diabetes mellitus in a transgenic model: role of anti-self (virus) immune response," *Cell*, vol. 65, no. 2, pp. 319–331, 1991.

[22] D. N. Posnett and D. Yarilin, "Amplification of autoimmune disease by infection," *Arthritis Research and Therapy*, vol. 7, no. 2, pp. 74–84, 2005.

[23] K. C. Faé, D. D. Da Silva, S. E. Oshiro et al., "Mimicry in recognition of cardiac myosin peptides by heart-intralesional T cell clones from rheumatic heart disease," *Journal of Immunology*, vol. 176, no. 9, pp. 5662–5670, 2006.

[24] M. Blank, I. Krause, M. Fridkin et al., "Bacterial induction of autoantibodies to β2-glycoprotein-I accounts for the infectious etiology of antiphospholipid syndrome," *The Journal of Clinical Investigation*, vol. 109, no. 6, pp. 797–804, 2002.

[25] S. J. Richardson, A. Willcox, A. J. Bone, A. K. Foulis, and N. G. Morgan, "The prevalence of enteroviral capsid protein vp1 immunostaining in pancreatic islets in human type 1 diabetes," *Diabetologia*, vol. 52, no. 6, pp. 1143–1151, 2009.

[26] L. Yu, D. T. Robles, N. Abiru et al., "Early expression of antiinsulin autoantibodies of humans and the NOD mouse: evidence for early determination of subsequent diabetes," *Proceedings of the National Academy of Sciences of the United States of America*, vol. 97, no. 4, pp. 1701–1706, 2000.

[27] A. L. Notkins, "New predictors of disease," *Scientific American*, vol. 296, no. 3, pp. 72–79, 2007.

[28] D. R. Gamble, M. L. Kinsley, M. G. FitzGerald, R. Bolton, and K. W. Taylor, "Viral antibodies in diabetes mellitus," *British medical journal*, vol. 3, no. 671, pp. 627–630, 1969.

[29] G. Frisk, G. Friman, T. Tuvemo, J. Fohlman, and H. Diderholm, "Coxsackie B virus IgM in children at onset of Type 1 (insulin-dependent) diabetes mellitus: evidence for IgM induction by a recent or current infection," *Diabetologia*, vol. 35, no. 3, pp. 249–253, 1992.

[30] G. B. Clements, D. N. Galbraith, and K. W. Taylor, "Coxsackie B virus infection and onset of childhood diabetes," *The Lancet*, vol. 346, no. 8969, pp. 221–223, 1995.

[31] J. W. Yoon, T. Onodera, and A. L. Notkins, "Virus-induced diabetes mellitus. XV. Beta cell damage and insulin-dependent hyperglycemia in mice infected with Coxsackie virus B4," *Journal of Experimental Medicine*, vol. 148, no. 4, pp. 1068–1080, 1978.

[32] J. W. Yoon, M. Austin, T. Onodera, and A. L. Notkins, "Virus-induced diabetes mellitus. Isolation of a virus from the pancreas of a child with diabetic ketoacidosis," *The New England Journal of Medicine*, vol. 300, no. 21, pp. 1173–1179, 1979.

[33] D. L. Kaufman, M. G. Erlander, M. Clare-Salzler, M. A. Atkinson, N. K. Maclaren, and A. J. Tobin, "Autoimmunity to two forms of glutamate decarboxylase in insulin-dependent diabetes mellitus," *The Journal of Clinical Investigation*, vol. 89, no. 1, pp. 283–292, 1992.

[34] K. Sadeharju, M. Lönnrot, T. Kimpimäki et al., "Enterovirus antibody levels during the first two years of life in prediabetic autoantibody-positive children," *Diabetologia*, vol. 44, no. 7, pp. 818–823, 2001.

[35] F. Calcinaro, S. Dionisi, M. Marinaro et al., "Oral probiotic administration induces interleukin-10 production and prevents spontaneous autoimmune diabetes in the non-obese diabetic mouse," *Diabetologia*, vol. 48, no. 8, pp. 1565–1575, 2005.

[36] O. Vaarala, M. A. Atkinson, and J. Neu, "The "perfect storm" for type 1 diabetes: the complex interplay between intestinal microbiota, gut permeability, and mucosal immunity," *Diabetes*, vol. 57, no. 10, pp. 2555–2562, 2008.

[37] L. A. Sechi, V. Rosu, A. Pacifico, G. Fadda, N. Ahmed, and S. Zanetti, "Humoral immune responses of type 1 diabetes patients to *Mycobacterium avium* subsp. paratuberculosis lend support to the infectious trigger hypothesis," *Clinical and Vaccine Immunology*, vol. 15, no. 2, pp. 320–326, 2008.

[38] H. Park, A. B. Bourla, D. L. Kastner et al., "Lighting the fires within: the cell biology of autoinflammatory disease," *Nature Reviews Immunology*, vol. 12, pp. 571–580, 2012.

[39] S. Subramanian, "Etiopathogenesis of rheumatoid arthritis may be misunderstood of non-infectious—a review on infectious etiology of RA," *Asian Journal of Medical Sciences*, vol. 1, no. 2, pp. 1–9, 2009.

[40] D. Farquharson, J. P. Butcher, and S. Culshaw, "Periodontitis, porphyromonas, and the pathogenesis of rheumatoid arthritis," *Mucosal Immunology*, vol. 5, no. 2, pp. 112–120, 2012.

[41] H.-J. Wu, I. I. Ivanov, J. Darce et al., "Gut-residing segmented filamentous bacteria drive autoimmune arthritis via T helper 17 cells," *Immunity*, vol. 32, no. 6, pp. 815–827, 2010.

[42] J. S. H. Gaston and M. S. Lillicrap, "Arthritis associated with enteric infection," *Best Practice and Research*, vol. 17, no. 2, pp. 219–239, 2003.

[43] G. J. McColl, M. B. Diviney, R. F. Holdsworth et al., "HLA-B27 expression and reactive arthritis susceptibility in two patient cohorts infected with *Salmonella Typhimurium*," *Australian and New Zealand Journal of Medicine*, vol. 30, no. 1, pp. 28–32, 2000.

[44] T. Hannu, L. Mattila, A. Siitonen, and M. Leirisalo-Repo, "Reactive arthritis attributable to *Shigella* infection: a clinical and epidemiological nationwide study," *Annals of the Rheumatic Diseases*, vol. 64, no. 4, pp. 594–598, 2005.

[45] A. Ebringer and T. Rashid, "Rheumatoid arthritis is an autoimmune disease triggered by Proteus urinary tract infection," *Clinical and Developmental Immunology*, vol. 13, no. 1, pp. 41–48, 2006.

[46] J. E. Pope, A. Krizova, A. X. Garg, H. Thiessen-Philbrook, and J. M. Ouimet, "Campylobacter reactive arthritis: a systematic review," *Seminars in Arthritis and Rheumatism*, vol. 37, no. 1, pp. 48–55, 2007.

[47] M. L. Domínguez-López, M. E. Cancino-Díaz, L. Jiménez-Zamudio, J. Granados-Arreola, R. Burgos-Vargas, and E. García-Latorre, "Cellular immune response to Klebsiella pneumoniae antigens in patients with HLA-B27+ ankylosing spondylitis," *Journal of Rheumatology*, vol. 27, no. 6, pp. 1453–1460, 2000.

[48] A. Cope, J. Anderson, and E. Wilkins, "Clostridium difficile toxin-induced reactive arthritis in a patient with chronic Reiter's syndrome," *European Journal of Clinical Microbiology and Infectious Diseases*, vol. 11, no. 1, pp. 40–43, 1992.

[49] Z.-Q. Liu, G.-M. Deng, S. Foster, and A. Tarkowski, "Staphylococcal peptidoglycans induce arthritis," *Arthritis Research*, vol. 3, no. 6, pp. 375–380, 2001.

[50] K. C. Faé, D. D. Da Silva, S. E. Oshiro et al., "Mimicry in recognition of cardiac myosin peptides by heart-intralesional T cell clones from rheumatic heart disease," *Journal of Immunology*, vol. 176, no. 9, pp. 5662–5670, 2006.

[51] E. Hermann, W.-J. Mayet, O. Klein et al., "Candida arthritis: cellular immune responses of synovial fluid and peripheral blood lymphocytes to Candida albicans," *Annals of the Rheumatic Diseases*, vol. 50, no. 10, pp. 697–701, 1991.

[52] W. D. Sutliff, R. Shephard, and W. B. Dunham, "Acute Leptospira pomona arthritis and myocarditis," *Annals of internal medicine*, vol. 39, no. 1, pp. 134–140, 1953.

[53] J. D. Carter, L. R. Espinoza, R. D. Inman et al., "Combination antibiotics as a treatment for chronic Chlamydia-induced reactive arthritis: a double-blind, placebo-controlled, prospective trial," *Arthritis and Rheumatism*, vol. 62, no. 5, pp. 1298–1307, 2010.

[54] B. C. Cole and J. R. Ward, "Mycoplasmas as arthritogenic agents," in *The Mycoplasmas*, J. G. Tully and R. F. Whitcomb, Eds., pp. 367–398, Academic Press, New York, NY, USA, 1979.

[55] H. R. Kim, E. Y. Kim, J. Cerny, and K. D. Moudgil, "Antibody responses to mycobacterial and self heat shock protein 65 in

autoimmune arthritis: epitope specificity and implication in pathogenesis," *Journal of Immunology*, vol. 177, no. 10, pp. 6634–6641, 2006.

[56] D. Imai, K. Holden, E. M. Velasquez et al., "Influence of arthritis-related protein (BBF01) on infectivity of *Borrelia burgdorferi* B31," *BMC Microbiology*, vol. 13, no. 100, 2013.

[57] J. R. Kerr, J. P. Cartron, M. D. Curran, J. E. Moore, J. R. M. Elliott, and R. A. B. Mollan, "A study of the role of parvovirus B19 in rheumatoid arthritis," *British Journal of Rheumatology*, vol. 34, no. 9, pp. 809–813, 1995.

[58] F. Pratesi, C. Tommasi, C. Anzilotti, D. Chimenti, and P. Migliorini, "Deiminated Epstein-Barr virus nuclear antigen 1 is a target of anti-citrullinated protein antibodies in rheumatoid arthritis," *Arthritis and Rheumatism*, vol. 54, no. 3, pp. 733–741, 2006.

[59] K. Bech, O. Clemmensen, and J. H. Larsen, "Cell-mediated immunity to *Yersinia enterocolitica* serotype 3 in patients with thyroid diseases," *Allergy*, vol. 33, no. 2, pp. 82–88, 1978.

[60] I. Shimon, C. Pariente, J. Shlomo-David, Z. Grossman, and J. Sack, "Transient elevation of triiodothyronine caused by triiodothyronine autoantibody associated with acute Epstein-Barr-virus infection," *Thyroid*, vol. 13, no. 2, pp. 211–215, 2003.

[61] K. Mori, Y. Munakata, T. Saito et al., "Intrathyroidal persistence of human parvovirus B19 DNA in a patient with Hashimoto's thyroiditis," *Journal of Infection*, vol. 55, no. 2, pp. e29–e31, 2007.

[62] L. Fernandez-Soto, A. Gonzalez, F. Escobar-Jimenez et al., "Increased risk of autoimmune thyroid disease in hepatitis C vs hepatitis B before, during, and after discontinuing interferon therapy," *Archives of Internal Medicine*, vol. 158, no. 13, pp. 1445–1448, 1998.

[63] R. C. Parmar, S. B. Bavdekar, D. R. Sahu, S. Warke, and J. R. Kamat, "Thyroiditis as a presenting feature of mumps," *Pediatric Infectious Disease Journal*, vol. 20, no. 6, pp. 637–638, 2001.

[64] P. R. Ziring, G. Gallo, and M. Finegold, "Chronic lymphocytic thyroiditis: identification of rubella virus antigen in the thyroid of a child with congenital rubella," *Journal of Pediatrics*, vol. 90, no. 3, pp. 419–420, 1977.

[65] P. Brouqui, D. Raoult, and B. Conte-Devolx, "Coxsackie thyroiditis," *Annals of Internal Medicine*, vol. 114, no. 12, pp. 1063–1064, 1991.

[66] H. Kawai, T. Inui, S. Kashiwagi et al., "HTLV-I infection in patients with autoimmune thyroiditis (Hashimoto's thyroiditis)," *Journal of Medical Virology*, vol. 38, no. 2, pp. 138–141, 1992.

[67] J. L. Leite, N. E. Bufalo, R. B. Santos et al., "Human herpes virus type 6 (HHV6) and human herpes virus type 7 (HHV7) may increase the susceptibility to Graves disease in individuals with inherited diminished TP53 apoptotic function," in *Proceedings of the 33rd annual meeting of the European Thyroid Association*, Thessalonique, 2008.

[68] T. F. Davies, "Infection and autoimmune thyroid disease," *Journal of Clinical Endocrinology and Metabolism*, vol. 93, no. 3, pp. 674–676, 2008.

[69] S. Ray, N. Sonthalia, S. Kundu et al., "Autoimmune disorders: an overview of molecular and cellular basis in today's perspective," *Journal of Clinical & Cellular Immunology*, 2012.

[70] M. E. Gershwin, "The mosaic of autoimmunity," *Autoimmunity Reviews*, vol. 7, no. 3, pp. 161–163, 2008.

[71] V. K. Tuohy, M. Yu, B. Weinstock-Guttman, and R. P. Kinkel, "Diversity and plasticity of self recognition during the development of multiple sclerosis," *The Journal of Clinical Investigation*, vol. 99, no. 7, pp. 1682–1690, 1997.

[72] R. C. Duke, "Self recognition by T cells. I. Bystander killing of target cells bearing syngeneic MHC antigens," *Journal of Experimental Medicine*, vol. 170, no. 1, pp. 59–71, 1989.

[73] K. W. Wucherpfennig, "Mechanisms for the induction of autoimmunity by infectious agents," *The Journal of Clinical Investigation*, vol. 108, no. 8, pp. 1097–1104, 2001.

[74] N. Agmon-Levin, M. Ram, O. Barzilai et al., "Prevalence of hepatitis C serum antibody in autoimmune diseases," *Journal of Autoimmunity*, vol. 32, no. 3-4, pp. 261–266, 2009.

[75] I. J. Brown, I. Tzoulaki, V. Candeias, and P. Elliott, "Salt intakes around the world: implications for public health," *International Journal of Epidemiology*, vol. 38, no. 3, pp. 791–813, 2009.

[76] G. Rose, J. Stamler, R. Stamler et al., "Intersalt: an international study of electrolyte excretion and blood pressure. Results for 24 hour urinary sodium and potassium excretion," *British Medical Journal*, vol. 297, no. 6644, pp. 319–328, 1988.

[77] E. Elliott, "Change in salt intake affects blood pressure of chimpanzees: implications for human populations," *Circulation*, vol. 116, no. 14, pp. 1563–1568, 2007.

[78] F. M. Sacks, L. P. Svetkey, W. M. Vollmer et al., "Effects on blood pressure of reduced dietary sodium and the dietary approaches to stop hypertension (dash) diet," *The New England Journal of Medicine*, vol. 344, no. 1, pp. 3–10, 2001.

[79] N. A. Graudal, A. M. Galløe, and P. Garred, "Effects of sodium restriction on blood pressure, renin, aldosterone, catecholamines, cholesterols, and triglyceride: a meta-analysis," *Journal of the American Medical Association*, vol. 279, no. 17, pp. 1383–1391, 1998.

[80] N. R. Cook, J. A. Cutler, E. Obarzanek et al., "Long term effects of dietary sodium reduction on cardiovascular disease outcomes: observational follow-up of the trials of hypertension prevention (TOHP)," *British Medical Journal*, vol. 334, no. 7599, pp. 885–888, 2007.

[81] J. X. Xie, S. Sasaki, J. V. Joossens, and H. Kesteloot, "The relationship between urinary cations obtained from the INTERSALT study and cerebrovascular mortality," *Journal of Human Hypertension*, vol. 6, no. 1, pp. 17–21, 1992.

[82] N. Sasaki, "High blood pressure and the salt intake of the Japanese," *International Heart Journal*, vol. 3, pp. 313–324, 1962.

[83] A. MacHnik, W. Neuhofer, J. Jantsch et al., "Macrophages regulate salt-dependent volume and blood pressure by a vascular endothelial growth factor-C-dependent buffering mechanism," *Nature Medicine*, vol. 15, no. 5, pp. 545–552, 2009.

[84] E. Cretney, A. Kallies, and S. L. Nutt, "Differentiation and function of $FOXP3^+$ effector regulatory T cells," *Trends in Immunology*, vol. 34, no. 2, pp. 74–80, 2013.

[85] T. Korn, E. Bettelli, M. Oukka, and V. K. Kuchroo, "IL-17 and Th17 cells," *Annual Review of Immunology*, vol. 27, pp. 485–517, 2009.

[86] M. Kleinewietfeld, A. Manzel, J. Titze et al., "Sodium chloride drives autoimmune disease by the induction of pathogenic T_H17 cells," *Nature*, vol. 496, pp. 518–522, 2013.

[87] C. Wu, N. Yosef, T. Thalhamer et al., "Induction of pathogenic T_H17 cells by inducible salt-sensing kinase SGK1," *Nature*, pp. 513–517, 2013.

[88] J. J. O' Shea and R. G. Jones, "Autoimmunity: rubbing salt in the wound," *Nature*, vol. 496, pp. 437–439, 2013.

[89] Institute of Medicine, *Dietary Reference Intakes For Water, Potassium, Sodium, Chloride, and Sulphate*, National Academies Press, Washington, DC, USA, 2004.

[90] A. Vojdani, A. W. Campbell, E. Anyanwu, A. Kashanian, K. Bock, and E. Vojdani, "Antibodies to neuron-specific antigens in children with autism: possible cross-reaction with encephalitogenic proteins from milk, *Chlamydia pneumoniae* and Streptococcus group A," *Journal of Neuroimmunology*, vol. 129, no. 1-2, pp. 168–177, 2002.

[91] A. Vojdani and I. Tarash, "Cross-reaction between gliadin and different food and tissue antigens," *Food and Nutrition Sciences*, vol. 4, pp. 20–32, 2013.

[92] A. Stefferl, A. Schubart, M. Storch et al., "Butyrophilin, a milk protein, modulates the encephalitogenic T cell response to myelin oligodendrocyte glycoprotein in experimental autoimmune Encephalomyelitis," *Journal of Immunology*, vol. 165, no. 5, pp. 2859–2865, 2000.

[93] Ø. Molberg and L. M. Sollid, "A gut feeling for joint inflammation—using coeliac disease to understand rheumatoid arthritis," *Trends in Immunology*, vol. 27, no. 4, pp. 188–194, 2006.

[94] J. Karjalainen, J. M. Martin, M. Knip et al., "A bovine albumin peptide as a possible trigger of insulin-dependent diabetes mellitus," *The New England Journal of Medicine*, vol. 327, no. 5, pp. 302–307, 1992.

[95] T. L. Van Belle, K. T. Coppieters, and M. G. Von Herrath, "Type 1 diabetes: etiology, immunology, and therapeutic strategies," *Physiological Reviews*, vol. 91, no. 1, pp. 79–118, 2011.

[96] M. G. Cavallo, D. Fava, L. Monetini, F. Barone, and P. Pozzilli, "Cell-mediated immune response to β casein in recent-onset insulin-dependent diabetes: implications for disease pathogenesis," *The Lancet*, vol. 348, no. 9032, pp. 926–928, 1996.

[97] S. M. Virtanen, E. Laara, E. Hypponen et al., "Cow's milk consumption, HLA-DQB1 genotype, and type 1 diabetes: a nested case-control study of sibling of children with diabetes," *Diabetes*, vol. 49, no. 9, p. 1617, 2000.

[98] U. Volta, C. Bonazzi, E. Pisi, S. Salardi, and E. Cacciari, "Antigliadin and antireticulin antibodies in coeliac disease and at onset of diabetes in children," *The Lancet*, vol. 2, no. 8566, pp. 1034–1035, 1987.

[99] A. J. MacFarlane, K. M. Burghardt, J. Kelly et al., "A type 1 diabetes-related protein from wheat (*Triticum aestivum*): cDNA clone of a wheat storage globulin, Glb1, linked to islet damage," *The Journal of Biological Chemistry*, vol. 278, no. 1, pp. 54–63, 2003.

[100] A. Vojdani, "The characterization of the repertoire of wheat antigens and peptides involved in the humoral immune responses in patients with gluten sensitivity and Crohn's disease," *ISRN Allergy*, vol. 2011, Article ID 950104, 12 pages, 2011.

[101] Z. Sumnik, S. Kolouskova, H. Malcova et al., "High prevalence of coeliac disease in siblings of children with type 1 diabetes," *European Journal of Pediatrics*, vol. 164, no. 1, pp. 9–12, 2005.

[102] M. Hvatum, L. Kanerud, R. Hällgren, and P. Brandtzaeg, "The gut-joint axis: cross reactive food antibodies in rheumatoid arthritis," *Gut*, vol. 55, no. 9, pp. 1240–1247, 2006.

[103] E. Sugai, A. Cherñavsky, S. Pedreira et al., "Bone-specific antibodies in Sera from patients with celiac disease: characterization and implications in osteoporosis," *Journal of Clinical Immunology*, vol. 22, no. 6, pp. 353–362, 2002.

[104] A. Frustaci, L. Cuoco, C. Chimenti et al., "Celiac disease associated with autoimmune myocarditis," *Circulation*, vol. 105, no. 22, pp. 2611–2618, 2002.

[105] M. Hadjivassiliou, M. Mäki, D. S. Sanders et al., "Autoantibody targeting of brain and intestinal transglutaminase in gluten ataxia," *Neurology*, vol. 66, no. 3, pp. 373–377, 2006.

[106] A. Vojdani, T. O'Bryan, J. A. Green et al., "Immune response to dietary proteins, gliadin and cerebellar peptides in children with autism," *Nutritional Neuroscience*, vol. 7, no. 3, pp. 151–161, 2004.

[107] A. Alaedini, H. Okamoto, C. Briani et al., "Immune cross-reactivity in celiac disease: anti-gliadin antibodies bind to neuronal synapsin I," *Journal of Immunology*, vol. 178, no. 10, pp. 6590–6595, 2007.

[108] L. C. Chin, M. K. Jones, and J. G. C. Kingham, "Celiac disease and autoimmune thyroid disease," *Clinical Medicine and Research*, vol. 5, no. 3, pp. 184–192, 2007.

[109] S. Bodvarsson, I. Jonsdottir, J. Freysdottir, J. N. Leonard, L. Fry, and H. Valdimarsson, "Dermatitis herpetiformis—an autoimmune disease due to cross-reaction between dietary glutenin and dermal elastin?" *Scandinavian Journal of Immunology*, vol. 38, no. 6, pp. 546–550, 1993.

[110] D. B.-A. Shor, O. Barzilai, M. Ram et al., "Gluten sensitivity in multiple sclerosis: experimental myth or clinical truth," *Annals of the New York Academy of Sciences*, vol. 1173, pp. 343–349, 2009.

[111] C. O' Leary, C. H. Walsj, P. Wieneke et al., "Coeliac disease and autoimmune Addison's disease: a clinical pitfall," *Quarterly Journal of Medicine*, vol. 95, no. 2, pp. 79–82, 2002.

[112] A. J. Naiyer, J. Shah, L. Hernandez et al., "Tissue transglutaminase antibodies in individuals with celiac disease bind to thyroid follicles and extracellular matrix and may contribute to thyroid dysfunction," *Thyroid*, vol. 18, no. 11, pp. 1171–1178, 2008.

[113] G. Zanoni, R. Navone, C. Lunardi et al., "In celiac disease, a subset of autoantibodies against transglutaminase binds toll-like receptor 4 and induces activation of monocytes," *PLoS Medicine*, vol. 3, no. 9, pp. 1637–1653, 2006.

[114] C. Sategna-Guidetti, E. Franco, S. Martini, and M. Bobbio, "Binding by serum IgA antibodies from patients with coeliac disease to monkey heart tissue," *Scandinavian Journal of Gastroenterology*, vol. 39, no. 6, pp. 540–543, 2004.

[115] E. V. Marietta, M. J. Camilleri, L. A. Castro, P. K. Krause, M. R. Pittelkow, and J. A. Murray, "Transglutaminase autoantibodies in dermatitis herpetiformis and celiac sprue," *Journal of Investigative Dermatology*, vol. 128, no. 2, pp. 332–335, 2008.

[116] V. Toscano, F. G. Conti, E. Anastasi et al., "Importance of gluten in the induction of endocrine autoantibodies and organ dysfunction in adolescent celiac patients," *American Journal of Gastroenterology*, vol. 95, no. 7, pp. 1742–1748, 2000.

[117] O. Rozenberg, A. Lerner, A. Pacht et al., "A new algorithm for the diagnosis of celiac disease," *Cellular and Molecular Immunology*, vol. 8, no. 2, pp. 146–149, 2011.

[118] O. Meyer, "Is the celiac disease model relevant to rheumatoid arthritis?" *Joint Bone Spine*, vol. 71, no. 1, pp. 4–6, 2004.

[119] H. Burkhardt, B. Sehnert, R. Bockermann, Å. Engström, J. R. Kalden, and R. Holmdahl, "Humoral immune response to citrullinated collagen type II determinants in early rheumatoid arthritis," *European Journal of Immunology*, vol. 35, no. 5, pp. 1643–1652, 2005.

[120] C. Masson-Bessière, M. Sebbag, E. Girbal-Neuhauser et al., "The major synovial targets of the rheumatoid arthritis-specific antifilaggrin autoantibodies are deiminated forms of the α-and β-chains of fibrin," *Journal of Immunology*, vol. 166, no. 6, pp. 4177–4184, 2001.

[121] E. R. Vossenaar, N. Després, E. Lapointe et al., "Rheumatoid arthritis specific anti-Sa antibodies target citrullinated vimentin," *Arthritis research & therapy*, vol. 6, no. 2, pp. R142–150, 2004.

[122] A. Kinloch, V. Tatzer, R. Wait et al., "Identification of citrullinated alpha-enolase as a candidate autoantigen in rheumatoid arthritis," *Arthritis research & therapy*, vol. 7, no. 6, pp. R1421–1429, 2005.

[123] J. B. Weinberg, A. M. M. Pippen, and C. S. Greenberg, "Extravascular fibrin formation and dissolution in synovial tissue of patients with osteoarthritis and rheumatoid arthritis," *Arthritis and Rheumatism*, vol. 34, no. 8, pp. 996–1005, 1991.

[124] J. G. Routsias, J. D. Goules, A. Goules, G. Charalampakis, and D. Pikazis, "Autopathogenic correlation of periodontitis and rheumatoid arthritis," *Rheumatology*, vol. 50, no. 7, Article ID ker090, pp. 1189–1193, 2011.

[125] J. A. Hill, S. Southwood, A. Sette, A. M. Jevnikar, D. A. Bell, and E. Cairns, "Cutting edge: the conversion of arginine to citrulline allows for a high-affinity peptide interaction with the rheumatoid arthritis-associated HLA-DRB1∗0401 MHC class II molecule," *Journal of Immunology*, vol. 171, no. 2, pp. 538–541, 2003.

[126] K. Lundberg, N. Wegner, T. Yucel-Lindberg, and P. J. Venables, "Periodontitis in RA-the citrullinated enolase connection," *Nature Reviews Rheumatology*, vol. 6, no. 12, pp. 727–730, 2010.

[127] K. Lundberg, A. Kinloch, B. A. Fisher et al., "Antibodies to citrullinated α-enolase peptide 1 are specific for rheumatoid arthritis and cross-react with bacterial enolase," *Arthritis and Rheumatism*, vol. 58, no. 10, pp. 3009–3019, 2008.

[128] A. J. Kinloch, S. Alzabin, W. Brintnell et al., "Immunization with porphyromonas gingivalis enolase induces autoimmunity to mammalian α-enolase and arthritis in DR4-IE-transgenic mice," *Arthritis and Rheumatism*, vol. 63, no. 12, pp. 3818–3823, 2011.

[129] J. A. Hill, D. A. Bell, W. Brintnell et al., "Arthritis induced by posttranslationally modified (citrullinated) fibrinogen in DR4-IE transgenic mice," *Journal of Experimental Medicine*, vol. 205, no. 4, pp. 967–979, 2008.

[130] American Autoimmune Related Disease Association, http://www.aarda.org.

3

Immunosenescence, Aging, and Systemic Lupus Erythematous

Gladis Montoya-Ortiz

Center for Autoimmune Diseases Research (CREA), School of Medicine and Health Sciences, Universidad del Rosario, Carrera 24 No. 63C-69, Bogota, Colombia

Correspondence should be addressed to Gladis Montoya-Ortiz; gladis.montoya@gmail.com

Academic Editor: Yehuda Shoenfeld

Senescence is a normal biological process that occurs in all organisms and involves a decline in cell functions. This process is caused by molecular regulatory machinery alterations, and it is closely related to telomere erosion in chromosomes. In the context of the immune system, this phenomenon is known as immunosenescence and refers to the immune function deregulation. Therefore, functions of several cells involved in the innate and adaptive immune responses are severely compromised with age progression (e.g., changes in lymphocyte subsets, decreased proliferative responses, chronic inflammatory states, etc.). These alterations make elderly individuals prone to not only infectious diseases but also to malignancy and autoimmunity. This review will explore the molecular aspects of processes related to cell aging, their importance in the context of the immune system, and their participation in elderly SLE patients.

1. Introduction

Aging can be defined as the progressive decay of tissue functions which eventually results in organ dysfunction and death. This decline may be the result of the loss of postmitotic cell function or the lack of replacement of such cells due to a decreased stem cell ability to maintain cell division and replication [1]. If the organism suffers damage and it is irreparable, the senescence or aging process will take place by limiting the cells' proliferative potential. Some control mechanisms include differential gene expression which may be detrimental [2]. However, there is a renewal mechanism that ensures damaged cell replacement. This singular mechanism corresponds to a set of proliferating precursor cells that provide a source of cell replacement within the tissues. The immune system provides an interesting case of replacement: cells that die by apoptosis are replaced by new ones, a process which is essential for immune system longevity and for adequate functionality. This review will describe main molecular mechanisms implicated in immunosenescence and their relationship with autoimmune disease, particularly related to systemic lupus erythematous (SLE).

2. Aging Molecular Mechanisms

One of the most striking features of cell aging is its close relationship with telomere length [3]. There is an inverse relationship between telomere length and cellular aging; for example, very short telomeres force their cells to enter senescence. Human telomeres contain guanine-rich repetitive sequences (i.e., TTAGGG) which are gradually lost in each mitotic division. This occurs by the fact that the DNA polymerase is unable to replicate linear chromosomes in a process known as telomere erosion (Figure 1) [4–6]. This process functions as a mitotic clock for which the length of the telomeres represents the number of cell divisions sustained by the cells [7].

There is also a significant variability with respect to the speed and quality of aging between and within populations [8]. This heterogeneity results from interaction between genetic, environmental, and stochastic factors. In this regard, several epigenetic alterations have been associated with aging and diseases caused by aging (e.g., DNA methylation state, histone modification, miRNA, etc.) [9]. Several studies about DNA methylation have shown loss of methylcytosines with age, especially in CpG islands within Alu repetitive sequences

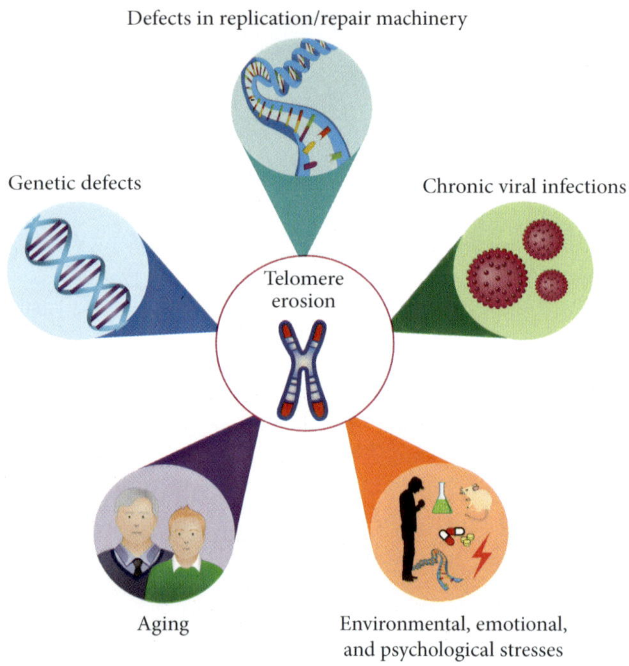

FIGURE 1: Factors related to telomere erosion. The mechanisms contributing to the loss of telomere length include genetic defects, chronic viral infections, defects in repair machinery, aging, and stress.

and endogenous retroviral sequences. On top of this, a study of monozygotic twins showed that, for other young people, they retain similar methylation profiles while other twins who were between 50 and 60 years old had different methylation profiles and an H3 and H4 differential acetylation state [10].

Another mechanism related to epigenetic changes in aging involves chromatin remodeling. This includes H3K9, H3K27, and H4K20 trimethylation, decreased H3K9 acetylation, and increased H3S10 phosphorylation [11]. A decrease in H3K27 methylation together with an augmentation in H3S10 phosphorylation supports the idea of a change in the heterochromatin and euchromatin dynamics in aging cells. In addition, there are several chromatin remodeling-related proteins that suffer alterations during aging. These include the histone deacetylases (HDACs), the sirtuin 1 (SIRT1) protein, and the histone methyltransferases [12].

Finally, several studies in both murine and humans have shown that miRNAs may influence aging and longevity. Recently, multiple miRNAs related to aging have been described including lin-4, miR-1, miR-145, miR-140, miR-34a, and miR-449th, and some of them modulate cell senescence critical molecules such as class I HDAC, SIRT1, p21, p53, and pRb. Another important miRNA related to TCR signaling (miR181a) has serious implications in elderly people and autoimmunity (this topic will be discussed later). Recently, Liu et al. summarized the miRNAs involved in cell senescence [13].

3. Immunosenescence

One characteristic of elderly people is their inability to respond properly to vaccines and infections. This condition could be the result of their low immune system efficiency [14] and occurs because of thymic involution in which the thymus loses its ability to produce and replace naïve T cells on the periphery. As a result, thymic dysfunction produces a decrease in cell-mediated response to foreign antigens, self-tolerance, and naïve T-cell population. In turn, it could increase the autoproliferation of T cells and eventually the induction of premature T-cell maturation which would also conduce to tolerance reduction [15]. These alterations lead to not only modifications in lymphocyte subsets but also to functional changes in cell population subsets. For instance, longitudinal studies have demonstrated an association between immunosenescence and an increase in cytomegalovirus (CMV) anergic CD8 T cells [16].

One of the main characteristics of the immune system is the constant renewal of its cells. At the same time, this renewal is highly dependent on the efficiency of telomere maintenance. Immune system cells are derived from hematopoietic progenitor cells that come from myeloid and lymphoid lineages. These cells are constantly dividing and differentiating throughout their lifespan and that leads to changes in their telomere length. Note that a high rate of telomere loss in the first years of life has been observed, perhaps because of their high rate of mitotic division. However, this telomere loss is not a linear process over time since, in older people, it is possible to find significant telomere erosion. In fact, several studies have shown a decline in the length of telomeres with aging [17]. A lot has been written regarding the relationship between aging, thymic degeneration, and changes in the bone marrow cells [18–20]. However, we will focus only on immune senescence with an emphasis on circulating cell populations.

There are reports about age-related changes in peripheral blood cell populations: increase in monocytes, decreased lymphocytes, decrease in naïve cells, and increase in memory cells (Table 1) [21]. Curiously, memory T cells ($CD4^+$-$CD45RO^+$ and $CD8^+$-$CD45RO^+$) increase with age and are preferentially located in tissue, whereas there is a similar proportion of $CD45RA^+$ and $CD45RO^+$ subsets in peripheral blood [22]. Unlike somatic cells, lymphocytes have a robust capability to proliferate given their clonal expansion and present an overexpression in the telomerase. This process ensures no significant telomere shortening during each division. Interestingly, T cells possess several special features regarding their phenotype and their telomere length. T-cell memory cells have shorter telomeres than naïve T cells, and $CD28^+$ T cells have longer telomeres than $CD28^-$ T cells.

Immune aging or immunosenescence not only affects adaptive response but also has implications in the innate response (Table 1) [23]. It has been found that older individuals who exhibit a breakdown of their innate immune barriers such as epithelial skin barriers, lungs, and gastrointestinal tract could be vulnerable to a pathogen attack. Among the cell types involved in innate response, there are neutrophils, macrophages, and natural killer (NK) cells, which also suffer

Table 1: Age-associated changes in immune cell populations and functions.

Cell type	Characteristics	References
	Innate immunity	
Neutrophils	↓ Phagocytic chemotaxis capability ↓ Superoxide anion production ↓ Ability to respond to soluble factors (GM-CSF) and bacteria (LPS and fMLP) ↓ Molecule recruitment into lipid raft, apoptosis, and signal transduction	[23, 70, 87, 140]
Dendritic cells	↓ Cell number, antigen presentation, TLR-mediated signaling, IFN I/III production, chemotaxis, and endocytosis ↓ Ability to stimulate lymphocytes in the ill elderly ↑ Function in the healthy elderly	[23, 102, 141]
Macrophages	↓ Phagocytic activity and chemotaxis ↑ Synthesis of proinflammatory cytokines (IL-6, IL-8, TNF-α, and IL-1β) ↓ Apoptosis, superoxide production, and signal transduction ↓ TLR expression and function ↑ PGE2 production ↓ MCH class II production	[23, 87, 142]
NK cells	↑ CD56dimCD57$^+$ population ↓ Function of cytotoxicity ↓ Secretion of IFN-γ induced by Interleukin 2 (IL-2) ↓ HLA-DR, IFN-α, CD57, and CD95 ↓ Cell proliferation ↑ Production of IL-1, IL-4, IL-6, IL-8, and TNF-α	[72, 143, 144]
	Adaptive immunity	
Cellular response		
Thymus	Involution from age of 9 months, thymic remnant after 50 years	[20, 145]
T Cells	Variable number (↓ proliferation to PHA, varying age, and health status)—HLA B8/DR3 associated with high proliferative responses ↑ Proportion of memory cells (CD45RO$^+$), especially tissue CD8$^+$ ↓ Proportion of naïve cells (CD45RA$^+$) ↓ Proliferative capacity ↓ Synthesis of IL-2 receptor and IL-2 in memory cells ↓ CD28$^+$ ↑ CD28$^-$ T cells—mainly CD8$^+$ CD28$^-$ (characterized by oligoclonal expansion, shortening of telomeres, potentially decreased proliferation, resistance to apoptosis, and increased production of TNF-α and IL-6) ↓ CD4 T lymphocytes Change from Th1 response to Th2 response with ↓ cell-mediated responses directed against intracellular bacteria (Th1 function) and relative preservation of humoral response (Th2 function) ↓ Treg population (CD4$^+$ CD25$^+$) that plays a role in the manifestations of autoimmunity Impaired immunological synapse formation and signaling pathways (calcium response and phosphorylations) ↓ CD4/CD8 rate	[14, 145–147]
Humoral response		
B Cells	↓ Pre-B lymphocytes with peripheral B lymphocyte count unchanged ↑ CD5$^+$ B cells (CD19$^+$ CD5$^+$ clones B) that produce low affinity antibodies without cooperation of T cell ↓ Naïve B cells Accumulation of memory B cells with ↓ diversity and affinity of antibodies Reaching primary humoral response (dependent T cell cooperation). Conserved secondary humoral response	[14, 33, 50, 53, 145, 148]

Table 1: Continued.

Cell type	Characteristics	References
Immunoglobulins	↑ Serum levels of IgA and IgG (IgG1, IgG2, and IgG4). Monoclonal immunoglobulin production by $CD19^+$ $CD5^+$ clones. Secretion of non-organ-specific self-antibodies (rheumatoid factor, antinuclear antibodies, antiphospholipid antithyroglobulines, and parietal cells).	[51, 113]
Interleukins	↓ IL-2 production because of the following: ↓ cooperation of T cells with antibody producer B cells, ↑ production of IL-4, IL-6, IL-8, IL-10, and TNF-α, ↓ production of IL-1 and IFN-γ.	[14, 106, 145]

functional alterations through aging (Table 1). Immunosenescence also affects the response to immunization. There are several reports indicating low response to infectious agents in elderly individuals [24, 25]. Latent proinflammatory status in old subjects is due to involution of thymus with subsequent alteration of function and balance of naïve, effector, and memory cells. This status combined with the presence of common and cumulative viral infections in the elderly (such as cytomegalovirus and Epstein-Barr virus) produces overall responses, loss of ability to control infectious diseases, and decreased response to vaccinations. The cytokine environmental balance (i.e., decline in the INFγ : IL-10 ratio) in challenge condition (i.e., influenza or other viral infections) could decline the $CD8^+$ cytotoxic ability, thus conducing to high IL-10 response to virus challenge. Therefore, vaccines that arouse inflammatory cytokines would be expected to enhance protection in elderly subjects.

3.1. Adaptive Immune Response

3.1.1. T Cells. T lymphocytes suffer alterations due to aging. Most of the observed changes are attributed to alterations during the initial activation step of the T-cell receptor (TCR). There is evidence of alteration in the downstream signaling of the TCR in the case of elderly people. This includes a decrease in intracellular free calcium, deficiencies in protein kinase C translocation, low Lck, ZAP70 activation, NFAT impairment, NF-κB translocation, low ras-mitogen activated protein kinase (MAPK) pathways, and a decrease in proteasome activity, [26]. These alterations have been demonstrated in both naïve and memory T cells [27].

TCR has the function to discriminate between self-antigens and respond to foreign peptides. This is caused by its activation threshold level, and therefore, the loss of TCR sensitivity is closely related to aging. As mentioned before, there is an important microRNA—named miR-181a—implicated in this phenomenon which controls the expression of several phosphatases related to the negative regulation of proximal CD4 TCR signaling events. Indeed, in a murine model, miR181a overexpression lowers TCR activation threshold and restores TCR ability to respond to autoantigens [28]. Note that miR-181a expression declines throughout life and shows a significant loss after the age of 70 [29].

Another interesting point is that there are reports indicating changes in gene expression of surface molecules on T cells. Changes in surface molecules may have a negative impact on T-cell activation by increasing phosphatase expression such as DUSP family. Furthermore, a study evaluated the effect of aging on surface molecule gene expression and found that IL-6R, CD8, CD27, and CD28 are downregulated while ILT2 (CD85j), KLRG, KIR, CD44, CD96, Klrf1, and CD94 are upregulated [30, 31]. Some of these molecules (ILT, KLRG, and KIR) function as negative regulators of TCR activation and proliferation (at least in murine models) or as specific molecules of particular T cells such as cytomegalovirus (CMV) peptide-specific T cells (KIR and ILT2). They also appear to be related to T-cell exhaustion although the relationship between aging, senescent, and exhausted T-cell gene expressions seems to be different (Figure 2). An excellent review of this topic was done by Cavanagh et al. [32].

In addition to surface molecule gene expression alteration, there are other processes related to TCR signaling alteration and aging. For instance, it is well known that a cell-intrinsic environment (ROS species, DNA damage) and a cell-extrinsic environment (cytokines) both modulate TCR responses, and they are also altered in the elderly. Moreover, studies have shown that increased oxidative stress produces displacement of LAT from the cell membrane, thus inhibiting TCR signaling. Along with this, activated CD4 T cells from aging humans express increased levels of metallothoineins, which are an important redox system [34]. Additionally, there are alterations in molecules that participate in nuclear and cytoplasmic signaling pathways such as DNA repair kinases (ATM, ATR, and DNA-PKCs), which are activated not only by DNA double-strand breaks (DSB) but also by telomere attrition (as we will see later). Both of them are related to activation of DNA repair kinases (ATM, ATR and DNA-PKcs) [35].

Host environment and specific cytokine profiles have enormous implications in the T-cell signaling threshold. Some cytokines such as IL-7, IL-21, and IL15 have been studied in this regard. These cytokines signal through PI3K, STAT3, and STAT5 [36] and participate in ERK pathway activation. Note that IL-7 and IL-15 have profound implications in lymphopenia development in RA animal models. This has been shown through the fact that when animals are primed with IL-7 or IL-15, T-cell response to autoantigens is enabled. In addition, another cytokine implicated in signaling alteration during aging is the IL-6. This cytokine has implications in the JAK-STAT pathway through activation of

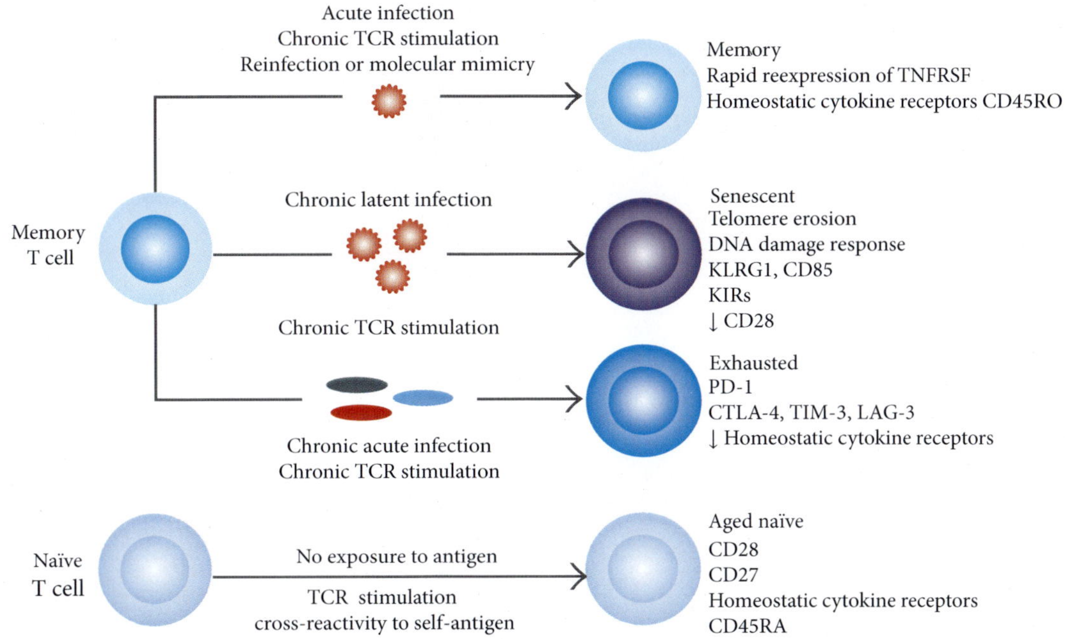

FIGURE 2: Changes in the T-cell pool and individual cells during aging. A Proportion of T subsets depends on individual infection antecedents and the environment. Memory T-cell subset can change to senescence by a chronic latent infection and chronic TCR stimulation. Meanwhile, exhausted T cells are produced by the same type of stimulation and the chronic acute infection. Aged naïve cells are generated from naïve cells stimulated by self-antigen exposure (adapted from [32]).

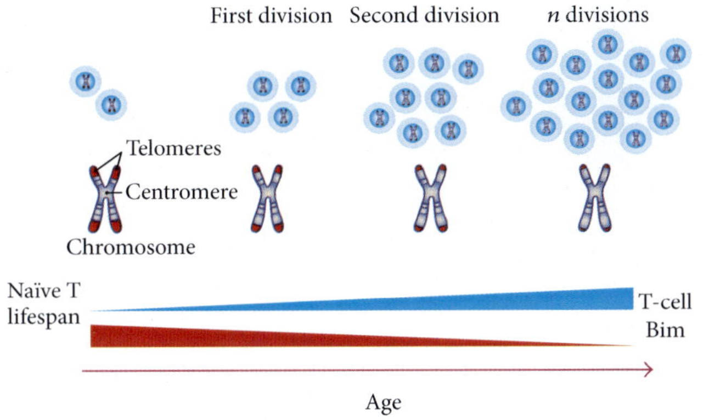

FIGURE 3: Schematic representation of T-cell divisions and their implication in telomere erosion and aging. Constantly dividing cells are accompanied by a decrease in their telomere length, which is related to aging phenotype: decreased Bim expression, increased naïve lifespan, and important functional changes.

SOCS3 transcription. Note that STAT molecules are highly phosphorylated in elderly humans, a phenomenon that also occurs through type I interferon T-cell activation [35].

As was discussed previously, telomere attrition is very frequent in elderly people and it is also known that T-cell replication is important for maintaining lymphocyte function. This suggests that T-cells employ the best mechanisms for telomere maintenance during clonal expansion. Indeed, there is evidence that telomerase activity is highly regulated during T lymphocyte development and differentiation [37]. The resting $CD4^+$ and $CD8^+$ and naïve T cells recorded no telomerase activity on the periphery. However, the telomerase is activated by lymphocyte stimulation. The level of telomerase activity decreases during successive stimulations of the lymphocyte (Figure 3) [38]. The rate of telomere shortening seems to be different among $CD4^+$ and $CD8^+$ cells, and it has been estimated to be 33 bp/year for $CD4^+$ T cells and 26 bp/year for $CD8^+$ T cells. One of the most outstanding features of aged $CD4^+$ naïve T cells is their inability to produce significant levels of IL-2 after stimulation of their T-cell receptor (TCR). This inability subsequently leads to poor Th1/Th2 polarization. However, these cells may retain their ability to suffer Th17 differentiation [39, 40], which, in turn, could favor an inflammatory and autoimmune phenotype development. On the other hand, the number of $CD4^+CD25^+FOXP3^+$ regulatory T cells (Treg) increases (2.4-fold), and they retain and gain functions during aging. Nonetheless, their ability to produce IL-10 is low. They may also contribute to Th17 bias (production of high levels of IL-17, IL-21, and IL-22) and show a decrease in antitumor responses too [40]. Meanwhile, aging $CD8^+$ lymphocytes show a reduction in the diversity of the TCR repertoire, low antitumor response, and marked clonal expansion development but without the ability to replicate after stimulation [26]. Note that Th2 inflammatory cytokines favor antibody production by B cells, and this condition could explain autoantibodies in the aged population.

One of the most important traits of immune aging is the loss of the CD28 surface marker. CD28 is one of the molecules expressed in T cells that provide costimulatory signals that are required for T-cell activation, T-cell proliferation, cytokine production, and T-cell survival promotion. Loss of CD28

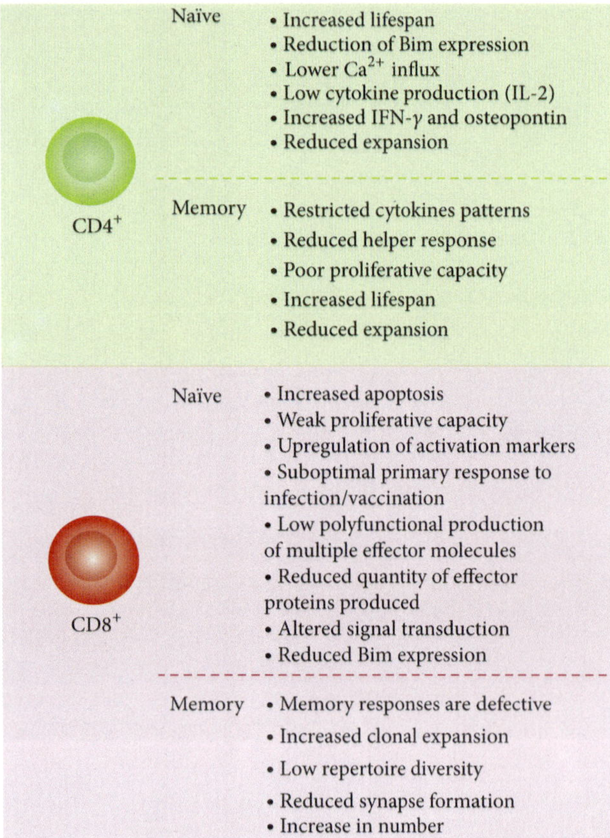

FIGURE 4: Aged-related functional changes in T-cell subsets. Alterations are produced in both memory and naïve subsets. These alterations depend on T-cell microenvironmental history, exposures to stressor agents, and stochastic events. There are differences in changes between $CD4^+$ and $CD8^+$ concerning aging, but in both cases, there is reduction of naïve subtype, increase in lifespan, and defective immune response.

expression is a phenotypic change associated with senescence in T lymphocytes, and it has been associated with functional alterations such as enhanced cytotoxicity, suppressive functions, and resistance of $CD4^+$ T cells to apoptosis. Loss of CD28 expression is characterized by telomere shortening and reduced proliferative ability, both *ex vivo* and *in vitro* [41, 42]. At birth, virtually all T cells express CD28, but with age, the marker decreases about 40 to 50% for $CD8^+$ T cells and 85 to 90% for $CD4^+$. This reduction in the markers is attributed to repeated antigenic stimulation in peripheral blood [43]. However, when the CD28 is lost, cells suffer reprograming and, as a consequence, they express new receptors such as KIR, CD70, and perforin. Moreover, phenotypic $CD28^-$ T-cell characteristics include interferon gamma (IFN-γ) production, potent cytotoxic capability, and CD158, CD158b, CD158J, DAP12, CD94, and CD244 receptor expression (similar to NK cell characteristics). These receptors give them the potential to interact with accessory cells such as mesenchymal cells, which include the fibroblasts of inflamed joints [44]. Furthermore, in elderly individuals with chronic viral infections and autoimmune diseases (e.g., multiple sclerosis (MS), rheumatoid arthritis (RA), and Wegener's disease), an increase in the frequency of $CD28^-$ T cells has been detected [43]. It has been suggested that autoantigens can lead to clonal expansion of these cells. Thus, there are reports [45, 46] indicating how they can, for instance, show reactivity to myelin basic protein (MBP). The presence of $CD4^+$ $CD28^-$ T cells in both elderly individuals and patients with autoimmune diseases (ADs) has supported the concept that ADs are closely related to the cell aging process. In this regard, the loss of CD28 molecule could favor CTLA-4 interaction with their ligands (CD80 and CD86), which are implicated in autoimmune phenotype too.

The main differential and functional alterations of $CD4^+$ and $CD8^+$ T-cell subsets are summarized in Figure 4.

3.1.2. B Cells. It is known that with aging, there is a decrease in not only the frequency and absolute number of pro-B cells but also in their ability to differentiate into pre-B (between 60 and 90%). Nevertheless, in healthy individuals, mature peripheral B-cell numbers do not change with aging; instead the relationship between naïve and memory cells is altered; that is, there is an increase in long-lived memory cells (homeostatic expansion of antigen-experienced or activated B cells) and a decrease in naïve cells [47]. This condition seems to depend on different factors other than genetic ones. A study comparing old individuals with healthy centenarian offspring could determine that centenarian offspring have more IgD^+ $CD27^-$ naïve B cells than older people. Nevertheless, the double negative memory cells (IgD^- $CD27^-$ B cells) are only found in healthy elderly individuals, and there are no differences between groups [48]. Recently, studies have reported a novel peripheral B-cell subset in the elderly named aging-associated B-cell (ABC) subset ($CD19^+CD11b^+CD11c^+$) [49]. *In vitro*, the ABC subset responds only to innate stimuli producing secretion of autoantibodies and cytokines, and this subset also has the ability to potentiate Th17 polarization, thus relating it to an autoimmune phenotype.

Another important fact is the presence of alterations in the repertoire of the B-cell receptor (BCR), which exhibits a decreased affinity and diversity to the antibody response with aging [33]. Indeed, elderly patients have impaired B-cell proliferation and activation, possibly as a result of defects in their threshold of activation [26]. Also, there is a loss of precision in distinguishing self- from non-self-antigens due to the oligoclonal expansion of the B lymphocyte subpopulation with a high proportion of antigen-experienced cells [50]. This subpopulation expresses CD5 on their surface, thus giving them the ability to produce low affinity antibodies independently of T cells. In the context of autoantibody generation, this is important for triggering an autoimmune response.

Moreover, the germinal centers (GC) from elderly people are small and have few cells producing IgM. In these individuals, levels of immunoglobulins, especially IgA and IgG, are increased [51]. Furthermore, it has been shown that IgG^+/IgA^+ B-cell subsets (both $CD27^+$ and $CD27^-$) express Ig mutated genes in their variable regions and high levels of CD80 and CD86 on their surface, thus exhibiting a similar B-cell memory phenotype [52]. According to the reports,

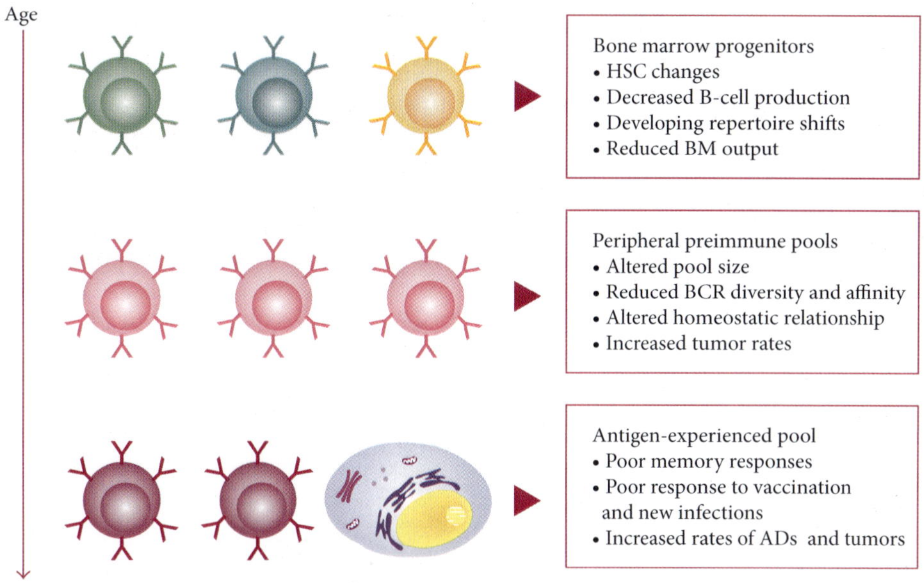

FIGURE 5: Age-related changes in the generation and function of B cells. There is a reduced output of B cells in the bone marrow, which induces accumulations in the periphery of antigen-experienced subsets with poor immune response and low diversity. HSC: hematopoietic stem cell; BCR: B-cell receptor; BM: bone marrow (adapted from [33]).

this subtype of cells declines with aging [51]. Finally, aging B cells have been observed to produce antibodies with low avidity because of their somatic hypermutation deterioration which leads to a gradual decline in the humoral response. Nevertheless, repertory changes are not synchronous with aging, and decreased diversity has been related to poor health status [53].

An interesting study [54] done to evaluate naïve ($CD19^+CD27^-$) and memory ($CD19^+CD27^+$) switch B-cell subsets in elderly individuals showed a decrease in total B cells, and, although the quantity of naïve cells increased in percentage, they decreased or remained constant in number. Moreover, another striking result is that the B-cell memory ($CD27^+$) increased in percentage but not significantly. In contrast, memory cells producing IgM subtype decreased in number but not in percentage. Finally, the memory switch cells decreased both in number and percentage with aging. An interesting point about memory B cells is that they have a hyporesponsive state to antigen-induced activation with less clonal expansion or less ability to differentiate into antibody secreting cells [55]. This condition may be caused by the decreasing number of antibody high affinity B cells that elderly people have.

Taken together, these results indicate that there is an accumulation of antigen-experienced B subsets in aging individuals. In these cases, overall B-cell numbers are unchanged, but they vary in their functional abilities (Figure 5).

3.2. Innate Immune Response

3.2.1. Dendritic Cells. Dendritic cells (DCs) are important because they function as a checkpoint between immunity and tolerance. DCs from aging individuals display a basal level of activation, increased secretion of proinflammatory cytokines such as TNF-α and IL-6 [56], and high levels of NF-κB activation. However, they do not exhibit upregulation of CD86 and CD80 molecules on their surface, which suggests that they are partially activated. Another important characteristic is that they are more reactive to self-antigens compared with their young counterparts and display an impaired clearance of apoptotic cells and antigens [57]. This could produce a higher presentation of self-antigens and, consequently, an activation of autoreactive lymphocytes. An interesting point is that these partially activated DCs have a greater ability to stimulate T cells, thus indicating that their ability to induce tolerance to self-antigens is affected.

Some explanations have been given regarding partially activated DCs: (1) an increased age-associated level of proinflammatory mediators and (2) age-associated modifications in autoantigens, which increase their immunogenicity [58].

Note that the functions of myeloid DCs (mDCs) such as IL-12 production, chemotaxis, and their ability to activate naïve CD4 T cells via antigen presentation appear to be altered in elderly individuals [57]. This inability is due to decreased PI3K activation [59], which leads to activation of NF-κB, as it was previously mentioned. This subtype of DCs also shows decreased capability in their antigen processing and increased expression of CD86.

Plasmacytoid DCs (pDCs) from elderly people, in turn, have reduced IFN I and IFN III production after stimulation via Toll-like receptor (TLR) [60]. Additionally, they have an impaired ability for antigen presentation to CD4 and CD8 T cells.

3.2.2. Neutrophils. Neutrophils are the first immune cells that are recruited to the site of infection or to the tissue damage [61]. Besides, there is a debate about whether the numbers of neutrophils change with age, but a variety of studies suggest that there are no number changes. However, there are reports indicating several functional defects in neutrophils from the elderly [62, 63]. The main function decreased in neutrophils is the chemotaxis, followed by the phagocytic activity. Both of them affect the time needed for the neutrophils to reach the infection site and their ability to control the infections, respectively [62, 64, 65]. These two alterations are closely related to increased infections in elderly subjects.

Low phagocytic activity has been associated with reduced surface expression of the Fcγ receptor CD16 [64]. Signaling function of other receptors involved in activation such as fMLp, TLR, retinoic-acid-inducible-gene-1-protein- (RIG-1-) like helicases (RLRs), nucleotide binding domain and leucine-rich-repeat-containing proteins (NLRs), and C3b has been reported to be significantly altered. This alteration is due to changes in signaling molecules but not in the number of their receptors [66, 67]. Some downstream signaling events include phosphoinositide-3 kinase (PI-3 K), MAP kinase, Calcium, protein kinase B, and SHP-1 and Jak-STAT pathways [68]. Interestingly, these alterations are produced by changes in membrane composition including lipid rafts distribution and their structure [69, 70].

3.2.3. NK and NKT Cells. NK cells participate in the innate immune defense against intracellular pathogens and tumor cells, and they mediate MHC-independent cytotoxicity. There are several studies indicating a remodeling of these cells in elderly individuals. The percentage and absolute number of NK cells are increased in healthy aging, and they are characterized by the increment of CD57 expression and expansion of CD56dim NK cells (mature and highly differentiated cells) [71, 72]. Other important features of these cells from aging subjects are decreased proliferative response to cytokines, altered expression of some NK receptors such as natural cytotoxicity receptors (NCRs) [73], CD226 [74], and KLRG-1 [75], and increased expression of HLA-specific killer immunoglobulin-like receptor [73].

At functional level, cytotoxic and proliferation ability and cytokines/chemokines (such as INFγ, RANTES, MIP1a, and IL8) production of NK cells are reduced [76].

NKT cells are important in the clearance of bacterial and viral infections as well as in regulation of immune tolerance and autoimmunity [77]. NKT cells are characterized by expression of a TCR encoded by Vα14/Vβ8.2 gene segments.

The effects of aging on NKT cell number and function have been little studied. In general, nowadays, it is accepted that the absolute number of NKTs within the lymphoid organ increases [78]. In addition, there are reports that show a decrease of proliferative ability and low number of CD1d-restricted NKT cells in the peripheral blood [79]. Studies of inhibition of NKT cell activation demonstrated age-associated decay of proliferative response and retarded type hypersensitivity responses [80]; in addition, results showed that NKT cells contribute to increments of IL-4 and IL-10 production and decreased IFN-γ in aging subjects [81].

3.2.4. Monocyte/Macrophages. Other essential components of innate immune response are macrophages and monocytes. Monocytes respond to inflammation by their differentiation into macrophages and dendritic cells. Studies have demonstrated that CD56$^+$ monocytes subpopulation (high producers of TNF-α via TLRs 2 and 4) is increased with age while their counterpart (CD56$^-$) is decreased [82]. The increment of CD56$^+$ monocytes is paradoxical with the alteration in macrophage TLR function. A study revealed a decrease in IL-6 and TNF-α via TLR1/2 in the elderly, and this fact was related to the decrease of TLR1 on monocyte surface [83]. These results are contradictory with another report which indicates substantial increase of the same cytokines [21]. Thus, this issue required further confirmation, which can be accomplished by the study of phenotype subpopulations (according to the expression levels of the receptors and proteins). In this regard, age-associated changes in TLRs expression on monocytes have been performed [84]. A particular study showed that old patients infected with West Nile virus have a persistent TLR3 expression on macrophages' surface while young patients have reduced expression of this receptor [85]. This feature may produce a higher inflammatory response with the subsequent increased morbidity of elderly subjects.

Furthermore, there are reports about age-related upregulation of CD80 molecule on monocytes after TLR activation [86] which is associated with production of a protective response to influenza vaccination.

Another important age-associated feature of both monocytes and macrophages is that several of their receptors become altered, thus producing cells dysfunction. This produces that clearance of free radical production and phagocytosis are reduced in monocyte/macrophages in the elderly [87]. Also, these alterations may lead to deregulation in clearing of apoptotic cells by macrophages, thus precipitating the exacerbation of inflammatory-aging condition.

4. Infection and Immunosenescence

To produce an adequate response to large numbers of pathogens throughout life, there are homeostatic mechanisms guaranteeing competent memory and a naïve cell pool for prolonging the survival of memory cells. However, under the conditions of advanced age, these mechanisms are seriously affected. As we have seen, during aging, many changes occur in the immune system, which means that immunosenescence becomes a factor contributing significantly to a higher risk and severity of infections. The most important diseases in the elderly are urinary tract infections, influenza and pneumonia, chronic viral infection reactivation (herpes virus and varicella-zoster virus), as well as bacterial (tuberculosis), fungal (candidiasis), or parasitic infections, and, more rarely, opportunistic infections such as *Clostridium* and *Staphylococcus* [88, 89]. Although the immune response to antigens may be preserved in elderly individuals, their ability to be immunized against new antigens is reduced. This may be the result of an increase in the proportion of memory cells and progressive decrease in naïve cells from the thymus [90].

While it is true that aging is associated with the emergence of infectious diseases, it is also true that these infectious events will promote aging. It is well known that viral infections (particularly the herpes virus family) are strong stressors which alter the lymphocyte phenotype and functionality, altered cytokine profile, resistance to apoptosis, and shortened telomeres [91]. These features are similar to those found in the elderly; thus it is possible that viral infections could represent an important extrinsic factor for aging by the repeated antigen stimulation characteristic of persistent latent infections [92]. Furthermore, it has been suggested that latent herpes virus infections are primarily responsible for *in vivo* generation of senescent $CD8^+$ T cells, perhaps due to constant and prolonged virus-specific T-cell proliferation [93]. Additionally, the Epstein-Barr virus (EBV) latent infection has also been associated with telomere shortening in antigen-specific $CD8^-$ T cells because EBV antigens cause a decrease in telomerase activity associated with T-cell proliferation [94]. In contrast (and related to telomere erosion and its relationship with CD28 molecule expression), the majority of T cells in a study done by Vescocini were $CD28^+$ unlike what was found for CMV, which were mainly $CD28^-$ [95]. During human immunodeficiency virus (HIV) infection, in turn, it has been reported that early presence of $CD8^+$ $CD28^-$ T cells is a predictive characteristic of rapid disease progression [96].

These data indicate that chronic infections during aging produce significant changes in the $CD8^+$ cell subset. Additionally, this shows that expansion of $CD28^-$ T cells is age dependent, and they have a positive correlation with proinflammatory cytokines. At the same time, these cytokines are heavily involved in the pathogenesis of immunological disorders which could favor the emergence of different pathologies including ADs.

5. Autoimmune Disease

Currently, it is clear that changes occurring in the immune system during aging affect the onset of ADs. This is due to the fact that aging is related to increased reactivity to self-antigens and loss of tolerance. The overall tendency supports this hypothesis because elderly people experience general systemic inflammation and, at the same time, they aggravate degenerative diseases [97], which, in turn, increase the risk of developing ADs [98, 99]. Proinflammatory cytokines on general systemic inflammation (produced by viral infection) lead to a state called inflammaging, which corresponds to the loss of equilibrium between adequate inflammatory response and efficient anti-inflammatory control in the elderly condition. Later, in normal aging, this control fails to fully neutralize the inflammatory processes.

In addition to this, it is important to remember (as we have seen previously) the epigenetic changes occurring in elderly people and how these may affect important genes involved in autoimmune disorder development [100]. In this regard, there are reports in which some genes associated with ADs are hypermethylated but others are hypomethylated. For instance, FoxP3, a hypermethylated gene, is a member of the forkhead transcription regulator family [101] and is associated with the development of multiple ADs. In contrast, the gene coding for the CD11a chain of lymphocyte function-associated antigen 1 (LFA-1)—a protein which is associated with certain ADs—is hypomethylated with age and thus overexpressed in aging cells [100]. Furthermore, there are other reports on elderly subjects indicating DNA hypomethylation states which could lead to an increase in the immunogenicity [58]

Another important aspect of aging that is closely related to autoimmunity in general and ADs in particular is the increase in inflammatory cytokines and chemokines such as TNF-α, C-reactive protein, IL-8, MCP1, and RANTES [102–104]. There is a substantial amount of evidence of age-associated alterations in the T-cell cytokine profile which could contribute to development of ADs. Studies have shown that there is a change from Th1 to Th2 molecules (mainly IL-4 and IL-6) in the cytokine profile as age advances [105]. IL-6 is a potent proinflammatory cytokine closely related to disability in patients with RA; therefore, IL-6 represents a therapeutic target for this disease [106]. In addition, there are reports of an imbalance between Th17 and Treg cells. A considerable number of IL-17-secreting naïve $CD4^+$ T helper cells have been detected in the elderly in contrast to reduced IL-17-secreting memory $CD4^+$ T helper cells [107].

Some ADs are very frequent in younger patients and are not limited to elderly people although the occurrence or presence of autoantibodies is greater at advanced age [108–111]. Autoantibody production such as rheumatoid factor, as well as antinuclear, antiphospholipid, and antithyroglobulin antibodies, is present during aging [109, 112]. Autoantibody production has been attributed to altered T- and B-cell functions [113], especially to the decrease in antibody affinity maturation. This evidence supports the idea that autoantibody levels may be closely related to the clinical characteristics of the elderly and to patients with ADs.

One of the important causes of dysfunctional immune responses is telomere abnormalities which may lead to autoimmunity. This observation is significant since numerous studies have shown an association between mean telomere length in peripheral blood mononuclear cells (PBMCs) and different diseases [91]. This evidence suggests an increase in $CD8^+$ $CD28^-$ T-cell proportions in several pathologies such as in the case of some ADs.

Moreover, there are reports of telomere length alteration in patients with ADs such as RA [114, 115], scleroderma (SSc) [116], systemic lupus erythematosus (SLE) [117], polyangiitis with granulomatosis [118], psoriasis, and atopic dermatitis [119], suggesting an excessive cell replication with their corresponding telomere erosion. These findings have been interpreted as evidence of T-cell accelerated proliferation in the autoimmune process.

At present, it is believed that there are differences among telomere abnormalities and various ADs. Some of these differences could be explained by the genetic background of the individuals studied. For example, a study performed in patients with SSc and their family members reported short telomeres [116]. The idea of a genetic predisposition to telomere shortening is also suggested in patients with RA, who exhibit telomere erosion in not only memory cells but also in naïve cells. Moreover, this evidence shows acceleration in telomere erosion occurring at the precursor cell level [120].

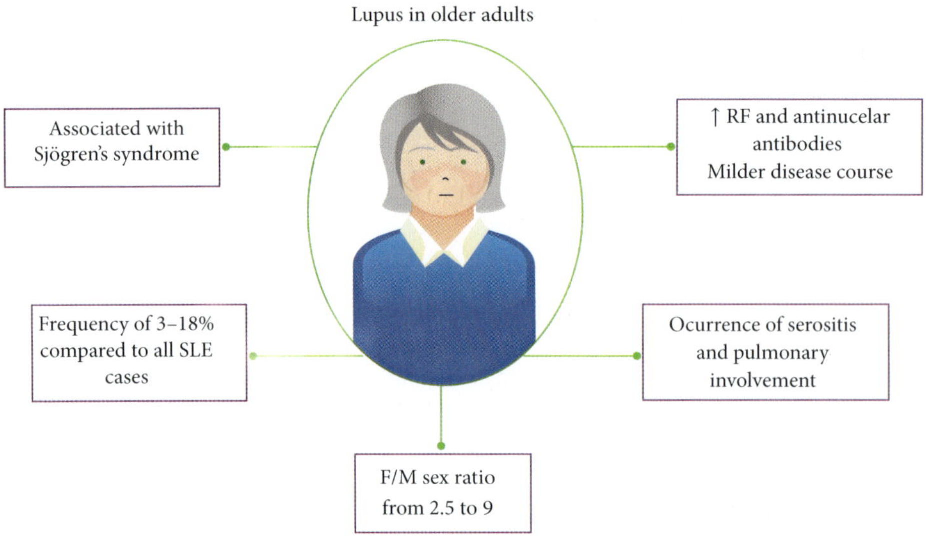

FIGURE 6: General characteristics of late-onset SLE. There are different manifestations of older SLE patients compared to young patients. RF: rheumatoid factor; F/M: female/male.

Another striking fact is that the genetic predisposition to short telomeres is strongly related to HLA-DR4 haplotype which is shared by RA and T1D in some individuals [121, 122].

5.1. Late-Onset Systemic Lupus Erythematous. Although SLE is considered a disease of the reproductive stage of women, there is evidence that it occurs between 3 and 18% in individuals older than 50 years [123]. Despite that there are aged SLE patients, their clinical manifestations, response to treatment, prognosis, and course of the disease are different in these individuals (Figure 6). For example, clinical manifestations such as malar rash, renal disease, arthritis, and photosensitivity are less frequent in them, while serositis, cytopenias, and pulmonary involvement are more frequent [124–127]. In addition, it has been shown that female/male (F/M) sex ratio declines with age. Studies report F/M ratio from 2.5 to 9 in elderly individuals compared to from 9.1 to 14.4 in young people [126, 128].

A striking feature of these patients is the differential diagnosis due to the SLE overlapping with other diseases. Late-onset rheumatoid arthritis, endocarditis, tuberculosis, neoplasia, polymyalgia rheumatica, temporal arteritis, and Sjögren's Syndrome (SS) had been described is these patients [124, 127]. In the particular case of SS, elderly patients with SLE and without SS have low frequency of compromising renal disease, lymphadenopathy, and thrombocytopenia and high frequency of Raynaud's phenomenon [129].

Besides changes in clinical and serological profiles, serological profiles of aged SLE patients also exhibit alterations [124]. Compared to younger individuals, elderly patients with SLE have high frequency of rheumatoid factor (33% versus 20%) and antinuclear antibodies but low frequency of antiribonucleoprotein (anti-RNP, 10% versus 21%) and anti-Sm (9% versus 17%). There are reports that indicate contradictory results [130], but these differences can be explained by different reasons: ethnicity, sample size, methodology, and so forth.

An important fact is that the severity of the disease appears to decrease with age. It has been reported that late-onset SLE patients have milder disease course which is reflected in a small number of relapses per patient. Additionally, it was found that the prevalence of lupus nephritis and nephrotic syndrome also is lower in elderly patients.

Currently, it is not clear if there is a relationship between telomere loss and SLE. Some studies have shown an increased telomere erosion in SLE patients [100, 101, 131, 132], while others report normal telomere length when compared with healthy controls [102, 103]. Nevertheless, it is clear that there is a reduction in telomerase activity in naïve $CD4^+$ T cells and an increased activity in B cells [101, 103]. In this regard, a recent study showed a differential expression of shelterin complex molecules in patients with lupus [104], but, unfortunately, it was not done cell specific.

According to the report of [132], shorter telomeres are associated with Ro antibodies while longer ones with steroid therapy and increased body mass index. However this study also showed that short telomeres are not related to disease activity or immune cell turnover, but they could be good predictors of premature aging.

Related to this topic, previous studies have indicated that bone marrow mesenchymal stem cells (BMSCs) from SLE patients exhibit not only increased apoptosis and senescence but also impaired capacity of differentiation, immune modulation, proliferation, and secretion of cytokines. Apoptosis and senescence in BMSCs from SLE patients appear, to be due to increased favorable conditions for these processes. There were described increased levels of p16INK4A, Bax, caspase 8, Fas and tumor necrosis factor-a receptor 1, and the respective ligands of the two last. There is also a decreased expression of Bcl-2, CDK4, CDK6, and p-Rb [133, 134].

Programmed cell death (PCD) is an essential mechanism of homeostasis and development and it is very important as an immune response regulator. Hence appropriate clearance of apoptotic cells in the immune system is necessary for regulating inflammation and maintaining self-tolerance. Impaired clearance of apoptotic cells in patients with SLE is considered an important process in the etiology of lupus [135]. This phenomenon is exacerbated in older age, and its deficiencies may account for the development of autoimmunity by the loss of tolerance in lymphoid tissues. This process is mediated by phagocytes and, as it was mentioned before, in elderly subjects; phagocytic functions of macrophages are altered. This functional deregulation may generate danger signals, followed by concomitant exposure of autoantigens and the subsequent autoimmune reaction.

Another mechanism that is related to development of lupus is the molecular mimicry in which B and T cells are activated as a result of an infection. This mechanism makes cells able to recognize self-molecules that are similar to infectious agent molecules, thus originating an autoimmune response [136–139]. In SLE, this response is associated with high levels of anti-Sm autoantibodies due to similar molecular sequence of pathogenic molecules of CMV and EBV, which develop the initial immune response. Although anti-Sm autoantibodies are less frequent in the elderly than in younger individuals, it may be possible that EBV infection—exacerbated with age—can contribute not only to inflammaging development but also to induction, by molecular mimicry, of an immune response towards itself. Further studies in this topic could be interesting.

Abnormalities in TCR signaling which have been documented in SLE patients are similar to those in RA patients. This may also be related to the elderly; for instance, TCR zeta chain expression is defective in these patients [105].

6. Concluding Remarks

Aging is a natural physiological process that could eventually conduce to increases in some pathological conditions. A lot of changes are detected in the immune system of elderly individuals which could contribute to the occurrence of complications such as infection, autoimmunity, and autoimmune disorders. In this regard, it is important to remember that elderly patients with SLE have different clinical and serological manifestations and poorer prognosis comparing with young patients (less insidious onset disease, more occurrences of severe manifestations, and higher frequency of comorbid conditions). Thus it is necessary to implement a proper immunological recognition of these patients in order to produce adequate therapeutic management which must be different because the treatment itself may cause long-term damage.

References

[1] G. Aubert and P. M. Lansdorp, "Telomeres and aging," *Physiological Reviews*, vol. 88, no. 2, pp. 557–579, 2008.

[2] A. N. Vallejo, C. M. Weyand, and J. J. Goronzy, "T-cell senescence: a culprit of immune abnormalities in chronic inflammation and persistent infection," *Trends in Molecular Medicine*, vol. 10, no. 3, pp. 119–124, 2004.

[3] J. J. Goronzy, H. Fujii, and C. M. Weyand, "Telomeres, immune aging and autoimmunity," *Experimental Gerontology*, vol. 41, no. 3, pp. 246–251, 2006.

[4] K. D. Jacob, N. N. Hooten, A. R. Trzeciak, and M. K. Evans, "Markers of oxidant stress that are clinically relevant in aging and age-related disease," *Mechanisms of Ageing and Development*, vol. 134, no. 3-4, pp. 139–157, 2013.

[5] R. Holliday, "Telomeres and telomerase: the commitment theory of cellular ageing revisited," *Science Progress*, vol. 95, no. 2, pp. 199–205, 2012.

[6] P. M. Lansdorp, "Role of telomerase in hematopoietic stem cells," *Annals of the New York Academy of Sciences*, vol. 1044, pp. 220–227, 2005.

[7] O. Samassekou, M. Gadji, R. Drouin, and J. Yan, "Sizing the ends: normal length of human telomeres," *Annals of Anatomy*, vol. 192, no. 5, pp. 284–291, 2010.

[8] A. Montesanto, S. Dato, D. Bellizzi, G. Rose, and G. Passarino, "Epidemiological, genetic and epigenetic aspects of the research on healthy ageing and longevity," *Immunity & Ageing*, vol. 9, no. 1, article 6, 2012.

[9] D. Gentilini, D. Castaldi, D. Mari et al., "Age-dependent skewing of X chromosome inactivation appears delayed in centenarians' offspring. Is there a role for allelic imbalance in healthy aging and longevity?" *Aging Cell*, vol. 11, no. 2, pp. 277–283, 2012.

[10] M. F. Fraga, E. Ballestar, M. F. Paz et al., "Epigenetic differences arise during the lifetime of monozygotic twins," *Proceedings of the National Academy of Sciences of the United States of America*, vol. 102, no. 30, pp. 10604–10609, 2005.

[11] E. Bártová, J. Krejcí, A. Harnicarová, G. Galiová, and S. Kozubek, "Histone modifications and nuclear architecture: a review," *The Journal of Histochemistry and Cytochemistry*, vol. 56, no. 8, pp. 711–721, 2008.

[12] A. Salminen and K. Kaarniranta, "SIRT1 regulates the ribosomal DNA locus: epigenetic candles twinkle longevity in the Christmas tree," *Biochemical and Biophysical Research Communications*, vol. 378, no. 1, pp. 6–9, 2009.

[13] F.-J. Liu, T. Wen, and L. Liu, "MicroRNAs as a novel cellular senescence regulator," *Ageing Research Reviews*, vol. 11, no. 1, pp. 41–50, 2012.

[14] S. K. Dewan, S.-B. Zheng, S.-J. Xia, and K. Bill, "Senescent remodeling of the immune system and its contribution to the predisposition of the elderly to infections," *Chinese Medical Journal*, vol. 125, no. 18, pp. 3325–3331, 2012.

[15] A. Globerson and R. B. Effros, "Ageing of lymphocytes and lymphocytes in the aged," *Immunology Today*, vol. 21, no. 10, pp. 515–521, 2000.

[16] G. Pawelec, E. Derhovanessian, A. Larbi, J. Strindhall, and A. Wikby, "Cytomegalovirus and human immunosenescence," *Reviews in Medical Virology*, vol. 19, no. 1, pp. 47–56, 2009.

[17] N. Rufer, T. H. Brümmendorf, S. Kolvraa et al., "Telomere fluorescence measurements in granulocytes and T lymphocyte subsets point to a high turnover of hematopoietic stem cells and memory T cells in early childhood," *The Journal of Experimental Medicine*, vol. 190, no. 2, pp. 157–167, 1999.

[18] S. Ferrando-Martínez, M. de la Fuente, J. M. Guerrero, M. Leal, and M. Á. Muñoz-Fernández, "Impact of thymic function in age-related immune deterioration," *Revista Española de Geriatría y Gerontología*, 2013.

[19] P. L. F. Johnson, A. J. Yates, J. J. Goronzy, and R. Antia, "Peripheral selection rather than thymic involution explains sudden contraction in naïve CD4 T-cell diversity with age," *Proceedings of the National Academy of Sciences of the United States of America*, vol. 109, no. 52, pp. 21432–21437, 2012.

[20] I. K. Chinn, C. C. Blackburn, N. R. Manley, and G. D. Sempowski, "Changes in primary lymphoid organs with aging," *Seminars in Immunology*, vol. 24, no. 5, pp. 309–320, 2012.

[21] P. Sansoni, R. Vescovini, F. Fagnoni et al., "The immune system in extreme longevity," *Experimental Gerontology*, vol. 43, no. 2, pp. 61–65, 2008.

[22] T. Sathaliyawala, M. Kubota, N. Yudanin et al., "Distribution and compartmentalization of human circulating and tissue-resident memory T cell subsets," *Immunity*, vol. 38, no. 1, pp. 187–197, 2013.

[23] R. Solana, R. Tarazona, I. Gayoso, O. Lesur, G. Dupuis, and T. Fulop, "Innate immunosenescence: effect of aging on cells and receptors of the innate immune system in humans," *Seminars in Immunology*, vol. 24, no. 5, pp. 331–341, 2012.

[24] G. Pfister and W. Savino, "Can the immune system still be efficient in the elderly? An immunological and immunoendocrine therapeutic perspective," *NeuroImmunoModulation*, vol. 15, no. 4–6, pp. 351–364, 2008.

[25] J. E. McElhaney, X. Zhou, H. K. Talbot et al., "The unmet need in the elderly: how immunosenescence, CMV infection, co-morbidities and frailty are a challenge for the development of more effective influenza vaccines," *Vaccine*, vol. 30, no. 12, pp. 2060–2067, 2012.

[26] A. Larbi, T. Fülöp, and G. Pawelec, "Immune receptor signaling, aging and autoimmunity," *Advances in Experimental Medicine and Biology*, vol. 640, pp. 312–324, 2008.

[27] G. G. Garcia and R. A. Miller, "Age-dependent defects in TCR-triggered cytoskeletal rearrangement in $CD4^+$ T cells," *The Journal of Immunology*, vol. 169, no. 9, pp. 5021–5027, 2002.

[28] Q.-J. Li, J. Chau, P. J. R. Ebert et al., "miR-181a is an intrinsic modulator of T cell sensitivity and selection," *Cell*, vol. 129, no. 1, pp. 147–161, 2007.

[29] G. Li, M. Yu, W.-W. Lee et al., "Decline in miR-181a expression with age impairs T cell receptor sensitivity by increasing DUSP6 activity," *Nature Medicine*, vol. 18, no. 10, pp. 1518–1524, 2012.

[30] J.-N. Cao, S. Gollapudi, E. H. Sharman, Z. Jia, and S. Gupta, "Age-related alterations of gene expression patterns in human $CD8^+$ T cells," *Aging Cell*, vol. 9, no. 1, pp. 19–31, 2010.

[31] M. Czesnikiewicz-Guzik, W.-W. Lee, D. Cui et al., "T cell subset-specific susceptibility to aging," *Clinical Immunology*, vol. 127, no. 1, pp. 107–118, 2008.

[32] M. M. Cavanagh, Q. Qi, C. M. Weyand, and J. J. Goronzy, "Finding balance: T cell regulatory receptor expression during aging," *Aging and Disease*, vol. 2, no. 5, pp. 398–413, 2011.

[33] M. P. Cancro, Y. Hao, J. L. Scholz et al., "B cells and aging: molecules and mechanisms," *Trends in Immunology*, vol. 30, no. 7, pp. 313–318, 2009.

[34] W.-W. Lee, D. Cui, M. Czesnikiewicz-Guzik et al., "Age-dependent signature of metallothionein expression in primary CD4 T cell responses is due to sustained zinc signaling," *Rejuvenation Research*, vol. 11, no. 6, pp. 1001–1011, 2008.

[35] J. J. Goronzy, G. Li, M. Yu, and C. M. Weyand, "Signaling pathways in aged T cells—a reflection of T cell differentiation, cell senescence and host environment," *Seminars in Immunology*, vol. 24, no. 5, pp. 365–372, 2012.

[36] P. Deshpande, M. M. Cavanagh, S. Le Saux, K. Singh, C. M. Weyand, and J. J. Goronzy, "IL-7- and IL-15-mediated TCR sensitization enables T cell responses to self-antigens," *The Journal of Immunology*, vol. 190, no. 4, pp. 1416–1423, 2013.

[37] L. Kaszubowska, "Telomere shortening and ageing of the immune system," *Journal of Physiology and Pharmacology*, vol. 59, supplement 9, pp. 169–186, 2008.

[38] A. Chebel, S. Bauwens, L.-M. Gerland et al., "Telomere uncapping during in vitro T-lymphocyte senescence," *Aging Cell*, vol. 8, no. 1, pp. 52–64, 2009.

[39] A. C. Maue, E. J. Yager, S. L. Swain, D. L. Woodland, M. A. Blackman, and L. Haynes, "T-cell immunosenescence: lessons learned from mouse models of aging," *Trends in Immunology*, vol. 30, no. 7, pp. 301–305, 2009.

[40] A. C. Maue and L. Haynes, "$CD4^+$ T cells and immunosenescence—a mini-review," *Gerontology*, vol. 55, no. 5, pp. 491–495, 2009.

[41] S. T. Parish, J. E. Wu, and R. B. Effros, "Sustained CD28 expression delays multiple features of replicative senescence in human CD8 T lymphocytes," *Journal of Clinical Immunology*, vol. 30, no. 6, pp. 798–805, 2010.

[42] R. B. Effros, M. Dagarag, and H. F. Valenzuela, "In vitro senescence of immune cells," *Experimental Gerontology*, vol. 38, no. 11-12, pp. 1243–1249, 2003.

[43] N.-P. Weng, A. N. Akbar, and J. Goronzy, "$CD28^-$ T cells: their role in the age-associated decline of immune function," *Trends in Immunology*, vol. 30, no. 7, pp. 306–312, 2009.

[44] A. E. R. Fasth, N. K. Björkström, M. Anthoni, K.-J. Malmberg, and V. Malmström, "Activating NK-cell receptors co-stimulate $CD4^+CD28^-$ T cells in patients with rheumatoid arthritis," *European Journal of Immunology*, vol. 40, no. 2, pp. 378–387, 2010.

[45] M. J. Pinto-Medel, J. A. García-León, B. Oliver-Martos et al., "The $CD4^+$ T-cell subset lacking expression of the CD28 costimulatory molecule is expanded and shows a higher activation state in multiple sclerosis," *Journal of Neuroimmunology*, vol. 243, no. 1-2, pp. 1–11, 2012.

[46] S. Markovic-Plese, I. Cortese, K.-P. Wandinger, H. F. McFarland, and R. Martin, "$CD4^+CD28^-$ costimulation-independent T cells in multiple sclerosis," *The Journal of Clinical Investigation*, vol. 108, no. 8, pp. 1185–1194, 2001.

[47] S. Buffa, M. Bulati, M. Pellicanò et al., "B cell immunosenescence: different features of naïve and memory B cells in elderly," *Biogerontology*, vol. 12, no. 5, pp. 473–483, 2011.

[48] G. Colonna-Romano, S. Buffa, M. Bulati et al., "B cells compartment in centenarian offspring and old people," *Current Pharmaceutical Design*, vol. 16, no. 6, pp. 604–608, 2010.

[49] A. V. Rubtsov, K. Rubtsova, A. Fischer et al., "Toll-like receptor 7 (TLR7)-driven accumulation of a novel $CD11c^+$ B-cell population is important for the development of autoimmunity," *Blood*, vol. 118, no. 5, pp. 1305–1315, 2011.

[50] S. A. Johnson, S. J. Rozzo, and J. C. Cambier, "Aging-dependent exclusion of antigen-inexperienced cells from the peripheral B cell repertoire," *The Journal of Immunology*, vol. 168, no. 10, pp. 5014–5023, 2002.

[51] D. Frasca and B. B. Blomberg, "Aging affects human B cell responses," *Journal of Clinical Immunology*, vol. 31, no. 3, pp. 430–435, 2011.

[52] S. G. Tangye and K. L. Good, "Human IgM^+CD27^+ B cells: memory B cells or "memory" B cells?" *The Journal of Immunology*, vol. 179, no. 1, pp. 13–19, 2007.

[53] K. L. Gibson, Y.-C. Wu, Y. Barnett et al., "B-cell diversity decreases in old age and is correlated with poor health status," *Aging Cell*, vol. 8, no. 1, pp. 18–25, 2009.

[54] D. Frasca, A. M. Landin, S. C. Lechner et al., "Aging down-regulates the transcription factor E2A, activation-induced cytidine deaminase, and Ig class switch in human b cells," *The Journal of Immunology*, vol. 180, no. 8, pp. 5283–5290, 2008.

[55] S. Sasaki, M. Sullivan, C. F. Narvaez et al., "Limited efficacy of inactivated influenza vaccine in elderly individuals is associated with decreased production of vaccine-specific antibodies," *The Journal of Clinical Investigation*, vol. 121, no. 8, pp. 3109–3119, 2011.

[56] A. Agrawal, J. Tay, S. Ton, S. Agrawal, and S. Gupta, "Increased reactivity of dendritic cells from aged subjects to self-antigen, the human DNA," *The Journal of Immunology*, vol. 182, no. 2, pp. 1138–1145, 2009.

[57] A. Agrawal and S. Gupta, "Impact of aging on dendritic cell functions in humans," *Ageing Research Reviews*, vol. 10, no. 3, pp. 336–345, 2011.

[58] A. Agrawal, J. Tay, G.-E. Yang, S. Agrawal, and S. Gupta, "Age-associated epigenetic modifications in human DNA increase its immunogenicity," *Aging*, vol. 2, no. 2, pp. 93–100, 2010.

[59] A. Agrawal, S. Agrawal, J.-N. Cao, H. Su, K. Osann, and S. Gupta, "Altered innate immune functioning of dendritic cells in elderly humans: a role of phosphoinositide 3-kinase-signaling pathway," *The Journal of Immunology*, vol. 178, no. 11, pp. 6912–6922, 2007.

[60] A. Sridharan, M. Esposo, K. Kaushal et al., "Age-associated impaired plasmacytoid dendritic cell functions lead to decreased CD4 and CD8 T cell immunity," *Age*, vol. 33, no. 3, pp. 363–376, 2011.

[61] V. Kumar and A. Sharma, "Neutrophils: cinderella of innate immune system," *International Immunopharmacology*, vol. 10, no. 11, pp. 1325–1334, 2010.

[62] C. Wenisch, S. Patruta, F. Daxböck, R. Krause, and W. Hörl, "Effect of age on human neutrophil function," *Journal of Leukocyte Biology*, vol. 67, no. 1, pp. 40–45, 2000.

[63] A. Fortin, D. Harbour, M. Fernandes, P. Borgeat, and S. Bourgoin, "Differential expression of adenosine receptors in human neutrophils: up-regulation by specific Th1 cytokines and lipopolysaccharide," *Journal of Leukocyte Biology*, vol. 79, no. 3, pp. 574–585, 2006.

[64] S. K. Butcher, H. Chahal, L. Nayak et al., "Senescence in innate immune responses: reduced neutrophil phagocytic capacity and CD16 expression in elderly humans," *Journal of Leukocyte Biology*, vol. 70, no. 6, pp. 881–886, 2001.

[65] B. Simell, A. Vuorela, N. Ekström et al., "Aging reduces the functionality of anti-pneumococcal antibodies and the killing of *Streptococcus pneumoniae* by neutrophil phagocytosis," *Vaccine*, vol. 29, no. 10, pp. 1929–1934, 2011.

[66] T. Fulop, A. Larbi, N. Douziech et al., "Signal transduction and functional changes in neutrophils with aging," *Aging Cell*, vol. 3, no. 4, pp. 217–226, 2004.

[67] A. C. Shaw, A. Panda, S. R. Joshi, F. Qian, H. G. Allore, and R. R. Montgomery, "Dysregulation of human toll-like receptor function in aging," *Ageing Research Reviews*, vol. 10, no. 3, pp. 346–353, 2011.

[68] A. Larbi, N. Douziech, C. Fortin, A. Linteau, G. Dupuis, and T. Fulop Jr., "The role of the MAPK pathway alterations in GM-CSF modulated human neutrophil apoptosis with aging," *Immunity & Ageing*, vol. 2, no. 1, article 6, 2005.

[69] C. F. Fortin, A. Larbi, O. Lesur, N. Douziech, and T. Fulop Jr., "Impairment of SHP-1 down-regulation in the lipid rafts of human neutrophils under GM-CSF stimulation contributes to their age-related, altered functions," *Journal of Leukocyte Biology*, vol. 79, no. 5, pp. 1061–1072, 2006.

[70] C. F. Fortin, O. Lesur, and T. Fulop Jr., "Effects of aging on triggering receptor expressed on myeloid cells (TREM)-1-induced PMN functions," *FEBS Letters*, vol. 581, no. 6, pp. 1173–1178, 2007.

[71] S. M. Chidrawar, N. Khan, Y. L. T. Chan, L. Nayak, and P. A. H. Moss, "Ageing is associated with a decline in peripheral blood $CD56^{bright}$ NK cells," *Immunity & Ageing*, vol. 3, article 10, 2006.

[72] M. Le Garff-Tavernier, V. Béziat, J. Decocq et al., "Human NK cells display major phenotypic and functional changes over the life span," *Aging cell*, vol. 9, no. 4, pp. 527–535, 2010.

[73] A. Almeida-Oliveira, M. Smith-Carvalho, L. C. Porto et al., "Age-related changes in natural killer cell receptors from childhood through old age," *Human Immunology*, vol. 72, no. 4, pp. 319–329, 2011.

[74] B. Sanchez-Correa, I. Gayoso, J. M. Bergua et al., "Decreased expression of DNAM-1 on NK cells from acute myeloid leukemia patients," *Immunology and Cell Biology*, vol. 90, no. 1, pp. 109–115, 2012.

[75] R. P. G. Hayhoe, S. M. Henson, A. N. Akbar, and D. B. Palmer, "Variation of human natural killer cell phenotypes with age: identification of a unique KLRG1-negative subset," *Human Immunology*, vol. 71, no. 7, pp. 676–681, 2010.

[76] E. Mocchegiani, R. Giacconi, C. Cipriano, and M. Malavolta, "NK and NKT cells in aging and longevity: role of zinc and metallothioneins," *Journal of Clinical Immunology*, vol. 29, no. 4, pp. 416–425, 2009.

[77] A. Bendelac, P. B. Savage, and L. Teyton, "The biology of NKT cells," *Annual Review of Immunology*, vol. 25, pp. 297–336, 2007.

[78] D. P. Dubey, Z. Husain, E. Levitan et al., "The MHC influences NK and NKT cell functions associated with immune abnormalities and lifespan," *Mechanisms of Ageing and Development*, vol. 113, no. 2, pp. 117–134, 2000.

[79] E. Peralbo, C. Alonso, and R. Solana, "Invariant NKT and NKT-like lymphocytes: two different T cell subsets that are differentially affected by ageing," *Experimental Gerontology*, vol. 42, no. 8, pp. 703–708, 2007.

[80] D. E. Faunce, J. L. Palmer, K. K. Paskowicz, P. L. Witte, and E. J. Kovacs, "CD1d-restricted NKT cells contribute to the age-associated decline of T cell immunity," *The Journal of Immunology*, vol. 175, no. 5, pp. 3102–3109, 2005.

[81] Y. Jing, S. Gravenstein, N. Rao Chaganty et al., "Aging is associated with a rapid decline in frequency, alterations in subset composition, and enhanced Th2 response in CD1d-restricted NKT cells from human peripheral blood," *Experimental Gerontology*, vol. 42, no. 8, pp. 719–732, 2007.

[82] J. Nyugen, S. Agrawal, S. Gollapudi, and S. Gupta, "Impaired functions of peripheral blood monocyte subpopulations in aged humans," *Journal of Clinical Immunology*, vol. 30, no. 6, pp. 806–813, 2010.

[83] D. van Duin, S. Mohanty, V. Thomas et al., "Age-associated defect in human TLR-1/2 function," *The Journal of Immunology*, vol. 178, no. 2, pp. 970–975, 2007.

[84] L. Alvarez-Rodriguez, M. Lopez-Hoyos, M. Garcia-Unzueta, J. A. Amado, P. M. Cacho, and V. M. Martinez-Taboada, "Age and low levels of circulating vitamin D are associated with impaired innate immune function," *Journal of Leukocyte Biology*, vol. 91, no. 5, pp. 829–838, 2012.

[85] K.-F. Kong, K. Delroux, X. Wang et al., "Dysregulation of TLR3 impairs the innate immune response to West Nile virus in the elderly," *Journal of Virology*, vol. 82, no. 15, pp. 7613–7623, 2008.

[86] D. van Duin, H. G. Allore, S. Mohanty et al., "Prevaccine determination of the expression of costimulatoiy B7 molecules in activated monocytes predicts influenza vaccine responses in young and older adults," *The Journal of Infectious Diseases*, vol. 195, no. 11, pp. 1590–1597, 2007.

[87] C. R. Gomez, V. Nomellini, D. E. Faunce, and E. J. Kovacs, "Innate immunity and aging," *Experimental Gerontology*, vol. 43, no. 8, pp. 718–728, 2008.

[88] A. Panda, A. Arjona, E. Sapey et al., "Human innate immunosenescence: causes and consequences for immunity in old age," *Trends in Immunology*, vol. 30, no. 7, pp. 325–333, 2009.

[89] K. P. High, "Infection as a cause of age-related morbidity and mortality," *Ageing Research Reviews*, vol. 3, no. 1, pp. 1–14, 2004.

[90] H. E. Lynch, G. L. Goldberg, A. Chidgey, M. R. M. van den Brink, R. Boyd, and G. D. Sempowski, "Thymic involution and immune reconstitution," *Trends in Immunology*, vol. 30, no. 7, pp. 366–373, 2009.

[91] R. B. Effros, "Telomere/telomerase dynamics within the human immune system: effect of chronic infection and stress," *Experimental Gerontology*, vol. 46, no. 2-3, pp. 135–140, 2011.

[92] J. Nikolich-Žugich, "Ageing and life-long maintenance of T-cell subsets in the face of latent persistent infections," *Nature Reviews Immunology*, vol. 8, no. 7, pp. 512–522, 2008.

[93] G. Pawelec, A. Akbar, C. Caruso, R. Effros, B. Grubeck-Loebenstein, and A. Wikby, "Is immunosenescence infectious?" *Trends in Immunology*, vol. 25, no. 8, pp. 406–410, 2004.

[94] H. F. Valenzuela and R. B. Effros, "Divergent telomerase and CD28 expression patterns in human CD4 and CD8 T cells following repeated encounters with the same antigenic stimulus," *Clinical Immunology*, vol. 105, no. 2, pp. 117–125, 2002.

[95] R. Vescovini, A. Telera, F. F. Fagnoni et al., "Different contribution of EBV and CMV infections in very long-term carriers to age-related alterations of $CD8^+$ T cells," *Experimental Gerontology*, vol. 39, no. 8, pp. 1233–1243, 2004.

[96] W. Cao, B. D. Jamieson, L. E. Hultin, P. M. Hultin, R. B. Effros, and R. Detels, "Premature aging of T cells is associated with faster HIV-1 disease progression," *Journal of Acquired Immune Deficiency Syndromes*, vol. 50, no. 2, pp. 137–147, 2009.

[97] C. Franceschi, M. Capri, D. Monti et al., "Inflammaging and anti-inflammaging: a systemic perspective on aging and longevity emerged from studies in humans," *Mechanisms of Ageing and Development*, vol. 128, no. 1, pp. 92–105, 2007.

[98] S. V. Mohan, Y. J. Liao, J. W. Kim, J. J. Goronzy, and C. M. Weyand, "Giant cell arteritis: immune and vascular aging as disease risk factors," *Arthritis Research & Therapy*, vol. 13, no. 4, article 231, 2011.

[99] J. J. Goronzy, L. Shao, and C. M. Weyand, "Immune aging and rheumatoid arthritis," *Rheumatic Disease Clinics of North America*, vol. 36, no. 2, pp. 297–310, 2010.

[100] Z. Zhang, C. Deng, Q. Lu, and B. Richardson, "Age-dependent DNA methylation changes in the ITGAL (CD11a) promoter," *Mechanisms of Ageing and Development*, vol. 123, no. 9, pp. 1257–1268, 2002.

[101] B. C. Richardson, "Role of DNA methylation in the regulation of cell function: autoimmunity, aging and cancer," *The Journal of Nutrition*, vol. 132, no. 8, supplement, pp. 2401S–2405S, 2002.

[102] A. Agrawal, A. Sridharan, S. Prakash, and H. Agrawal, "Dendritic cells and aging: consequences for autoimmunity," *Expert Review of Clinical Immunology*, vol. 8, no. 1, pp. 73–80, 2012.

[103] M. Maggio, J. M. Guralnik, D. L. Longo, and L. Ferrucci, "Interleukin-6 in aging and chronic disease: a magnificent pathway," *The Journals of Gerontology A*, vol. 61, no. 6, pp. 575–584, 2006.

[104] C. Perricone, N. Agmon-Levin, and Y. Shoenfeld, "Novel pebbles in the mosaic of autoimmunity," *BMC Medicine*, vol. 11, article 101, 2013.

[105] A. Desai, A. Grolleau-Julius, and R. Yung, "Leukocyte function in the aging immune system," *Journal of Leukocyte Biology*, vol. 87, no. 6, pp. 1001–1009, 2010.

[106] M. Murakami and N. Nishimoto, "The value of blocking IL-6 outside of rheumatoid arthritis: current perspective," *Current Opinion in Rheumatology*, vol. 23, no. 3, pp. 273–277, 2011.

[107] J. S. Lee, W.-W. Lee, S. H. Kim et al., "Age-associated alteration in naïve and memory Th17 cell response in humans," *Clinical Immunology*, vol. 140, no. 1, pp. 84–91, 2011.

[108] E. P. Nagele, M. Han, N. K. Acharya, C. DeMarshall, M. C. Kosciuk, and R. G. Nagele, "Natural IgG autoantibodies are abundant and ubiquitous in human sera, and their number is influenced by age, gender, and disease," *PLoS ONE*, vol. 8, no. 4, Article ID e60726, 2013.

[109] P. Hasler and M. Zouali, "Immune receptor signaling, aging, and autoimmunity," *Cellular Immunology*, vol. 233, no. 2, pp. 102–108, 2005.

[110] Y. Tomer and Y. Shoenfeld, "Ageing and autoantibodies," *Autoimmunity*, vol. 1, no. 2, pp. 141–149, 1988.

[111] C. Perricone, N. Agmon-Levin, F. Ceccarelli, G. Valesini, J.-M. Anaya, and Y. Shoenfeld, "Genetics and autoantibodies," *Immunologic Research*, vol. 56, no. 2-3, pp. 206–219, 2013.

[112] T. E. Johnson, "Recent results: biomarkers of aging," *Experimental Gerontology*, vol. 41, no. 12, pp. 1243–1246, 2006.

[113] S. Agarwal and P. J. Busse, "Innate and adaptive immunosenescence," *Annals of Allergy, Asthma & Immunology*, vol. 104, no. 3, pp. 183–190, 2010.

[114] K. Koetz, E. Bryl, K. Spickschen, W. M. O'Fallon, J. J. Goronzy, and C. M. Weyand, "T cell homeostasis in patients with rheumatoid arthritis," *Proceedings of the National Academy of Sciences of the United States of America*, vol. 97, no. 16, pp. 9203–9208, 2000.

[115] S. O. Schönland, C. Lopez, T. Widmann et al., "Premature telomeric loss in rheumatoid arthritis is genetically determined and involves both myeloid and lymphoid cell lineages," *Proceedings of the National Academy of Sciences of the United States of America*, vol. 100, no. 23, pp. 13471–13476, 2003.

[116] C. M. Artlett, C. M. Black, D. C. Briggs, C. O. Stevens, and K. I. Welsh, "Telomere reduction in scleroderma patients: a possible cause for chromosomal instability," *British Journal of Rheumatology*, vol. 35, no. 8, pp. 732–737, 1996.

[117] M. Honda, E. Mengesha, S. Albano et al., "Telomere shortening and decreased replicative potential, contrasted by continued proliferation of telomerase-positive $CD8^+$ $CD28^{lo}$ T cells in patients with systemic lupus erythematosus," *Clinical Immunology*, vol. 99, no. 2, pp. 211–221, 2001.

[118] S. Vogt, C. Iking-Konert, F. Hug, K. Andrassy, and G. M. Hänsch, "Shortening of telomeres: evidence for replicative senescence of T cells derived from patients with Wegener's granulomatosis," *Kidney International*, vol. 63, no. 6, pp. 2144–2151, 2003.

[119] K. Wu, N. Higashi, E. R. Hansen, M. Lund, K. Bang, and K. Thestrup-Pedersen, "Telomerase activity is increased and telomere length shortened in T cells from blood of patients with

atopic dermatitis and psoriasis," *The Journal of Immunology*, vol. 165, no. 8, pp. 4742–4747, 2000.

[120] H. Fujii, L. Shao, I. Colmegna et al., "Telomerase insufficiency in rheumatoid arthritis," *Proceedings of the National Academy of Sciences of the United States of America*, vol. 106, no. 11, pp. 4360–4365, 2009.

[121] C. M. Weyand and J. J. Goronzy, "Stem cell aging and autoimmunity in rheumatoid arthritis," *Trends in Molecular Medicine*, vol. 10, no. 9, pp. 426–433, 2004.

[122] M. Salmon and A. N. Akbar, "Telomere erosion: a new link between *HLA DR4* and rheumatoid arthritis?" *Trends in Immunology*, vol. 25, no. 7, pp. 339–341, 2004.

[123] R. K. Maddock, "Incidence of systemic lupus erythematosus by age and sex," *The Journal of the American Medical Association*, vol. 191, pp. 137–138, 1965.

[124] J. Boddaert, D. L. T. Huong, Z. Amoura, B. Wechsler, P. Godeau, and J.-C. Piette, "Late-onset systemic lupus erythematosus: a personal series of 47 patients and pooled analysis of 714 cases in the literature," *Medicine*, vol. 83, no. 6, pp. 348–359, 2004.

[125] S. Jacobsen, J. Petersen, S. Ullman et al., "A multicentre study of 513 Danish patients with systemic lupus erythematosus. II. Disease mortality and clinical factors of prognostic value," *Clinical Rheumatology*, vol. 17, no. 6, pp. 478–484, 1998.

[126] R. Cervera, M. A. Khamashta, J. Font et al., "Systemic lupus erythematosus: clinical and immunologic patterns of disease expression in a cohort of 1,000 patients. The European working party on systemic lupus erythematosus," *Medicine*, vol. 72, no. 2, pp. 113–124, 1993.

[127] A. Tomic-Lucic, R. Petrovic, M. Radak-Perovic et al., "Late-onset systemic lupus erythematosus: clinical features, course, and prognosis," *Clinical Rheumatology*, vol. 32, no. 7, pp. 1053–1058, 2013.

[128] J. Font, L. Pallares, R. Cervera et al., "Systemic lupus erythematosus in the elderly: clinical and immunological characteristics," *Annals of the Rheumatic Diseases*, vol. 50, no. 10, pp. 702–705, 1991.

[129] M. N. Manoussakis, C. Georgopoulou, E. Zintzaras et al., "Sjögren's syndrome associated with systemic lupus erythematosus: clinical and laboratory profiles and comparison with primary Sjögren's syndrome," *Arthritis & Rheumatism*, vol. 50, no. 3, pp. 882–891, 2004.

[130] M. Ramos-Casals, M. García-Carrasco, M. P. Brito, A. López-Soto, and J. Font, "Autoimmunity and geriatrics: clinical significance of autoimmune manifestations in the elderly," *Lupus*, vol. 12, no. 5, pp. 341–355, 2003.

[131] S. Georgin-Lavialle, A. Aouba, L. Mouthon et al., "The telomere/telomerase system in autoimmune and systemic immune-mediated diseases," *Autoimmunity Reviews*, vol. 9, no. 10, pp. 646–651, 2010.

[132] S. Haque, C. Rakieh, F. Marriage et al., "Shortened telomere length in patients with systemic lupus erythematosus," *Arthritis & Rheumatism*, vol. 65, no. 5, pp. 1319–1323, 2013.

[133] X. Li, L. Liu, D. Meng et al., "Enhanced apoptosis and senescence of bone-marrow-derived mesenchymal stem cells in patients with systemic lupus erythematosus," *Stem Cells and Development*, vol. 21, no. 13, pp. 2387–2394, 2012.

[134] Z. Gu, X. Cao, J. Jiang et al., "Upregulation of $p16^{INK4A}$ promotes cellular senescence of bone marrow-derived mesenchymal stem cells from systemic lupus erythematosus patients," *Cellular Signalling*, vol. 24, no. 12, pp. 2307–2314, 2012.

[135] U. S. Gaipl, R. E. Voll, A. Sheriff, S. Franz, J. R. Kalden, and M. Herrmann, "Impaired clearance of dying cells in systemic lupus erythematosus," *Autoimmunity Reviews*, vol. 4, no. 4, pp. 189–194, 2005.

[136] K. W. Wucherpfennig, "Mechanisms for the induction of autoimmunity by infectious agents," *The Journal of Clinical Investigation*, vol. 108, no. 8, pp. 1097–1104, 2001.

[137] B. D. Poole, R. H. Scofield, J. B. Harley, and J. A. James, "Epstein-Barr virus and molecular mimicry in systemic lupus erythematosus," *Autoimmunity*, vol. 39, no. 1, pp. 63–70, 2006.

[138] A. Perl, G. Nagy, A. Koncz et al., "Molecular mimicry and immunomodulation by the HRES-1 endogenous retrovirus in SLE," *Autoimmunity*, vol. 41, no. 4, pp. 287–297, 2008.

[139] P. Sfriso, A. Ghirardello, C. Botsios et al., "Infections and autoimmunity: the multifaceted relationship," *Journal of Leukocyte Biology*, vol. 87, no. 3, pp. 385–395, 2010.

[140] T. Peters, J. M. Weiss, A. Sindrilaru et al., "Reactive oxygen intermediate-induced pathomechanisms contribute to immunosenescence, chronic inflammation and autoimmunity," *Mechanisms of Ageing and Development*, vol. 130, no. 9, pp. 564–587, 2009.

[141] G. Pawelec and A. Larbi, "Immunity and ageing in man: annual review 2006/2007," *Experimental Gerontology*, vol. 43, no. 1, pp. 34–38, 2008.

[142] J. Plowden, M. Renshaw-Hoelscher, S. Gangappa, C. Engleman, J. M. Katz, and S. Sambhara, "Impaired antigen-induced $CD8^+$ T cell clonal expansion in aging is due to defects in antigen presenting cell function," *Cellular Immunology*, vol. 229, no. 2, pp. 86–92, 2004.

[143] R. Solana and E. Mariani, "NK and NK/T cells in human senescence," *Vaccine*, vol. 18, no. 16, pp. 1613–1620, 2000.

[144] X. Camous, A. Pera, R. Solana, and A. Larbi, "NK cells in healthy aging and age-associated diseases," *Journal of Biomedicine and Biotechnology*, vol. 2012, Article ID 195956, 8 pages, 2012.

[145] S. Ponnappan and U. Ponnappan, "Aging and immune function: molecular mechanisms to interventions," *Antioxidants & Redox Signaling*, vol. 14, no. 8, pp. 1551–1585, 2011.

[146] J. Nikolich-Žugich, G. Li, J. L. Uhrlaub, K. R. Renkema, and M. J. Smithey, "Age-related changes in CD8 T cell homeostasis and immunity to infection," *Seminars in Immunology*, vol. 24, no. 5, pp. 356–364, 2012.

[147] L. Haynes and S. L. Swain, "Aged-related shifts in T cell homeostasis lead to intrinsic T cell defects," *Seminars in Immunology*, vol. 24, no. 5, pp. 350–355, 2012.

[148] G. R. Kolar, D. Mehta, P. C. Wilson, and J. D. Capra, "Diversity of the Ig repertoire is maintained with age in spite of reduced germinal centre cells in human tonsil lymphoid tissue," *Scandinavian Journal of Immunology*, vol. 64, no. 3, pp. 314–324, 2006.

4

Serology of Lupus Erythematosus: Correlation between Immunopathological Features and Clinical Aspects

Emanuele Cozzani, Massimo Drosera, Giulia Gasparini, and Aurora Parodi

Di.S.Sal, Section of Dermatology, IRCCS Azienda Ospedaliera, Universitaria San Martino-IST, 16132 Genoa, Italy

Correspondence should be addressed to Emanuele Cozzani; emanuele.cozzani@unige.it

Academic Editor: Juan-Manuel Anaya

Systemic lupus erythematosus (SLE) is an autoimmune disease characterized by the aberrant production of a broad and heterogenous group of autoantibodies. Even though the presence of autoantibodies in SLE has been known, for more than 60 years, still nowadays a great effort is being made to understand the pathogenetic, diagnostic, and prognostic meaning of such autoantibodies. Antibodies to ds-DNA are useful for the diagnosis of SLE, to monitor the disease activity, and correlate with renal and central nervous involvements. Anti-Sm antibodies are highly specific for SLE. Anti-nucleosome antibodies are an excellent marker for SLE and good predictors of flares in quiescent lupus. Anti-histone antibodies characterize drug-induced lupus, while anti-SSA/Ro and anti-SSB/La antibodies are associated with neonatal lupus erythematosus and photosensitivity. Anti-ribosomal P antibodies play a role in neuropsychiatric lupus, but their association with clinical manifestations is still unclear. Anti-phospholipid antibodies are associated with the anti-phospholipid syndrome, cerebral vascular disease, and neuropsychiatric lupus. Anti-C1q antibodies amplify glomerular injury, and the elevation of their titers may predict renal flares. Anti-RNP antibodies are a marker of Sharp's syndrome but can be found in SLE as well. Anti-PCNA antibodies are present in 5–10% of SLE patients especially those with arthritis and hypocomplementemia.

1. Introduction

Systemic lupus erythematosus (SLE) is an autoimmune disease characterized by the presence of autoreactive B and T cells, responsible for the aberrant production of a broad and heterogeneous group of autoantibodies (Table 1). Indeed, in 2004 Sherer et al. reported that one hundred sixteen autoantibodies have been described in SLE patients [1]. In SLE, especially in its systemic form (SLE), autoantibodies directed to nuclear (ANAs), cytoplasmtic, and cellular membrane antigens are considered the serological hallmark. ANAs consist of various types of autoantibodies characterized by different antigen specificities. These nuclear antigens include single strand (ss) and double strand (ds) DNA (deoxyribonucleic acid), histone proteins, nucleosome (histone-DNA complex), centromere proteins, and extractable nuclear antigens (ENA) (Smith antigen (Sm), Ro, La, ribonucleoprotein (RNP), etc.). ANAs are present in about 95% of SLE patients with an active disease. In patients with prevalent cutaneous lesions, ANAs have been found positive in 75% of cases.

Therefore, considering the very wide spectrum of discovered autoantibodies, the aim of the present paper is to highlight the most promising and significant ones from both immunopathologic and clinical perspectives.

The presence of autoantibodies in SLE was envisaged when lupus phenomenon was described by Hargraves et al. in 1948 [2] and then proven when it was understood that it was due to neutrophil phagocytosis of cell nuclei opsonised by autoantibodies. In 1957, antibodies to DNA were identified [3] and in 1966 Tan and Kunkel found autoantibodies directed to antigens different from DNA and described the anti-Sm antibodies [4].

Even though the presence of autoantibodies in SLE has been known for more than 60 years, still nowadays a great effort is being made to understand the pathogenetic, diagnostic, and prognostic meaning of such autoantibodies. In particular, studies have focused on ANAs, anti-C1q antibodies, and anti-phospholipid antibodies.

Demonstrating the pathogenic role of autoantibodies is an arduous task; nevertheless recent data from murine, and

Table 1: Correlation between antibodies reactivity lupus subtypes and diagnostic utility.

Antibody	Target	Diagnostic utility	Associated lupus subtypes (prevalence)	Other associated diseases	References
ANAs	The cell nucleus	High sensitivity, but specificity is low	SLE (98%) LN (100%) MCTD Drug-induced lupus Discoid lupus (35%)	Hepatic diseases (autoimmune hepatitis A), malignancies, chronic infections, thyroid diseases, elderly people, SS, SSc, PM, DM, juvenile chronic arthritis, Felty's syndrome, relapsing polychondritis, and rheumatoid arthritis	[12, 21, 22]
Anti-dsDNA	Double strand DNA	High sensitivity and specificity for SLE. Correlate with disease activity	SLE (70–98%) LN (70%) NPSLE (44, 4–81, 6%)	RA, HIV and parvovirus B19 infections, myeloma, and type 1 autoimmune hepatitis	[12, 21, 23–26]
Anti-Sm	Sm[1]	Low sensitivity, but high specificity for SLE	SLE (20–40%) LN (14%) MCTD (8%)	EBV infections	[12, 21, 27, 28]
Anti-nucleosome	Nuclesome[2]	High sensitivity and specificity for SLE. Correlate with disease activity	SLE (61–85%) LN (60–90%) MTCD (41%)	RA, SSc, and SS	[14, 21, 29, 30]
Anti-histone	Histone	Low IgM Higher IgG	SLE (70%) LN (37%) Anti-H2A and Anti-H2b specific for SLE induced by drugs (96–100%)	Rheumatoid arthritis, SSc, PBC[3], Alzheimer's disease, dementia, and infections	[12, 21, 31, 32]
Anti-SSA/Ro	SSA/Ro (proteins 60/52 kD)[4]	High prognostic value for NLE in pregnant women	SLE (30%) LN (31%) NLE (especially CHB) (90%) SCLE (70–80%) Discoid Lupus (5–20%)	SSc, IIM[5], PBC, RA, and SS	[12, 21, 33–36]
Anti-SSB/La	SSB/La[6]	Moderate	SLE (10%) LN (14%) Protective for LN SCLE (30%) NLE (90%)	SS	[12, 21, 35, 36]
Anti-ribosomal P	Ribosomes[7]	Moderate	SLE (13–40%) LN (6%) NPSLE (especially psychosis and depression) (21%)	Hepatic diseases, malignancies, and RA	[12, 21, 37, 38]

Table 1: Continued.

Antibody	Target	Diagnostic utility	Associated lupus subtypes (prevalence)	Other associated diseases	References
Anti-phospholipid	Phospholipids[8] (of cardiolipin, LACs are the most important ones)	High if Anti-PL syndrome is suspected	SLE (30–40%) LN (20–80%) Anti-PL syndrome: venous thrombosis, arterial thrombosis, recurrent pregnancy loss, thrombocytopenia and haemolytic anaemia, livedo reticularis, and skin ulcers.	Other autoimmune diseases, infections, malignancies, and drug-induced disorders, rheumatoid arthritis	[12, 21, 39]
Anti-Clq	Clq[9]	Low but useful to monitor evolution of LE nephritis	SLE (17–46%) LN (40–100%) CLE (44%)	Hypocomplementemic urticarial vasculitis syndrome, rheumatoid arthritis, and renal disease	[21, 40, 41]
Anti-RNP	RNP[10]	Unclear	SLE (20–30%) MCTD (100%)	Sharp's syndrome scleroderma, polymyositis, rheumatoid arthritis, SSc, Sjögren's syndrome	[12, 42, 43]
Anti-PCNA	PCNA[11]	Low	SLE (5–10%)	Chronic hepatitis B and C	[44, 45]

[1] In biology, Sm proteins are a family of RNA-binding proteins found in virtually every cellular organism.
[2] A nucleosome is the basic unit of DNA packaging in eukaryotes, consisting of a segment of DNA wound in sequence around eight histone protein cores.
[3] Primary biliary cirrhosis.
[4] Ro60 is a ribonuclear protein containing small uridine-rich nucleic acids known. Protein 60 KD is located into the nucleus and nucleolus, while protein 52 is located into the cytoplasm.
[5] Idiopathic inflammatory myopathies.
[6] SSB/La particle is a 48–50 kDa nuclear phosphoprotein composed of 2 distinct regions of 28 and 23 kDa.
[7] P0, P1, and P2 of 38, 19, and 17 kDa, respectively, of the 60S subunit.
[8] Anionic phospholipis including cardiolipin (CL), LA, phophatidylserine (PS), phsphatidylinositol (PI), and phosphatidic acid (PA).
[9] Clq is a cationic glycoprotein of 410–450 kDa which binds to the Fc portions of immunoglobulins in immune complexes to initiate complement activation via the classical pathway.
[10] 3 ribonucleoproteins: of 70 kDa (U1), 33 kDa (protein A), and 22 kDa (protein C), respectively.
[11] Anti-proliferating cell nuclear antigen.

human models have clarified the key role of autoantibodies in severe organ involvements, such as nephritis and neuropsychiatric dysfunctions [5]. Common autoantibody-mediated mechanisms of damage in SLE include immune complex-mediate damage, cell surface binding and cytotoxicity, reactivity with autoantigens expressed on apoptotic or activated cell surface, penetration into living cells, and binding to cross-reactive extracellular molecules [6].

Beyond elucidating the mechanisms behind the disease, understanding the pathogenetic role of autoantibodies, might have therapeutic implications. Indeed, in a recent article Diamond et al., after discovering the antigenic specificity of a subset of anti-DNA antibodies, hypothesized a potential therapeutic strategy, using peptides to block the antigen-binding site of the pathogenetic antibody [7].

Pisetsky gives another extremely interesting perspective, based on different sources [8–10], on the role of ANAs in autoimmune diseases, hypothesizing a protective role of such antibodies [11]. ANAs would prevent the disease by inhibiting the immunological activity of nuclear antigens, promoting their clearance in a nonphlogistic way or blocking the formation of immune complexes. Indeed, in SLE anti-SSA/Ro and anti-SSB/La antibodies seem to exert a protective role from lupus nephritis [12]. This hypothesis requires further investigations but could translate into other interesting findings in SLE as well.

However, the biggest effort was made to understand the clinical implications of antibodies found in the sera of patients affected by SLE. Indeed, the diagnostic and prognostic values of such antibodies are well known and no less than two of the American College of Rheumatology (ACR) criteria for SLE [13] regard immunological abnormalities:

"10. Immunologic disorder:

1. Anti-DNA: antibody to native DNA in abnormal titer or
2. Anti-Sm: presence of antibody to Sm nuclear antigen or
3. Positive finding of antiphospholipid antibodies on:
    - An abnormal serum level of IgG or IgM anticardiolipin antibodies,
    - A positive test result for lupus anticoagulant using a standard method,
    - A false-positive test result for at least 6 months confirmed by treponema pallidum immobilization or fluorescent treponemal antibody absorption test

11. Positive antinuclear antibody: An abnormal titer of antinuclear antibody by immunofluorescence or an equivalent assay at any point in time and in the absence of drugs"

Many authors have recently questioned the validity of these criteria, for example, Bizzaro et al. demonstrated through a study of meta analysis that the anti-nucleosome antibodies (AnuA) test is superior for diagnostics than the test for anti-dsDNA antibodies [14]. Furthermore Doria et al. underline that the test for anti-ribosomal P protein antibodies has a sensitivity and specificity for the classification of SLE similar to that of anti-Sm antibodies and that it could possibly substitute anti-Sm antibodies in the ACR criteria [15, 16].

Furthermore, anti-ribosomal P protein antibodies correlate with the activity of the disease and are associated with neuropsychiatric manifestations of SLE, while anti-Sm antibodies are frequently static over the disease course and it is difficult to link them with clinical manifestations. Nevertheless, the Systemic Lupus International Collaborating Clinics (SLICC) group recently revised and validated the ACR SLE classification criteria, maintaining and further emphasizing the same immunological criteria [17]. Indeed, according to the SLICC rules, patients must satisfy at least 4 criteria, including at least one immunologic criterion, or the patient must have biopsy-proven lupus nephritis in the presence of antinuclear antibodies or anti-double stranded DNA antibodies.

ANAs can be useful to identify particular subsets of LE: Anti-dsDNA is associated with renal involvement, anti-Ro/SSA antibodies with photosensitive rash especially subacute lupus erythematosus (SCLE) as well as with serositis and haematological manifestations, anti-P ribosomal protein with neuropsychiatric disorders, and anti-RNP with arthritis, Raynaud's, and puffy fingers. In this regard, another interesting point of view is given by Shivastava and Khanna [18], who propose the cluster theory: according to which distinct autoantibody clustering correlates to particular clinical syndromes. Cluster 1 (anti-Sm and anti-RNP) is characterized by the lowest incidence of proteinuria, anaemia, lymphopenia, and thrombocythemia. Cluster 2 (anti-dsDNA, anti-Ro and anti-La) is associated with a higher rate of nephritic syndrome and leukopenia. Cluster 3 (anti-ds-DNA, LAC and aCL) is expectedly associated with thrombotic events [19]. Moreover, Ching et al. [20] studied the serological profiles of SLE patients, finding that most of them segregated into one of two distinct clusters defined by autoantibodies against Sm/anti-RNP or Ro/La autoantigens. The Sm/RNP cluster was associated with a higher prevalence of serositis in comparison to the Ro/La cluster.

2. Techniques

ANAs can be detected by various assays: indirect immunofluorescence (IIF) using cultured cells as substrates, enzyme-linked immunosorbent assay (ELISA), and farr radioimmunoassay (RIA).

IIF and ELISA are most popular in routine work. ELISA is more sensitive but less specific while IIF is sensitive, reproducible, and easy to perform. ELISA is preferable when the exact titration of ANAs is needed in the follow-up of SLE.

Lately, multiplexed ELISA assays have been used for ANAs titration and these new sophisticated techniques are able to detect simultaneously multiple autoantibodies from a single sample. Until now, various studies report overall agreement between the detection of lupus autoantibodies by conventional ELISA and by multiplexed ELISA assays [46–48].

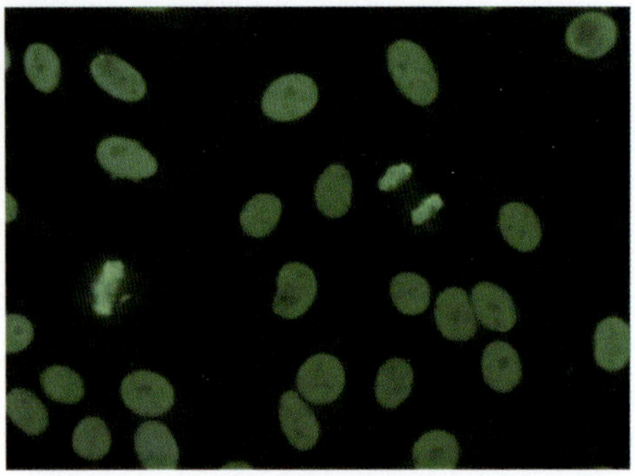

Figure 1: IIF on Hep2 cells: homogeneous pattern. Dilution 1 : 40.

Monolayer of cultured cells, particularly HEp2 (a human laryngeal carcinoma cell line), is now considered the gold standard for IIF. In cultured cells used for IIF, the antigens are in the native location and form, undenatured or minimally denatured, and the nuclei and nucleoli are clearly visible in dividing cells.

About 40 different fluoroscopic patterns have been described in IIF, related to different antibody specificities. The most common are homogeneous, peripheral or ring, speckled, nucleolar, pleomorphic speckled, nuclear dots, and nuclear membrane. Generally, the homogenous pattern is linked to SLE (Figure 1). ANA pattern has some correlation with clinical subsets, such as a shrunken peripheral pattern with renal disease, a fine particulate pattern in SCLE, and a homogeneous pattern with anti-histone antibodies [49]. However, the homogenous pattern can be found in many other autoimmune diseases and, in contrast, various ANA patterns may coexist in the same disease. For these reasons, more specific tests, such as the anti-dsDNA test or anti-ENA test are necessary for a precise diagnosis, according to the well-known "cascade testing" as suggested by guidelines [50]. Indeed, it must be kept in mind that ANAs may be found not only in autoimmune diseases, but also hepatic diseases, malignancies, chronic infections, thyroid diseases, and even in individuals with no medical condition, particularly elderly people [51, 52].

Ippolito et al. [53] report the results of current serologic tests for SLE are generally consistent with the historical ones. However, probably due to their better sensitivity, current serological tests yield a certain percentage of additional positives. Further, due to a lower sensitivity in the past tests for C3 and C4 detected more frequently the depletion of these factors.

3. Anti-DNA Antibodies

Anti-DNA antibodies constitute a subgroup of antinuclear antibodies that bind to either single-stranded or double-stranded DNA [54]. Both subtypes of DNA-binding antibodies may be found in SLE. Nonetheless, while some authors highlighted a possible role of anti-ssDNA antibodies in the diagnosis and follow-up of SLE, especially when anti-dsDNA antibodies were negative [55, 56], others doubted the specificity and utility of this test [57–60]. Instead, because of their high specificity, anti-dsDNA antibodies are universally used as a diagnostic criterion for SLE (70–98% of patients are positive for such antibodies) [12] and for monitoring the clinical course of the patient [61] (every 6 weeks, for example), especially in the presence of an immunosuppressive treatment that reduces their production. IIF on *Crithidia luciliae* (Figure 1), RIA, and ELISA is the most commonly used assays to detect anti-dsDNA antibodies. IIF-based *Crithidia* assay is probably the most specific technique, but ELISA is the most practical and clinically relevant method. In IIF anti-dsDNA antibodies correlate with a shrunken peripheral ANA pattern [49]. It is generally accepted that anti-dsDNA antibodies, in particular of the IgG isotype, have an important pathogenetic role in SLE. A clear-cut relationship exists, for example, between anti-dsDNA antibodies (R4A antibody) [7] and disease activity in nephritis [62]. Anti-DNA-DNA immune complexes can deposit in the mesangial matrix and their subsequent complement activation leads to inflammation and mesangial nephritis. Moreover, anti-dsDNA antibodies also contribute to the end-stage lupus nephritis by directly binding exposed chromatine fragments in glomerular basement membrane [5]. On the other hand, IgM-class anti-dsDNA antibodies seem to have a protective role for nephropathy [63, 64]. Furthermore De Giorgio et al. demonstrated that a subset of anti-DNA antibodies cross-reacts with N-methyl-D-aspartate receptors (NMDAR), and through an excitotoxic mechanism, could induce neuronal apoptosis. Anti-NMDAR antibodies are present in 40% of lupus patients and some reports have supported the correlation between such antibodies and the presence of neuropsychiatric lupus [23, 65, 66], while others have not [67]. More recently, Franchin et al. have demonstrated that anti-NMDAR antibodies also bind C1q; therefore, they hypothesized that this subset of anti-DNA antibodies contributes in lupus pathogenesis through direct targeting of C1q on glomeruli and also through removal of soluble C1q thereby limiting the ability of C1q to suppressor of immune activation [68].

4. Anti-Sm Antibodies

Sm antigen consists of at least 4 proteins: B (28 kDa), B1 (29 kDa), D (19 kDa), and E (13 kDa). Anti-Sm antibodies are a highly specific marker for SLE and Anti-Sm reactivity is not described in other diseases. Their sensitivity is however low. In fact, anti-Sm antibodies are detectable only in 20% of SLE white patients, but 30–40% in black and Asian people. Clinical correlations of these autoantibodies remain unclear [12] and generally show persistent expression over time [11]. In some studies anti-Sm titers were found to fluctuate with disease activity and treatment [69], but it is unclear whether serial monitoring predicts relapse [70].

5. Anti-Nucleosome Antibodies

The antigen consists of pairs of 4 core histones: H2A, H2B, H3, and H4, forming the histone octamer around which 200 pairs of basis of DNA are wound twice, with H1 bound

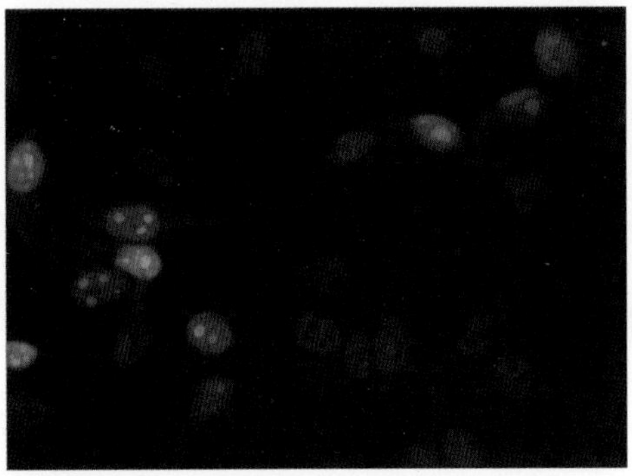

Figure 2: IIF on HEp2 cells: speckeld and nuclear and nucleolar staining (anti-SSA/Ro antibodies). Dilution 1 : 40.

on the outside. Anti-nucleosomes antibodies (ANuA) react exclusively to nucleosomes and not to individual histones or native non-protein-complexed DNA [71].

Although anti-nucleosome antibodies can be seen in IIF as homogeneous pattern (Figure 2), only ELISA detects them.

They represent the first serological marker of SLE described and, at present, nucleosomes are considered a major autoantigen in SLE in which they are positive in about 85% of patients and probably play an important pathogenetic role [29]. There is major evidence that nucleosome antibodies play an important role in the pathogenesis of SLE, being the first ones to appear in murine lupus models before the onset of any other autoantibodies, which are only later produced by B cells, stimulated by nucleosome-specific T cells through epitope spreading [72]. In glomerulonephritis, nucleosomes facilitate binding of autoantibodies to glomerular basement membranes with an increased permeability and inflammatory response [5, 73].

According to Bizzaro's meta-analysis ANuA test appears to have an adequate level of diagnostic accuracy for SLE, with equal specificity, but higher sensitivity, positive likelihood ratio, and diagnostic odds ratio than anti-dsDNA antibodies test [14]. Indeed, they could be one of the most sensitive markers in the diagnosis of SLE, especially in anti-ds-DNA-negative patients [74]. Furthermore, there is a strong correlation between the level of anti-nucleosome antibodies and lupus disease severity [23, 75, 76]. ANuAs are probably better to predict flares in quiescent lupus [77].

6. Anti-Histone Antibodies

The target antigens are 5 major classes of histones (H1, H2A, H2B, H3, and H4), which organize and constrain the topology of DNA.

ELISA is the only reliable method for detection of anti-histone antibodies. It is important to use IgG-specific antibodies and not IgM that are not specifically related to the disease. Using IIF on standard substrates anti-histone antibodies produces a homogeneous, chromosome-positive staining of the nucleus.

These autoantibodies are characteristic of particular subset of SLE. In fact, anti-H2A-H2b antibodies are a sensitive test in drug-induced SLE. About 96% of patients with SLE induced by procainamide [31] and 100% of patients with SLE induced by penicillamine, isoniazid [32], and methyldopa have anti-histone antibodies. Nonetheless, they are also present in idiopathic SLE (70% of patients with SLE [12]), in rheumatoid arthritis, Felty's syndrome, Sjögren's syndrome (SS), systemic sclerosis (SSc) [78], primary biliary cirrhosis, infectious diseases (including HIV infection), and even neurological disorders such as Alzheimer's disease and dementia. In our experience, anti-histone antibodies are found in 10% of SLE patients and in 40% of SSc patients [79]. However, because of their low specificity these anti-histone antibodies albeit more prevalent, are not pathognomonic of drug-induce SLE [80]. This apparent paradox might be explained by the fact that the metabolites of offending drugs probably have the capacity to disrupt nonspecifically central immune tolerance to chromatin [81]. From a pathogenetic point of view, the histone-anti-histone antibody system might play a role in the perpetuation of murine lupus nephritis [82] and recently Sui et al. demonstrate in their study a strong association between simultaneous positivity to anti-DNA, anti-nucleosome, and anti-histone antibodies and renal disease activities, especially in proliferative glomerulonephritis [83].

7. Anti-SSA/Ro Antibodies

SSA/Ro antigen is a ribonucleoprotein containing small uridine-rich nucleic acids known as hY1, hY3, hY4, and hY5 (hY is the abbreviation of human cytoplasmic). SSA/Ro antigen consists of at least of 4 proteins: 45, 52, 54, and 60 kDa, respectively, with the best known of them being the 52 and 60 kDa proteins [84].

The most sensitive and specific method for detection of anti-SSA/Ro antibodies is ELISA. Using tumoral cell lines transfected with SSA/Ro antigen (HEp 2000) as a substrate, IIF is useful too, showing a typical speckled nuclear and nucleolar staining (Figure 2).

Anti-SSA/Ro antibodies might have a pathogenetic role in the initiation of tissue damage especially in photosensitive SLE, for ultraviolet radiation has been shown to induce *de novo* synthesis and the expression on the cell surface of SSA/Ro polypeptides in keratinocytes [85, 86].

Since the 1980s, it was known that anti-SSA/Ro and anti-SSB/La antibodies can cross the maternal placenta and determine neonatal lupus erythematosus (NLE). Indeed, anti-SSA/Ro as well as also anti-SSB/La antibodies bind to fetal heart conduction tissue and inhibit cardiac repolarization [87], determining isolated complete atrioventricular block (CHB). Other frequently observed manifestations of NLE are cutaneous rash, haematological disorders (thrombocytopenia, anemia, and leukopenia), and liver dysfunction [88], all of which tend to resolve within the time of clearance of maternal antibodies from the infant's circulation.

In a recent paper, it was reported that newborns from mothers with high to moderate titers of anti-SSA/Ro antibodies are more likely to develop cardiac manifestations of NLE, independently from the anti-SSB/La titers, while infants with prenatal exposure to high titers of anti-SSB/La antibodies were most likely to present non-cardiac manifestations [89].

Anti-SSA/Ro antibodies can be detected in 70–100% of patients with SS, in 30–70% of patients in particular in SCLE and NLE (70–80%) and with a lower frequency also in discoid LE (5–20%). Antibodies to the 52 kDa subunit are more specific for SS while antibodies to the 60 kDa subunit are more frequent in SLE patients. Anti-Ro and Anti-La antibodies are found earlier than other SLE-related autoantibodies and are present on average 6.6 years before the the diagnosis of SLE [33]. A close association between anti-SSA/Ro antibodies and late onset of SLE (average age of 50) was suggested [34]. Anti-SSA/Ro antibodies correlate with photosensitivity, SCLE, cutaneous vasculitis (palpable purpura), and haematological disorders (anemia, leukopenia, and thrombocytopenia) [35, 90–92].

There are discordant data regarding the association between anti-SSA/Ro titers and the disease activity, but it seems that anti-SSA/Ro antibody levels tend to decline when patients are treated with cytotoxic drugs [93–97].

Recently, greater attention is being paid toward distinguishing the two subtypes of anti-SSA/Ro: anti-SSA/Ro60 and anti-Ro52/TRIM21. A recent retrospective study conducted by Menendez et al. supports their routine distinction in clinical practice, since the two subtypes show different associations with different clinical subtypes of SLE. Indeed, anti-SSA/Ro60 are more frequently reported in association with SLE and CLE. Nevertheless, the pattern with both anti-SSA/Ro60 and anti-Ro52/TRIM21 is more frequent in SCLE and anti-Ro52/TRIM21 is more strongly associated with CHB [98]. In particular, the antibodies that seem to be strictly linked to CHB are directed against peptide aa 200–239 of subunit 52 kDa of Ro/SSA antigen [99].

8. Anti-SSB/La Antibodies

The SSB/La particle is a 48–50 kDa nuclear phosphoprotein composed of 2 distinct regions of 28 and 23 kDa [100]. The larger domain contains a RNA binding site that binds RNA polymerase III transcripts. Although anti-SSB/La antibodies were originally detected by immunodiffusion and counter-immunoelectrophoresis, they are now commonly detected by ELISA and immunoblotting.

Even though there is no direct evidence of a pathogenetic role of anti-SSB/La antibodies in SS and SLE, their presence in maternal blood is strongly associated with NLE and congenital heart block. In fact, both SSB/La and SSA/Ro antibodies bind to the surface of the fibres of the heart suggesting that the maternal anti-SSB/La and anti-SSA/Ro antibodies bind to the surface of cardiac muscle cells and damage them. Anti-SSB/La antibodies are the serological marker of SS [101]: if detected by ELISA, anti-SSB/La antibodies are present in 90% of patients with primary SS and 50% with secondary SS. In SLE, anti-SSB/La antibodies are instead present only in about 10% of patients with lower prevalence of renal disease. About 30% of patients with SCLE have anti-SSB/La antibodies.

9. Anti-Ribosomal P Antibodies

Ribosomes are complex macromolecular structures incorporating both protein and ribonucleic acid (RNA) elements. Mammalian ribosomes are formed by the 60S and 40S subunit. The 40S subunit is a ribonucleoprotein complex containing a single 18S species of RNA and 33 different basic proteins. The 60S subunit incorporates 3 distinct species of RNA, 46 different basic proteins, and 3 phosphoproteins named P0, P1, and P2 of 38, 19 and 17 kDa, respectively, that are the most important antigen targets of anti-ribosomal antibodies [102].

The specificity of autoantibodies directed against ribosomal components is evaluated by immunoblotting, but their presence is already suggested in IIF by a cytoplasmatic pattern. In the routine work, however, they are usually detected by ELISA. In comparative studies immunoblotting and ELISA seem to give the same diagnostic accuracy [103]. More recently, the international multicentre evaluation of the clinical accuracy of a new ELISA based on recombinant P polypeptides demonstrated that a combination of all three P proteins resembling the native heterocomplex P0 $(P1/P2)_2$ as antigen gives the best accuracy [104].

Anti-ribosomal P antibodies seem to have an intriguing pathogenetic potential that needs further investigations. Indeed, anti-ribosomal P antibodies may exert different cellular effects by binding to the surface of T cells, monocytes, and endothelial cells [21].

They are able to penetrate into living cells by binding a cell-surface 38 kDa protein, which is the corresponding surface version of P0 ribosomal protein. In this way, they can cause cellular dysfunction and tissue damage by inhibiting protein synthesis, inducing apoptosis or proinflammatory cytokine production [105]. More recently, two independent groups elucidated the neuropathogenic potential of anti-ribosamal P antibodies [106, 107]. Moreover, Caponi et al. demonstrated that anti-ribosomal P antibodies in some cases can cross react with cardiolipin, ssDNA, dsDNA, and also nucleosomes. Such data indicate a partial overlapping of anti-ribosmal P antibodies with the other autoantibody populations detected frequently in SLE. For this reason anti-ribosomal P might have a similar pathogenetic role, for instance, in NPSLE [108].

The autoimmune response to ribosomal components is quite specific for SLE. Anti-ribosomal P antibodies occur in 13–20% of Caucasian SLE patients and in more than 40% of Asian patients [37].

Since the first prospective study in 1987 by Bonfa et al. [52] reporting a strong association between anti-ribosomal P antibodies and lupus psychosis, many other studies tried to confirm the utility of such antibodies in predicting NPSLE. However, the results were contrasting [38, 109]. Anyhow, many studies report associations with psychosis and especially depression.

10. Anti-Phospholipid Antibodies

The study of anti-phospholipid antibodies (aPL) antibodies began in 1906 when Wasserman introduced his serological test for syphilis [110]. In 1941, the active component was found to be a phospholipid, which was called cardiolipin [111]. After the 1950s, it became clear that people with positive Wasserman-test did not necessarily have syphilis but that they may have instead an autoimmune disorder, including

SLE [112]. The term *lupus anticoagulant* (LAC) first used in 1972 should be abandoned because LA can be found in patients without SLE and it is associated with thrombosis and not with bleeding [113].

Anti-PL antibodies recognize a number of anionic negatively charged phospholipids, including cardiolipin (CL), LAC, phosphatidylserine (PS), phosphatidylinositol (PI), phosphatidylglycerol, and phosphatidic acid (PA). Neutrally charged autoantigen targets include phosphatidyl ethanolamine, phosphatidyl choline, platelet activating factor and sphingomyelin. These antibodies are usually detected with radioimmunoassay and ELISA. CL remains the most commonly used antigen for detecting anti-PL antibodies with ELISA. It is now clear, however, that the optimal binding of anti-PL antibodies depends on cofactors; the best known of them is termed Beta2-Glycoprotein I (Beta2GP1), that is, a 50 kDa B2 globulin involved in the regulation of blood coagulation [114]. ELISA testing for Beta2GP1 is also available [12].

As mentioned before, anti-PL antibodies are not confined to SLE patients but can be found in other autoimmune diseases, infections, malignant, and drug-induced disorders as well as in some apparently healthy individuals. In addition, anti-PL antibodies are positive in 30–40% of SLE patients, but only 1/3 of them develop clinical features of anti-PL syndrome, namely, venous thrombosis, arterial thrombosis, recurrent pregnancy loss, thrombocytopenia and haemolytic anaemia, *livedo reticularis,* and skin ulcers [39]. Furthermore, aPL antibodies are involved in cerebral vascular disease and are also implied in the pathogenesis of focal damage in NPSLE. In particular, anti-beta2GPI antibodies are the most thrombogenic and may exert a pathogenetic potential either as a strong procoagulant factor in the cerebral circulation or by directly interacting with neuronal tissue [5].

11. Anti-C1q Antibodies

C1q is a cationic glycoprotein of 410–450 kDa, which binds to the Fc portions of immunoglobulins in immune complexes to initiate complement activation via the classical pathway [115]. C1q is produced by macrophages, monocytes, dendritic cells, fibroblasts, and epithelial cells and acts like a binding molecule between debris from cellular apoptosis (apoptotic blebs) and macrophages. Therefore, anti-C1q antibody development seems to be related to a deficiency in apoptotic cell clearance, as suggested by the fact that such antibodies from SLE patients specifically bind to C1q on apoptotic cells [116].

Anti-C1q antibodies are commonly detected by ELISA. From a pathogenic point of view anti-C1q antibodies probably amplify glomerular injury but only when C1q has already been brought to the site by other types of glomerular-reactive autoantibodies [117]. Furthermore, Hegazy et al. recently reported in their study a strong correlation between anti-C1q antibodies and cutaneous lupus and hypothesised a potential pathogenetic role in such context [40].

They are found in SLE with a prevalence ranging from 17% to 46%, especially in patients with nephritis [41]. Moroni suggests that the elevation of their titers may predict renal flares even better than anti-dsDNA antibody levels [118]. Elevated titres of anti-C1q antibodies are usually associated with the proliferative forms of lupus nephritis and with subendothelial deposits of immune complexes. They are therefore a useful marker for assessing both disease activity and progression of the renal disease [118]. Anti-C1q antibodies can be found also in other autoimmune diseases such as hypocomplementemic urticarial vasculitis syndrome, rheumatoid arthritis, Felty's syndrome, rheumatoid vasculitis, Sjögren's syndrome, membranoproliferative glomerulonephritis (MPGN), and IgA nephropathy [119, 120].

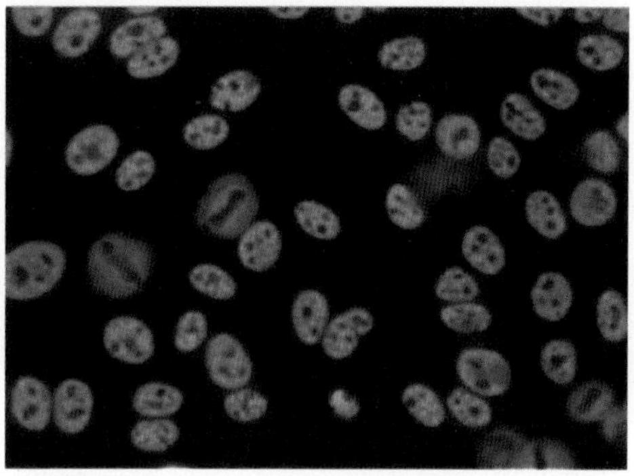

Figure 3: IIF on Hep2 cells: speckled pattern (anti-RNP antibodies). Dilution 1 : 40.

12. Anti-RNP Antibodies

Anti-RNP antibodies are directed to at least 3 proteins of 70 kDa (U1), 33 kDa (protein A), and 22 kDa (protein C), respectively. In IIF anti-RNP antibodies produce a fine speckled staining (Figure 3). Anti-U1small nuclear (sn) RNP antibodies are considered pathognomonic for Sharp's syndrome (mixed connective tissue disease or MCTD), but they can be found in 20–30% of patients with SLE as well [42]. Their presence is associated with HLA DR4 and their prevalence is higher in African American patients [12]. Other diseases in which anti-U1snRNP activity is described include rheumatoid arthritis, polymyositis, SSc, and Sjögren's syndrome (SS). Data from recent experimental studies promote the hypothesis that U1snRNP antibodies participate in both innate and adaptive immune responses, implicating them in the pathogenesis of connective tissue disease [121]. According to some authors anti-RNP antibodies are more prevalent in patients with Raynaud's phenomenon and are associated with milder renal involvement [122]. Although, ultimately anti-U1 RNP antibodies do not reflect the disease activity and their utility in monitoring the latter remains unclear.

13. Anti-Proliferating Cell Nuclear Antigen (PCNA) Antibodies

Anti-PCNA antibodies can be detected by using IIF on cultured cells in which they show a characteristic nuclear speckled pattern of varying intensity (Figure 4). ELISA kits are also available. PCNA is an auxiliary protein for DNA polymerase delta. PCNA expression increases proportionally to DNA synthesis and/or cell growth, beginning in late G1, increasing in S, and decreasing in G2 cellular phases.

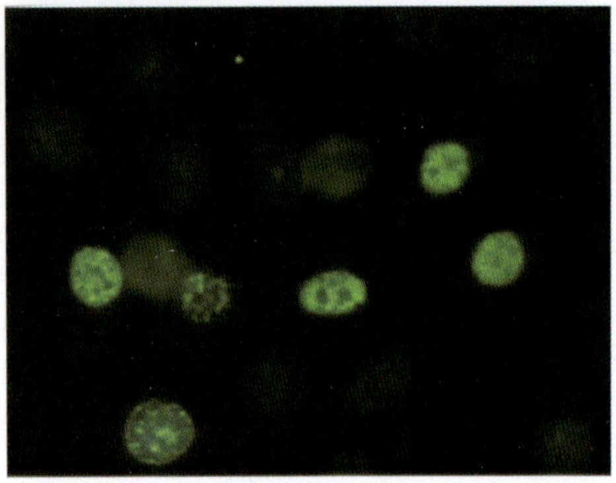

Figure 4: IIF on Hep2 cells: speckled pattern of varying intensity (anti-PCNA antibodies). Diluition 1 : 40.

Anti-PCNA antibodies are present in 5–10% of SLE patients especially those with arthritis and hypocomplementemia [44]. After treatment with steroids or cytotoxic drugs, anti-PCNA antibodies become undetectable.

14. Serology of SLE in Overlap Syndromes

SLE can be associated with other autoimmune diseases such as Sjögren's syndrome (SS), systemic sclerosis (SSc), rheumatoid arthritis (RA), dermatomyositis (DM)/polymyositis (PM), and determining overlap syndromes (OSs). OSs share clinical and immunological features of two or more distinct autoimmune diseases and might also have their own peculiar features. From a serological point of view OSs can be associated with a specific antibody profile (MCTD and SLE/SS) or not associated with a specific antibody profile (rhupus syndrome, SLE/SSc). MCTD has mixed features of SLE, SSc, DM/PM, and RA, in which anti-U1snRNP antibodies are the specific antibodies of the disease (see above). Anti-Ro/SS-A, anti-ssDNA, anti-Sm, anti-dsDNA [123], and anti-PL antibodies [124] have also been detected; nevertheless, they are not specific of MCTD. Recently, autoantibodies to angiotensin-converting enzyme 2 (ACE2) [125] were also reported in MCTD. SLE/SS patients have a higher frequency of SS-related immunological markers, such as rheumatoid factor (RF), polyclonal hypergammaglobulinemia, anti-Ro/SSA, and anti-La/SSB, while SLE-related antibodies are less frequent [126]. Anti-La/SSB antibodies are considered the serological markers of this OS. Most authors define rhupus syndrome as a condition characterized by signs and symptoms of both SLE and RA [127, 128]. In patients affected by such OS no specific antibody is identifiable and specific autoantibodies for SLE (anti-dsDNA and anti-Sm) and RA (anti-citrullinated peptides ACPA) coexist [126]. SLE/SSc overlap is a rare condition, in which a specific serological marker has not been identified yet, but a high incidence of anti-dsDNA and anti-Scl70 antibodies has been reported [126].

15. Conclusions

The comprehension of pathogenetic mechanisms is the starting point for the development of new and better laboratory tests, with various clinical implications. For example, the discovery of the cross-reactivity of certain types of anti-dsDNA antibodies with the NMDA receptor helped to comprehend the pathogenesis of NPSLE, but the detection of such antibodies in patients' sera could also be a potential predictive marker of the risk of developing NP disorders in SLE. Furthermore, distinguishing between the two different subtypes of anti-SSA/Ro antibodies might have interesting clinical implications. A better knowledge of the specificities of the antibodies might be a useful tool to subclassify patients with lupus and to predict which clinical manifestations they might develop. Detecting simultaneously a battery of various antibodies with multiplexed ELISA could be helpful for this purpose.

For the diagnosis of lupus certainly ds-DNA antibodies are an excellent biomarker, but we believe that perhaps ANuAs might be a better one, in accordance with Bizzaro's meta analysis, and considering that from a pathogenetic point of view these autoantibodies are the first ones to appear.

The role played by autoantibodies in the pathogenesis of lupus is yet to be revealed in many respects and the strive to find new and more valid biomarkers for a better management of the disease is constant, being lupus such a complex disease. Therefore, we believe there is still room for improvement as far as lupus serology is concerned.

Conflict of Interests

The authors declare that there is no conflict of interests regarding the publication of this paper.

References

[1] Y. Sherer, A. Gorstein, M. J. Fritzler, and Y. Shoenfeld, "Autoantibody explosion in systemic lupus erythematosus: more than 100 different antibodies found in SLE patients," *Seminars in Arthritis and Rheumatism*, vol. 34, no. 2, pp. 501–537, 2004.

[2] M. Hargraves, H. Richmond, and R. Morton, "Presentation of two bone marrow components, the tart cell and the LE cell," *Mayo Clinic Proceedings*, vol. 21, pp. 25–28, 1948.

[3] R. Ceppellini, E. Polli, and F. Celada, "A DNA-reacting factor in serum of a patient with lupus erythematosus diffusus," *Proceedings of the Society for Experimental Biology and Medicine*, vol. 96, no. 3, pp. 572–574, 1957.

[4] E. M. Tan and H. G. Kunkel, "Characteristics of a soluble nuclear antigen precipitating with sera of patients with systemic lupus erythematosus," *Journal of Immunology*, vol. 96, no. 3, pp. 464–471, 1966.

[5] O. P. Rekvig, C. Putterman, C. Casu et al., "Autoantibodies in lupus: culprits or passive bystanders?" *Autoimmunity Reviews*, vol. 11, no. 8, pp. 596–603, 2012.

[6] R. Gualtierotti, M. Biggioggero, A. E. Penatti, and P. L. Meroni, "Updating on the pathogenesis of systemic lupus erythematosus," *Autoimmunity Reviews*, vol. 10, no. 1, pp. 3–7, 2010.

[7] B. Diamond, O. Bloom, Y. Al Abed, C. Kowal, P. T. Huerta, and B. T. Volpe, "Moving towards a cure: blocking pathogenic antibodies in systemic lupus erythematosus," *Journal of Internal Medicine*, vol. 269, no. 1, pp. 36–44, 2011.

[8] B. Wittemann, G. Neuer, H. Michels, H. Truckenbrodt, and F. A. Bautz, "Autoantibodies to nonhistone chromosomal proteins

HMG-1 and HMG-2 in sera of patients with juvenile rheumatoid arthritis," *Arthritis & Rheumatism*, vol. 33, no. 9, pp. 1378–1383, 1990.

[9] D. A. Abdulahad, J. Westra, J. Bijzet, P. C. Limburg, C. G. M. Kallenberg, and M. Bijl, "High mobility group box 1 (HMGB1) and anti-HMGB1 antibodies and their relation to disease characteristics in systemic lupus erythematosus," *Arthritis Research & Therapy*, vol. 13, no. 3, article R71, 2011.

[10] H. Schierbeck, P. Lundbäck, K. Palmblad et al., "Monoclonal anti-HMGB1 (high mobility group box chromosomal protein 1) antibody protection in two experimental arthritis models," *Molecular Medicine*, vol. 17, no. 9-10, pp. 1039–1044, 2011.

[11] D. S. Pisetsky, "Antinuclear antibodies in rheumatic disease: a proposal for a function-based classification," *Scandinavian Journal of Immunology*, vol. 76, no. 3, pp. 223–228, 2012.

[12] A. Fauci, D. Kasper, D. Longo, E. Braunwald, S. Hauser, and J. L. Jameson, *Harrison's Principles of Internal Medicine*, McGraw-Hill, 17th edition, 2008.

[13] M. C. Hochberg, "Updating the American College of Rheumatology revised criteria for the classification of systemic lupus erythematosus," *Arthritis & Rheumatism*, vol. 40, no. 9, p. 1725, 1997.

[14] N. Bizzaro, D. Villalta, D. Giavarina, and R. Tozzoli, "Are anti-nucleosome antibodies a better diagnostic marker than anti-dsDNA antibodies for systemic lupus erythematosus? A systematic review and a study of metanalysis," *Autoimmunity Reviews*, vol. 12, no. 2, pp. 97–106, 2012.

[15] A. Ghirardello, L. Caponi, F. Franceschini et al., "Diagnostic tests for antiribosomal P protein antibodies: a comparative evaluation of immunoblotting and ELISA assays," *The Journal of Autoimmunity*, vol. 19, no. 1-2, pp. 71–77, 2002.

[16] A. Doria, M. Zen, M. Canova et al., "SLE diagnosis and treatment: when early is early," *Autoimmunity Reviews*, vol. 10, no. 1, pp. 55–60, 2010.

[17] J. G. Hanly, M. B. Urowitz, F. Siannis et al., "Derivation and validation of the Systemic Lupus International Collaborating Clinics classification criteria for systemic lupus erythematosus," *Arthritis & Rheumatism*, vol. 64, no. 8, pp. 2677–2686, 2012.

[18] A. Shivastava and D. Khanna, "Autoantibodies in systemic lupus erythematosus: revisited," *Indian Journal of Rheumatology*, vol. 6, no. 3, pp. 138–142, 2011.

[19] C. H. To and M. Petri, "Is antibody clustering predictive of clinical subsets and damage in systemic lupus erythematosus?" *Arthritis & Rheumatism*, vol. 52, no. 12, pp. 4003–4010, 2005.

[20] K. H. Ching, P. D. Burbelo, C. Tipton et al., "Two major autoantibody clusters in systemic lupus erythematosus," *PLoS ONE*, vol. 7, no. 2, Article ID e32001, 2012.

[21] S. D. Marks and K. Tullus, "Autoantibodies in systemic lupus erythematosus," *Pediatric Nephrology*, vol. 27, no. 10, pp. 1855–1868, 2012.

[22] A. S. Wiik, M. Høier-Madsen, J. Forslid, P. Charles, and J. Meyrowitsch, "Antinuclear antibodies: a contemporary nomenclature using HEp-2 cells," *The Journal of Autoimmunity*, vol. 35, no. 3, pp. 276–290, 2010.

[23] Y. Arinuma, T. Yanagida, and S. Hirohata, "Association of cerebrospinal fluid anti-NR2 glutamate receptor antibodies with diffuse neuropsychiatric systemic lupus erythematosus," *Arthritis & Rheumatism*, vol. 58, no. 4, pp. 1130–1135, 2008.

[24] K. E. Hansen, J. Arnason, and A. J. Bridges, "Autoantibodies and common viral illnesses," *Seminars in Arthritis and Rheumatism*, vol. 27, no. 5, pp. 263–271, 1998.

[25] D. A. Isenberg, J. J. Manson, M. R. Ehrenstein, and A. Rahman, "Fifty years of anti-ds DNA antibodies: are we approaching journey's end?" *Rheumatology*, vol. 46, no. 7, pp. 1052–1056, 2007.

[26] R. Maya, M. E. Gershwin, and Y. Shoenfeld, "Hepatitis B virus (HBV) and autoimmune disease," *Clinical Reviews in Allergy and Immunology*, vol. 34, no. 1, pp. 85–102, 2008.

[27] G. W. Zieve and P. R. Khusial, "The anti-Sm immune response in autoimmunity and cell biology," *Autoimmunity Reviews*, vol. 2, no. 5, pp. 235–240, 2003.

[28] K. D. Pagana and T. J. Pagana, *Mosby's Diagnostic and Laboratory Test Reference*, 9th edition, 2013.

[29] A. Bruns, S. Bläss, G. Hausdorf, G. R. Burmester, and F. Hiepe, "Nucleosomes are major T and B cell autoantigens in systemic lupus erythematosus," *Arthritis & Rheumatism*, vol. 43, no. 10, pp. 2307–2315, 2000.

[30] P. Quattrocchi, A. Barrile, D. Bonanno et al., "The role of anti-nucleosome antibodies in systemic lupus erythematosus. Results of a study of patients with systemic lupus erythematosus and other connective tissue diseases," *Reumatismo*, vol. 57, no. 2, pp. 109–113, 2005.

[31] R. L. Rubin, R. W. Burlingame, J. E. Arnott, M. C. Totoritis, E. M. McNally, and A. D. Johnson, "IgG but not other classes of anti-[(H2A-H2B)-DNA] is an early sign of procainamide-induced lupus," *Journal of Immunology*, vol. 154, no. 5, pp. 2483–2493, 1995.

[32] M. Salazar-Paramo, R. L. Rubin, and I. Garcia-De La Torre, "Systemic lupus erythematosus induced by isoniazid," *Annals of the Rheumatic Diseases*, vol. 51, no. 9, pp. 1085–1087, 1992.

[33] C. Eriksson, H. Kokkonen, M. Johansson, G. Hallmans, G. Wadell, and S. Rantapää-Dahlqvist, "Autoantibodies predate the onset of systemic lupus erythematosus in northern Sweden," *Arthritis Research & Therapy*, vol. 13, no. 1, article R30, 2011.

[34] E. K. L. Chan, J. C. Hamel, J. P. Buyon, and E. M. Tan, "Molecular definition and sequence motifs of the 52-kD component of human SS-A/Ro autoantigen," *The Journal of Clinical Investigation*, vol. 87, no. 1, pp. 68–76, 1991.

[35] R. Yoshimi, A. Ueda, K. Ozato, and Y. Ishigatsubo, "Clinical and pathological roles of Ro/SSA autoantibody system," *Clinical and Developmental Immunology*, vol. 2012, Article ID 606195, 12 pages, 2012.

[36] T. L. Rivera, P. M. Izmirly, B. K. Birnbaum et al., "Disease progression in mothers of children enrolled in the Research Registry for Neonatal Lupus," *Annals of the Rheumatic Diseases*, vol. 68, no. 6, pp. 828–835, 2009.

[37] A. Ghirardello, A. Doria, S. Zampieri, P. F. Gambari, and S. Todesco, "Autoantibodies to ribosomal P proteins in systemic lupus erythematosus," *Israel Medical Association Journal*, vol. 3, no. 11, pp. 854–857, 2001.

[38] J. G. Hanly, M. B. Urowitz, F. Siannis et al., "Autoantibodies and neuropsychiatric events at the time of systemic lupus erythematosus diagnosis: results from an international inception cohort study," *Arthritis & Rheumatism*, vol. 58, no. 3, pp. 843–853, 2008.

[39] P. Chu, K. Pendry, and T. E. Blecher, "Detection of lupus anticoagulant in patients attending an anticoagulation clinic," *British Medical Journal*, vol. 297, no. 6661, p. 1449, 1988.

[40] A. Hegazy, A. F. Barakat, M. A. E. Gayyar, and L. F. Arafa, "Prevalence and clinical significance of anti-C1q antibodies in cutaneous and systemic lupus erythematosus," *The Egyptian Journal of Medical Human Genetics*, vol. 13, pp. 167–171, 2012.

[41] M. H. Wener, M. Mannik, M. M. Schwartz, and E. J. Lewis, "Relationship between renal pathology and the size of circulating immune complexes in patients with systemic lupus erythematosus," *Medicine*, vol. 66, no. 2, pp. 85–97, 1987.

[42] G. C. Williamson, J. Pennebaker, and J. A. Boyle, "Clinical characteristics of patients with rheumatic disorders who possess antibodies against ribonucleoprotein particles," *Arthritis & Rheumatology*, vol. 26, no. 4, pp. 509–515, 1983.

[43] G. C. Williamson, A. Mary, L. M. Snyder, and J. B. Wallach, "Autoimmune and miscellaneous diseases," in *Wallach's Interpretation of Diagnostic Tests*, p. 1035, Wolters Kluwer, Lippincott Williams & Wilkins, Philadelphia, Pa, USA, 2011.

[44] J. Wenzel, R. Bauer, T. Bieber, and I. Böhm, "Autoantibodies in patients with lupus erythematosus: spectrum and frequencies," *Dermatology*, vol. 201, no. 3, pp. 282–283, 2000.

[45] T.-C. Hsu, G. J. Tsay, T.-Y. Chen, Y.-C. Liu, and B.-S. Tzang, "Anti-PCNA autoantibodies preferentially recognize C-terminal of PCNA in patients with chronic hepatitis B virus infection," *Clinical & Experimental Immunology*, vol. 144, no. 1, pp. 110–116, 2006.

[46] J. G. Hanly, L. Su, V. Farewell, and M. J. Fritzler, "Comparison between multiplex assays for autoantibody detection in systemic lupus erythematosus," *Journal of Immunological Methods*, vol. 358, no. 1-2, pp. 75–80, 2010.

[47] N. Bardin, S. Desplat-Jego, L. Daniel, N. Jourde Chiche, and M. Sanmarco, "BioPlexe 2200 multiplexed system: simultaneous detection of anti-dsDNA and anti-chromatin antibodies in patients with systemic lupus erythematosus," *Autoimmunity*, vol. 42, no. 1, pp. 63–68, 2009.

[48] J. G. Hanly, K. Thompson, G. McCurdy, L. Fougere, C. Theriault, and K. Wilton, "Measurement of autoantibodies using multiplex methodology in patients with systemic lupus erythematosus," *Journal of Immunological Methods*, vol. 352, no. 1-2, pp. 147–152, 2010.

[49] W. D. James, T. G. Berger, and D. M. Elston, *Andrews' Diseases of the Skin. Clinical Dermatology*, Saunders Elsevier, 11th edition, 2011.

[50] D. H. Solomon, A. J. Kavanaugh, P. H. Schur et al., "Evidence-based guidelines for the use of immunologic tests: antinuclear antibody testing," *Arthritis & Rheumatism*, vol. 47, no. 4, pp. 434–444, 2002.

[51] N. Bizzaro and A. Wiik, "Appropriateness in anti-nuclear antibody testing: from clinical request to strategic laboratory practice," *Clinical and Experimental Rheumatology*, vol. 22, no. 3, pp. 349–355, 2004.

[52] E. Bonfa, S. J. Golombek, L. D. Kaufman et al., "Association between lupus psychosis and anti-ribosomal P protein antibodies," *The New England Journal of Medicine*, vol. 317, no. 5, pp. 265–271, 1987.

[53] A. Ippolito, D. J. Wallace, D. Gladman et al., "Autoantibodies in systemic lupus erythematosus: comparison of historical and current assessment of seropositivity," *Lupus*, vol. 20, no. 3, pp. 250–255, 2011.

[54] B. H. Hahn, "Antibodies to DNA," *The New England Journal of Medicine*, vol. 338, no. 19, pp. 1359–1368, 1998.

[55] M. Teodorescu, "Clinical value of anti-ssDNA (denatured DNA) autoantibody test: beauty is in the eyes of the beholder," *Clinical and Applied Immunology Reviews*, vol. 2, no. 2, pp. 115–128, 2002.

[56] J. D. Reveille, "Predictive value of autoantibodies for activity of systemic lupus erythematosus," *Lupus*, vol. 13, no. 5, pp. 290–297, 2004.

[57] C.-L. Yu, M.-H. Huang, C.-Y. Tsai et al., "The reactivity of sera from patients with systemic lupus erythematosus to seven different species of single and double stranded deoxyribonucleic acids," *Clinical and Experimental Rheumatology*, vol. 14, no. 2, pp. 137–144, 1996.

[58] S. Albani, M. Massa, S. Viola, G. Pellegrini, and A. Martini, "Antibody reactivity against single stranded DNA of various species in normal children and in children with diffuse connective tissue diseases," *Autoimmunity*, vol. 8, no. 1, pp. 77–80, 1990.

[59] R. Misra, A. N. Malaviya, R. Kumar, and A. Kumar, "Clinical relevance of the estimation of antibodies to single stranded DNA in systemic lupus erythematosus," *The Indian Journal of Medical Research*, vol. 87, pp. 463–467, 1988.

[60] D. Koffler, V. Agnello, R. Winchester, and H. G. Kunkel, "The occurrence of single-stranded DNA in the serum of patients with systemic lupus erythematosus and other diseases," *The Journal of Clinical Investigation*, vol. 52, no. 1, pp. 198–204, 1973.

[61] H. Bootsma, P. Spronk, R. Derksen et al., "Prevention of relapses in systemic lupus erythematosus," *The Lancet*, vol. 345, no. 8965, pp. 1595–1599, 1995.

[62] S. Yung and T. M. Chan, "Autoantibodies and resident renal cells in the pathogenesis of lupus nephritis: getting to know the unknown," *Clinical and Developmental Immunology*, vol. 2012, Article ID 139365, 13 pages, 2012.

[63] Y. Shoenfeld and E. Toubi, "Protective autoantibodies: role in homeostasis, clinical importance, and therapeutic potential," *Arthritis & Rheumatism*, vol. 52, no. 9, pp. 2599–2606, 2005.

[64] T. Witte, "IgM antibodies against dsDNA in SLE," *Clinical Reviews in Allergy and Immunology*, vol. 34, no. 3, pp. 345–347, 2008.

[65] E. S. Husebye, Z. M. Sthoeger, M. Dayan et al., "Autoantibodies to a NR2A peptide of the glutamate/NMDA receptor in sera of patients with systemic lupus erythematosus," *Annals of the Rheumatic Diseases*, vol. 64, no. 8, pp. 1210–1213, 2005.

[66] T. Yoshio, K. Onda, H. Nara, and S. Minota, "Association of IgG anti-NR2 glutamate receptor antibodies in cerebrospinal fluid with neuropsychiatric systemic lupus erythematosus," *Arthritis & Rheumatism*, vol. 54, no. 2, pp. 675–678, 2006.

[67] J. G. Hanly, J. Robichaud, and J. D. Fisk, "Anti-NR2 glutamate receptor antibodies and cognitive function in systemic lupus erythematosus," *Journal of Rheumatology*, vol. 33, no. 8, pp. 1553–1558, 2006.

[68] G. Franchin, M. Son, S. J. Kim, I. Ben-Zvi, J. Zhang, and B. Diamond, "Anti-DNA antibodies cross-react with C1q," *The Journal of Autoimmunity*, vol. 44, pp. 34–39, 2013.

[69] E. J. ter Borg, G. Horst, P. C. Limburg, and C. G. M. Kallenberg, "Shifts of anti-Sm-specific antibodies in patients with systemic lupus erythematosus: analysis by counter-immunoelectrophoresis, immunoblotting and RNA-immunoprecipitation," *The Journal of Autoimmunity*, vol. 4, no. 1, pp. 155–164, 1991.

[70] W. J. Habets, D. J. de Rooij, M. H. Hoet, L. B. van de Putte, and W. J. van Venrooij, "Quantitation of anti-RNP and anti-Sm antibodies in MCTD and SLE patients by immunoblotting," *Clinical & Experimental Immunology*, vol. 59, no. 2, pp. 457–466, 1985.

[71] Z. Amoura, H. Chabre, J. F. Bach, and S. Koutouzov, "Antinucleosome antibodies and systemic lupus erythematosus," *Advances in Nephrology from the Necker Hospital*, vol. 26, pp. 303–316, 1997.

[72] J. van der Vlag and J. H. M. Berden, "Lupus nephritis: role of antinucleosome antibodies," *Seminars in Nephrology*, vol. 31, no. 4, pp. 376–389, 2011.

[73] A. J. Ullal, C. F. Reich III, M. Clowse et al., "Microparticles as antigenic targets of antibodies to DNA and nucleosomes in systemic lupus erythematosus," *The Journal of Autoimmunity*, vol. 36, no. 3-4, pp. 173–180, 2011.

[74] S. Saisoong, S. Eiam-Ong, and O. Hanvivatvong, "Correlations between antinucleosome antibodies and anti-double-stranded DNA antibodies, C3, C4, and clinical activity in lupus patients," *Clinical and Experimental Rheumatology*, vol. 24, no. 1, pp. 51–58, 2006.

[75] Z. Amoura, J. C. Piette, J. F. Bach, and S. Koutouzov, "The key role of nucleosomes in lupus," *Arthritis & Rheumatism*, vol. 42, pp. 833–843, 1999.

[76] R. W. Burlingame, M. L. Boey, G. Starkebaum, and R. L. Rubin, "The central role of chromatin in autoimmune responses to histones and DNA in systemic lupus erythematosus," *The Journal of Clinical Investigation*, vol. 94, no. 1, pp. 184–192, 1994.

[77] K. P. Ng, J. J. Manson, A. Rahman, and D. A. Isenberg, "Association of antinucleosome antibodies with disease flare in serologically active clinically quiescent patients with systemic lupus erythematosus," *Arthritis & Rheumatism*, vol. 55, no. 6, pp. 900–904, 2006.

[78] D. J. Wallace, H. C. Lin, G. Q. Shen, and J. B. Peter, "Antibodies to histone (H2a-H2b)-DNA complexes in the absence of antibodies to double-stranded DNA or to (Ha-H2b) complexes are more sensitive and specific for scleroderma-related disorders than for lupus," *Arthritis & Rheumatism*, vol. 37, no. 12, pp. 1795–1797, 1994.

[79] A. Parodi, M. Drosera, L. Barbieri, and A. Rebora, "Antihistone antibodies in scleroderma," *Dermatology*, vol. 191, no. 1, pp. 16–18, 1995.

[80] S. Vasoo, "Drug-induced lupus: an update," *Lupus*, vol. 15, no. 11, pp. 757–761, 2006.

[81] R. L. Rubin, "Drug-induced lupus," *Toxicology*, vol. 209, no. 2, pp. 135–147, 2005.

[82] S. Minota, T. Yoshio, M. Iwamoto et al., "Selective accumulation of anti-histone antibodies in glomeruli of lupus-prone Ipr mice," *Clinical Immunology and Immunopathology*, vol. 80, no. 1, pp. 82–87, 1996.

[83] M. Sui, Q. Lin, Z. Xu et al., "Simultaneous positivity for anti-DNA, anti-nucleosome and anti-histone antibodies is a marker for more severe lupus nephritis," *Journal of Clinical Immunology*, vol. 33, no. 2, pp. 378–387, 2013.

[84] M. Reichlin, "Significance of the Ro antigen system," *Journal of Clinical Immunology*, vol. 6, no. 5, pp. 339–348, 1986.

[85] F. Furukawa, M. Kashihara-Sawami, M. B. Lyons, and D. A. Norris, "Binding of antibodies to the extractable nuclear antigens SS-A/Ro and SS-B/La is induced on the surface of human keratinocytes by ultraviolet light (UVL): implications for the pathogenesis of photosensitive cutaneous lupus," *Journal of Investigative Dermatology*, vol. 94, no. 1, pp. 77–85, 1990.

[86] T. D. Golan, K. B. Elkon, A. E. Gharavi, and J. G. Krueger, "Enhanced membrane binding of autoantibodies to cultured keratinocytes of systemic lupus erythematosus patients after ultraviolet B/ultraviolet A irradiation," *The Journal of Clinical Investigation*, vol. 90, no. 3, pp. 1067–1076, 1992.

[87] E. Alexander, J. P. Buyon, T. T. Provost, and T. Guarnieri, "Anti-Ro/SS-A antibodies in the pathophysiology of congenital heart block in neonatal lupus syndrome, an experimental model: in vitro electrophysiologic and immunocytochemical studies," *Arthritis & Rheumatism*, vol. 35, no. 2, pp. 176–189, 1992.

[88] R. Cimaz, D. L. Spence, L. Hornberger, and E. D. Silverman, "Incidence and spectrum of neonatal lupus erythematosus: a prospective study of infants born to mothers with anti-ro autoantibodies," *Journal of Pediatrics*, vol. 142, no. 6, pp. 678–683, 2003.

[89] E. Jaeggi, C. Laskin, R. Hamilton, J. Kingdom, and E. Silverman, "The importance of the level of maternal Anti-Ro/SSA antibodies as a prognostic marker of the development of cardiac neonatal lupus erythematosus. A prospective study of 186 antibody-exposed fetuses and infants," *Journal of the American College of Cardiology*, vol. 55, no. 24, pp. 2778–2784, 2010.

[90] C. B. Mond, M. G. E. Peterson, and N. F. Rothfield, "Correlation of anti-Ro antibody with photosensitivity rash in systemic lupus erythematosus patients," *Arthritis & Rheumatism*, vol. 32, no. 2, pp. 202–204, 1989.

[91] D. P. McCauliffe, "Cutaneous diseases in adults associated with Anti-Ro/SS-A autoantibody production," *Lupus*, vol. 6, no. 2, pp. 158–166, 1997.

[92] M. V. Fukuda, S. C. Lo, C. S. de Almeida, and S. K. Shinjo, "Anti-Ro antibody and cutaneous vasculitis in systemic lupus erythematosus," *Clinical Rheumatology*, vol. 28, no. 3, pp. 301–304, 2009.

[93] S. Praprotnik, B. Bozic, T. Kveder, and B. Rozman, "Fluctuation of anti-Ro/SS-A antibody levels in patients with systemic lupus erythematosus and Sjogren's syndrome: a prospective study," *Clinical and Experimental Rheumatology*, vol. 17, no. 1, pp. 63–68, 1999.

[94] E. Scopelitis, J. J. Biundo Jr., and M. A. Alspaugh, "Anti-SS-A antibody and other antinuclear antibodies in systemic lupus erythematosus," *Arthritis & Rheumatism*, vol. 23, no. 3, pp. 287–293, 1980.

[95] R. H. W. M. Derksen and J. F. Meilof, "Anti-Ro/SS-A and anti-La/SS-B autoantibody levels in relation to systemic lupus erythematosus disease activity and congenital heart block: a longitudinal study comprising two consecutive pregnancies in a patient with systemic lupus erythematosus," *Arthritis & Rheumatism*, vol. 35, no. 8, pp. 953–959, 1992.

[96] M. Wahren, P. Tengnér, I. Gunnarsson et al., "Ro/SS-A and La/SS-B antibody level variation in patients with Sjogren's syndrome and systemic lupus erythematosus," *The Journal of Autoimmunity*, vol. 11, no. 1, pp. 29–38, 1998.

[97] A. B. Hassan, I. E. Lundberg, D. Isenberg, and M. Wahren-Herlenius, "Serial analysis of Ro/SSA and La/SSB antibody levels and correlation with clinical disease activity in patients with systemic lupus erythematosus," *Scandinavian Journal of Rheumatology*, vol. 31, no. 3, pp. 133–139, 2002.

[98] A. Menendez, J. Gomez, E. Escanlar, L. Caminal-Montero, and L. Mozo, "Clinical associations of anti-SSA/Ro60 and anti-Ro52/TRIM21 antibodies: diagnostic utility of their separate detection," *Autoimmunity*, vol. 46, no. 1, pp. 32–39, 2013.

[99] N. Costedoat-Chalumeau, Z. Amoura, E. Villain, L. Cohen, and J.-C. Piette, "Anti-SSA/Ro antibodies and the heart: more than complete congenital heart block? A review of electrocardiographic and myocardial abnormalities and of treatment options," *Arthritis Research & Therapy*, vol. 7, no. 2, pp. 69–73, 2005.

[100] W. J. van Venrooij, R. L. Slobbe, and G. J. M. Pruijn, "Structure and function of La and Ro RNPs," *Molecular Biology Reports*, vol. 18, no. 2, pp. 113–119, 1993.

[101] J. B. Harley, "Autoantibodies in Sjögren's syndrome," *The Journal of Autoimmunity*, vol. 2, no. 4, pp. 383–394, 1989.

[102] K. Elkon, S. Skelly, and A. Parnassa, "Identification and chemical synthesis of a ribosomal protein antigenic determinant

in systemic lupus erythematosus," *Proceedings of the National Academy of Sciences of the United States of America*, vol. 83, no. 19, pp. 7419–7423, 1986.

[103] C. Briani, M. Lucchetta, A. Ghirardello et al., "Neurolupus is associated with anti-ribosomal P protein antibodies: an inception cohort study," *The Journal of Autoimmunity*, vol. 32, no. 2, pp. 79–84, 2009.

[104] M. Mahler, K. Kessenbrock, M. Szmyrka et al., "International multicenter evaluation of autoantibodies to ribosomal P proteins," *Clinical and Vaccine Immunology*, vol. 13, no. 1, pp. 77–83, 2006.

[105] E. Toubi and Y. Shoenfeld, "Clinical and biological aspects of anti-P-ribosomal protein autoantibodies," *Autoimmunity Reviews*, vol. 6, no. 3, pp. 119–125, 2007.

[106] A. Katzav, I. Solodeev, O. Brodsky et al., "Induction of autoimmune depression in mice by anti-ribosomal P antibodies via the limbic system," *Arthritis & Rheumatism*, vol. 56, no. 3, pp. 938–948, 2007.

[107] S. Matus, P. V. Burgos, M. Bravo-Zehnder et al., "Antiribosomal-P autoantibodies from psychiatric lupus target a novel neuronal surface protein causing calcium influx and apoptosis," *The Journal of Experimental Medicine*, vol. 204, no. 13, pp. 3221–3234, 2007.

[108] L. Caponi, C. Anzilotti, G. Longombardo, and P. Migliorini, "Antibodies directed against ribosomal P proteins cross-react with phospholipids," *Clinical & Experimental Immunology*, vol. 150, no. 1, pp. 140–143, 2007.

[109] F. B. Karassa, A. Afeltra, A. Ambrozic et al., "Accuracy of anti-ribosomal P protein antibody testing for the diagnosis of neuropsychiatric systemic lupus erythematosus: an international meta-analysis," *Arthritis & Rheumatism*, vol. 54, no. 1, pp. 312–324, 2006.

[110] V. A. Wasserman, A. Niesser, and C. Bruck, "Eine sierdiagnostische Reaction bei Syphilis," *Deutsche Medizinische Wochenschrift*, vol. 19, pp. 745–776, 1906.

[111] M. D. Pangbor, "A new serologically active phospholipid from beef heart," *Proceedings of the Society for Experimental Biology and Medicine*, vol. 48, pp. 484–486, 1941.

[112] C. L. Conley and R. C. Hartmann, "A hemorrhagic disorder caused by circulating anticoagulant in patients with disseminated lupus erythematosus," *The Journal of Clinical Investigation*, vol. 31, pp. 621–623, 1952.

[113] D. I. Feinstein and S. I. Rapaport, "Acquired inhibitors of blood coagulation," *Progress in Hemostasis and Thrombosis*, vol. 1, pp. 75–95, 1972.

[114] J. E. Hunt, H. P. McNeil, G. J. Morgan, R. M. Crameri, and S. A. Krilis, "A phospholipid-beta 2-glycoprotein I complex is an antigen for anticardiolipin antibodies occurring in autoimmune disease but not with infection," *Lupus*, vol. 1, no. 2, pp. 75–81, 1992.

[115] K. B. M. Reid, "C1q," *Methods in Enzymology*, vol. 82, pp. 319–324, 1982.

[116] C. Bigler, M. Schaller, I. Perahud, M. Osthoff, and M. Trendelenburg, "Autoantibodies against complement C1q specifically target C1q bound on early apoptotic cells," *Journal of Immunology*, vol. 183, no. 5, pp. 3512–3521, 2009.

[117] V. M. Holers, "Anti-C1q autoantibodies amplify pathogenic complement activation in systemic lupus erythematosus," *The Journal of Clinical Investigation*, vol. 114, no. 5, pp. 616–619, 2004.

[118] G. Moroni, M. Trendelenburg, N. Del Papa et al., "Anti-C1q antibodies may help in diagnosing a renal flare in lupus nephritis," *American Journal of Kidney Diseases*, vol. 37, no. 3, pp. 490–498, 2001.

[119] M. A. Seelen, L. A. Trouw, and M. R. Daha, "Diagnostic and prognostic significance of anti-C1q antibodies in systemic lupus erythematosus," *Current Opinion in Nephrology and Hypertension*, vol. 12, no. 6, pp. 619–624, 2003.

[120] C. G. M. Kallenberg, "Anti-C1q autoantibodies," *Autoimmunity Reviews*, vol. 7, no. 8, pp. 612–615, 2008.

[121] M. P. Keith, C. Moratz, and G. C. Tsokos, "Anti-RNP immunity: implications for tissue injury and the pathogenesis of connective tissue disease," *Autoimmunity Reviews*, vol. 6, no. 4, pp. 232–236, 2007.

[122] P. Migliorini, C. Baldini, V. Rocchi, and S. Bombardieri, "Anti-Sm and anti-RNP antibodies," *Autoimmunity*, vol. 38, no. 1, pp. 47–54, 2005.

[123] Y. Tokano, M. Yasuma, S. Harada et al., "Clinical significance of IgG subclasses of anti-Sm and U1 ribonucleoprotein antibodies in patients with systemic lupus erythematosus and mixed connective tissue disease," *Journal of Clinical Immunology*, vol. 11, no. 6, pp. 317–325, 1991.

[124] A. Doria, A. Ruffatti, A. Calligaro et al., "Antiphospholipid antibodies in mixed connective tissue disease," *Clinical Rheumatology*, vol. 11, no. 1, pp. 48–50, 1992.

[125] Y. Takahashi, S. Haga, Y. Ishizaka, and A. Mimori, "Autoantibodies to angiotensin-converting enzyme 2 in patients with connective tissue diseases," *Arthritis Research & Therapy*, vol. 12, no. 3, article R86, 2010.

[126] L. Iaccarino, M. Gatto, S. Bettio et al., "Overlap connective tissue disease syndromes," *Autoimmunity Reviews*, vol. 12, no. 3, pp. 363–373, 2013.

[127] L. M. Amezcua-Guerra, R. Springall, R. Marquez-Velasco, L. Gómez-García, A. Vargas, and R. Bojalil, "Presence of antibodies against cyclic citrullinated peptides in patients with "rhupus": a cross-sectional study," *Arthritis Research & Therapy*, vol. 8, no. 5, article R144, 2006.

[128] J. A. Simón, J. Granados, J. Cabiedes, J. R. Morales, and J. A. Varela, "Clinical and immunogenetic characterization of Mexican patients with 'rhupus'," *Lupus*, vol. 11, no. 5, pp. 287–292, 2002.

5

Role of HLA-B Alleles and Clinical Presentation of B27 Negative Spondyloarthritis Patients from Mumbai, Western India

Devaraj J. Parasannanavar,[1] Anjali Rajadhyaksha,[2] and Kanjaksha Ghosh[3]

[1] *Microbiology and Immunology Division, National Institute of Nutrition (ICMR), Jamai-Osmania, Tarnaka, Hyderabad, Andhra Pradesh 500007, India*
[2] *Department of Medicine, King Edward Memorial Hospital, Parel, Mumbai 400 012, India*
[3] *National Institute of Immunohaematology (ICMR), King Edward Memorial Hospital, 13th Floor, N.M.S. Building, Parel, Mumbai 400 012, India*

Correspondence should be addressed to Kanjaksha Ghosh; kanjakshaghosh@hotmail.com

Academic Editor: Edmond J. Yunis

Seronegative spondyloarthritis (SpA) are variably associated with HLA-B*27 antigen. HLA-B*27 negative SpA has also been reported from different parts of the world. There is paucity of data on this entity from Indian subcontinent. We studied 100 consecutively diagnosed HLA-B27 negative spondyloarthritis patients from a tertiary care center in India. Modified New York Criteria for ankylosing spondylitis (AS) and ESSG criteria for SpA were used for diagnosing patients. HLA-B*27 typing was done by an in-house PCR-SSP technique in SpA patients to exclude B*27 positive patients and PCR-SSOP technique was used to type 100 B*27 negative SpA patients and 100 controls from the same ethnicity. Frequency of B*07 was significantly increased (B*07: % PF 54 versus 18; OR 5.348; 95% CI 2.808–10.186; P value 1.14E − 07), whereas frequency of B*40 was significantly decreased (B*40: % PF 17 versus 32; OR 0.435; 95% CI 0.222–0.850; P value 0.013) when compared with B*27 negative controls. Among 100 SpA patients, 47 were undifferentiated spondyloarthritis and 33 patients were reactive arthritis patients. 40% of the patients were suffering from polyarticular arthritis, 35% had pauciarticular arthritis with knee joint, hip joint, ankle joint, and SI joint involvement. We conclude that B*07 was significantly associated with B27 negative spondyloarthropathy from Western India and majority of B*27 negative patients were uSpA.

1. Introduction

The spondyloarthritis (SpA) is a group of diseases which include mainly ankylosing spondylitis (AS), Reiter's syndrome/reactive arthritis (RS/ReA), enteropathic spondylitis (Crohn's disease and ulcerative colitis), Psoriatic Arthropathy (PsA), and undifferentiated spondylitis (uSpA). AS is a chronic inflammatory disease that begins primarily in the sacroiliac joints and goes on to involve the spine and other large joints. Reactive arthritis (ReA) is an acute nonporulant arthritis complicating an infection elsewhere in the body, usually genitourinary infection with *Chlamydia trachomatis* and enteritis due to gram negative enterobacteria such as *Shigella, Salmonella, Yersinia,* or *Campylobacter* species [1]. Psoriatic arthritis (PsA) refers to an inflammatory arthritis that typically occurs in individuals with Psoriasis [2]. Many patients, usually young adults, present with some features of one or more of the spondyloarthritis but lack criteria for these diagnosis; for example, a patient may present with inflammatory synovitis of one knee, achilles tendonitis, and dactylitis of one digit or sacroiliitis in the absence of other criteria for AS. Such patients are said to have undifferentiated spondyloarthritis (uSpA).

An association between HLA-B27 and AS was first reported in 1973 [3] and this was confirmed later [4–8]. The frequency of HLA-B27 ranges from 88 to 90% among patients as compared to 4–8% in controls. However, different races show different rates of association. The frequency of HLA-B27 with AS or other related SpA among Indian population varies from 30 to 94% as compared to 1.4–8% of

Table 1: Distribution of HLA-B alleles among B27 negative SpA patients and controls from Western India (patients (n = 100); controls (n = 100)).

Serial number	HLA-B	%PF	%P.F	OR	95% CI	χ^2Y	P value
1	B*51	10	13	0.743	0.309–1.785	0.196	0.506
2	B*52	7	8	0.865	0.301–2.485	0.072	0.788
3	**B*07**	**54**	**18**	**5.348**	**2.808–10.186**	**26.584**	**1.14E − 07**
4	B*15	19	12	1.720	0.785–3.765	1.374	0.171
5	B*08	12	14	0.837	0.366–1.914	0.044	0.674
6	B*18	6	9	0.645	0.220–1.887	0.288	0.420
7	B*13	4	3	1.347	0.293–6.183	0.148	0.700
8	**B*40**	**17**	**32**	**0.435**	**0.222–0.850**	**5.298**	**0.013**
9	B*35	33	44	0.626	0.353–1.113	2.112	0.109
10	B*57	9	7	1.314	0.469–3.678	0.067	0.602
11	B*58	8	4	2.080	0.607–7.169	0.797	0.233
12	B*44	9	15	0.560	0.232–1.348	1.184	0.191
13	B*47	3	6	0.484	0.117–1.995	0.465	0.306
14	B*48	2	0	5.102	0.241–107.70	0.505	0.155
15	B*53	1	1	1.000	0.061–16.224	0.000	1.000
16	B*49	1	3	0.326	0.033–3.196	0.255	0.312
17	B*38	0	1	0.330	0.013–8.205	1.005	0.316
18	B*78	0	2	0.196	0.009–4.138	0.505	0.155
19	B*81	1	3	0.326	0.333–3.196	0.255	0.312
20	B*37	1	3	0.326	0.333–3.196	0.255	0.312
21	B*42	0	1	0.330	0.013–8.205	1.005	0.316
22	B*56	3	1	3.062	0.312–29.965	0.255	0.312

N+: number positive, PF: phenotype frequency, OR: odds ratio, χ^2Y: chi-square with Yates' correction.

the general population [8]. However, a more number of B27 negative individuals could develop SpA with typical clinical and radiological findings. There are reports which reveal that other HLA-B locus alleles have also be involved in B27 negative SpA patients from India [9] and worldwide [10–21]. Association of HLA-B7 CREG antigens (B7, B22, B27, B40, and B42) with AS patients among American Blacks was studied by Khan et al. [10, 11]. Subsequently these findings were confirmed among ReA and uSpA patients from different parts of the world [12–15]. The association of HLA-B40 with AS was reported by Robinson et al. for the first time, who found that HLA-B60 (Split of B40) was increased in B27 positive AS patients [16]. Later these findings were confirmed by other investigators among B27 positive as well as negative SpA patients [14, 16–18]. Earlier studies also showed the association between HLA-B16 (currently B38 and B39) and HLA-B35CREG (B18, B35, B51, and B62) with HLA-B27 negative Caucasian, Japanese, and German AS patients [19–21]. Hence, our aim was to study the role of HLA-B alleles and their clinical presentation in B*27 negative SpA patients from Western India.

2. Materials and Methods

2.1. Selection Criteria for Patients and Controls. In the present study, a total of 100 consecutive B*27 negative SpA patients were selected according to the revised New York criteria for AS [22] and ESSG for SpA [23]. Patients were evaluated by rheumatologist at K.E.M. and various hospitals from Mumbai and reevaluated by one of us (K.G). As per the selection criteria, SpA patients fulfilled at least any 4 of the following criteria: (1) insidious onset, (2) duration > 3 months, (3) radiological bilateral or unilateral sacroiliitis, (4) limitation of motion of the lumbar spine and chest expansion, and (5) improvement of morning stiffness with exercise and not relieved by rest. All patients were negative for B*27 typed by in-house PCR-SSP to exclude B*27 positivity [8]. These patients had undergone various tests including radiology of affected joints, sacroiliac joints, lumbar spine, cervical spine, full blood count with ESR, rheumatoid factor, anticitrullinated antibody (anti-CCP), and other autoimmune parameters like ANA and ds DNA. The study was carried out over a period of three years from April 2009 to March 2011. The study was approved by Ethics Committees of the institute. 100 age- and sex-matched healthy individuals which were negative for B*27 belonging to the same socioeconomic status and ethnic background during the same period comprised the controls for this study.

2.2. HLA Typing

2.2.1. Molecular Typing. Genomic DNA extracted standard phenol-chloroform-isoamyl alcohol method from 5 mL of EDTA blood. B27 negative patients and controls were typed for B locus by polymerase chain reaction reverse line strip sequence-specific oligonucleotide hybridization (PCR-RLS-SSOP) strips (Dynal-Reli-SSO typing). Each strip for HLA-B typing carried a total of 62 immobilized SSOs. Genomic DNA was amplified using HLA-B locus specific biotinylated primers and hybridized with the SSO strips. Streptavidin-horseradish peroxidase (SA-HRP) conjugates for positive color development using hydrogen peroxide (H_2O_2) and tetramethylbenzidine (TMB) as substrate. The alleles were determined using the pattern interpretation software (PMP) supplied with the kit [24].

2.3. Statistical Analysis. The allele frequencies, odds ratio, 95% confidence interval, and chi-square with Yates' correction were estimated using SPSS software.

3. Results

Rheumatoid factor, anti-CCP antibody, ANA, and ds DNA were negative for all patients. Distribution of HLA-B alleles among 100 B*27 negative SpA patients and 100 controls is as shown in Table 1. The frequency of HLA-B*07 was significantly increased among patients as compared to the controls (B*07: %PF **54** versus **18;** OR **5.348;** 95% CI **2.808–10.186;** χ^2Y **26.584;** *P* value **1.14*E* − 07**), whereas frequency of B*40 was significantly decreased (B*40: **%PF 17** versus **32;** OR **0.435;** 95% CI **0.222–0.850;** χ^2Y **5.298;** *P* value **0.013**). Clinical presentation of B*27 negative SpA patients is as shown in Table 2; when 52% of patients who are analyzed had the onset of clinical symptom between the age of 16 to 30 years, 30% showed the onset between the age between 31 to 45 years of age and male to female ratio of 4 : 1. Subgroup classification among B*27 negative SpA patients revealed that 47% patients had undifferentiated spondyloarthritis, 33% were ReA, 14% were AS, and JSpA were 4%. Analysis of the type of arthritis showed that 40% of the patients were suffering from polyarticular arthritis, 35% had pauciarticular arthritis, and 25% had monoarticular. Further analysis of the involvent of joints showed that 54% had knee joints affected, 46% had hip joint pain, 30% had ankle joints, and 25% of patients had SI joints involvement. When Scober's test results were analyzed, 50% of the patients had restricted spine flexion and 25% had diminished chest expansion. Enthesitis was present in 84% of the patients.

Table 2: Clinical presentation of B27 negative SpA patients.

Serial number	Character	B27 negative $n = 100$	Normal controls $n = 100$
	Age of onset	%	%
	≤15	11	14
1	16–30	52	21
	31–45	30	58
	>45	7	7
	Sex:		
2	M	80	56
	F	20	44
3	Fam H/O arthritis	13	0
4	Polyarticular arthritis >3 Jts	40	0
5	Pauciarticular	35	0
6	Monoarticular	25	0
7	Chest exp ≤5 cm	25	0
8	Spine flx ≤5 cm	50	0
9	Tend SI JT	25	0
10	Knee jt	54	0
11	Ankle jt	30	0
12	L-spine	38	0
13	C-spine	43	0
14	Hip jt	46	0
15	SI jt	25	0
16	Shoulder jt	7	0
17	Wrist jt	11	0
18	Foot jt	7	0
19	Hand jt	9	0
20	Enthesitis	84	0

4. Discussion

The association between HLA-B27 with AS and related arthropathies has been known for a long time. But it is thought that in addition to B27, other HLA-B and DR alleles may increase susceptibility to the development of AS and related arthropathies [16]. The present study revealed the role of other HLA-B locus alleles and their clinical presentation among B27 negative SpA patients from Western India. In this study, HLA-B*07 was significantly increased among B27 negative SpA patients from Western India, which confirms earlier reports [9–15]. B*07 may be associated with AS either directly or because of linkage disequilibrium with further MHC gene. Our findings suggest that in addition to HLA-B*27, B*07 may also play a significant role in the development of SpA in Western Indian population.

Several studies have suggested that association of HLA-B*40 with B*27 positive as well as negative AS patients from various populations [16–18]. However, in our study B*40 was decreased among patients when compared with controls. An earlier study reported that even though B*40 frequency was increased marginally, no association was found between B*40 and SpA from north Indian population [24]. As HLA-B*27 and B*07 are more strongly associated with the disease, hence in our cohort of SpA patients where HLA-B*27 and B*07 are present in significant numbers, impact of B*40 has become statistically less. However, there are quite a few studies where B*40 was found to have stronger association with rheumatoid arthritis than with SpA [25], and these patients have higher tendency to have an associated pulmonary involvement. In our cohort such patients who were rheumatoid factor positive or were diagnosed with rheumatoid arthritis were meticulously excluded providing another reason for lower B*40 prevalence in our series.

Spondyloarthritis patients presented, either singly or in combination, with sacroiliitis with spondylitis; polyarticular arthritis; persistent pain and tenderness in the tendo-Achillis or heel; or pauciarticular arthritis associated with recent history (three months previously) of dysentery, together with high (ESR > 40 mm/h) and negative autoimmune parameters (ANA, dsDNA, and ANCA). The disease lasted for more than three months and responded to nonsteroidal anti-inflammatory drugs (NSAIDS) even before the diagnosis. Some patients showed systemic symptoms such as weight loss and low grade fever, 5 patients had uveitis, 4 patients had urethritis, and 2 patients had psoriatic arthropathies. Diseases at different duration revealed that majority of the patients were between age 16 to 30 years group in all durations. Chest expansion of ≤5 cm was present alone or together in 64% of the patients studied. Hence even in HLA-B*27 negative SpA patients, and this test is clinically useful. Undifferentiated form of SpA (47%), enthesitis (84%), and polyarticular arthritis was significantly over represented than in B*27 associated SpA as reported in the literature [15]. Hence HLA-B*27 negative SpA resembles classical HLA-B*27 positive variety of SpA in showing male preponderance and seronegativity (for both rheumatoid factor and anti-CCP antibodies). However, it differs substantially in clinical presentation by older age of presentation, high frequency of enthesitis, and polyarticular arthritis, but much lower frequency of sacroiliitis which corroborates earlier study on American pediatric SpA patients suggests that clinician needs look closely for enthesitis to diagnose SpA [26]. In our study HLA-B*40 was significantly underrepresented in our patients when compared to other reported studies elsewhere in the world [14–18] which suggests that environmental precipitating factors are likely to be varied in different parts of the world, explaining the differential presentation of HLA-B*07 and HLA-B*40 in these groups of patients.

Conflict of Interests

The authors declare that there is no conflict of interests regarding the publication of this paper.

Acknowledgments

This study was presented as poster presentation at 1st Meeting of Asian-Pacific Federation of Inflammation and Regeneration: APFIR-2011 which was held on June 2-3, 2011, at Kyoto, Japan. The authors acknowledge Professor (Dr.) N. K. Mehra, Department of Transplant Immunology and Immunogenetics, All India Institute of Medical Sciences, New Delhi, for his critical comments, valuable suggestions, and recommendations.

References

[1] R. A. Hughes and A. C. Keat, "Reiter's syndrome and reactive arthritis: a current view," *Seminars in Arthritis and Rheumatism*, vol. 24, no. 3, pp. 190–210, 1994.

[2] J. M. H. Moll and V. Wright, "Psoriatic arthritis," *Seminars in Arthritis and Rheumatism*, vol. 3, no. 1, pp. 55–78, 1973.

[3] D. A. Brewerton, F. D. Hart, A. Nicholls, M. Caffrey, D. C. James, and R. D. Sturrock, "Ankylosing spondylitis and HL-A 27," *The Lancet*, vol. 301, no. 7809, pp. 904–907, 1973.

[4] C. Lopez-Larrea, K. Sujirachato, N. K. Mehra et al., "HLA-B27 subtypes in Asian patients with ankylosing spondylitis: evidence for new associations," *Tissue Antigens*, vol. 45, no. 3, pp. 169–176, 1995.

[5] S. R. Kankonkar, S. C. Raikar, S. V. Joshi, and S. J. Tijoriwala, "Association of HLA-B27 antigen in Indian patients of ankylosing spondylitis and other autoimmune diseases," *Journal of Association of Physicians of India*, vol. 46, no. 4, pp. 345–350, 1998.

[6] U. Shankarkumar, J. P. Devraj, K. Ghosh, and D. Mohanty, "Seronegative spondarthritis and human leucocyte antigen association," *British Journal of Biomedical Science*, vol. 59, no. 1, pp. 38–41, 2002.

[7] U. Shankarkumar, K. Ghosh, and D. Mohanty, "Novel HLA B*2714 and B*2708 allele associations in seronegative spondarthritis patients and haemophilia patients with chronic synovitis in India," *Tissue Antigens*, vol. 62, no. 2, pp. 175–178, 2003.

[8] J. P. Devraj, A. Rajyadhaksha, and K. Ghosh, "Application of a simple in-house PCR-SSP technique for HLA-B*27 typing in Spondyloarthropathies (SpA) patients," *Arthritis*, vol. 2013, Article ID 504109, 4 pages, 2013.

[9] J. P. Devraj, U. Shankarkumar, and K. Ghosh, "Increased frequency of HLA-B7 among B27-negative seronegative spondarthritis patients from Mumbai, Western India," *British Journal of Biomedical Science*, vol. 66, no. 1, pp. 25–27, 2009.

[10] M. A. Khan, I. Kushner, and W. E. Braun, "A subgroup of ankylosing spondylitis associated with HLA-B7 in American blacks," *Arthritis and Rheumatism*, vol. 21, no. 5, pp. 528–530, 1978.

[11] M. A. Khan, "B7-CREG and ankylosing spondylitis," *British Journal of Rheumatology*, vol. 22, no. 4, supplement 2, pp. 129–133, 1983.

[12] F. C. Arnett Jr., M. C. Hochberg, and W. B. Bias, "Cross-reactive HLA antigens in B27-negative Reiter's syndrome and sacroiliitis," *The Johns Hopkins Medical Journal*, vol. 141, no. 4, pp. 193–197, 1977.

[13] E. Ben-Chetrit, C. Brautbar, and A. Rubinow, "HLA antigens in Reiter's syndrome in Israeli patients," *The Journal of Rheumatology*, vol. 12, no. 5, pp. 964–966, 1985.

[14] J.-P. Cedoz, D. Wendling, and J.-F. Viel, "The B7 cross reactive group and spondyloarthropathies: an epidemiological approach," *The Journal of Rheumatology*, vol. 22, no. 10, pp. 1884–1890, 1995.

[15] P. D. Sampaio-Barros, R. A. Conde, E. A. Donadi et al., "Undifferentiated spondyloarthropathies in Brazilians: importance of HLA-B27 and the B7-CREG alleles in characterization and disease progression," *The Journal of Rheumatology*, vol. 30, no. 12, pp. 2632–2637, 2003.

[16] W. P. Robinson, S. M. van der Linden, M. A. Khan et al., "HLA-Bw60 increases susceptibility to ankylosing spondylitis in HLA-B27+ patients," *Arthritis and Rheumatism*, vol. 32, no. 9, pp. 1135–1141, 1989.

[17] J. C. C. Wei, W. C. Tsai, H. S. Lin, C. Y. Tsai, and C. T. Chou, "HLA-B60 and B61 are strongly associated with ankylosing spondylitis in HLA-B27-negative Taiwan Chinese patients," *Rheumatology*, vol. 43, no. 7, pp. 839–842, 2004.

[18] M. A. Khan, I. Kushner, and W. E. Braun, "B27-negative HLA-BW16 in ankylosing spondylitis," *The Lancet*, vol. 311, no. 8078, pp. 1370–1371, 1978.

[19] A. Yamaguchi, N. Tsuchiya, H. Mitsui et al., "Association of HLA-B39 with HLA-B27-negative ankylosing spondylitis and pauciarticular juvenile rheumatoid arthritis in Japanese patients: evidence for a role of the peptide-anchoring B pocket," *Arthritis and Rheumatism*, vol. 38, no. 11, pp. 1672–1677, 1995.

[20] P. Wagener, H. Zeidler, G. Eckert, and H. Deicher, "Increased frequency of HLA-Bw35 CREG antigens in HLA-B27 negative ankylosing spondylitis," *British Journal of Rheumatology*, vol. 22, no. 4, pp. 134–135, 1983.

[21] S. van der Linden, H. A. Valkenburg, and A. Cats, "Evaluation of diagnostic criteria for ankylosing spondylitis. A proposal for modification of the New York criteria," *Arthritis and Rheumatism*, vol. 27, no. 4, pp. 361–368, 1984.

[22] M. Dougados, S. van der Linden, R. Juhlin et al., "The European spondylarthropathy study group preliminary criteria for the classification of spondylarthropathy," *Arthritis and Rheumatism*, vol. 34, no. 10, pp. 1218–1227, 1991.

[23] V. Agrawal, R. M. Gupta, U. Usha, and S. V. Sharma, "HLA class-I and class-II antigen association in rheumatoid arthritis at Varanasi, India," *Indian Journal of Pathology and Microbiology*, vol. 39, no. 1, pp. 19–25, 1996.

[24] U. Shankarkumar, D. Prasanavar, K. Ghosh, and D. Mohanty, "HLA-A*02 allele frequencies and B haplotype associations in Western Indians," *Human Immunology*, vol. 64, no. 5, pp. 562–566, 2003.

[25] J. Seignalet, F. Blotman, L. Simon, and B. Soustelle, "HLA-A, B, C, and DR typing in rheumatoid arthritis," *La Revue de Médecine Interne*, vol. 5, no. 2, pp. 128–135, 1984.

[26] M. L. Stoll, R. Bhore, M. Dempsey-Robertson, and M. Punaro, "Spondyloarthritis in a pediatric population: risk factors for sacroiliitis," *The Journal of Rheumatology*, vol. 37, no. 11, pp. 2402–2408, 2010.

6

Gender and Ethnicity Based Differences in Clinical and Laboratory Features of Myasthenia Gravis

Fawzi Abukhalil,[1] Bijal Mehta,[1,2] Erin Saito,[1] Sejal Mehta,[1] and Aaron McMurtray[1,2]

[1]*Neurology Department, Los Angeles Biomedical Research Institute, 1124 West Carson Street, Building E5, Torrance, CA 90502, USA*
[2]*Department of Neurology, Harbor-UCLA Medical Center, 1000 West Carson Street, Torrance, CA 90509, USA*

Correspondence should be addressed to Aaron McMurtray; amcmurtray@hotmail.com

Academic Editor: Corrado Betterle

Background. Previous reports describe ethnicity based differences in clinical and laboratory features between Caucasians and African Americans with myasthenia gravis. However, it is not known whether these findings apply to other ethnicities. *Methods.* Retrospective analysis of all patients treated for myasthenia gravis during a three-year period at a community based medical center. *Results.* A total of 44 patients were included, including 19 of Hispanic, 16 of African American, 6 of Caucasian, and 3 of Asian ethnicities. Female gender was more common among those with Hispanic, Asian, and African American ethnicities compared to Caucasian ethnicity ($p = 0.029$). Anti-acetylcholine receptor antibody subtypes demonstrated no significant ethnicity based differences in either generalized or ocular myasthenia gravis. A trend was noted towards greater frequency of blocking antibodies among Hispanics (52.6%) compared to African American (37.5%) and Caucasian (33.3%) patients ($p = 0.059$). Generalized but not ocular myasthenia patients showed greater frequency of anti-muscle specific kinase antibodies in Asians and Hispanics compared to African Americans and Caucasians ($p = 0.041$). *Conclusions.* The results of this study support the existence of ethnicity based differences in clinical and laboratory features of myasthenia gravis. Further study of genetic factors influencing clinical features of myasthenia gravis is indicated.

1. Introduction

Myasthenia gravis (MG) is the most common autoimmune disorder affecting the neuromuscular junction and is caused by production of autoantibodies that target postsynaptic acetylcholine receptors or associated protein kinases [1, 2]. One striking and well known clinical feature is the complex relationship between gender and onset age, with increased prevalence found in women younger than the third decade of life and men older than the sixth decade of life, with an overall female-to-male ratio of 3 : 2 [3, 4]. While the underlying etiology for gender based differences in onset age is not yet determined, it is likely that this finding relates to yet unidentified gender based genetic differences in regulation of immune system functioning, which serves to highlight the potential role that yet undetermined genetic factors may play in the clinical features of this disease.

In this study, we used ethnicity as a surrogate marker for the existence of possible underlying genetic differences influencing clinical characteristics of MG, with differences in clinical and laboratory features of MG between ethnic groups taken as evidence for the existence of underlying genetic factors that influence or control expression of clinical features. For example, previous studies have shown that the incidence of anti-acetylcholine receptor- (AChR-) negative MG, including those with muscle specific kinase (MuSK) positive antibodies, varies considerably according to ethnic background, with a reported frequency in Norwegian populations near 0% but as high as 49% in Turkey [5, 6]. Another recent study also reported the existence of ethnicity based differences between Caucasians and African Americans with MG in the United States and identified ethnicity based differences in the rates of anti-AChR antibody positivity, anti-MuSK positivity, frequency of abnormalities on repetitive nerve stimulation results, and differences in rates of clinical severity, as well as gender based differences in age of onset [7].

We hypothesized that since the proposed etiology for ethnicity based differences in clinical and laboratory features of MG between Caucasians and African Americans is underlying genetic differences [7], we would be able to detect similar ethnicity based differences in clinical and laboratory features among additional ethnicity groups as well. In particular, we were interested in ethnicity based differences affecting Hispanic patients, as this group represents one of the fastest growing segments of the population in the United States and has displayed an increasing prevalence of MG in recent years [8]. Identification of ethnicity based differences in clinical and laboratory features in MG is important since the genetic background differences inherently present between ethnicity based groups allow ethnicity to serve as a surrogate marker for the existence of genetic differences that underlie or control phenotypic expression. Identification of underlying genetic factors may eventually lead to new or improved treatments for patients of all ethnicities suffering from MG.

2. Materials and Methods

2.1. Participant Characteristics. This is a retrospective cross-sectional study of all adults diagnosed with or treated for MG in a community based neurology clinic during a three-year period between January 1, 2010, and January 1, 2013. Demographic data including ethnicity, age, gender, presence of comorbid medical conditions, presence of thymoma, and tobacco, alcohol, and illicit substance use was collected and analyzed through retrospective chart review. Institutional Review Board approval was obtained.

2.2. Diagnosis of Myasthenia Gravis. Diagnoses of generalized and ocular MG were determined by ICD-9 code and retrospective chart review. In brief, all patients met standard clinical diagnostic criteria for MG as determined by presence of one or more of the following characteristic symptoms or signs: diplopia, ptosis, dysarthria, difficulty in chewing, difficulty in swallowing, muscle weakness with preserved deep tendon reflexes or increased weakness during exercise, and dramatic improvement in signs and symptoms following administration of an anticholinesterase medication [9]. In addition to one of the above characteristic findings, all participants displayed positive results on at least one of the following serum based laboratory tests: anti-AChR antibodies (blocking, binding, or modulating) or anti-MuSK antibodies [10].

2.3. Statistical Analysis. Categorical demographic, clinical, and laboratory features were compared between groups using Pearson's Chi-Square tests or Fisher's exact test as appropriate. Continuous demographic, clinical, and laboratory features were compared between groups using analysis of variance (ANOVA). p values less than 0.05 were considered statistically significant and no correction for multiple comparisons was performed.

3. Results

A total of forty-four patients were included in the study, including 19 (43.2%) with Hispanic, 16 (36.4%) with African American, 6 (13.6%) with Caucasian, and 3 (6.8%) with Asian ethnicities. Overall, there were more women than men and the age of the participants ranged from 20 to 82 years but did not differ significantly between ethnicity groups (see Table 1). Gender ratios differed significantly by ethnicity, with the greatest percentage of females being among the Asian group (3/3, 100%), compared to 16 of 19 (84%) Hispanic participants, 8 of 16 (50%) African American participants, and 2 of 6 (33.3%) Caucasian participants ($p = 0.029$; see Table 1). No significant differences were detected between ethnicity groups for presence of comorbid medical conditions, psychiatric symptoms, prevalence of thymoma, or tobacco, alcohol, or illicit substance use (see Table 1). Disease severity was similar between ethnicity groups, with the majority of the patients having Myasthenia Gravis Foundation of America (MGFA) scale classification scores of 2a and 3a, and there were no MGFA class 4 or class 5 patients (see Table 1). Additionally, there were a total of three MGFA class 1 patients identified among the MuSK positive antibody patients (see Table 1).

Overall, an anti-AChR antibody test was positive in 63.64% of all MG patients and was positive more often among those with ocular MG (87.50%) compared to those with generalized MG (58.33%, $p = 0.049$). The anti-AChR antibody most likely to be positive was the binding type, which was positive in 59.09% of all patients and accounted for 41.94% of all anti-AChR antibodies identified (see Table 2). The AChR antibody that was least likely to be positive was the modulating type, which was present in 36.36% of all patients and accounted for 25.81% of all positive anti-AChR antibodies detected (see Table 2). While no significant ethnicity based differences were detected for anti-AChR subtypes among MG patients, there was a trend ($p = 0.059$) towards greater frequency of blocking antibodies among Hispanic patients (52.6%) compared to African American (37.5%) and Caucasian (33.3%) patients, and it is notable that the three Asian participants displayed only anti-MuSK antibodies and no anti-AChR antibodies (see Table 2). Overall, among the 18 patients who were tested for the presence of anti-MuSK antibodies, 5 (27.78%) tested positive, including 2 (10.52%) of those with Hispanic ethnicity and 3 (100%) with Asian ethnicity, compared to none (0.0%) in both African American and Caucasian groups ($p = 0.041$; see Table 2).

Ocular MG was present in 8 (18.18%) of the participants, and frequency of ocular MG did not differ significantly among the different ethnicity groups. However, none of the Asian participants were diagnosed with ocular MG (see Table 2). Also, no significant ethnicity based differences were detected for rates of positive anti-AChR antibodies or positive anti-MuSK antibodies for those with ocular MG (see Table 2).

4. Discussion

In this study, we confirmed the existence of ethnicity based differences in gender distribution and serum antibody

TABLE 1: Ethnicity and clinical features in myasthenia gravis.

	Hispanic	African American	Caucasian	Asian	Sig.
Number (%)	19 (43.2%)	16 (36.4%)	6 (13.6%)	3 (6.8%)	N/A
Mean age in years (S.D.)	42.05 (16.02)	48.31 (17.51)	49.67 (11.48)	44.67 (6.51)	$p = 0.610$
Female gender	16 (84.2%)	8 (50.0%)	2 (33.3%)	3 (100%)	**p = 0.029**
Hypertension	7 (36.8%)	6 (37.5%)	3 (50.0%)	0 (0.0%)	$p = 0.822$
Diabetes	2 (10.5%)	2 (12.50%)	0 (0.0%)	0 (0.0%)	$p = 0.862$
Tobacco	0 (0.0%)	2 (12.50%)	0 (0.0%)	0 (0.0%)	$p = 0.585$
Alcohol	1 (5.3%)	3 (18.8%)	1 (16.7%)	0 (0.0%)	$p = 0.658$
Illicit substance	0 (0.0%)	0 (0.0%)	0 (0.0%)	0 (0.0%)	$p = 0.279$
Depression	1 (5.3%)	2 (12.50%)	1 (16.7%)	0 (0.0%)	$p = 0.602$
Anxiety	0 (0.0%)	1 (6.3%)	1 (16.7%)	0 (0.0%)	$p = 0.218$
Thymoma present	6 (31.6%)	2 (12.50%)	2 (33.3%)	0 (0.0%)	$p = 0.381$
Myasthenia Gravis Foundation of America scale score					
1	1 (5.3%)	0 (0.0%)	0 (0.0%)	2 (66.6%)	$p = 0.107$
2a	12 (63.2%)	12 (75.0%)	4 (66.6%)	1 (33.3%)	$p = 0.247$
2b	0 (0.0%)	0 (0.0%)	0 (0.0%)	0 (0.0%)	$p = 0.279$
3a	6 (31.6%)	4 (25.0%)	2 (33.3%)	0 (0.0%)	$p = 0.463$
3b	0 (0.0%)	0 (0.0%)	0 (0.0%)	0 (0.0%)	$p = 0.279$
4	0 (0.0%)	0 (0.0%)	0 (0.0%)	0 (0.0%)	$p = 0.279$
5	0 (0.0%)	0 (0.0%)	0 (0.0%)	0 (0.0%)	$p = 0.279$

TABLE 2: Ethnicity and laboratory features in myasthenia gravis.

	Hispanic	African American	Caucasian	Asian	Sig.
		All myasthenia gravis			
Anti-AChR antibodies positive (%)					
Blocking	10 (52.6%)	6 (37.5%)	2 (33.3%)	0 (0.0%)	**p = 0.059**
Binding	13 (68.4%)	9 (56.3%)	3 (50.0%)	0 (0.0%)	$p = 0.622$
Modulating	7 (36.8%)	5 (31.3%)	3 (50.0%)	0 (0.0%)	$p = 0.877$
Anti-MUSK antibodies positive (%)	2 (10.5%)	0 (0.0%)	0 (0.0%)	3 (100%)	**p = 0.017**
		Generalized myasthenia gravis			
Anti-AChR antibodies positive (%)					
Blocking	7 (46.67%)	5 (38.5%)	2 (40.0%)	0 (0.0%)	$p = 0.514$
Binding	9 (60.0%)	7 (53.9%)	3 (60.0%)	0 (0.0%)	$p = 0.363$
Modulating	4 (26.7%)	4 (30.8%)	2 (40.0%)	0 (0.0%)	$p = 0.391$
MUSK antibodies positive (%)	2 (13.3%)	0 (0.0%)	0 (0.0%)	3 (100%)	**p = 0.041**
		Ocular myasthenia gravis			
Anti-AChR antibodies positive (%)					
Blocking	3 (75.0%)	1 (33.3%)	1 (100%)	n/a	$p = 0.376$
Binding	4 (100%)	2 (66.7%)	0 (0.0%)	n/a	$p = 0.108$
Modulating	3 (75.0%)	1 (33.3%)	1 (100%)	n/a	$p = 0.376$
Anti-MUSK antibodies positive (%)	0 (0.0%)	0 (0.0%)	0 (0.0%)	n/a	n/a

distribution among MG patients. These results support the presence of underlying genetic differences that affect aspects of phenotypic expression in MG, such as anti-AChR antibody type. It is possible that other aspects of the disease may show ethnicity based differences that were not detected in this study due to the small sample size and limited availability of data from patients of several ethnicities. A larger population based study, including data from a more diverse sample of participants, may help to elucidate additional clinical features that are similarly affected by ethnicity or demonstrate further evidence of genetic influences on phenotypic expression in MG.

Previous studies have reported the existence of ethnicity based differences in clinical and laboratory features of MG [5, 7]. A recent report by Oh et al. [7] described racial differences in clinical and laboratory features of MG between

Caucasians and African Americans [7]. As discussed by Oh et al. [7], anti-AChR antibodies were more frequently positive in Caucasians (71%) compared to African Americans (59%). This is in agreement with the results from our sample, where anti-AChR antibodies demonstrated nonsignificant ethnicity related differences and were positive more frequently among Hispanics and Caucasians compared to African Americans and Asians. Their study also reported greater frequency of ocular myasthenia and positive repetitive nerve stimulation testing among African Americans compared to Caucasians, as well as differences in gender and age distributions between Caucasians and African Americans, with Caucasians having greater frequency of male gender and later age of onset [7]. In this study, we confirmed the greater frequency of male gender among Caucasians, but we did not have reliable age of onset information to either confirm or dispute this finding and we did not have information about repetitive nerve stimulation results. Additionally, while we did not detect any statistically significant differences in frequency of ocular MG between ethnicity groups, this may have been due to the small sample size of our study, and while not statistically significant, ocular MG occurred more frequently among those with Hispanic and African American ethnicities compared to Caucasians and Asians.

Anti-MuSK antibodies are also reported to vary between ethnic groups in MG. As discussed by Deymeer et al. [5], they found an overall rate of 49% for MuSK positive antibodies among MG patients, which is greater than the 27.78% rate of MuSK positive antibodies among the patients in this study. Previous reports of ethnicity based variation in MuSK antibodies showed greater frequency of positivity among African Americans (14%) compared to Caucasians (4%); and among patients with seronegative generalized MG the rates were 50% in African Americans and 16.7% in Caucasians [7]. The lower rate of MuSK positivity among Caucasians described in their study [7] also compares well to the rates identified in our study, in which 23.5% of patients overall were found to be MuSK positive, and although the differences were not statistically significant, the rates of MuSK positivity were greater among Hispanic and Asian participants than the Caucasian participants. However, we did not find a greater rate of MuSK positivity among African Americans compared to Caucasians, possibly related to the small sample size of our study.

This study has several limitations. First, the data was obtained exclusively from participants who visited an outpatient clinic and we were not able to obtain data from inpatients who may display more active disease. Consequently, this may have underestimated the true anti-AChR antibody positivity rates. Additionally, antibody positivity rates may have been underestimated due to the cross-sectional study design, since some patients that are initially anti-AChR antibody negative may seroconvert over time. However, these factors would be expected to have affected all ethnicity groups equally, so this is unlikely to have affected the overall results of the study and we feel confident that the ethnicity based differences identified in this study are indeed accurate. Another limitation of this study is the relatively small sample size with limited representation of some ethnicity groups which may have prevented detection of additional ethnicity based differences. Furthermore, clinical features were documented based on self-report and chart review, which also may have contributed to underreporting, especially regarding presence of comorbid psychiatric symptoms and use of tobacco, alcohol, or illicit substances. However, this type of underreporting error would also be expected to have affected all ethnicity groups equally and consequently also would not likely adversely affect the results of the study.

5. Conclusions

The results of this study confirm the existence of ethnicity based differences in clinical and laboratory features of MG. These results suggest a need for further study of genetic and biological factors involved in the pathogenesis of the disease, clinical features, disease course, and response to treatment. Identification of genetic factors underlying ethnicity based differences in clinical and laboratory features of MG may lead to development of new or improved treatments for this disorder and benefit patients of all ethnicities suffering from MG.

Conflict of Interests

The authors declare that they have no conflict of interests or financial support.

References

[1] W. L. Nastuk, O. J. Plescia, and K. E. Osserman, "Changes in serum complement activity in patients with myasthenia gravis," *Proceedings of the Society for Experimental Biology and Medicine*, vol. 105, pp. 177–184, 1960.

[2] L. Padua, E. Stalberg, M. Lomonaco, A. Evoli, A. Batocchi, and P. Tonali, "SFEMG in ocular myasthenia gravis diagnosis," *Clinical Neurophysiology*, vol. 111, no. 7, pp. 1203–1207, 2000.

[3] J. C. Keesey, "Clinical evaluation and management of myasthenia gravis," *Muscle and Nerve*, vol. 29, no. 4, pp. 484–505, 2004.

[4] D. Grob, N. Brunner, T. Namba, and M. Pagala, "Lifetime course of myasthenia gravis," *Muscle and Nerve*, vol. 37, no. 2, pp. 141–149, 2008.

[5] F. Deymeer, O. Gungor-Tuncer, V. Ylmaz et al., "Clinical comparison of anti-MuSK- vs anti-AChR-positive and seronegative myasthenia gravis," *Neurology*, vol. 68, no. 8, pp. 609–611, 2007.

[6] F. Romi, J. A. Aarli, and N. E. Gilhus, "Seronegative myasthenia gravis: disease severity and prognosis," *European Journal of Neurology*, vol. 12, no. 6, pp. 413–418, 2005.

[7] S. J. Oh, M. B. Morgan, L. Lu et al., "Racial differences in myasthenia gravis in Alabama," *Muscle & Nerve*, vol. 39, no. 3, pp. 328–332, 2009.

[8] L. H. Phillips, "The epidemiology of myasthenia gravis," *Seminars in Neurology*, vol. 24, no. 1, pp. 17–20, 2004.

[9] J. C. Keesey, "A history of treatments for myasthenia gravis," *Seminars in Neurology*, vol. 24, no. 1, pp. 5–16, 2004.

[10] S. J. Oh, D. E. Kim, R. Kuruoglu, R. J. Bradley, and D. Dwyer, "Diagnostic sensitivity of the laboratory tests in myasthenia gravis," *Muscle and Nerve*, vol. 15, no. 6, pp. 720–724, 1992.

7

The Role of Decay Accelerating Factor in Environmentally Induced and Idiopathic Systemic Autoimmune Disease

Christopher B. Toomey,[1] David M. Cauvi,[2] and Kenneth M. Pollard[3]

[1] *Department of Ophthalmology, Duke University School of Medicine, Albert Eye Research Institute, Durham, NC 27710, USA*
[2] *Department of Surgery and Center for Investigations of Health and Education Disparities, University of California, San Diego, La Jolla, CA 92037, USA*
[3] *Department of Molecular and Experimental Medicine, The Scripps Research Institute, La Jolla, CA 92037, USA*

Correspondence should be addressed to Kenneth M. Pollard; mpollard@scripps.edu

Academic Editor: Aristo Vojdani

Decay accelerating factor (DAF) plays a complex role in the immune system through complement-dependent and -independent regulation of innate and adaptive immunity. Over the past five years there has been accumulating evidence for a significant role of DAF in negatively regulating adaptive T-cell responses and autoimmunity in both humans and experimental models. This review discusses the relationship between DAF and the complement system and highlights major advances in our understanding of the biology of DAF in human disease, particularly systemic lupus erythematosus. The role of DAF in regulation of idiopathic and environmentally induced systemic autoimmunity is discussed including studies showing that reduction or absence of DAF is associated with autoimmunity. In contrast, DAF-mediated T cell activation leads to cytokine expression consistent with T regulatory cells. This is supported by studies showing that interaction between DAF and its molecular partner, CD97, modifies expression of autoimmunity promoting cytokines. These observations are used to develop a hypothetical model to explain how DAF expression may impact T cell differentiation via interaction with CD97 leading to T regulatory cells, increased production of IL-10, and immune tolerance.

1. Introduction

Decay accelerating factor (DAF) was first described in 1969 in human erythrocytes that inhibited complement activation *in vitro* [1]. (The gene and protein designations used for decay accelerating factor in this paper are *DAF* for the human gene and DAF for the human protein. The mouse genes are *Daf1* and *Daf2* and the protein is DAF1.) However, its biological significance was not appreciated until 1982 when the human protein was isolated and deficiency of DAF was found in patients with paroxysmal nocturnal hemoglobinuria (PNH) [1–3]. The major function of DAF is to protect self-cells from complement-mediated attack by inhibiting the cleavage of C3 and C5, blocking the formation of C3 and C5 convertases, and accelerating their decay [4]. In humans, DAF is expressed as a posttranslationally modified glycosylphosphatidylinositol-(GPI-) anchored molecule [5, 6]. In mice, functionally equivalent, GPI-anchored, and transmembrane-anchored DAF proteins are produced, which are derived from two different genes, *Daf1* and *Daf2*, respectively [7]. *Daf1* is ubiquitously expressed, whereas, *Daf2* is mostly present in the testis and splenic dendritic cells [8]. DAF is also found in soluble form in plasma, cerebrospinal fluid, saliva, synovial fluid, and urine [9]. In humans, *DAF* is encoded by a single gene which maps to q32 on chromosome 1 [10]. It is widely expressed on the surface of all major circulating blood cells as well as epithelial and endothelial cells [9, 11]. Constitutive expression can vary depending on tissue and cell type [8, 12]. In human cells, *DAF* expression is modulated by cytokines such as IL-1, IL-6, TNF-α, TGF-β1, and IFN-γ, prostaglandins, and tissue-specific factors and controlled by the transcription factor SP1 [13–17]. In 1988, DAF was found to be rapidly expressed in T-cells activated by mitogens and *in vitro* stimulation with anti-DAF antibodies led to phosphatidylinositol-specific phospholipase C dependent T-cell proliferation [18]. This led to the hypothesis that an alternative function of DAF may be to regulate T-cell tolerance. Subsequently, DAF has been shown to negatively regulate a variety of autoimmune diseases including animal models of antiglomerular basement membrane glomerulonephritis, experimental autoimmune myasthenia gravis (EAMG), experimental autoimmune encephalomyelitis (EAE), cardiac allograft rejection, and idiopathic and induced models of systemic lupus erythematosus (SLE) [19–24].

2. Complement System and DAF

The complement system is among the oldest evolutionary components of the immune system. It was discovered in 1896 as a heat-labile fraction of serum that led to opsonization of bacteria. Biochemical characterization showed that the complement system is composed of over 30 proteins that function to mediate removal of apoptotic cells and eliminate pathogens. Three separate pathways (i.e., classical, alternative, and lectin pathways) converge to convert C3 to C3 convertase, an enzyme capable of initiating a cascade that results in cell membrane pore formation and subsequent cell lysis known as the membrane attack complex (MAC) (Figure 1). To protect host cells from complement activation four plasma membrane complement regulatory proteins are expressed, CD59 (membrane inhibitor of reactive lysis (MIRL)), CD35 (type 1 complement receptor (CR1)), CD46 (membrane cofactor protein (MCP)), and CD55 (decay accelerating factor (DAF)), that interrupt the complement cascade on self-cells. CD59 blocks MAC complex formation [25], CD35 acts as a cofactor to inactivate C3b and C4b by factor I and interacts with C3b and C4b to promote immune-complex removal [9], and CD46 acts as a cofactor to inactivate C3b and C4b through factor I [9]. DAF inhibits the cleavage of C3 and C5 by blocking the formation of C3 and C5 convertases and accelerating their decay [4]. The original premise of the complement system as a member of the innate immune system, however, was redefined three decades ago when it was shown that complement participates in B- and T-cell responses especially the induction and regulation of type I helper (T_h1) $CD4^+$ T-cell responses [26].

3. DAF in Human Autoimmune Diseases

Deficiency of DAF is found in PNH patients, a GPI linked protein deficiency, which leads to systemic complications particularly through intravascular hemolysis and platelet activation [27–30]. Interestingly, however, it has been reported that DAF (CD55) deletion, also known as the Inab phenotype, hardly alters the sensitivity of cells to lysis by complement and only with inhibition of CD59 does hemolysis occur *in vitro* [31–34]. Deficient expression of the complement regulatory proteins CD55 and CD59 has been found in a variety of human diseases (Table 1) [35–61], however, most prevalently in autoimmune hemocytopenia,

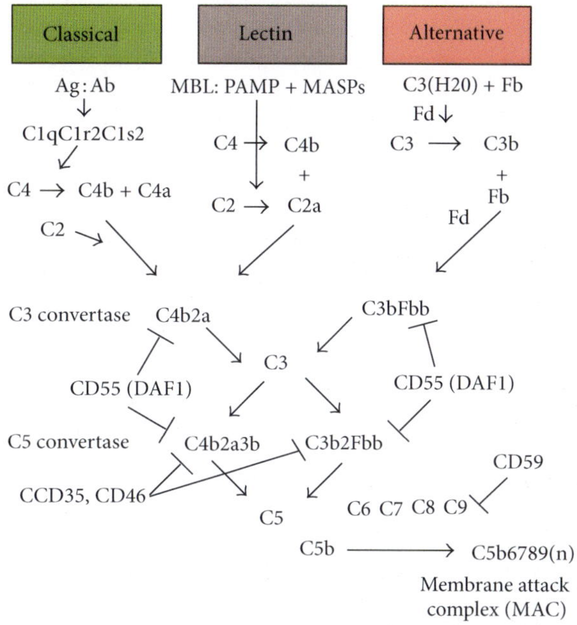

FIGURE 1: Overview of the complement system. Stimulated by antigen : antibody complexes, bacterial cell surfaces, and spontaneous hydrolysis, respectively, the classical, lectin, and alternative pathways converge to convert C3 to C3 convertase, an enzyme capable of initiating a cascade that results in cell membrane pore formation and subsequent cell lysis known as the membrane attack complex (MAC). To protect host cells from complement activation four main plasma membrane complement regulatory proteins are expressed, CD59 (membrane inhibitor of reactive lysis (MIRL)), CD35 (type 1 complement receptor (CR1)), CD46 (membrane cofactor protein, (MCP)), and CD55 (decay accelerating factor (DAF)), that interrupt the complement cascade on self-cells. CD59 blocks MAC complex formation, CD35 acts as a cofactor to inactivate C3b and C4b by factor I, and interacts with C3b and C4b to promote immune-complex removal, CD46 acts as a cofactor to inactivate C3b and C4b through factor I and DAF inhibits the cleavage of C3 and C5 by blocking the formation of C3 and C5 convertases and accelerating their decay. MBL: mannose-binding lectin; MASPs: MBL-associated serine proteases; PAMP: pathogen-associated molecular pattern; Fb: factor B.

autoimmune vasculitis, and other diseases involving dysregulated immune responses [41, 44, 62–68]. It is important to note that deficient expression seen in these diseases does not always mimic the PNH pattern of deficiency on specific cell populations but instead shows decreased expression of all cells, suggesting the nonclonal nature of the deficiency [44].

A paradox exists in SLE where complement activation is associated with tissue injury, yet deficiencies in the early classical complement component pathways predispose to SLE [69, 70]. C1q deficiency due to either gene deletion or anti-C1q autoantibodies has been shown to be related to disease activity; in fact between 53 and 93% of SLE patients have been reported to have low C1q during active disease [71]. This has been reconciled by studies demonstrating the protective role of classical complement pathway components (C1, C2, and C4) in facilitating the clearance of immune complexes as well as autoantigens in apoptotic debris [70, 72]. However,

Table 1: Decreased DAF expression in human disease.

Disease	Cell surface DAF deficiency	Citation
Immune dysregulation		
Sjogren's Syndrome	T-lymphocytes	[36]
SLE with lymphopenia and anemia	T-lymphocytes (CD8+), endothelium, lymphocytes, and anemia	[38, 41, 73]
Psoriatic skin	Epithelium and endothelium	[39]
Systemic sclerosis	Endothelium	[37]
Vasculitic skin lesions	Endothelium	[35]
Recurrent pregnancy loss in aPL	Endometrium	[42]
Autoimmune hemocytopenia	Platelets, lymphocytes, and RBC	[43, 44]
Rheumatoid arthritis	Neutrophils and RBC	[45, 46]
Myasthenia gravis	SNP with decreased expression	[47]
Vitiligo	Whole epidermis	[48]
Asthma	Bronchial epithelial cells and SNP	[49, 50]
Proliferative disorders		
Myelodysplastic syndrome	Granulocytes and RBC	[51, 52]
Plasma cell dyscrasias	RBC	[53]
Lymphoproliferative disorders	RBC	[54]
Anemias		
Anemia of malaria	RBC	[55–59]
Aplastic anemia	RBC	[51]
HIV	RBC, lymphocytes, and PBMC	[60, 61]

RBC: red blood cell; SNP: single-nucleotide polymorphism; aPL: antiphospholipid; PBMC: peripheral blood mononuclear cell.

decreased complement regulatory components on lymphocytes and erythrocytes, including CD55 and CD59, have been shown to be associated with lymphopenia and autoimmune hemolytic anemia (AHIA). In 2003, it was shown that AIHA patients with SLE had decreased levels of DAF compared to SLE patients without AIHA but similar levels to patients with AIHA but without SLE [73]. No correlation was seen, however, between IgG or IgM antiphospholipid antibodies [73]. In a follow-up study an analysis of 40 SLE patients with and without lymphopenia showed that mean fluorescence intensities (MFI) of CD55 and CD59 were diminished on T- and B-cells in lymphopenic patients compared to nonlymphopenic patients [41]. These results were unrelated to disease activity [41]. In two recent studies Alegretti et al. conducted a peripheral blood flow cytometric analysis of SLE patients and healthy controls [67, 68]. They found a decrease in the percent of DAF high peripheral lymphocytes and decreased DAF MFI in peripheral lymphocytes in patients with lymphopenia; however, no difference was seen in non-lymphopenic SLE patients compared to controls [67, 68]. Mean DAF levels were also shown to be decreased on red blood cells and granulocytes but not on monocytes; however, no relationship between disease activity and DAF lymphocyte levels was seen [67, 68]. Collectively, these studies suggest a role for complement regulatory proteins in the pathophysiology of a subset of SLE patients with lymphopenia and AIHA. The most plausible explanation is antibody-dependent cellular cytotoxicity and complement-mediated cell lysis which would explain the correlation between reduced CD55 and CD59 in AIHA and lymphopenic SLE populations. An alternative hypothesis that decreased CD55 lymphocyte levels predispose a subset of SLE patients to lymphopenia should not be ignored.

Not nearly as many studies have investigated the relationship between DAF and other systemic autoimmune diseases. One study found that percentages of DAF negative $CD4^+$ and $CD8^+$ T-cell subsets were higher in Sjogren's Syndrome (SS) patients [36]. The DAF expression observed in other circulating blood cells was not changed [36]. However, these results were not thought to be due to increases in DAF low cells but rather a decrease in DAF high cells [36]. In patients with systemic sclerosis (Scleroderma or SSc), DAF was found to be decreased or undetectable in endothelium of both lesional skin and nonlesional skin compared to controls [37]. Interestingly this result was later reproduced in morphea lesions, suggesting a link between systemic autoimmune disease skin lesions and low DAF levels, although low DAF levels are also seen in psoriatic skin lesions [38, 39]. These studies, however, are limited by their power and lack of supporting follow-up studies.

4. DAF in Animal Models of Systemic Autoimmune Disease

DAF1 has been shown to play a role in the maintenance of immune tolerance in mouse models of autoimmune disease. Deletion of *Daf1* was shown to increase susceptibility to antiglomerular basement membrane disease and to markedly enhance susceptibility in a mouse model of myasthenia gravis [20, 23]. This increased susceptibility was later shown to result from the influence of DAF1 on T-cell hypersensitivity, when it was demonstrated that $Daf1^{-/-}$ T-cells displayed a C3 dependent enhanced response to antigen restimulation resulting in increased IFN-γ [24, 74, 75]. Similar results were found in MRL-Fas^{lpr} mice, an idiopathic SLE model, where deletion of *Daf1* resulted in exacerbated lymphadenopathy and splenomegaly, increased serum antichromatin autoantibody, and aggravated dermatitis [21]. In a follow-up study it was shown that, aside from local skin inflammation, these effects were largely complement independent [76].

These observations stimulated us to investigate the role of DAF1 in murine mercury-induced autoimmunity (mHgIA). Mice exposed to mercury develop lymphadenopathy, hypergammaglobulinemia, humoral autoimmunity, and immune-complex disease, which are consistent with the systemic features observed in SLE [77, 78]. All forms of inorganic mercury tested, including $HgCl_2$, vapor, or dental amalgam, elicit the same disease [79–81] as do different routes of administration [82, 83]. Sensitivity to mHgIA is influenced by both MHC and non-MHC genes and covers the spectrum from nonresponsiveness to overt systemic autoimmunity [82, 84–86]. Disease expression is influenced by TCR costimulatory molecules including CD28 and CD40L [87, 88], proinflammatory cytokines, including IFN-γ [80, 89] and IL-6 [90], and modulators of innate immunity, including endosomal Toll-like receptors (TLR) [91, 92], demonstrating that multiple checkpoints and pathways are implicated in the regulation of the disease. In addition lupus prone strains exhibit accelerated and more severe systemic autoimmunity following mercury exposure [93–95]. Environmental factors have been associated with systemic autoimmune diseases in humans [96, 97]. Exposure to mercury has been implicated as an environmental trigger in the induction of autoimmunity [98–100] including production of autoantibodies and proinflammatory cytokines, such as IL-1β, TNF-α, and IFN-γ [101], and membranous nephropathy [102].

We found that autoimmune-prone NZB mice had low endogenous levels of DAF1 while mHgIA-resistant DBA/2 animals have high endogenous levels [103]. Furthermore, we showed that induction of mHgIA in B10.S mice was associated with reduction of DAF1 on activated $CD4^+$ T cells [103]. Both these observations, reduction of DAF1 in autoimmune-prone mice and reduction upon induction of mHgIA, support the argument that DAF1 is required to maintain immune tolerance. In a follow-up study the absence of *Daf1* in C57BL/6 mice was shown to cause increased serum autoantibodies and exacerbated hypergammaglobulemia following mercury exposure (Table 2) [19]. This response, however, could not be explained by increased T-cell activation but rather was explained by increased levels of IFN-γ, IL-2, IL-4, and IL-10 (Table 2) [19]. Furthermore, depletion of C3 was found to have no major effects on development of mHgIA suggesting that the role of DAF1 in mHgIA is independent of an intact complement system [104]. This is supported by results showing that C3 levels are not affected following mercury exposure of mHgIA sensitive or resistant strains (Pollard, unpublished results). Thus our findings and those of others [76] suggest that DAF1 may regulate idiopathic and induced models of systemic autoimmunity in a complement-independent fashion.

Table 2: Effect of *Daf1* deletion on mHgIA*.

Serum autoantibodies	
ANA	↑↑↑
AntiChromatin abs	↑↑↑
Serum immunoglobulins	
IgG	↑
IgG1	NC
IgG2a	NC
T-cell activation	
$CD4^+CD44^{high}$	NC
Cytokines	
IFN-γ	↑
IL-4	↑
IL-2	↑
IL-10	↑
IL-17	NC
IL-22	NC
TGF-β	NC

*Data from Toomey et al., 2010 [19].
↑: $P < 0.05$; ↑↑↑: $P < 0.0001$; NC: no change.

5. How Does DAF1 Regulate Immune Tolerance?

Several models of systemic autoimmunity exhibit disease independent of an intact complement system, yet an exacerbated phenotype is observed by DAF1 deletion [19, 21, 76, 104, 105]. This suggests that complement-independent effects of DAF1 are the major contributors to tolerance induction via the interaction of DAF (CD55) with its natural ligand, CD97. CD97 is a member of the epidermal growth factor-like, seven span transmembrane (EGF-TM7) family of proteins, is expressed on macrophages, granulocytes, dendritic cells, and smooth muscle cells, and is rapidly upregulated on activated T- and B-cells [106, 107]. In the mouse alternative RNA splicing produces two isoforms with three or four epidermal growth factor-like (EGF) domains (namely CD97(EGF1,2,4) and CD97(EGF1,2,3,4)) and a third isoform with a protein module inserted between EGF domains 2 and 3 (namely, CD97(EGF1,2,X,3,4)) [108]. DAF (CD55) binds to both CD97(EGF1,2,4) and CD97(EGF1,2,3,4) but not to CD97(EGF1,2,X,3,4) [108].

Structural studies of a model of the CD55-CD97 complex reveal that the sites of interaction of CD97 and complement components occur on opposite faces of CD55 arguing that CD55 can bind to CD97 and complement independently [106]. Activation of human $CD4^+$ T cells in the presence of anti-CD3 and recombinant CD97 (rCD97) results in increased IL-10 production that is IL-2 dependent [109]. Costimulation of naïve human $CD4^+$ T-cells via interaction

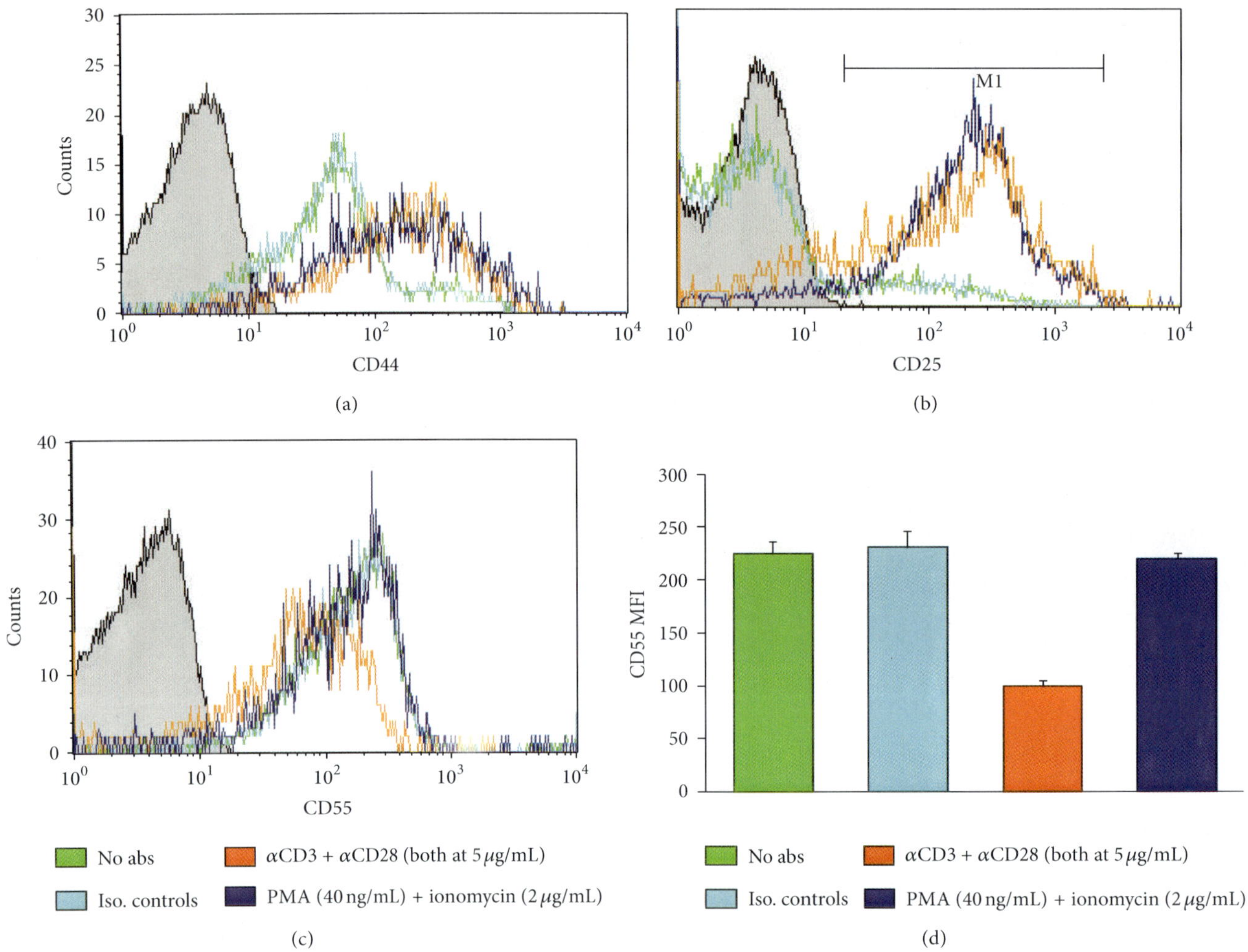

FIGURE 2: Anti-CD3/anti-CD28 but not phorbol 12-myristate 13-acetate (PMA)/ionomycin lowers CD55 expression of $CD4^+$ T-cells. Lymph node cells from B10.S mice were cultured with no additives (green), Ig isotype controls (light blue), anti-CD3/anti-CD28 (5 μg/mL each) (orange), or phorbol 12-myristate 13-acetate (PMA) (40 ng/mL) and ionomycin (2 μg/mL) (dark blue). Cells were incubated at 37°C and 5% CO_2 for 72 hr and then analyzed by flow cytometry to determine activation status ($CD44^{hi}$, $CD25^{hi}$) and then CD55 expression of activated cells. $n = 4$/group.

of CD97/CD55 leads to T regulatory type 1 (Tr1) activation, expansion, and function [110]. Antibody mediated blockade of CD97-CD55 interaction inhibits proliferation and IFN-γ production [106]. These properties of CD97-CD55 costimulation, particularly IL-2 dependent IL-10, are consistent with stimulation of human $CD4^+$ T cells by another complement regulatory protein, CD46. Activation via CD3/CD46 induces a T_h1 phenotype with significant IFN-γ production [111]. However in the presence of IL-2, immunoregulatory IL-10 is produced resulting in a T regulatory phenotype [111, 112] capable of suppressing antigen-specific T cells [113]. We hypothesize that the immunosuppressive potential of CD55 [24, 75] lies in its interaction with CD97 leading to a T regulatory cell phenotype under appropriate conditions of increasing IL-2, as would happen in an inflammatory response [114]. Thus, like CD46 activation, CD97 mediated activation of CD55 acts to switch T_h1 effector $CD4^+$ T cells toward IL-10 producing immunosuppressive cells [112]. We have shown that activation of murine $CD4^+$ T cells with anti-CD3 and rCD97 leads to a cytokine profile with increased IL-10 and reduced IL-17 and IL-21 compared to a more proinflammatory profile of elevated IFN-γ, IL-2, IL-4, IL-10, IL-17, and IL-21 elicited by conventional costimulation by anti-CD3/anti-CD28 [19]. Increased IL-10 and reduced IFN-γ and IL-17 suggest that rCD97 may be driving T cells to differentiate into T regulatory cells rather than autoimmune promoting T_h1 and T_h17 cells, but it remains to be determined whether rCD97 activated $CD4^+$ T cells have immunoregulatory activity.

Our previous studies had established that activated $CD4^+$ T cells have reduced CD55 expression [103, 115]. However it was unclear if conventional activation of $CD4^+$ T cells with anti-CD3/anti-CD28 could mimic the *in vivo* reduction of CD55 in idiopathic SLE or mHgIA [103].

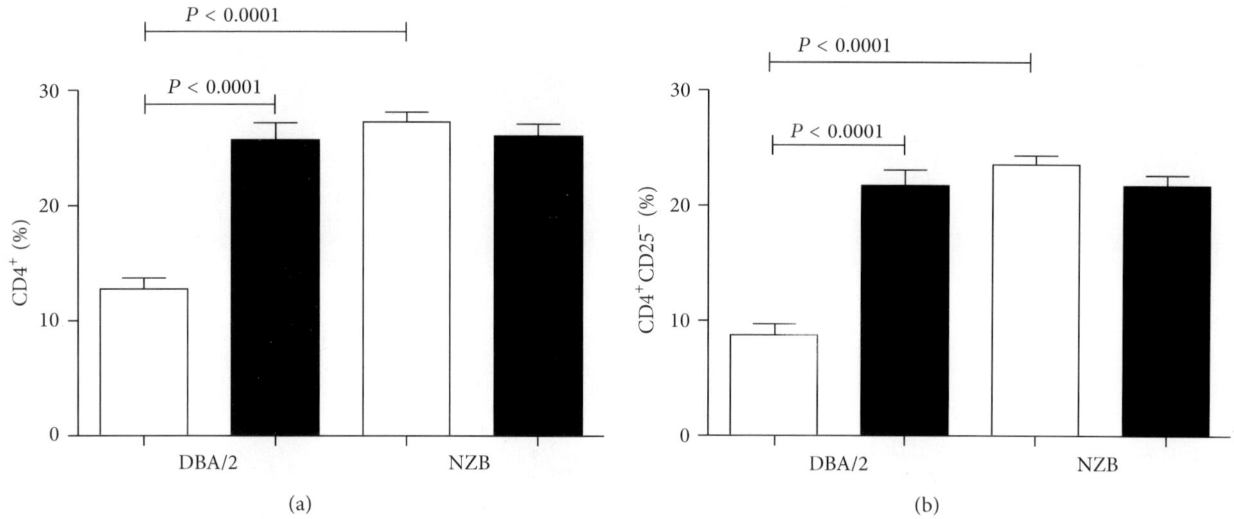

Figure 3: $CD4^+$ T-cell expansion in mHgIA-resistant DBA/2 consists of CD25 negative cells. NZB and DBA/2 mice were exposed to PBS (white bar) or $HgCl_2$ (black bar) for 5 weeks. Splenocytes were then cultured in the presence of PMA/ionomycin and analyzed for percent $CD4^+$ T cells (a) and $CD4^+CD25^-$ T cells (b). Percentages represent cells in total spleen cells. $n = 4$/group.

Experimental comparison between anti-CD3/anti-CD28 and PMA/ionomycin activation (Figure 2) revealed that anti-CD3/anti-CD28 activation does indeed reduce CD55 expression of $CD4^+$ T-cells by about 50% in B10.S mice which is very similar to the reduction found in mercury-exposed B10.S mice and constitutively in autoimmune prone NZB mice [103]. Unexpectedly, PMA/ionomycin activation of $CD4^+$ T cells did not affect CD55 expression (Figure 2) indicating that direct intracellular signaling of protein kinase C (PKC) does not impact CD55 expression and that CD55 reduction is mediated by events occurring at the cell surface. Whether $CD4^+$ T cell activation in the presence of anti-CD3/rCD97 also reduces CD55 remains to be determined.

The increased expression of IL-10 in human and murine $CD4^+$ T cells stimulated by anti-CD3 and rCD97 [19, 109] suggests a regulatory T-cell phenotype [110, 116, 117]. As CD55 is required for this response, we asked whether a difference in CD55 expression might affect the generation of regulatory T cells. NZB and DBA/2 mice have reduced and elevated CD55, respectively, and exposure to $HgCl_2$ exacerbates autoimmunity in NZB while DBA/2 mice are resistant [103]. Thus regulatory T cells may be more common in DBA/2 than NZB mice. To examine this possibility NZB and DBA/2 mice were exposed to $HgCl_2$ and splenocytes were then cultured *in vitro* in the presence of PMA/ionomycin and analyzed for the presence of markers of T regulatory type 1 (Tr1) ($CD4^+CD25^-IL\text{-}10^+IL\text{-}4^-$) cells [118]. This protocol increased $CD4^+$ T cells in $HgCl_2$ exposed DBA/2 mice but not in NZB mice (Figure 3(a)). This was an unexpected finding given that DBA/2 mice are resistant to mHgIA, however these cells were primarily of the $CD4^+CD25^-$ type (Figure 3(b)) indicating that they were not conventionally activated $CD4^+$ T cells which can express CD25 [103]. $CD4^+CD25^-$ T cells were then examined for expression of both IL-10 and IL-4 to identify Tr1-like cells (Figure 4). In total spleen, Tr1-like cells were dramatically increased following $HgCl_2$ in DBA/2 mice but were reduced in NZB mice (Figure 4(a)). A similar situation was found when only $CD4^+$ cells in the spleen were analyzed (Figure 4(b)). Finally we asked what percentage of $CD4^+CD25^-$ cells were $IL\text{-}10^+IL\text{-}4^-$ and found that the vast majority in the DBA/2 mice possessed the cytokine phenotype of T regulatory cells while such cells were much fewer in number in the NZB mice (Figure 4(c)). The greater percentage of putative Tr1 cells in PBS treated DBA/2 mice compared to NZB mice and the changing percentages of Tr1-like cells following mercury exposure are consistent with the sensitivity of these strains to mercury-induced autoimmunity. We hypothesize that the constitutively reduced CD55 expression in NZB mice [103] reduces CD55-CD97 interaction and the generation of Tr1 cells but favors T_h1 responses. In contrast, DBA/2 mice, with a higher level of CD55 that is not impacted by mercury exposure [103], are able to maintain a higher level of CD55-CD97 interaction which favors regulatory T-cell generation and tolerance to mHgIA.

Our hypothesis is supported by studies comparing CD28 and CD55 mediated T cell activation. CD28 and GPI-anchored proteins, like DAF1, exist in detergent-resistant microdomains or lipid rafts, and their engagement leads to redistribution and clustering at the site of the T cell receptor (TCR) [119]. Moreover, CD28 cross-linking leads to the formation of lipid raft clusters which exclude CD55 and vice versa [120]. It has also been argued that recruitment and crosslinking of GPI-anchored proteins, such as CD55, are less efficient at T cell activation than that elicited by crosslinking of CD28 [119–121]. These observations raise the possibility that the cell surface density of DAF influences T cell activation by competing with other costimulatory molecules. Thus reduced levels of DAF favor more efficient T cell activation via CD28 crosslinking (Figure 5). Conversely increasing the surface density of DAF1 would affect the effectiveness of CD28-mediated T cell activation. This supports observations

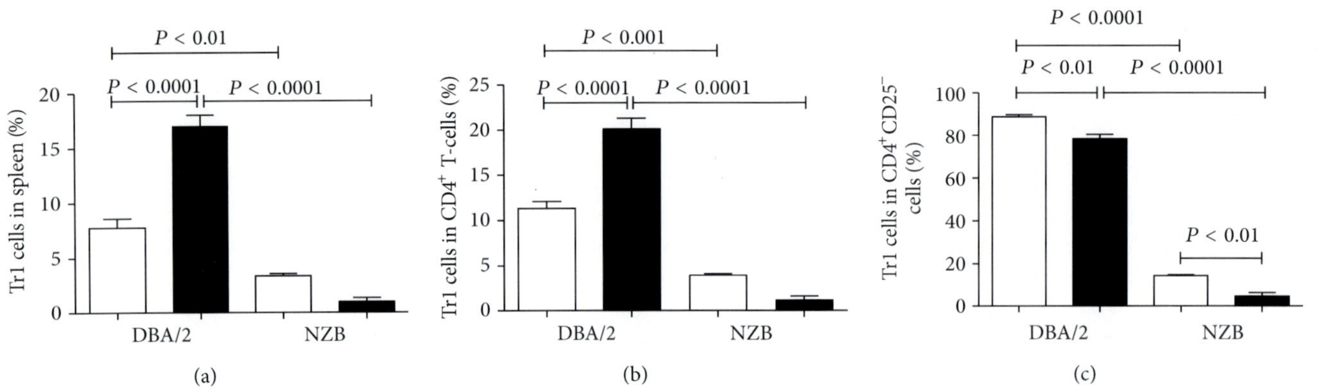

FIGURE 4: $CD4^+CD25^-$ T cells in mHgIA-resistant DBA/2 possess the cytokine phenotype of regulatory T-cells. NZB and DBA/2 mice were exposed to PBS (white bar) or $HgCl_2$ (black bar) for 5 weeks. Splenocytes were then cultured in the presence of PMA/ionomycin and $CD4^+CD25^-$ T-cells analyzed for the cytokine phenotype of $IL\text{-}10^+IL\text{-}4^-$ (Trl cells). (a) shows the percent of Trl cells in total spleen. (b) shows the percent of Trl cells in $CD4^+$ cells. (c) shows the percent of Trl cells in $CD4^+CD25^-$ cells. $n = 4$/group.

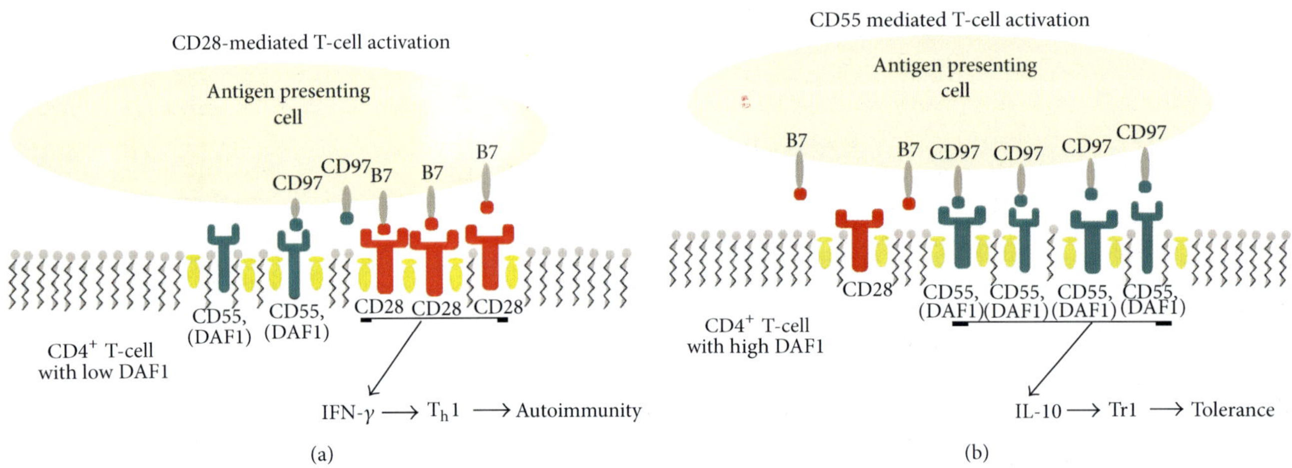

FIGURE 5: Hypothetical DAF function during T-cell costimulation. Conventional T-cell activation via CD28 cross-linking leads to the formation of lipid raft clusters which exclude CD55 (a) resulting in proinflammatory (i.e., IFN-γ) cytokine production which, under suitable conditions, may lead to T_h1-mediated autoimmunity such as mHgIA. Conversely, increasing the surface density of DAF leads to less efficient CD28-mediated T cell activation (b) and in the presence of CD97 potentiates CD55 signaling leading to increased production of IL-10, a T regulatory cell phenotype and immune tolerance.

by us [19] and others [109] that preferential costimulation via CD28 elicits a different cytokine profile than that produced by costimulation via DAF1 (CD55).

6. Conclusion

DAF serves a complex role in the immune system through complement-dependent and -independent functions in the regulation of innate and adaptive immunity. Initial reports on DAF1 in systemic autoimmune disease models suggested that it played a role in regulating adaptive immune responses. In the context of mHgIA our lab has shown that (1) DAF1 is constitutively reduced in mice prone to systemic autoimmune disease, (2) mHgIA is associated with reduced DAF1 expression on T-cells, and (3) interaction of DAF1 with its natural ligand, CD97, can regulate cytokine expression. These results suggest that understanding how mercury exposure reduces DAF1 expression may lead to approaches to regulate DAF in SLE. Evidence in patients shows that decreased levels of DAF on lymphocytes are associated with lymphopenia in SLE as well as in T cells of SS and the endothelial skin lesions of SLE, SSc, and other vasculitic diseases. DAF1 has both complement-dependent and- independent effects by regulating T-cell pro-inflammatory cytokine production *in vivo*. In systemic autoimmune disease models, such as mHgIA, complement-independent effects of DAF1 appear to be the major contributors regulating disease. Based on our mHgIA studies, we hypothesize that CD55 : CD97 interaction at the immunological synapse can regulate CD28 crosslinking and promote a Trl-like phenotype, either by direct CD55 signal transduction or possibly through blocking of CD28 costimulation, and expression of a Treg cytokine profile.

Conflict of Interests

The authors declare that there is no conflict of interests regarding the publication of this paper.

Acknowledgments

This work was supported by NIH Research Grants ES014847, ES020388, and ES021464. This is publication number 25088 from The Scripps Research Institute.

References

[1] E. M. Hoffmann, "Inhibition of complement by a substance isolated from human erythrocytes—I. Extraction from human erythrocyte stromata," *Immunochemistry*, vol. 6, no. 3, pp. 391–403, 1969.

[2] A. Nicholson-Weller, D. B. Spicer, and K. F. Austen, "Deficiency of the complement regulatory protein, "decay-accelerating factor", on membranes of granulocytes, monocytes, and platelets in paroxysmal nocturnal hemoglobinuria," *The New England Journal of Medicine*, vol. 312, no. 17, pp. 1091–1097, 1985.

[3] A. Nicholson-Weller, J. Burge, D. T. Fearon, P. F. Weller, and K. F. Austen, "Isolation of a human erythrocyte membrane glycoprotein with decay-accelerating activity for C3 convertases of the complement system," *Journal of Immunology*, vol. 129, no. 1, pp. 184–189, 1982.

[4] D. M. Lublin and J. P. Atkinson, "Decay-accelerating factor: biochemistry, molecular biology, and function," *Annual Review of Immunology*, vol. 7, pp. 35–58, 1989.

[5] M. E. Medof, E. I. Walter, W. L. Roberts, R. Haas, and T. L. Rosenberry, "Decay accelerating factor of complement is anchored to cells by a C-terminal glycolipid," *Biochemistry*, vol. 25, no. 22, pp. 6740–6747, 1986.

[6] M. A. Davitz, M. G. Low, and V. Nussenzweig, "Release of decay-accelerating factor (DAF) from the cell membrane by phosphatidylinositol-specific phospholipase C (PIPLC). Selective modification of a complement regulatory protein," *Journal of Experimental Medicine*, vol. 163, no. 5, pp. 1150–1161, 1986.

[7] D. M. Lublin and K. E. Coyne, "Phospholipid-anchored and transmembrane versions of either decay-accelerating factor or membrane cofactor protein show equal efficiency in protection from complement-mediated cell damage," *Journal of Experimental Medicine*, vol. 174, no. 1, pp. 35–44, 1991.

[8] F. Lin, Y. Fukuoka, A. Spicer et al., "Tissue distribution of products of the mouse decay-accelerating factor (DAF) genes. Exploitation of a Daf1 knock-out mouse and site-specific monoclonal antibodies," *Immunology*, vol. 104, no. 2, pp. 215–225, 2001.

[9] M. E. Medof, E. I. Walter, J. L. Rutgers, D. M. Knowles, and V. Nussenzweig, "Identification of the complement decay-accelerating factor (DAF) on epithelium and glandular cells and in body fluids," *Journal of Experimental Medicine*, vol. 165, no. 3, pp. 848–864, 1987.

[10] T. W. Post, M. A. Arce, M. K. Liszewski, E. S. Thompson, J. P. Atkinson, and D. M. Lublin, "Structure of the gene for human complement protein decay accelerating factor," *Journal of Immunology*, vol. 144, no. 2, pp. 740–744, 1990.

[11] A. Nicholson-Weller, J. P. March, and C. E. Rosen, "Surface membrane expression by human blood leukocytes and platelets of decay-accelerating factor, a regulatory protein of the complement system," *Blood*, vol. 65, no. 5, pp. 1237–1244, 1985.

[12] D. J. Thomas and D. M. Lublin, "Identification of 5′-flanking regions affecting the expression of the human decay accelerating factor gene and their role in tissue-specific expression," *Journal of Immunology*, vol. 150, no. 1, pp. 151–160, 1993.

[13] D. M. Cauvi, G. Cauvi, and K. M. Pollard, "Constitutive expression of murine decay-accelerating factor 1 is controlled by the transcription factor Sp1," *Journal of Immunology*, vol. 177, no. 6, pp. 3837–3847, 2006.

[14] O. B. Spiller, O. Criado-Garcia, S. R. de Cordoba, and B. P. Morgan, "Cytokine-mediated up-regulation of CD55 and CD59 protects human hepatoma cells from complement attack," *Clinical and Experimental Immunology*, vol. 121, no. 2, pp. 234–241, 2000.

[15] E. T. Cocuzzi, D. Bardenstyein, A. Stavitsky, N. Sudarraj, and M. E. Medof, "Upregulation of DAF (CD55) on orbital fibroblasts by cytokines. Differential effects of TNF-β and TNF-α," *Current Eye Research*, vol. 23, no. 2, pp. 86–92, 2001.

[16] S. R. Ahmad, E. A. Lidington, R. Ohta et al., "Decay-accelerating factor induction by tumour necrosis factor-α, through a phosphatidylinositol-3 kinase and protein kinase C-dependent pathway, protects murine vascular endothelial cells against complement deposition," *Immunology*, vol. 110, no. 2, pp. 258–268, 2003.

[17] V. R. Holla, D. Wang, J. R. Brown, J. R. Mann, S. Katkuri, and R. N. DuBois, "Prostaglandin E2 regulates the complement inhibitor CD55/decay-accelerating factor in colorectal cancer," *The Journal of Biological Chemistry*, vol. 280, no. 1, pp. 476–483, 2005.

[18] L. S. Davis, S. S. Patel, J. P. Atkinson, and P. E. Lipsky, "Decay-accelerating factor functions as a signal transducing molecule for human T cells," *Journal of Immunology*, vol. 141, no. 7, pp. 2246–2252, 1988.

[19] C. B. Toomey, D. M. Cauvi, W. Song, and K. M. Pollard, "Decay-accelerating factor 1 (Daf1) deficiency exacerbates xenobiotic-induced autoimmunity," *Immunology*, vol. 131, no. 1, pp. 99–106, 2010.

[20] H. Sogabe, M. Nangaku, Y. Ishibashi et al., "Increased susceptibility of decay-accelerating factor deficient mice to anti-glomerular basement membrane glomerulonephritis," *Journal of Immunology*, vol. 167, no. 5, pp. 2791–2797, 2001.

[21] T. Miwa, M. A. Maldonado, L. Zhou et al., "Deletion of decay-accelerating factor (CD55) exacerbates autoimmune disease development in MRL/lpr mice," *The American Journal of Pathology*, vol. 161, no. 3, pp. 1077–1086, 2002.

[22] J. Liu, F. Lin, M. G. Strainic et al., "IFN-γ and IL-17 production in experimental autoimmune encephalomyelitis depends on local APC-T cell complement production," *Journal of Immunology*, vol. 180, no. 9, pp. 5882–5889, 2008.

[23] F. Lin, H. J. Kaminski, B. M. Conti-Fine, W. Wang, C. Richmonds, and M. E. Medof, "Markedly enhanced susceptibility to experimental autoimmune myasthenia gravis in the absence of decay-accelerating factor protection," *Journal of Clinical Investigation*, vol. 110, no. 9, pp. 1269–1274, 2002.

[24] J. Liu, T. Miwa, B. Hilliard et al., "The complement inhibitory protein DAF (CD55) suppresses T cell immunity in vivo," *Journal of Experimental Medicine*, vol. 201, no. 4, pp. 567–577, 2005.

[25] D. D. Kim and W. C. Song, "Membrane complement regulatory proteins," *Clinical Immunology*, vol. 118, no. 2-3, pp. 127–136, 2006.

[26] M. Kolev, G. Le Friec, and C. Kemper, "The role of complement in CD4+ T cell homeostasis and effector functions," *Seminars in Immunology*, vol. 25, no. 1, pp. 12–19, 2013.

[27] P. Hillmen, J. M. Hows, and L. Luzzatto, "Two distinct patterns of glycosylphosphatidylinositol (GPI) linked protein deficiency in the red cells of patients with paroxysmal nocturnal haemoglobinuria," *The British Journal of Haematology*, vol. 80, no. 3, pp. 399–405, 1992.

[28] T. Masuda, Y. Yonemura, K. Fujimoto et al., "Establishment of a human T-cell line with deficient surface expression of glycosylphosphatidylinositol (GPI)-anchored proteins from a patient with paroxysmal nocturnal haemoglobinuria," *The British Journal of Haematology*, vol. 87, no. 1, pp. 24–30, 1994.

[29] J. Schubert, P. Uciechowski, P. Delany, H. J. Tischler, W. Kolanus, and R. E. Schmidt, "The PIG-anchoring defect in NK lymphocytes of PNH patients," *Blood*, vol. 76, no. 6, pp. 1181–1187, 1990.

[30] A. Hill, R. Kelly, and P. Hillmen, "Thrombosis in paroxysmal nocturnal hemoglobinuria," *Blood*, vol. 121, no. 25, pp. 4985–4996, 2013.

[31] M. E. Medof, A. Gottlieb, T. Kinoshita et al., "Relationship between decay accelerating factor deficiency, diminished acetylcholinesterase activity, and defective terminal complement pathway restriction in paroxymal nocturnal hemoglobinuria erythrocytes," *Journal of Clinical Investigation*, vol. 80, no. 1, pp. 165–174, 1987.

[32] M. E. Reid, G. Mallinson, R. B. Sim et al., "Biochemical studies on red blood cells from a patient with the Inab phenotype (decay-accelerating factor deficiency)," *Blood*, vol. 78, no. 12, pp. 3291–3297, 1991.

[33] M. J. Telen and A. M. Green, "The Inab phenotype: characterization of the membrane protein and complement regulatory defect," *Blood*, vol. 74, no. 1, pp. 437–441, 1989.

[34] G. L. Daniels, C. A. Green, G. Mallinson et al., "Decay-accelerating factor (CD55) deficiency phenotypes in Japanese," *Transfusion Medicine*, vol. 8, no. 2, pp. 141–147, 1998.

[35] B. W. Boom, A. M. Mommaas, M. R. Daha, and B. J. Vermeer, "Decreased expression of decay-accelerating factor on endothelial cells of immune complex-mediated vasculitic skin lesions," *Journal of Dermatological Science*, vol. 2, no. 4, pp. 308–315, 1991.

[36] Y. Ichikawa, A. Masumoto, M. Yoshida et al., "Decay-accelerating factor (DAF, CD55)-negative T lymphocytes in the peripheral blood of Sjogren's syndrome patients," *Tokai Journal of Experimental and Clinical Medicine*, vol. 21, no. 3, pp. 121–128, 1996.

[37] G. T. Venneker, F. H. J. van den Hoogen, A. M. T. Boerbooms, J. D. Bos, and S. S. Asghar, "Aberrant expression of membrane cofactor protein and decay-accelerating factor in the endothelium of patients with systemic sclerosis: a possible mechanism of vascular damage," *Laboratory Investigation*, vol. 70, no. 6, pp. 830–835, 1994.

[38] G. T. Venneker, P. K. Das, B. Naafs, A. J. Tigges, J. D. Bos, and S. S. Asghar, "Morphoea lesions are associated with aberrant expression of membrane cofactor protein and decay accelerating factor in vascular endothelium," *The British Journal of Dermatology*, vol. 131, no. 2, pp. 237–242, 1994.

[39] G. T. Venneker, P. K. Das, M. M. H. M. Meinardi et al., "Glycosylphosphatidylinositol (GPI)-anchored membrane proteins are constitutively down-regulated in psoriatic skin," *Journal of Pathology*, vol. 172, no. 2, pp. 189–197, 1994.

[40] Y. Richaud-Patin, J. Piedras, E. Carrillo-Maravilla, X. López-Karpovitch, and L. Llorente, "CD8+ chronic lymphocytic leukemia: an extensive characterization of a bizarre hybrid neoplasia," *European Journal of Haematology*, vol. 71, no. 3, pp. 224–230, 2003.

[41] I. García-Valladares, Y. Atisha-Fregoso, Y. Richaud-Patin et al., "Diminished expression of complement regulatory proteins (CD55 and CD59) in lymphocytes from systemic lupus erythematosus patients with lymphopenia," *Lupus*, vol. 15, no. 9, pp. 600–605, 2006.

[42] J. Francis, R. Rai, N. J. Sebire et al., "Impaired expression of endometrial differentiation markers and complement regulatory proteins in patients with recurrent pregnancy loss associated with antiphospholipid syndrome," *Molecular Human Reproduction*, vol. 12, no. 7, pp. 435–442, 2006.

[43] B. Zupanska, I. Bogdanik, J. Fabijanska-Mitek, and H. Pyl, "Autoimmune haemolytic anaemia with a paroxysmal nocturnal haemoglobinuria-like defect," *European Journal of Haematology*, vol. 62, no. 5, pp. 346–349, 1999.

[44] A. Ruiz-Argüelles and L. Llorente, "The role of complement regulatory proteins (CD55 and CD59) in the pathogenesis of autoimmune hemocytopenias," *Autoimmunity Reviews*, vol. 6, no. 3, pp. 155–161, 2007.

[45] J. Jones, I. Laffafian, A. M. Cooper, B. D. Williams, and B. P. Morgan, "Expression of complement regulatory molecules and other surface markers on neutrophils from synovial fluid and blood of patients with rheumatoid arthritis," *The British Journal of Rheumatology*, vol. 33, no. 8, pp. 707–712, 1994.

[46] M. Arora, A. Kumar, S. N. Das, and L. M. Srivastava, "Complement-regulatory protein expression and activation of complement cascade on erythrocytes from patients with rheumatoid arthritis (RA)," *Clinical and Experimental Immunology*, vol. 111, no. 1, pp. 102–106, 1998.

[47] J. M. Heckmann, H. Uwimpuhwe, R. Ballo, M. Kaur, V. B. Bajic, and S. Prince, "A functional SNP in the regulatory region of the decay-accelerating factor gene associates with extraocular muscle pareses in myasthenia gravis," *Genes and Immunity*, vol. 11, no. 1, pp. 1–10, 2010.

[48] R. M. J. G. J. van den Wijngaard, S. S. Asghar, A. C. L. M. Pijnenborg, A. J. Tigges, W. Westerhof, and P. K. Das, "Aberrant expression of complement regulatory proteins, membrane cofactor protein and decay accelerating factor, in the involved epidermis of patients with vitiligo," *The British Journal of Dermatology*, vol. 146, no. 1, pp. 80–87, 2002.

[49] A. Agrawal, A. Sinha, T. Ahmad et al., "Maladaptation of critical cellular functions in asthma: bioinformatic analysis," *Physiological Genomics*, vol. 40, no. 1, pp. 1–7, 2009.

[50] T. Kawai, S. Takeshita, Y. Imoto et al., "Associations between decay-accelerating factor polymorphisms and allergic respiratory diseases," *Clinical and Experimental Allergy*, vol. 39, no. 10, pp. 1508–1514, 2009.

[51] J. Meletis, E. Terpos, M. Samarkos et al., "Detection of CD55 and/or CD59 deficient red cell populations in patients with aplastic anaemia, myelodysplastic syndromes and myeloproliferative disorders," *Haematologia*, vol. 31, no. 1, pp. 7–16, 2001.

[52] G. Kaiafa, A. Papadopoulos, G. Ntaios et al., "Detection of CD55- and CD59-deficient granulocytic populations in patients with myelodysplastic syndrome," *Annals of Hematology*, vol. 87, no. 4, pp. 257–262, 2008.

[53] J. Meletis, E. Terpos, M. Samarkos et al., "Detection of CD55- and/or CD59-deficient red cell populations in patients with plasma cell dyscrasias," *International Journal of Hematology*, vol. 75, no. 1, pp. 40–44, 2002.

[54] J. Meletis, E. Terpos, M. Samarkos et al., "Detection of CD55- and/or CD59-deficient red cell populations in patients with lymphoproliferative syndromes," *Hematology Journal*, vol. 2, no. 1, pp. 33–37, 2001.

[55] J. N. Waitumbi, M. O. Opollo, R. O. Muga, A. O. Misore, and J. A. Stoute, "Red cell surface changes and erythrophagocytosis in children with severe *Plasmodium falciparum* anemia," *Blood*, vol. 95, no. 4, pp. 1481–1486, 2000.

[56] J. A. Stoute, A. O. Odindo, B. O. Owuor, E. K. Mibei, M. O. Opollo, and J. N. Waitumbi, "Loss of red blood cell-complement regulatory proteins and increased levels of circulating immune complexes are associated with severe malarial anemia," *Journal of Infectious Diseases*, vol. 187, no. 3, pp. 522–525, 2003.

[57] J. M. Waitumbi, B. Donvito, A. Kisserli, J. H. M. Cohen, and J. A. Stoute, "Age-related changes in red blood cell complement regulatory proteins and susceptibility to severe malaria," *Journal of Infectious Diseases*, vol. 190, no. 6, pp. 1183–1191, 2004.

[58] C. O. Odhiambo, W. Otieno, C. Adhiambo, M. M. Odera, and J. A. Stoute, "Increased deposition of C3b on red cells with low CR1 and CD55 in a malaria-endemic region of western Kenya: implications for the development of severe anemia," *BMC Medicine*, vol. 6, article 23, 2008.

[59] R. C. Mahajan, K. Narain, and J. Mahanta, "Anaemia & expression levels of CD35, CD55 & CD59 on red blood cells in *Plasmodium falciparum* malaria patients from India," *Indian Journal of Medical Research*, vol. 133, no. 6, pp. 662–664, 2011.

[60] J. N. Jarvis, H. Taylor, P. M. Long, P. V. Gutta, T. Pousak, and N. Fine, "Diminished expression of cell-surface complement regulatory proteins in HIV-infected children and with HIV infection of peripheral blood mononuclear cells in vitro," *Journal of Acquired Immune Deficiency Syndromes and Human Retrovirology*, vol. 9, no. 3, pp. 249–256, 1995.

[61] E. Terpos, A. Sarantopoulos, A. Kouramba et al., "Reduction of CD55 and/or CD59 in red blood cells of patients with HIV infection," *Medical Science Monitor*, vol. 14, no. 5, pp. CR276–CR280, 2008.

[62] M. Yamaguchi, T. Machii, Y. Azenishi et al., "Detection of small populations of CD59-deficient erythrocytes in patients with aplastic anemia or myelodysplastic syndrome and normal individuals," *Blood Cells, Molecules, and Diseases*, vol. 26, no. 3, pp. 247–254, 2000.

[63] H. Wang, T. Chuhjo, H. Yamazaki et al., "Relative increase of granulocytes with a paroxysmal nocturnal haemoglobinuria phenotype in aplastic anaemia patients: the high prevalence at diagnosis," *European Journal of Haematology*, vol. 66, no. 3, pp. 200–205, 2001.

[64] R. Hu, G. L. Mukhina, S. Piantadosi, J. P. Barber, R. J. Jones, and R. A. Brodsky, "PIG-A mutations in normal hematopoiesis," *Blood*, vol. 105, no. 10, pp. 3848–3854, 2005.

[65] U. Oelschlaegel, I. Besson, C. Arnoulet et al., "A standardized flow cytometric method for screening paroxysmal nocturnal haemoglobinuria (PNH) measuring CD55 and CD59 expression on erythrocytes and granulocytes," *Clinical and Laboratory Haematology*, vol. 23, no. 2, pp. 81–90, 2001.

[66] M. M. Lederman, S. F. Purvis, E. I. Walter, J. T. Carey, and M. E. Medof, "Heightened complement sensitivity of acquired immunodeficiency syndrome lymphocytes related to diminished expression of decay-accelerating factor," *Proceedings of the National Academy of Sciences of the United States of America*, vol. 86, no. 11, pp. 4205–4209, 1989.

[67] A. P. Alegretti, T. Mucenic, J. Merzoni, G. A. Faulhaber, L. M. Silla, and R. M. Xavier, "Expression of CD55 and CD59 on peripheral blood cells from systemic lupus erythematosus (SLE) patients," *Cellular Immunology*, vol. 265, no. 2, pp. 127–132, 2010.

[68] A. P. Alegretti, L. Schneider, A. K. Piccoli et al., "Diminished expression of complement regulatory proteins on peripheral blood cells from systemic lupus erythematosus patients," *Clinical and Developmental Immunology*, vol. 2012, Article ID 725684, 9 pages, 2012.

[69] K. B. Elkon and D. M. Santer, "Complement, interferon and lupus," *Current Opinion in Immunology*, vol. 24, no. 6, pp. 665–670, 2012.

[70] S. D. Webster, M. D. Galvan, E. Ferran, W. Garzon-Rodriguez, C. G. Glabe, and A. J. Tenner, "Antibody-mediated phagocytosis of the amyloid β-peptide in microglia is differentially modulated by C1q," *Journal of Immunology*, vol. 166, no. 12, pp. 7496–7503, 2001.

[71] D. M. Santer, A. E. Wiedeman, T. H. Teal, P. Ghosh, and K. B. Elkon, "Plasmacytoid dendritic cells and C1q differentially regulate inflammatory gene induction by lupus immune complexes," *Journal of Immunology*, vol. 188, no. 2, pp. 902–915, 2012.

[72] M. J. Walport, "Complement (second of two parts)," *The New England Journal of Medicine*, vol. 344, no. 15, pp. 1140–1144, 2001.

[73] Y. Richaud-Patin, B. Pérez-Romano, E. Carrillo-Maravilla et al., "Deficiency of red cell bound CD55 and CD59 in patients with systemic lupus erythematosus," *Immunology Letters*, vol. 88, no. 2, pp. 95–99, 2003.

[74] V. Pavlov, H. Raedler, S. Yuan et al., "Donor deficiency of decay-accelerating factor accelerates murine T cell-mediated cardiac allograft rejection," *Journal of Immunology*, vol. 181, no. 7, pp. 4580–4589, 2008.

[75] P. S. Heeger, P. N. Lalli, F. Lin et al., "Decay-accelerating factor modulates induction of T cell immunity," *Journal of Experimental Medicine*, vol. 201, no. 10, pp. 1523–1530, 2005.

[76] T. Miwa, M. A. Maldonado, L. Zhou et al., "Decay-accelerating factor ameliorates systemic autoimmune disease in MRL/lpr mice via both complement-dependent and -independent mechanisms," *The American Journal of Pathology*, vol. 170, no. 4, pp. 1258–1266, 2007.

[77] J. Vas and M. Monestier, "Immunology of mercury," *Annals of the New York Academy of Sciences*, vol. 1143, pp. 240–267, 2008.

[78] M. A. Lynes, A. P. Fontenot, D. A. Lawrence, A. J. Rosenspire, and K. M. Pollard, "Gene expression influences on metal immunomodulation," *Toxicology and Applied Pharmacology*, vol. 210, no. 1-2, pp. 9–16, 2006.

[79] P. Hultman, U. Johansson, S. J. Turley, U. Lindh, S. Eneström, and K. M. Pollard, "Adverse immunological effects and autoimmunity induced by dental amalgam and alloy in mice," *FASEB Journal*, vol. 8, no. 14, pp. 1183–1190, 1994.

[80] D. H. Kono, D. Balomenos, D. L. Pearson et al., "The prototypic Th2 autoimmunity induced by mercury is dependent on IFN-γ and not Th1/Th2 imbalance," *Journal of Immunology*, vol. 161, no. 1, pp. 234–240, 1998.

[81] K. Warfvinge, H. Hansson, and P. Hultman, "Systemic autoimmunity due to mercury vapor exposure in genetically susceptible mice: dose-response studies," *Toxicology and Applied Pharmacology*, vol. 132, no. 2, pp. 299–309, 1995.

[82] P. Hultman, S. J. Turley, S. Eneström, U. Lindh, and K. M. Pollard, "Murine genotype influences the specificity, magnitude

and persistence of murine mercury-induced autoimmunity," *Journal of Autoimmunity*, vol. 9, no. 2, pp. 139–149, 1996.

[83] P. Hultman and J. B. Nielsen, "The effect of dose, gender, and non-H-2 genes in murine mercury-induced autoimmunity," *Journal of Autoimmunity*, vol. 17, no. 1, pp. 27–37, 2001.

[84] M. Schiraldi and M. Monestier, "How can a chemical element elicit complex immunopathology? Lessons from mercury-induced autoimmunity," *Trends in Immunology*, vol. 30, no. 10, pp. 502–509, 2009.

[85] P. Hultman, L. J. Bell, S. Enestrom, and K. M. Pollard, "Murine susceptibility to mercury. I. Autoantibody profiles and systemic immune deposits in inbred, congenic, and intra-H-2 recombinant strains," *Clinical Immunology and Immunopathology*, vol. 65, no. 2, pp. 98–109, 1992.

[86] K. M. Pollard, P. Hultman, and D. H. Kono, "Immunology and genetics of induced systemic autoimmunity," *Autoimmunity Reviews*, vol. 4, no. 5, pp. 282–288, 2005.

[87] L. M. Bagenstose, R. Class, P. Salgame, and M. Monestier, "B7-1 and B7-2 co-stimulatory molecules are required for mercury-induced autoimmunity," *Clinical and Experimental Immunology*, vol. 127, no. 1, pp. 12–19, 2002.

[88] K. M. Pollard, M. Arnush, P. Hultman, and D. H. Kono, "Costimulation requirements of induced murine systemic autoimmune disease," *Journal of Immunology*, vol. 173, no. 9, pp. 5880–5887, 2004.

[89] L. M. Bagenstose, P. Salgame, and M. Monestier, "Mercury-induced autoimmunity in the absence of IL-4," *Clinical and Experimental Immunology*, vol. 114, no. 1, pp. 9–12, 1998.

[90] S. Havarinasab, K. M. Pollard, and P. Hultman, "Gold- and silver-induced murine autoimmunity—requirement for cytokines and CD28 in murine heavy metal-induced autoimmunity," *Clinical and Experimental Immunology*, vol. 155, no. 3, pp. 567–576, 2009.

[91] J. Vas, J. Mattner, S. Richardson et al., "Regulatory roles for NKT cell ligands in environmentally induced autoimmunity," *Journal of Immunology*, vol. 181, no. 10, pp. 6779–6788, 2008.

[92] K. M. Pollard and D. H. Kono, "Requirements for innate immune pathways in environmentally induced autoimmunity," *BMC Medicine*, vol. 11, article 100, 2013.

[93] K. M. Pollard, D. L. Pearson, P. Hultman, T. N. Deane, U. Lindh, and D. H. Kono, "Xenobiotic acceleration of idiopathic systematic autoimmunity in lupus-prone BXSB mice," *Environmental Health Perspectives*, vol. 109, no. 1, pp. 27–33, 2001.

[94] K. M. Pollard, D. L. Pearson, P. Hultman, B. Hildebrandt, and D. H. Kono, "Lupus-prone mice as models to study xenobiotic-induced acceleration of systemic autoimmunity," *Environmental Health Perspectives*, vol. 107, no. 5, pp. 729–735, 1999.

[95] M. Abedi-Valugerdi, H. Hu, and G. Möller, "Mercury-induced renal immune complex deposits in young (NZB × NZW)F1 mice: characterization of antibodies/autoantibodies," *Clinical and Experimental Immunology*, vol. 110, no. 1, pp. 86–91, 1997.

[96] F. W. Miller, L. Alfredsson, K. H. Costenbader et al., "Epidemiology of environmental exposures and human autoimmune diseases: findings from a national institute of environmental health sciences expert panel workshop," *Journal of Autoimmunity*, vol. 39, no. 4, pp. 253–258, 2012.

[97] S. C. L. Farhat, C. A. Silva, M. A. M. Orione, L. M. A. Campos, A. M. E. Sallum, and A. L. F. Braga, "Air pollution in autoimmune rheumatic diseases: a review," *Autoimmunity Reviews*, vol. 11, no. 1, pp. 14–21, 2011.

[98] I. A. Silva, J. F. Nyland, A. Gorman et al., "Mercury exposure, malaria, and serum antinuclear/antinucleolar antibodies in amazon populations in Brazil: a cross-sectional study," *Environmental Health*, vol. 3, article 11, 2004.

[99] G. S. Cooper, C. G. Parks, E. L. Treadwell, E. W. St Clair, G. S. Gilkeson, and M. A. Dooley, "Occupational risk factors for the development of systemic lupus erythematosus," *Journal of Rheumatology*, vol. 31, no. 10, pp. 1928–1933, 2004.

[100] A. M. Abréu Vélez, G. Warfvinge, W. L. Herrera et al., "Detection of mercury and other undetermined materials in skin biopsies of endemic pemphigus foliaceus," *The American Journal of Dermatopathology*, vol. 25, no. 5, pp. 384–391, 2003.

[101] R. M. Gardner, J. F. Nyland, I. A. Silva, A. Maria Ventura, J. M. de Souza, and E. K. Silbergeld, "Mercury exposure, serum antinuclear/antinucleolar antibodies, and serum cytokine levels in mining populations in Amazonian Brazil: a cross-sectional study," *Environmental Research*, vol. 110, no. 4, pp. 345–354, 2010.

[102] S. J. Li, S. H. Zhang, H. P. Chen et al., "Mercury-induced membranous nephropathy: clinical and pathological features," *Clinical Journal of the American Society of Nephrology*, vol. 5, no. 3, pp. 439–444, 2010.

[103] D. M. Cauvi, G. Cauvi, and K. M. Pollard, "Reduced expression of decay-accelerating factor 1 on CD4+ T cells in murine systemic autoimmune disease," *Arthritis and Rheumatism*, vol. 56, no. 6, pp. 1934–1944, 2007.

[104] D. M. Cauvi, C. B. Toomey, and K. M. Pollard, "Depletion of complement does not impact initiation of xenobiotic-induced autoimmune disease," *Immunology*, vol. 135, no. 4, pp. 333–343, 2012.

[105] H. Sekine, C. M. Reilly, I. D. Molano et al., "Complement component C3 is not required for full expression of immune complex glomerulonephritis in MRL/lpr mice," *Journal of Immunology*, vol. 166, no. 10, pp. 6444–6451, 2001.

[106] R. J. M. Abbott, I. Spendlove, P. Roversi et al., "Structural and functional characterization of a novel T cell receptor co-regulatory protein complex, CD97-CD55," *The Journal of Biological Chemistry*, vol. 282, no. 30, pp. 22023–22032, 2007.

[107] E. N. Kop, M. Matmati, W. Pouwels, G. Leclercq, P. P. Tak, and J. Hamann, "Differential expression of CD97 on human lymphocyte subsets and limited effect of CD97 antibodies on allogeneic T-cell stimulation," *Immunology Letters*, vol. 123, no. 2, pp. 160–168, 2009.

[108] J. Hamann, C. van Zeventer, A. Bijl, C. Molenaar, K. Tesselaar, and R. A. W. van Lier, "Molecular cloning and characterization of mouse CD97," *International Immunology*, vol. 12, no. 4, pp. 439–448, 2000.

[109] M. Capasso, L. G. Durrant, M. Stacey, S. Gordon, J. Ramage, and I. Spendlove, "Costimulation via CD55 on human CD4+ T cells mediated by CD97," *Journal of Immunology*, vol. 177, no. 2, pp. 1070–1077, 2006.

[110] R. V. Sutavani, R. G. Bradley, J. M. Ramage, A. M. Jackson, L. G. Durrant, and I. Spendlove, "CD55 costimulation induces differentiation of a discrete T regulatory type 1 cell population with a stable phenotype," *Journal of Immunology*, vol. 191, no. 12, pp. 5895–5903, 2013.

[111] C. Kemper, A. C. Chan, J. M. Green, K. A. Brett, K. M. Murphy, and J. P. Atkinson, "Activation of human CD4+ cells with CD3 and CD46 induces a T-regulatory cell 1 phenotype," *Nature*, vol. 421, no. 6921, pp. 388–392, 2003.

[112] C. M. Karsten and J. Köhl, "The complement receptor CD46 tips the scales in T H 1 self-control," *Nature Immunology*, vol. 11, no. 9, pp. 775–777, 2010.

[113] S. M. Truscott, G. Abate, J. D. Price, C. Kemper, J. P. Atkinson, and D. F. Hoft, "CD46 engagement on human CD4+ T cells produces T regulatory type 1-like regulation of antimycobacterial T cell responses," *Infection and Immunity*, vol. 78, no. 12, pp. 5295–5306, 2010.

[114] C. Hsieh and J. L. Bautista, "Sliding set-points of immune responses for therapy of autoimmunity," *Journal of Experimental Medicine*, vol. 207, no. 9, pp. 1819–1823, 2010.

[115] K. M. Pollard, P. Hultman, C. B. Toomey et al., "Definition of IFN-γ-related pathways critical for chemically-induced systemic autoimmunity," *Journal of Autoimmunity*, vol. 39, no. 4, pp. 323–331, 2012.

[116] H. Y. Wu, F. J. Quintana, A. P. da Cunha et al., "In vivo induction of Tr1 cells via mucosal dendritic cells and AHR signaling," *PLoS ONE*, vol. 6, no. 8, Article ID e23618, 2011.

[117] C. Pot, L. Apetoh, A. Awasthi, and V. K. Kuchroo, "Molecular pathways in the induction of interleukin-27-driven regulatory type 1 cells," *Journal of Interferon and Cytokine Research*, vol. 30, no. 6, pp. 381–388, 2010.

[118] H. Y. Wu, F. J. Quintana, and H. L. Weiner, "Nasal anti-CD3 antibody ameliorates lupus by inducing an IL-10-secreting CD4+CD25-LAP+ regulatory T Cell and is associated with down-regulation of IL-17+CD4+ICOS +CXCR5+ follicular helper T cells," *Journal of Immunology*, vol. 181, no. 9, pp. 6038–6050, 2008.

[119] A. Viola, S. Schroeder, Y. Sakakibara, and A. Lanzavecchia, "T lymphocyte costimulation mediated by reorganization of membrane microdomains," *Science*, vol. 283, no. 5402, pp. 680–682, 1999.

[120] P. Legembre, S. Daburon, P. Moreau, J. F. Moreau, and J. L. Taupin, "Cutting edge: modulation of Fas-mediated apoptosis by lipid rafts in T lymphocytes," *Journal of Immunology*, vol. 176, no. 2, pp. 716–720, 2006.

[121] M. P. Longhi, B. Sivasankar, N. Omidvar, B. P. Morgan, and A. Gallimore, "Cutting edge: murine CD59a modulates antiviral CD4+ T cell activity in a complement-independent manner," *Journal of Immunology*, vol. 175, no. 11, pp. 7098–7102, 2005.

8

Mercury, Autoimmunity, and Environmental Factors on Cheyenne River Sioux Tribal Lands

Jennifer Ong,[1] Esther Erdei,[1] Robert L. Rubin,[2] Curtis Miller,[1] Carlyle Ducheneaux,[3] Marcia O'Leary,[4] Bernadette Pacheco,[1] Michael Mahler,[5] Patricia Nez Henderson,[6] K. Michael Pollard,[7] and Johnnye L. Lewis[1]

[1] *College of Pharmacy, Community Environmental Health Program, University of New Mexico Health Sciences Center, 905 Vassar NE, Albuquerque, NM 87106, USA*
[2] *School of Medicine, University of New Mexico Health Sciences Center, 1 University of New Mexico, Albuquerque, NM 87131, USA*
[3] *Department of Natural Resources, Cheyenne River Sioux Tribe, P.O. Box 590, East Highway 212, Eagle Butte, SD 57625, USA*
[4] *Missouri Breaks Industries Research, Inc., Hc 64 Box 52, Timber Lake, SD 57656, USA*
[5] *INOVA Diagnostics, Inc., 9900 Old Grove Road, San Diego, CA 92131, USA*
[6] *Black Hills Center for American Indian Health, 701 St. Joseph Street, Suite 204, Rapid City, SD 57701, USA*
[7] *Scripps Research Institute, 10550 North Torrey Pines Road, La Jolla, CA 92037, USA*

Correspondence should be addressed to Johnnye L. Lewis; jlewis@cybermesa.com

Academic Editor: Aristo Vojdani

Mercury (Hg), shown to induce autoimmune disease in rodents, is a ubiquitous toxicant throughout Cheyenne River Sioux Tribe (CRST) lands. CRST members may be exposed to Hg through fish consumption (FC), an important component of native culture that may supplement household subsistence. Our goals were to ascertain whether total blood Hg levels (THg) reflect Hg exposure through FC and smoking, and determine whether THg is associated with the presence of anti-nuclear antibody (ANA) and specific autoantibodies (sAuAb). We recruited 75 participants who regularly consume fish from CRST waters. Hg exposure through FC and smoking were assessed via questionnaires. Whole blood samples were collected from participants, and THg was measured using ICP-MS. ANA and sAuAb in serum were modeled using demographic and exposure information as predictors. Female gender, age, and FC were significant predictors of THg and sAuAb; self-reported smoking was not. 31% of participants tested positive for ANA $\geq$ 2+. Although ANA was not significantly associated with Hg, the interactions of gender with Hg and proximity to arsenic deposits were statistically significant ($P < 0.05$). FC resulted in a detectable body burden of Hg, but THg alone did not correlate with the presence of ANA or sAuAb in this population.

1. Introduction

For more than a century, mining from greater than 900 mines in the Black Hills, including gold mines in which Hg was used for amalgamation purposes, has released contaminants into watersheds draining onto CRST lands [1]. Additionally, approximately one ton of airborne Hg is emitted per year from coal power plants in Montana, Wyoming, North Dakota, and South Dakota [2] and carried downwind to CRST lands where precipitation and dust wash this mercury out of the air into water and soil. Thus, Hg is virtually ubiquitous throughout the CRST reservation. Studies over the last decade conducted by the tribe, United States Environmental Protection Agency (USEPA), and University of Colorado [3] have documented high mercury concentrations in mid-flow water samples and sediment [4], invertebrates [5], and fish [5–7]. As a result of the widespread presence of Hg in the environment, fish consumption warnings have been posted along the Cheyenne River since 1974, yet no comprehensive health studies have ever been conducted in the CRST population to assess the health effects of consuming fish from tribal waters. In spite of posted warnings, CRST members still consume locally caught fish for complex reasons. Fishing and fish consumption are not only important in Lakota culture, but high rates of poverty (~50%) [8, 9] and unemployment (88%) [10] on the CRST reservation increase the community's likelihood of using fish to supplement household subsistence. Therefore, the safety of eating mercury-contaminated fish caught on tribal lands was a prime concern for CRST members. To address the CRST's environmental health concerns, a research partnership, *Environmental Justice on Cheyenne River*, was established in 2003 among the CRST Department of Environment and Natural Resources (DENR), the Black Hills Center for American Indian Health, and the University of New Mexico Community Environmental Health Program (UNM CEHP). Through community forums and discussions with tribal leaders, the partnership identified a major concern that a perceived increase in autoimmune disease (AD) prevalence in the CRST population might be related to Hg exposures through fish consumption, as well as a widespread frustration that actual health studies had not occurred in spite of Hg warnings posted for nearly 40 years. Although deidentified numbers of autoimmune cases were obtained from Indian Health Service (IHS) data sources, interpretation of the prevalence is difficult in identification of an appropriate denominator and determination of an appropriate comparison figure for Native American populations. Data on antinuclear antibody (ANA) prevalence in Native populations has not been evaluated. Prevalence of ANA in other US populations was recently derived from National Health and Nutrition Survey data (NHANES) [11, 12], but values for Native American populations could not be extracted due to no representation in that sample. Reference values for specific AD in tribal populations relative to the US total population are also not readily accessible.

Since tribal populations are comparatively more homogenous than other studied US populations, it may be tempting to ascribe any elevations in AD in the CRST merely to genetics. However, while genetic susceptibility has long been acknowledged as an important causative factor in the development of AD and evidence [13, 14] exists that genetic composition may predispose CRST members to AD, it is estimated that genetic factors only account for one-third of disease risk and that gene-environmental interactions play a vital role in the onset of autoimmunity [15]. The growing role of environmental factors, including aluminum metal compounds and thimerisol in vaccines, as adjuvants to the pathogenesis of autoimmunity has been studied extensively [16]. In addition, studies [17, 18] indicate that Hg toxicity and autoimmunity may be synergistically enhanced by various infectious and noninfectious triggers. It is reasonable that chronic stimulation of the immune system by environmental Hg may act through similar mechanisms. To address the community's concerns and begin to address existing gaps in knowledge about the effects of chronic low-level environmental exposures to metals, we sought to systematically examine the relationships among fish consumption, THg, and basic immune system markers in the CRST population in this study.

Existing knowledge about the effects of metals on the immune system comes mainly from the use of rodent models. In these models, relatively high doses of inorganic mercury administered to genetically susceptible mouse strains lead to the development of lupus-like autoimmune syndrome, which includes increased circulating antibodies to nuclear targets (antinuclear autoantibodies, ANA) [16, 17]. Further, exposure to inorganic *or* organic mercury exacerbates and accelerates the development of lupus-like disease in susceptible mouse strains [18–21]. Rodent models of mercury-induced autoimmunity [22–24], as well as their consistency with sex differences in autoimmune disease incidence observed in humans, suggest it is biologically plausible that Hg and other metals contribute to autoimmune pathogenesis in humans. Yet, with the exception of a few epidemiologic studies investigating the role of mercury amalgam fillings in multiple sclerosis [25, 26] and studies of ANA and cytokines in mercury-exposed Amazonian Brazil populations [27–30], too few [31, 32] have investigated the potential role of chronic environmental metal exposures as risk factors in the development of AD in humans. While relationships between metal exposure and immune dysfunction have been demonstrated in animals, limited data exist in humans. Since Hg has long been linked to development of AD-like symptoms in animal models [17], we hypothesized that increased mercury exposure, primarily through fish consumption, would be associated with higher levels of circulating autoantibodies in the CRST population. In order to test this hypothesis and respond to community concerns, we modeled ANA and specific autoantibody concentrations in blood collected from CRST community members using THg, fish consumption, smoking, age, gender, and proximity to high-concentration arsenic sediment deposits as predictors.

2. Materials and Methods

2.1. Human Subjects. The protocol and study design were approved by the Executive Committee of the Cheyenne River Sioux Tribe Tribal Council (Tribal Resolution number: E-302-08-CR and extended under E-343-2009-CR) and by the University of New Mexico Health Sciences Center Human Research Protection Office (HRPO number: 08-486). As deidentified serum samples were sent to the Scripps Research Institute Department of Molecular and Experimental Medicine, the Scripps Research Institute's Institutional Review Board provided approval for an analysis of serum ANA and specific autoantibodies.

Participants were recruited by using community-based communication tools and procedures previously developed by this team and applied in the *Environmental Justice on Cheyenne River* study. Outreach, enrollment, and sampling were conducted in conjunction with local collaborators, notably Missouri Breaks Industries Research, Inc. (MBIRI), who were crucial contributors in several previous federally funded research projects among Cheyenne River Tribal communities, and collaborating staff from the CRST DENR. The recruitment was targeted toward fishermen and their family members, who were known to local collaborators as regular consumers of fish caught from the Cheyenne River and its tributaries.

Written informed consent was obtained from a total of 75 adults living on the CRST Lands during the peak of fishing season. The study population includes members from

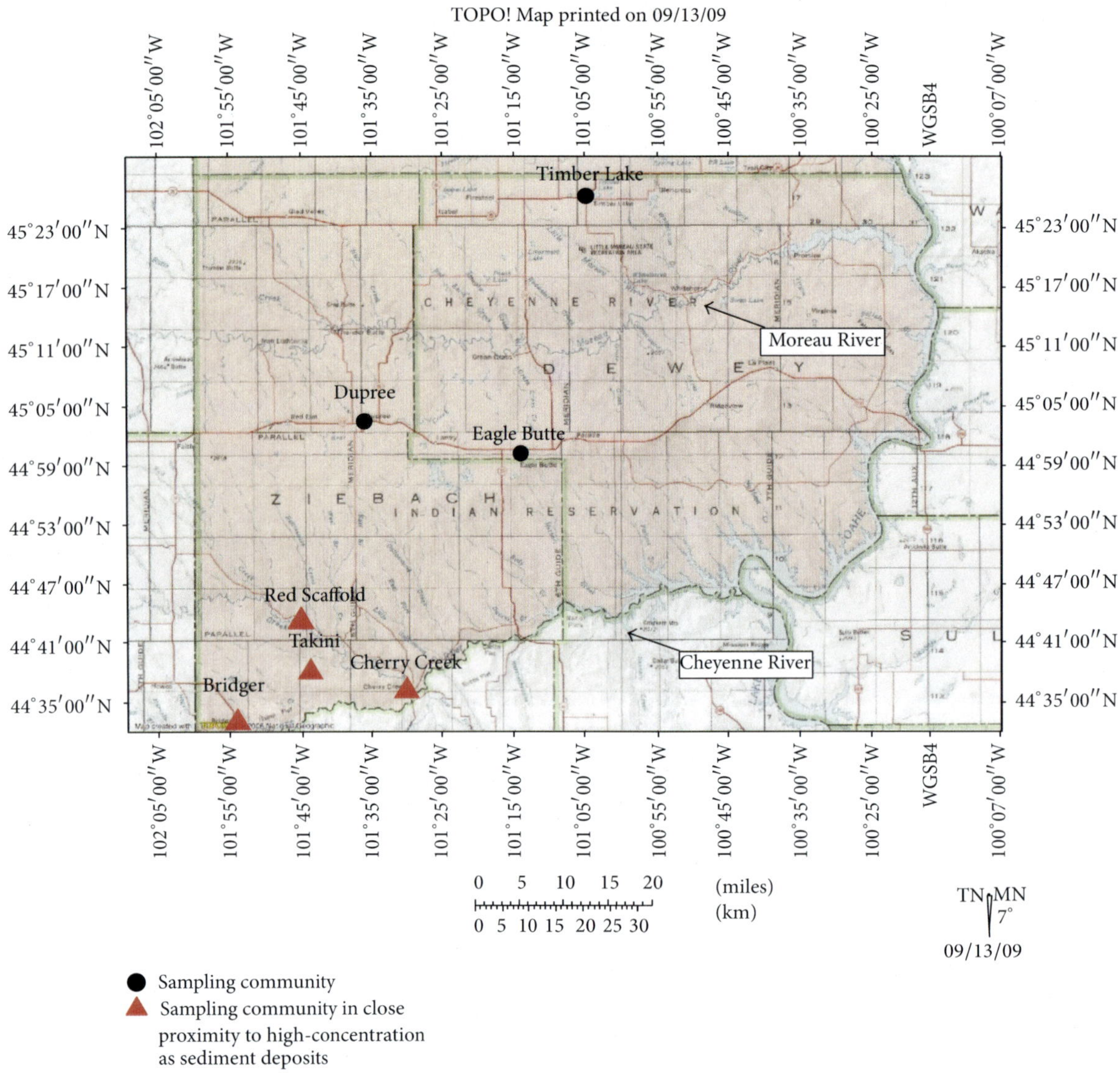

Figure 1: Map of Cheyenne River Sioux Tribal lands and sampling communities.

multiple communities including Eagle Butte, Cherry Creek, Dupree, Timber Lake, Red Scaffold, Bridger, Takini, and Howes (Figure 1). At each location, enrollment was conducted and biological samples were collected in community centers. These communities, some of which are in close proximity to rivers, lakes and ponds on CRST lands, encompass both commercial centers and rural areas, as well as members whose primary source of food is store-bought versus acquired from the local environment (subsistence lifestyle), and therefore reflect a wide range of potential exposures to Hg through fish consumption. Smoking status was a concern as an alternate contributor to THg based on previously reported increases in smoking on the CRST reservation [33] and the demonstrated contributions to THg from cigarette smoking [34, 35]. MBIRI team interviewers collected demographic (e.g., age, gender), health condition, fishing, and smoking habit information through personal interviews conducted in English using a Centers for Disease Control- (CDC-) developed fish consumption survey and our own short smoking exposure questionnaire. When participants needed information or clarification spoken in their native language, the community-certified nurse interviewers provided the answers.

2.2. Surveys Used in the Study

2.2.1. Fish Consumption. A CDC questionnaire, as well as local collaborators' knowledge of CRST community members' fishing habits, was used to assign a categorical rating of 1, 2, or 3 to each participant's fish consumption, with 1 designating minimal to no fish consumption, and 3 corresponding to high fish consumption. For reference to the local environment and consumption patterns, the safe amount of fish intake per month was previously recommended by our *Environmental Justice on Cheyenne River* study using DENR Hg measurements from local fish and USEPA guidelines [37].

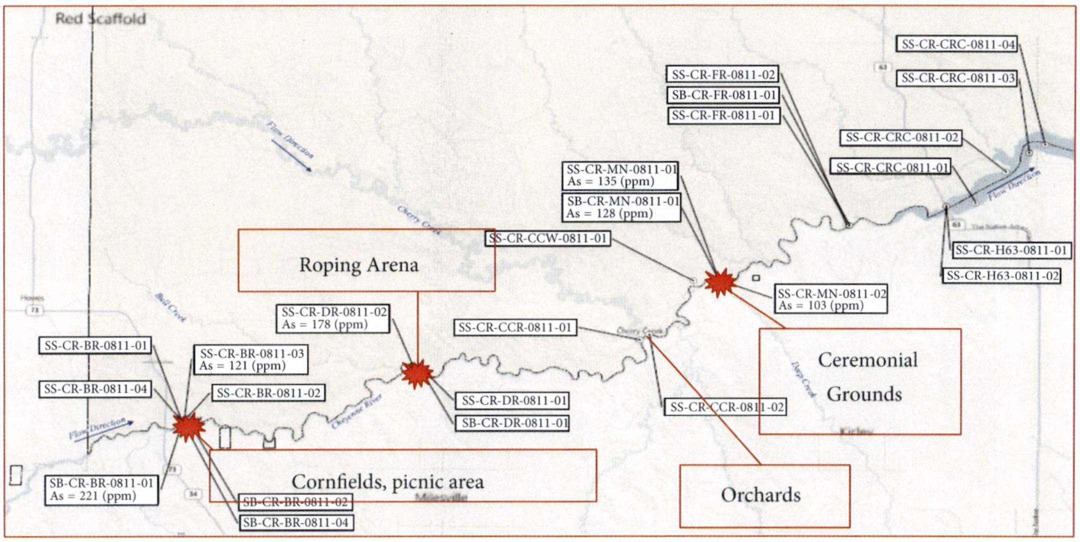

FIGURE 2: Map of arsenic sampling conducted by USEPA and CRST DENR. Concentrations of arsenic in sediment exceeding 100 ppm are marked with a burst pattern. Exposure-relevant sites are labeled with activities frequently conducted in those areas.

One monthly recommended serving was defined as one northern pike, two bass or perch, three walleye, or four catfish. A rating of (1) denotes consumption of <1 serving of fish per month; (2) denotes 1-2 servings/month; and (3) denotes >2 servings/month.

2.2.2. Smoking. To account for smoking as both a potential source of Hg and contributor to immune system effects, participant smoking data were collected via questionnaire. The questionnaire was based on coauthor PNH's previous work [33] on smoking among tribal members and was given to all participants in order to obtain self-reported information regarding smoking exposures. The questionnaire encompassed both direct and second-hand exposure to cigarette smoke. There were seven questions total; smoking score was coded as low (1) when fewer than two questions were answered affirmatively; medium (2) when 3-4 questions were answered affirmatively; and high (3) when greater than five questions were answered affirmatively. A participant was considered an "active smoker" if he/she answered "yes" to the included question, "Do you smoke currently?"

2.2.3. Arsenic Proximity. During the analytic phase of this study, elevated sedimentary arsenic deposits were discovered in land-use areas in close proximity to several of the sampling-site communities in this study (Figure 2). Ongoing collaborations among DENR, Dr. Lewis, and USEPA Region 8 are surveying residents and characterizing exposure pathways, frequencies, and duration. However, as these deposits were identified subsequent to consent for this study, no arsenic biomonitoring data were obtained from the population in the original design nor were exposure activities involving these sedimentary deposits identified. Due to studies in humans and animals indicating that arsenic suppresses autoimmunity [38, 39], while mercury may either suppress or increase autoimmune response [28, 32], a surrogate of participant arsenic exposure was incorporated into models to address potentially competing exposures. A binary surrogate for arsenic exposure was derived; the designations of "near" or "far" proximity to known quantified environmental arsenic deposits by USEPA were given according to self-reported participant residence data. The designation of "near" was given to participants who live in the communities of Cherry Creek, Takini, Bridger, and Red Scaffold (Figure 1). Surveys of residents have identified potential exposure pathways which include common land-use practices such as fishing; herb, fruit, and firewood gathering; inhalation of wood combustion products during sweat lodge and ceremonial practices; and roping/other horseback riding activities along the Cheyenne River near the identified alluvial arsenic deposits (Figure 2) (personal communication C. Ducheneaux and J. Lewis). Participants residing in the Eagle Butte, Dupree, and Timber Lake (Figure 1) communities more distal to the arsenic deposits were given a designation of "far" for arsenic proximity in this pilot assessment. This binary variable was incorporated to determine if further studies on the relationship of these exposures to AD were warranted.

2.3. Biological Sample Collection

2.3.1. Blood and Serum Samples. Venous blood samples were collected by venipuncture at community centers or during home visits by a trained and certified phlebotomist or registered nurse. One red top (9 mL) for serum collection and one purple top (7 mL) Vacutainer tube were collected for biomonitoring from each participant. After clotting, serum samples were spun at 2,500 rpm for 10 minutes and separated into cryovials and placed into a −80°C freezer. At a later time point, sera were shipped to the UNM HSC laboratory and subsequently to the Scripps Research Institute.

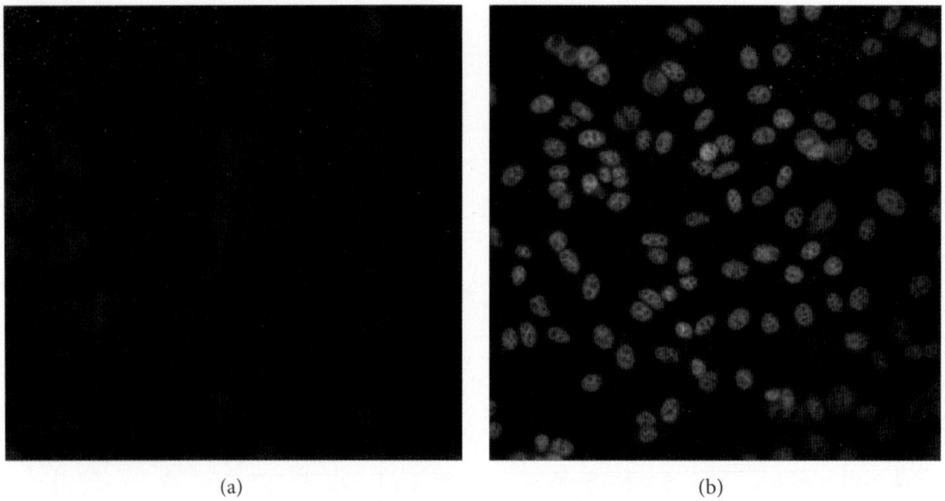

Figure 3: Examples of ANA determination by immunofluorescence. Human sera were incubated with HEp-2 cells followed by fluorescent anti-human IgG. The sample on the left (a) is ANA negative, while the sample on the right (b) was considered 2+ ANA positive, showing fine speckled nuclear staining sparing the nucleolus.

2.4. Experimental Use of Collected Biological Samples

2.4.1. Biomonitoring. The EDTA-containing whole blood samples were transported to the CDC ONDIEH/NCEH Environmental Health Laboratory where inductively coupled plasma mass spectrometry (ICP-MS) was used to determine THg concentrations. The limit of detection was 0.32 μg/L.

2.4.2. Detection of Autoantibodies

(1) Antinuclear Antibodies (ANA). The presence of ANA was determined by indirect immunofluorescence (IIF) microscopy using HEp-2 cells as substrate (MBL-BION, Des Plaines, IL) and Alexa Fluor 488 Goat Anti-Human IgG (H + L) (Life Technologies, NY, USA) as detecting reagent. Sera were diluted 1 : 100 in serum diluent, and detecting reagent 1 : 200 with anti-Ig diluent as previously described [40]. Slides were viewed by a single observer (KMP) blinded to participant identity on a BH2-RFCA fluorescence microscope (Olympus, Lake Success, NY). Intensity of fluorescence was graded on a scale of 0–4+. A reading of ≥2+ was considered significant and further used in our statistical modeling. This cut-off value reflects a stricter value based on the literature [36, 41]. Example immunofluorescence images for ANA determination can be found in Figure 3 for negative (0) and ANA ≥ 2+ readings.

(2) Specific Autoantibodies (sAuAb). Commercially available kits (INOVA Diagnostics, San Diego, CA) were used as described by the manufacturer to detect and quantify serum autoantibodies to the following antigens: chromatin, Sm, RNP, SSA, SSA-52, SSB, Scl-70, RNA Pol III, CENP-A/B, Ribo-P, Jo-1, M2 EP (MIT3), and primary biliary cirrhosis (PBC) screen, a panel of antigens (M2 EP, gp210 and sp100 IgG/IgA). Assay-specific positive controls were used to convert optical density values to units in order to determine whether the results of assays for Sm, RNP, SSA, SSA-52, SSB, Scl-70, RNA Pol III, Ribo-P, and Jo-1 were negative/equivocal (<20 units), weakly positive (20–39 units), moderately positive (40–80 units), or strongly positive (>80 units). The tests for M2 EP and the PBC screen were interpreted as being equivocal from 20.1 to 24.9 units and positive for >25 units. Centromere-A/B (CENP-A/B) has negative/equivocal results for <20 units, weak positive for 20–30 units, and strong positive for >30 units. Chromatin has a negative/equivocal reading <20 units, moderate positive between 20 and 60 units, and a strong positive >60 units.

Additional assays to chromatin, denatured DNA (single-stranded, dDNA), native DNA (nDNA), and histones were quantified by enzyme-linked immunosorbent assays (ELISA) as previously described in [42, 43]. Briefly, Immulon 2HB microtiter plates (Dynex Laboratories, Inc., Alexandria, VA) were coated with antigen at 2.5 μg/mL concentrations. For the antichromatin assays, in-house-prepared H1-stripped chromatin was used as the solid-phase antigen. S1-nuclease (Invitrogen-) treated DNA (Calbiochem) was used in the antinative DNA assay, and DNA was heated for 10 min and then quickly cooled for preparation of the dDNA antigen. Prior to coating plates with nDNA or dDNA, plates were pre-coated at 2 μg/mL with the synthetic 20–50 kDA polypeptide poly(lys-phe) (Sigma-Aldrich), comprising a co-polymer of lysine and phenylalanine at a 1:1 ratio as previously described [43]. Total histone was from Worthington. Serum samples were diluted 1 : 200 and incubated on the plate for 2 hours at room temperature with gentle shaking. Each sample was run in duplicate. The bound antibodies were detected with peroxidase-conjugated anti-human IgG (Southern Biotech, AL) and 2,2′-azino-bis(3-ethylbenzthiazoline-6-sulfonic acid) (MP Bioproducts) as the secondary substrate. Optical densities (OD) beyond the range of direct measurement at 1 h in the ELISA were extrapolated from OD at earlier time-points as described [44]. Positive and negative control sera were always included in each assay, and values determined in different assays were normalized by multiplying by the ratio of the reactivity of the positive control sera tested in each assay.

2.5. Statistical Analysis: Modeling. Total blood mercury results lower than the limit of detection (LOD = 0.32 μg/L) were analyzed with the value of LOD/$\sqrt{2}$, because fewer than 50% of participants had a biomonitoring value < LOD. Total blood mercury results are presented as median values with the interquartile range, since the median is a better indicator of the true population value for the distribution of the collected data. The mean and 95% confidence interval for THg are also presented for ease of comparison with published NHANES population data. When comparing groups (e.g., male versus female) in relation to THg and ANA status, Fisher's exact test was used.

To characterize the complex exposures on CRST lands and their relationships to immune system responses and autoantibody production, several statistical models incorporating biomonitoring data, fish consumption score, smoking exposure score, distance to arsenic contamination, and immune system markers were developed. The approaches included multiple linear, logistic, and Poisson regression models to evaluate relative contributions of environmental exposures to circulating autoantibodies. They also included accepted risk factors such as age and gender. Multiple linear regression was used to model THg in relation to environmental exposure and risk factors, while logistic regression was used to model ANA $\geq$ 2+ in relation to predictors. Poisson regression was used to model the numbers of specific autoantibodies (both determined via INOVA and additional assays) with environmental exposure and risk factors. Poisson models accommodate count information with nonnormal distribution, thereby enhancing the analytical capacity to understand the exposure factors' underlying contribution to risk. Full models were fitted using all demographic, biomonitoring, and exposure data as predictors. Reduced models were selected using the Akaike information criterion (AIC), which is a measure of the relative quality of a statistical model. The openly available statistical software R [45] and the stepAIC function from the package MASS [46] were used to complete this AIC model selection, where

$$\text{AIC} = 2k - 2\ln(L). \quad (1)$$

And $k = 2$ and L is the likelihood of each model. The AIC selection criterion minimizes the distance between the predicted values of the model and the true values while also favoring models with fewer parameters.

2.5.1. Specific Approach to Analyze Specific Autoantibody Results from INOVA Assays. Since positivity for individual-specific autoantibodies was expected to be lower in frequency, we pooled all participants who tested positive for any specific autoantibodies to examine an overall prevalence of specific autoantibodies and the contributing exposure factors by summing the number of specific autoantibodies for which each participant tested positive and then conducting Poisson regression on the count variable generated. Biomonitoring data and exposure data were incorporated as well. This count variable makes biological sense because it follows established clinical AD diagnosis criteria; individuals diagnosed with AD present with varying combinations of specific autoantibodies.

2.5.2. Specific Approach to Analyze Specific Autoantibodies Results from Additional Autoantibody Assays. Poisson regression was used to model several combinations of autoantibodies that would otherwise be rarely detected. The combinations modeled were selected in order to examine different possible scenarios of positive autoantibody response. Individuals with detectable autoantibody response were classified into groups according to the following scenarios based on the literature [42–44]:

(a) presence of any autoantibody response (nDNA, dDNA, histone, chromatin);

(b) detectable levels of potentially environmentally related autoantibodies (dDNA and histone);

(c) disease-associated autoantibodies (nDNA and chromatin).

Results of these models were summarized in several tables presented in the next section.

Because anti-chromatin autoantibodies were detected using both INOVA and in-house assays, we evaluated the reproducibility of this antigen. We applied a nonparametric correlation (Spearman r-value) and used a z-score.

2.5.3. Reporting of Significant Results. While our primary results will follow a more standard reporting cutoff of $P < 0.05$, we will report those with probabilities up to 0.1 to guard against Type 2 error and to ensure comprehensive consideration of predictors in designing follow-up investigations. This decision is warranted given (1) the importance of the results to the communities, (2) the lack of prior studies in this area and in this population, and (3) the lack of biomonitoring data at this time on other potential environmental exposures including arsenic resulting in imprecise measures for that variable.

3. Results

3.1. Mercury Exposure and Population Characteristics. Population characteristics, including gender, smoking score, fish consumption score, community size, and proximity to identified high-concentration sedimentary arsenic deposits, are summarized in Table 1. Total blood mercury concentrations (THg) ranged from below the limit of detection (LOD, 0.32 μg Hg/L) to 4.14 μg Hg/L, with a median lower than the LOD (Figure 4). For most population characteristic categories, the median THg was below the LOD, with the exception of males (0.37 μg Hg/L) and participants with "medium" or "high" fish consumption scores (0.35 and 0.54 μg Hg/L, resp.).

Total blood mercury in the CRST depended on gender, age, and fish consumption but not smoking. The reduced multiple linear regression modeling results for THg as a response with demographic and exposure information as

TABLE 1: Biomonitoring and ANA ≥2+ results linked with study participant characteristics.

Population characteristic	N	Participants with THg >LOD*	Hg biomarker median (interquartile range)	Hg biomarker mean (95% CI)	ANA reading ≥2+ (n, %)
All participants	75	36 (36%)	<LOD (<LOD–0.87)	0.75 (0.55–0.95)	23 (31%)
Gender					
Male	38	23 (61%)	0.37 (<LOD–1.81)	1.01 (0.67–1.37)	2 (5%)
Female	37	13 (35%)	<LOD (<LOD–0.56)	0.48 (0.32–0.63)	9 (24%)
Smoking score					
(1) Low	32	17 (53%)	0.37 (<LOD–0.74)	0.67 (0.41–0.92)	8 (25%)
(2) Medium	18	8 (44%)	<LOD (<LOD–1.24)	0.82 (0.36–1.28)	3 (17%)
(3) High	25	11 (44%)	<LOD (<LOD–1.21)	0.81 (0.39–1.23)	7 (28%)
Active smoker					
Yes	42	19 (45%)	<LOD (<LOD–0.96)	0.77 (0.49–1.05)	4 (10%)
No	31	16 (52%)	0.37 (<LOD–0.87)	0.76 (0.40–1.06)	7 (23%)
Fish score					
(1) Low	41	17 (59%)	<LOD (<LOD–0.60)	0.59 (0.36–0.82)	7 (17%)
(2) Medium	18	10 (56%)	0.35 (<LOD–1.53)	0.90 (0.38–1.43)	2 (11%)
(3) High	16	9 (56%)	0.54 (<LOD–1.89)	0.99 (0.51–1.48)	2 (13%)
Arsenic proximity					
Yes	23	7 (30%)	<LOD (<LOD–0.52)	0.45 (0.25–0.64)	7 (30%)
No	52	29 (56%)	0.37 (<LOD–1.27)	0.89 (0.62–1.16)	4 (8%)

*LOD = 0.32 μg/L.

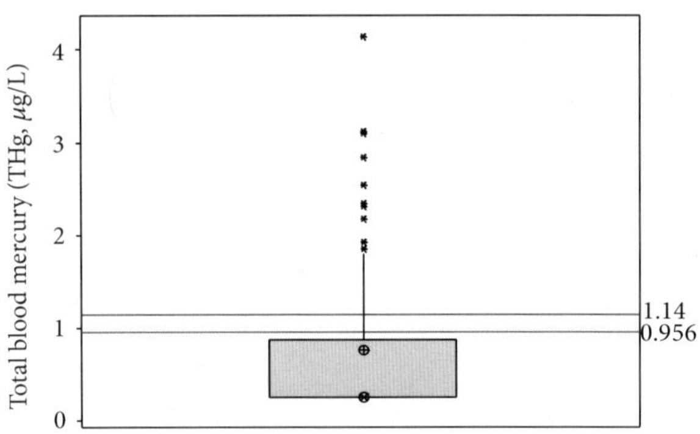

FIGURE 4: Scatterplot of total blood mercury (THg) for sample population with median denoted by an encircled "X" and mean denoted by an encircled cross. The reference lines at 0.956 μg/L and 1.14 μg/L indicate the 95% CI for THg in the US population from NHANES [36].

TABLE 2: Reduced model (multiple linear regression) for total blood mercury.

	Estimate	P value	Std. error
Intercept	0.412	0.46	0.56
Gender*	−0.545	*0.0084*	0.2
Age	0.0181	*0.022*	0.0077
Smoking score	−0.0127	0.91	0.12
Fish score	0.246	0.053	0.13
Arsenic proximity	−0.526	*0.020*	0.22

P values less than or equal to 0.05 are italicized.
*Male gender was used as the reference, so the estimate describes the effect of being a female.

predictors are summarized in Table 2. Male gender and older age were significant predictors of THg ($P = 0.0084$ and 0.022, resp.); fish consumption approached significance as a predictor for THg ($P = 0.053$).

3.2. Prevalence of ANA in the CRST Population. Anti-nuclear antibodies (ANA) were analyzed in serum samples from all participants. Data are presented in Table 1 and representative images of negative and ANA ≥ 2+ readings are shown in Figure 3. Approximately thirty-one percent of participants had an ANA reading of ≥2+. For readings ≥2+, ANA prevalence was significantly higher in women than in men (24% versus 5%; $P = 0.025$). ANA prevalence was also larger in community members living in proximity to high-concentration sedimentary arsenic deposits (30% versus 8%; $P = 0.028$).

Gender and fish consumption were significant predictors of ANA ≥2+, and gender modifies the effects of environmental exposures with respect to ANA. The logistic regression model information is shown in Table 3. Age and fish consumption are borderline predictors ($P < 0.10$) of ANA ≥ 2+ ($P = 0.081$ and $P = 0.092$, resp.), with age and fish consumption positively associated with the probability of ANA ≥ 2+ level of circulating ANA. Gender, THg, and proximity to arsenic, by themselves, do not strongly correlate with the probability of ANA ≥ 2+; however, the *interactions* of gender with THg and arsenic proximity are significant, and

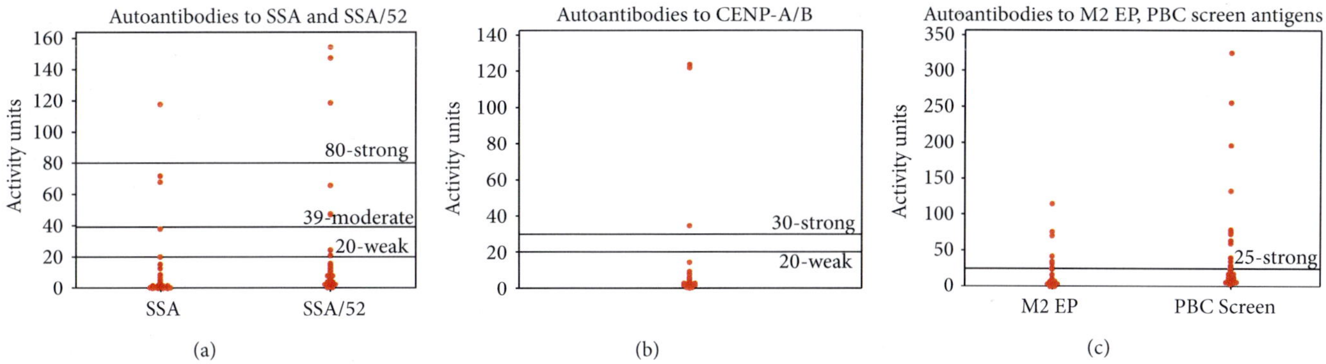

FIGURE 5: Dot plots of detectable autoantibodies in participant serum measured in activity units with labels for clinical cutoffs. Note: In clinical practice, there are no "moderate" positive readings for CENP-A/B; there are no "weak" or "moderate" positive readings for M2 EP and the PBC Screen.

TABLE 3: Point estimates and 95% confidence intervals (CI) for coefficients and odds ratios (OR) for fitting logistic regression models for ANA ≥2+.

	OR	95% CI	P value
Intercept	0.011	N/A	0.93
Age	1.1	0.96–1.17	0.081
Gender	2.4	0.046–645.5	0.37
THG	0.4	0.045–1.75	0.89
Fish score	2.9	0.56–20.70	0.092
Gender: THG	13.8	0.97–487.8	*0.026*
Gender: fish score	0.1	0.0013–1.12	0.97
Gender: arsenic proximity	27.1	0.68–2101	*0.040*
Arsenic proximity	0.3	0.015–4.26	0.82

P values less than or equal to 0.05 are italicized.

their odds ratios are greater than one (OR = 13.83, $P = 0.026$ and OR = 27.71, $P = 0.04$, resp.).

3.3. Specific Autoantibodies in the CRST Population. Of the specific autoantibodies for which participant sera were tested, SSA, SSA/52, CENP-A/B, M2 EP, and the autoantibodies detected by the primary biliary cirrhosis (PBC) panel were noteworthy. These results are summarized in Figure 5 and Table 4. Fifteen percent of participants tested positive for autoantibodies to M2 EP, while 24% were positive for autoantibodies to the PBC panel.

The number of specific autoantibodies detectable by INOVA kit increased with female gender and fish consumption score. Information for the reduced Poisson model for the number of detectable specific autoantibodies using INOVA assays can be found in Table 5(a). The number of specific autoantibodies detectable from INOVA assays was associated significantly with female gender ($P = 0.0064$). The model indicated that the mean number of specific autoantibodies detectable in serum is increased by a factor of 6.5 in female versus male community members. Age and fish consumption had significant ($P = 0.012$ and $P = 0.0073$, resp.) but smaller effects on the number of specific autoantibodies in the collected serum samples. In particular, the mean number of specific autoantibodies detectable by INOVA assay was 2.6 times greater in participants with a high (3) versus a low (1) fish consumption score. The number of participants positive for autoantibodies to native DNA, histone, and chromatin using in-house assays was small in our study. No significant associations were found between any demographic or exposure predictors, including smoking, and various combinations of in-house autoantibodies except in the case of dDNA and histone. The values for the reduced model can be seen in Table 5(b). Fish score was a significant predictor ($P = 0.035$) of the number of subjects with elevated anti-dDNA and anti-histone autoantibodies detectable using in-house assays. An increase of one fish score category predicts a 2.5-factor increase in the number of dDNA and histone autoantibodies. Smoking was a borderline predictor ($P = 0.065$) with a 0.4-factor decrease in the number of dDNA and histone autoantibodies for an increase of one smoking category.

Antichromatin positivity and reproducibility between INOVA and additional assays were confirmed in all positive serum samples (5/75); there was 100% agreement in detection using INOVA and in-house assays.

4. Discussion

We assumed that, due to consumption of locally caught fish, community members would have elevated levels of total blood mercury (THg). We hypothesized that THg would correspond to an increased level of autoantibodies, as has been shown in animal models [17]. Contrary to expectations, although Hg deposition in fish tissue had been documented in CRST sources by DENR, the detected THg levels in participants were low with a median THg < LOD, despite sampling during the middle of fishing season when fish consumption was considered to be maximal. The median THg for all participants (<LOD) was lower than the published results of the NHANES survey [47]. NHANES reported a mean THg of 0.944 μg/L for those 12 years and older [47]. Native American populations were not stratified in that study; the data were compiled under "other" ethnicity. The low levels of blood mercury among the CRST members

TABLE 4: Results of selected specific autoantibody results from the CRST population sample.

$n = 75$ Autoantibody	Negative	Moderate positive	Strong positive	Total positive
SSA	72 (96%)	2 (3%)	1 (1.3%)	3 (4%)
SSA-52	70 (93%)	2 (3%)	3 (4%)	5 (7%)
CENP-A/B	72 (96%)	0 (0%)	3 (4%)	3 (4%)
M2 EP	64 (85%)			11 (15%)
PBC panel	57 (76%)			18 (24%)

TABLE 5: (a) Model (Poisson regression) for the number of detected specific autoantibodies using INOVA assays. (b) Model (Poisson regression) for number of detected specific denatured DNA and histone autoantibodies from in-house assays.

(a)

	Factor of change	95% CI	P value
Intercept	0.0	0.00–0.18	0.0012
Gender*	6.5	1.69–24.78	*0.0064*
Age	1.0	1.01–1.04	*0.012*
Fish score	1.6	1.13–2.16	*0.0073*
Smoking score	1.9	0.60–5.77	0.29
Gender: smoking score	0.5	0.25–1.01	0.053

P values less than or equal to 0.05 are italicized. *Male gender was used as the reference, thus, the factor of change reflects the effect of being female.

(b)

	Factor of change	95% CI	P value
Intercept	0.2	0.004–9.831	0.406
Age	1	0.919–1.055	0.658
Smoking	0.4	0.127–1.064	0.065
Fish score	2.5	1.067–5.980	*0.035*
Arsenic proximity	0	0.000–3.752	0.117
Age: arsenic proximity	1.1	0.984–1.244	0.092

P values less than or equal to 0.05 are italicized.

found in our study confirmed the THg levels reported in a 2008 collaborative study between our team and CDC [48, 49]. Potential reasons for the observed low THg include variation due to race/ethnicity and possible physiological and metabolic changes among CRST community members, or possible alterations in deposition and clearance with repeated exposure in this population.

While gender, age, and fish consumption showed an impact on THg levels in the CRST population, smoking did not (Table 2). This finding is puzzling since 56% of the participants reported current smoking, yet only 45% of that group had THg above the detection level. The trends in our data parallel those seen in the NHANES survey [50]. Males have greater mean THg versus females, and THg increases with age. Males may consume larger quantities of locally caught fish or engage in activities that increase dust and particulate exposures to mercury (e.g., agricultural work, horse-tending). The age-dependent increase in THg found in this study, as well as in Wolkin et al. [48] and the NHANES survey [50], is likely due to the accumulation of metals in the body over time.

Thirty-one percent of participants had an ANA reading of ≥2+. ANA production could be associated with chronic toxicant exposure, which introduces self-antigens to antigen presenting cells, resulting in the breakdown of T-cell tolerance. While no single predictor was significantly associated ($P < 0.05$) with ANA ≥ 2+, fish score was a borderline predictor ($P = 0.092$). A larger proportion of ANA-positive participants were female, which concurs with the literature and clinical findings about autoimmune diseases [24], and may support a possible role for female hormones in AD and immune dysregulation. Although THg and proximity to high-concentration arsenic deposits, by themselves, did not correlate with the probability of ANA ≥ 2+, the *interactions* of female gender with THg and female gender with arsenic proximity are significant ($P = 0.026$ and $P = 0.040$, resp.) and the odds ratios were large (OR = 13.8 and 27.1, resp.). Gender differences may reflect alterations in the molecular mechanisms by which gender-specific detoxification occurs within the human body.

Another interesting finding is that current smokers were less likely to have ANA ≥ 2+ results (Table 1). Additionally, the specific autoantibody model estimates for smoking were negative with ORs less than one (Tables 5(a) and 5(b)), suggesting a protective effect of smoking. The fact that fewer autoantibodies were detected in this subgroup of smokers sheds light on probable molecular mechanisms by which smoking induces immunosuppressive effects.

There were significant associations between predictor exposure variables and the presence of autoantibodies to dDNA and histone (Table 5(b)). This is potentially similar to previously observed instances of xenobiotic-induced antibody responses such as drug-induced lupus [42]. Autoantibody production to dDNA and histone may also be linked to epigenetic changes triggered by environmental stimuli.

The CRST population exhibited strong positivity for M2 EP autoantibodies and autoantibodies detectable with the PBC screen, both of which are associated with liver diseases. It is possible that the medical problem of high rates of idiopathic liver cirrhosis in Sioux communities (personal communication J. Henderson) may have environmental etiology. Similar findings were reported among Alaskan Natives [51]. As with ANA ≥ 2+ models, fish score was a significant predictor of *specific* autoantibodies using both detection methods ($P < 0.01$ for INOVA kit detection and $P < 0.05$ for in-house ELISA).

As to the specific mechanisms responsible for mercury and metal/metalloid-induced autoimmune responses in the CRST population, several mechanisms should be considered. In susceptible individuals, environmental metals may behave as adjuvants that prolong or enhance antigen-specific immune response through various mechanisms such as molecular mimicry [52], polyclonal activation of B cells [53], bystander activation [54], and epitope spreading [55]. Additionally, chronic exposures to environmental metals, including Hg and arsenic, are well known to induce oxidative stress. As has been characterized with thimerisol [56], this oxidative stress could lead to sensitization of inositol 1,4,5-triphospate (IP3) receptors, resulting in enhanced intracellular calcium release and subsequently the dysregulation of immune cells and autoimmunity. Another possibility includes the role of chronic gut exposures to ingested dietary nanoparticles of soil and minerals, which induce inflammasome production and the breakdown of immune tolerance via enhanced gastrointestinal antigen presentation. Since fish consumption was an important predictor of antibody production in this study, dietary exposure may be one potential pathway through which molecular markers of autoimmunity are generated, especially among native community members who are more likely to inhale and ingest large quantities of dust and metals due to their rural location, cultural practices, and subsistence and agricultural activities.

We hypothesize that fish consumption reflects multiple exposures, including coexposures to mercury, arsenic, and other environmental toxicants, such as pesticides, pharmaceuticals, and infectious agents. In animal and cell studies, Hg toxicity and autoimmunity are synergistically enhanced by coexposure to additional xenobiotics. These ideas will be explored in future studies, and additional activities that increase inadvertent exposure to toxicants will also be examined. Future studies will include a larger sample size, participant AD medical record history, and biomonitoring for arsenic and cotinine (indicator of smoking exposures) in order to address this study's limitations. We also acknowledge that technical issues with indirect immunofluorescence assays (IIFA) for the detection of ANA limit the comparability of these data to other population information and previous publications. However, IIFA is the gold-standard technique for ANA detection [57], and we attempted to minimize variability by using only one evaluator of staining (KMP, coauthor).

In this study, compelling evidence that the CRST population exhibited elevated levels of both ANA and specific autoantibodies was found. The observed results highlighted environmental toxicants that may contribute to autoantibody production in this population and also underscored the need to characterize the CRST communities' lifestyles and behaviors to better understand how complex exposures contribute to autoimmune health effects. There is a large knowledge gap concerning environmental influences on the development of AD, and it is imperative that they be addressed within the context of environmental health disparities issues, particularly in tribal communities. Information will empower CRST community members and leaders by aiding them in making informed decisions about health, health services, the environment, and the preservation of their culture, in which fishing plays a vital role.

Conflict of Interests

The authors declare that there is no conflict of interests regarding the publication of this paper.

Authors' Contribution

Jennifer Ong and Esther Erdei contributed equally to this work.

Acknowledgments

Colleen Martin and the Centers for Disease Control are acknowledged for their help with data collection and biomonitoring. Dr. Jeffrey A. Henderson from the Black Hills Center for American Indian Health is acknowledged for his continuing support, close relationship with CRST community members, and clinical knowledge. Esther Erdei received Community Engaged Research Pilot Grant from University of New Mexico (UNM) (2008) Center for Participatory Research under the Institute for Public Heath, Department of Family and Community Medicine in partnership with the Community Engagement and Research Unit of the Clinical and Translational Science Center (CTSC). Johnnye Lewis received theUniversity of New Mexico Clinical and Translational Science Center Pilot Grant *NIEHS R25 ES013292* Environmental Justice on Cheyenne River (2010).

References

[1] H. Kirkemo, W. L. Newman, and R. P. Ashley, *Gold*, U.S. Geological Survey, Denver, Colo, USA, 2001.

[2] S. Vinyard and R. Lauren, "Dirty Energy's Assault on Our Health: Mercury," 2011.

[3] G. C. Bryner, "Coalbed methane development: the costs and benefits of an emerging energy resource," *Natural Resources Journal*, vol. 43, no. 2, pp. 519–560, 2003.

[4] T. W. May, R. H. Wiedmeyer, J. Gober, and S. Larson, "Influence of mining-related activities on concentrations of metals in water and sediment from streams of the Black Hills, South Dakota," *Archives of Environmental Contamination and Toxicology*, vol. 40, no. 1, pp. 1–9, 2001.

[5] J. BigEagle, "Development processes of consumption advisories for the Cheyenne River Sioux Indian Reservation," in *Proceedings of the National Forum on Contaminants in Fish*, pp. 142–144, Baltimore, Md, USA, 2005.

[6] J. M. Johnston, D. Hoff, R. Hoogerheide, R. Edgar, D. Wall, and C. Ducheneaux, *Mercury Risk Management in Livestock Ponds on the Cheyenne River Sioux Reservation*, Science Forum, Washington, DC, USA, 2003.

[7] A. T. Byrne, "Fish Consumption Survey for the Cheyenne River Basin within the Cheyenne River Indian Reservation, South Dakota," Eagle Butte, SD, USA, 2002.

[8] U.S. Census Bureau, "Distribution of Income by Family and Household," 2000.

[9] U.S. Department of Health & Human Services, "Poverty Guidelines, Research, and Measurement n.d.".

[10] United States Department of the Interior Bureau of Indian Affairs Office of Indian Services, "2005 American Indian Population and Labor Force Report," 2005.

[11] M. Satoh, E. K. L. Chan, L. A. Ho et al., "Prevalence and sociodemographic correlates of antinuclear antibodies in the United States," *Arthritis & Rheumatism*, vol. 64, no. 7, pp. 2319–2327, 2012.

[12] C. M. Gallagher, A. E. McElroy, D. M. Smith, M. G. Golightly, and J. R. Meliker, "Polychlorinated biphenyls, mercury, and antinuclear antibody positivity, NHANES 2003-2004," *International Journal of Hygiene and Environmental Health*, vol. 216, no. 6, pp. 721–727, 2013.

[13] M. S. Leffell, M. D. Fallin, W. H. Hildebrand, J. W. Cavett, B. A. Iglehart, and A. A. Zachary, "HLA alleles and haplotypes among the lakota sioux: report of the ASHI minority workshops, part III," *Human Immunology*, vol. 65, no. 1, pp. 78–89, 2004.

[14] R. C. Williams, L. T. H. Jacobsson, W. C. Knowler et al., "Meta-analysis reveals association between most common class II haplotype in full-heritage native Americans and rheumatoid arthritis," *Human Immunology*, vol. 42, no. 1, pp. 90–94, 1995.

[15] J. Heward and S. C. Gough, "Genetic susceptibility to the development of autoimmune disease," *Clinical Science*, vol. 93, no. 6, pp. 479–491, 1997.

[16] K. M. Pollard, P. Hultman, and D. H. Kono, "Immunology and genetics of induced systemic autoimmunity," *Autoimmunity Reviews*, vol. 4, no. 5, pp. 282–288, 2005.

[17] D. Germolec, D. H. Kono, J. C. Pfau, and K. M. Pollard, "Animal models used to examine the role of the environment in the development of autoimmune disease: findings from an NIEHS Expert Panel Workshop," *Journal of Autoimmunity*, vol. 39, no. 4, pp. 285–293, 2012.

[18] S. Havarinasab and P. Hultman, "Alteration of the spontaneous systemic autoimmune disease in (NZB × NZW)F1 mice by treatment with thimerosal (ethyl mercury)," *Toxicology and Applied Pharmacology*, vol. 214, no. 1, pp. 43–54, 2006.

[19] P. Hultman, A. Taylor, J. M. Yang, and K. M. Pollard, "The effect of xenobiotic exposure on spontaneous autoimmunity in (SWR × SJL)F1 hybrid mice," *Journal of Toxicology and Environmental Health A*, vol. 69, no. 6, pp. 505–523, 2006.

[20] K. M. Pollard, D. L. Pearson, P. Hultman, T. N. Deane, U. Lindh, and D. H. Kono, "Xenobiotic acceleration of idiopathic systematic autoimmunity in lupus-prone BXSB mice," *Environmental Health Perspectives*, vol. 109, no. 1, pp. 27–33, 2001.

[21] K. M. Pollard, D. L. Pearson, P. Hultman, B. Hildebrandt, and D. H. Kono, "Lupus-prone mice as models to study xenobiotic-induced acceleration of systemic autoimmunity," *Environmental Health Perspectives*, vol. 107, supplement 5, pp. 729–735, 1999.

[22] D. Fairweather, S. Frisancho-Kiss, and N. R. Rose, "Sex differences in autoimmune disease from a pathological perspective," *The American Journal of Pathology*, vol. 173, no. 3, pp. 600–609, 2008.

[23] J. B. Nielsen and P. Hultman, "Mercury-induced autoimmunity in mice," *Environmental Health Perspectives*, vol. 110, no. 5, pp. 877–881, 2002.

[24] K. M. Pollard, "Gender differences in autoimmunity associated with exposure to environmental factors," *Journal of Autoimmunity*, vol. 38, no. 2-3, pp. J177–J186, 2012.

[25] K. K. Aminzadeh and M. Etminan, "Dental amalgam and multiple sclerosis: a systematic review and meta-analysis," *Journal of Public Health Dentistry*, vol. 67, no. 1, pp. 64–66, 2007.

[26] M. N. Bates, J. Fawcett, N. Garrett, T. Cutress, and T. Kjellstrom, "Health effects of dental amalgam exposure: a retrospective cohort study," *International Journal of Epidemiology*, vol. 33, no. 4, pp. 894–902, 2004.

[27] J. F. Nyland, M. Fillion, F. Barbosa Jr. et al., "Biomarkers of methylmercury exposure immunotoxicity among fish consumers in amazonian Brazil," *Environmental Health Perspectives*, vol. 119, no. 12, pp. 1733–1738, 2011.

[28] R. M. Gardner, J. F. Nyland, I. A. Silva, A. M. Ventura, J. M. de Souza, and E. K. Silbergeld, "Mercury exposure, serum antinuclear/antinucleolar antibodies, and serum cytokine levels in mining populations in Amazonian Brazil: a cross-sectional study," *Environmental Research*, vol. 110, no. 4, pp. 345–354, 2010.

[29] E. K. Silbergeld, I. A. Silva, and J. F. Nyland, "Mercury and autoimmunity: implications for occupational and environmental health," *Toxicology and Applied Pharmacology*, vol. 207, no. 2, supplement, pp. 282–292, 2005.

[30] I. A. Silva, J. F. Nyland, A. Gorman et al., "Mercury exposure, malaria, and serum antinuclear/antinucleolar antibodies in amazon populations in Brazil: a cross-sectional study," *Environmental Health: A Global Access Science Source*, vol. 3, article 11, 2004.

[31] R. M. Gardner, J. F. Nyland, and E. K. Silbergeld, "Differential immunotoxic effects of inorganic and organic mercury species *in vitro*," *Toxicology Letters*, vol. 198, no. 2, pp. 182–190, 2010.

[32] R. M. Gardner, J. F. Nyland, S. L. Evans et al., "Mercury induces an unopposed inflammatory response in human peripheral blood mononuclear cells *in vitro*," *Environmental Health Perspectives*, vol. 117, no. 12, pp. 1932–1938, 2009.

[33] P. N. Henderson, S. Kanekar, Y. Wen et al., "Patterns of cigarette smoking initiation in two culturally distinct American Indian tribes," *American Journal of Public Health*, vol. 99, no. 11, pp. 2020–2025, 2009.

[34] F. Pragst and S. Leo, "Smoking trials with mercury contaminated cigarettes: studies of attempted poisoning," *Archiv für Kriminologie*, vol. 188, no. 3-4, pp. 77–86, 1991.

[35] M. R. Fresquez, R. S. Pappas, and C. H. Watson, "Establishment of toxic metal reference range in tobacco from US cigarettes," *Journal of Analytical Toxicology*, vol. 37, no. 5, pp. 298–304, 2013.

[36] J. S. Smolen, B. Butcher, M. J. Fritzler et al., "Reference sera for antinuclear antibodies: II. Further definition of antibody specificities in international antinuclear antibody reference sera by immunofluorescence and western blotting," *Arthritis & Rheumatism*, vol. 40, no. 3, pp. 413–418, 1997.

[37] United States Environmental Protection Agency, "Consumption Advice: Joint Federal Advisory for Mercury in Fish n.d.".

[38] A. S. Andrew, D. A. Jewell, R. A. Mason, M. L. Whitfield, J. H. Moore, and M. R. Karagas, "Drinking-water arsenic exposure modulates gene expression in human lymphocytes from a U.S. population," *Environmental Health Perspectives*, vol. 116, no. 4, pp. 524–531, 2008.

[39] R. Biswas, P. Ghosh, N. Banerjee et al., "Analysis of T-cell proliferation and cytokine secretion in the individuals exposed to arsenic," *Human and Experimental Toxicology*, vol. 27, no. 5, pp. 381–386, 2008.

[40] J.-M. Yang, B. Hildebrandt, C. Luderschmidt, and K. M. Pollard, "Human scleroderma sera contain autoantibodies to protein components specific to the U3 small nucleolar RNP complex," *Arthritis & Rheumatism*, vol. 48, no. 1, pp. 210–217, 2003.

[41] E. M. Tan, T. E. W. Feltkamp, J. S. Smolen et al., "Range of antinuclear antibodies in "healthy" individuals," *Arthritis & Rheumatism*, vol. 40, no. 9, pp. 1601–1611, 1997.

[42] R. L. Rubin, "Drug-induced lupus," *Toxicology*, vol. 209, no. 2, pp. 135–147, 2005.

[43] R. W. Burlingame and R. L. Rubin, "Subnucleosome structures as substrates in enzyme-linked immunosorbent assays," *Journal of Immunological Methods*, vol. 134, no. 2, pp. 187–199, 1990.

[44] G. Schett, J. Smolen, C. Zimmermann et al., "The autoimmune response to chromatin antigens in systemic lupus erythematosus: autoantibodies against histone H1 are a highly specific marker for SLE associated with increased disease activity," *Lupus*, vol. 11, no. 11, pp. 704–715, 2002.

[45] R Core Team, *R: A Language and Environment for Statistical Computing*, R Foundation for Statistical Computing, Vienna, Austria, 2013.

[46] B. D. Ripley, B. Venables, D. M. Bates, K. Hornik, A. Gebhardt, and D. Firth, "Support Functions and Datasets for Venables and Ripley's MASS," 2013.

[47] Centers for Disease Control, "Fourth National Report on Human Exposure to Environmental Chemicals: Updated Tables, September 2013," 2013.

[48] A. Wolkin, D. Hunt, C. Martin, K. L. Caldwell, and M. A. McGeehin, "Blood mercury levels among fish consumers residing in areas with high environmental burden," *Chemosphere*, vol. 86, no. 9, pp. 967–971, 2012.

[49] C. Martin, A. Wolkin, C. Ducheneaux, J. Lewis, and J. Henderson, *Blood Mercury (Hg) Levels Among Consumers of Locally Caught Fish Residing on the Cheyenne River Sioux Tribe (CRST) Reservation*, American Public Health Association, 2009.

[50] K. L. Caldwell, M. E. Mortensen, R. L. Jones, S. P. Caudill, and J. D. Osterloh, "Total blood mercury concentrations in the U.S. population: 1999–2006," *International Journal of Hygiene and Environmental Health*, vol. 212, no. 6, pp. 588–598, 2009.

[51] K. J. Hurlburt, B. J. McMahon, H. Deubner, B. Hsu-Trawinski, J. L. Williams, and K. V. Kowdley, "Prevalence of autoimmune liver disease in Alaska natives," *The American Journal of Gastroenterology*, vol. 97, no. 9, pp. 2402–2407, 2002.

[52] E. Israeli, N. Agmon-Levin, M. Blank, and Y. Shoenfeld, "Adjuvants and autoimmunity," *Lupus*, vol. 18, no. 13, pp. 1217–1225, 2009.

[53] O. Barzilai, M. Ram, and Y. Shoenfeld, "Viral infection can induce the production of autoantibodies," *Current Opinion in Rheumatology*, vol. 19, no. 6, pp. 636–643, 2007.

[54] K. Murali-Krishna, J. D. Altman, M. Suresh et al., "Counting antigen-specific CD8 T cells: a reevaluation of bystander activation during viral infection," *Immunity*, vol. 8, no. 2, pp. 177–187, 1998.

[55] P. V. Lehmanann, T. Forthuber, A. Miller, and E. E. Sercaz, "Spreading of T-cell autoimmunity to cryptic determinants of an antigen," *Nature*, vol. 358, no. 6382, pp. 155–157, 1992.

[56] D. Yeter and R. Deth, "ITPKC susceptibility in Kawasaki syndrome as a sensitizing factor for autoimmunity and coronary arterial wall relaxation induced by thimerosal's effects on calcium signaling via IP3," *Autoimmunity Reviews*, vol. 11, no. 12, pp. 903–908, 2012.

[57] N. Agmon-Levin, J. Damoiseaux, C. Kallenberg, U. Sack, T. Witte, M. Herold et al., "International recommendations for the assessment of autoantibodies to cellular antigens referred to as anti-nuclear antibodies," *Annals of the Rheumatic Diseases*, vol. 73, no. 1, pp. 17–23, 2014.

9

Updates on Morphea: Role of Vascular Injury and Advances in Treatment

Julio C. Sartori-Valinotti,[1] Megha M. Tollefson,[1] and Ann M. Reed[2]

[1] *The Department of Dermatology, Mayo Clinic College of Medicine, Rochester, MN 55905, USA*
[2] *The Department of Pediatrics, Mayo Clinic College of Medicine, Rochester, MN 55905, USA*

Correspondence should be addressed to Ann M. Reed; reed.ann18@mayo.edu

Academic Editor: Paulo Ricardo Criado

Morphea and systemic sclerosis are fibrosing disorders of the skin that share common inflammatory and immunologic pathways that are responsible for the vascular changes, increased collagen production, and extracellular matrix proliferation seen in both conditions. Recent advances in molecular biology techniques have furthered our knowledge of the potential underlying pathogenic mechanisms and offer new and provocative areas of research for novel diagnostic and therapeutic interventions. This review focuses on the role of vascular injury in the development of morphea, the use of ultrasonography as a diagnostic modality, and well-established and newly proposed treatments.

1. Introduction

Morphea is an inflammatory, fibrosing skin disorder that leads to sclerosis of the dermis and subcutaneous tissue but in some cases may also extend to the fascia, muscle, and underlying bone. Clinically, morphea has an asymmetric distribution and is usually confined to one body area; hence it is also referred to as localized scleroderma. Systemic sclerosis (SSc), however, in addition to symmetric skin changes is characterized by internal organ involvement, sclerodactyly, presence of Raynaud's phenomenon, and nailfold capillary abnormalities. Despite these differences, both entities share common inflammatory and immunologic pathways that are ultimately responsible for the vascular changes, increased collagen production, and extracellular matrix proliferation seen in both conditions. Although the etiology and precise mechanisms that trigger the cascade of molecular events that culminate in skin fibrosis are not fully understood, advances in molecular biology techniques have furthered our knowledge of the potential culprits and offer new and provocative areas of research for novel diagnostic and therapeutic interventions. This brief review will focus on the role of vascular injury in the development of morphea with emphasis on recent basic research data as well as use of ultrasonography as a diagnostic method. Lastly, well-established and newly proposed treatments will be discussed.

2. Clinical Features

Several classification systems have been developed in attempt to grasp the breath of the various forms of presentation of morphea [1, 2]. They are largely based on clinical findings and include, with minor differences, at least four major variants: plaque-type, linear, generalized and a miscellaneous group of morphologically distinct phenotypes.

Plaque-Type Morphea (Morphea en Plaque or Circumscribed). It is the most common subtype overall and the most common variant in adults. Most often located on the trunk, it begins as an erythematous-to-violaceous, edematous plaque of several centimeters that extends peripherally over a period of 3 to 5 years before it reaches a plateau phase. This is followed by an involution phase that leaves behind atrophic skin (Figure 1).

Linear Morphea (Including Morphea en Coup de Sabre (Figure 2) and Progressive Hemifacial Atrophy or Parry-Romberg Syndrome). Most common in children and adolescents, it presents as a linear induration on the scalp,

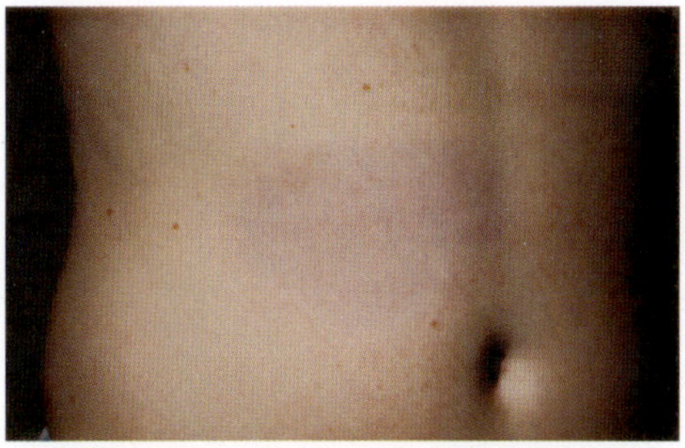

FIGURE 1: Plaque-type morphea.

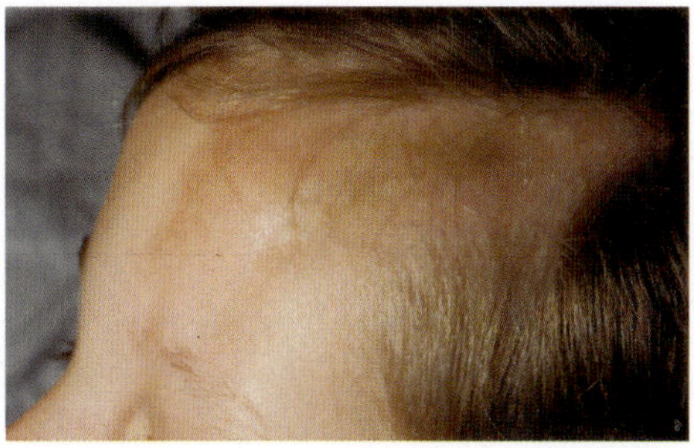

FIGURE 2: Morphea en coup de sabre.

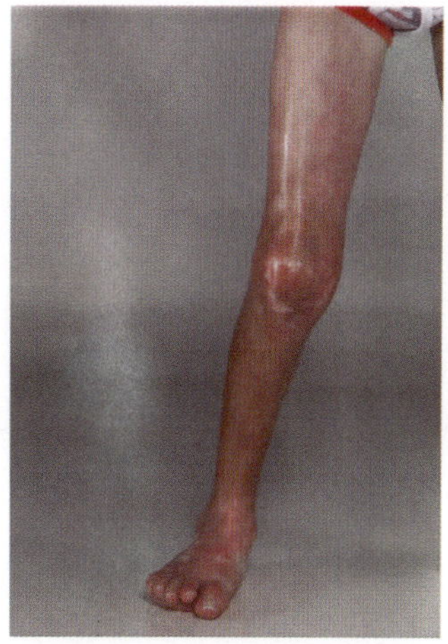

FIGURE 3: Linear morphea affecting the leg.

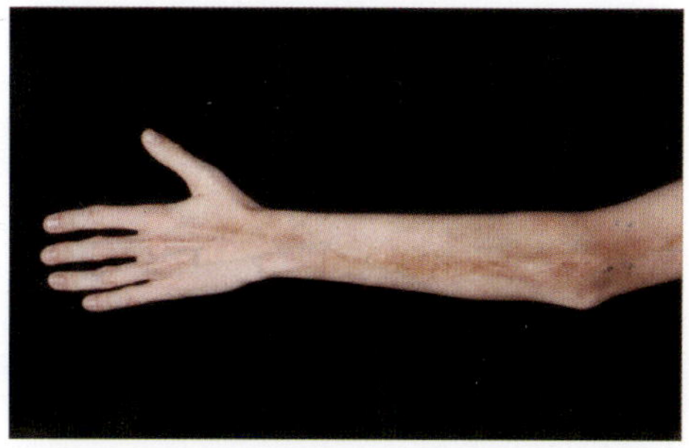

FIGURE 4: Linear morphea of the upper extremity.

forehead, trunk, or extremities (Figures 3 and 4), sometimes with involvement of the eye (in the case of facial lesions), underlying fascia, muscle, and bone. The latter may lead to limb atrophy and joint immobilization. Patients with Parry-Romberg syndrome and *en coup de sabre* morphea may also have seizures, headaches, and abnormal intracranial findings on magnetic resonance imaging (MRI) [3]. Linear morphea affecting the mouth has also been described (Figure 5). Antinuclear antibodies, ssDNA, and antihistones antibodies are usually positive.

Generalized Morphea. It is defined by the presence of four or more plaque-type lesions affecting two or more body sites or by the insidious onset of a slowly progressing plaque-type morphea on the trunk with eventual involvement of the entire trunk leading to progressive dyspnea due to mechanical restriction of chest cage expansion. Similar to linear morphea, patients in this subgroup have positive serology for antinuclear antibodies, ssDNA, and antihistones antibodies and are more likely to have constitutional symptoms.

Miscellaneous Group. Encompasses a variety of phenotypically different lesions including nodular, mixed (combination of two or more variants), guttate, bullous morphea and atrophoderma of Pasini and Pierini.

Irrespective of the clinical subgroup, morphea can be distinguished from SSc by the absence of internal organ involvement, Raynaud's phenomenon and nailfold capillary changes. On the other hand, SSc can be further subdivided into limited SSc (lSSc) and diffuse SSc (dSSC) on the basis of the extent and distribution pattern of skin disease. Sclerodermatous skin changes distal to the elbows or knees are referred to as lSSC whereas skin thickening proximal to these anatomic landmarks are characteristic of dSSC. A subset of patients with lSSc and calcinosis, Raynaud's phenomenon, esophageal dysmotility, sclerodactyly, and telangiectasias comprised the so-called CREST syndrome.

3. Pathogenesis

Vascular Injury as the Crucial Event. It has been proposed that endothelial cell damage may represent the initial and pivotal step in the development of soft tissue changes in morphea and systemic sclerosis. For example, using whole-field digital microscopy and transmission electron microscopy, Frech and coworkers demonstrated that 20 patients with SSc had increased skin interstitial edema, fibrosis, basal lamina lamellation, and endothelial swelling compared to normal controls, irrespective of disease duration, or appreciable clinical features [4]. This is consistent with the clinical findings of Raynaud's phenomenon and nail fold capillary changes seen in the early stages of the disease prior to the development of frank fibrosis. Infection, hypoxia, trauma, radiation, reactive oxygen species, and antiendothelial cell autoantibodies contribute to vascular injury and subsequent recruitment and activation of T and B lymphocytes and mononuclear cells, secretion of proinflammatory mediators and growth factors, endothelial cell apoptosis, and fibroblast activation which in

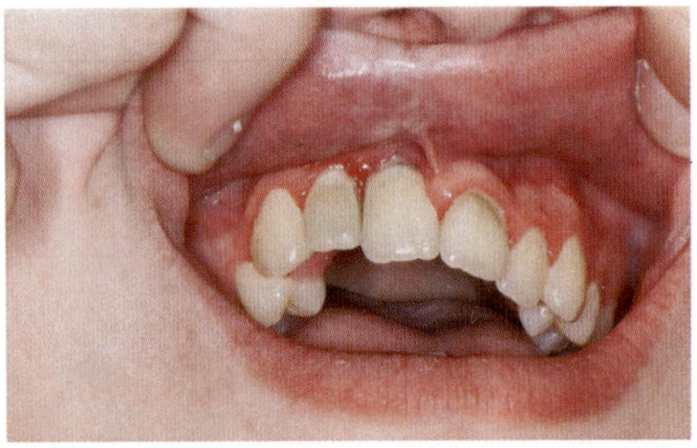

FIGURE 5: Linear morphea of the mouth. Note subtle changes of the inner upper lip and gingival mucosa around the maxillary right central incisor.

turn leads to vascular and tissue remodeling and fibrosis [5–9].

Under physiologic and pathologic conditions, disruption of the capillary network results in decreased blood flow and tissue ischemia. The ability to withstand hypoxia varies by tissue type and is tightly regulated by hypoxia inducible factors. One of the adaptive responses to diminished tissue oxygen delivery is the formation of new vessels via either angiogenesis and/or vasculogenesis. The former refers to the formation of new vessels from preexisting vessels whereas vasculogenesis represents de novo vessel formation from bone marrow derived endothelial precursor cells (EPC). Cumulative evidence suggests that both processes are defective in SSc despite strong proangiogenic stimuli [10].

Viruses may trigger vascular damage via neointimal proliferation and apoptosis likely through overproduction of profibrotic cytokines including TGF-beta, PDGF-alpha, and PDGF-beta [11]. Cytomegalovirus (CMV) RNA transcripts have been found in the endothelium of patients with sclerodermoid changes [12]. Similarly, parvovirus B19-infected endothelial cells, fibroblasts, and perivascular inflammatory cells of SSc patients have increased expression of TNF-alpha [13] which has been shown to participate in regulation of fibroblast function and endothelial activation [14]. A role for viral infection is further supported by the observation that molecular mimicry between human CMV late protein UL94 and NAG-2, a surface molecule present on endothelial cells and dermal fibroblasts, is responsible for cross-reactivity of human anti-CMV antibodies against the latter and may contribute to chronic sclerodermoid graft versus host disease (GVHD) [15, 16].

Endothelial cell apoptosis is a key feature of SSc and arguably the earliest event [17]. IL-6 and the Fas-pathway have been implicated in endothelial cell apoptosis [18, 19] via mechanisms dependent on the presence of neutrophils and antibody-induced cell-mediated toxicity, respectively. Circulating angiogenic cells are also prone to and undergo apoptosis in SSc through phagocytosis of microparticles and stimulation of acid sphingomyelinase activity [20]. Plasma samples of SSc patients have significantly higher levels of microparticles [21]. They are small, membrane-bound vesicles with altered surface lipids that participate in intercellular signaling [22]. Conversely, dermal fibroblasts are resistant to Fas-mediated apoptosis, perhaps due to deficiency in acid sphingomyelinase, and increased levels of anti-apoptotic proteins cFLIPs and cIAP, partially explaining their survival and contribution to increased extracellular matrix deposition in SSc [23, 24].

Antiendothelial cell autoantibodies (AECAs) likely promote vascular injury, endothelial cell apoptosis, generation of reactive oxygen species, and expression of adhesion molecules on endothelial cells in patients with SSc. They are a heterogeneous group of antibodies against endothelial cell-specific proteins and are present in 22–86% of patients with SSc [25]. Upon interaction with these antibodies, endothelial cells augment the expression of vascular cell adhesion molecule-1 (VCAM-1), intercellular adhesion molecule-1 (ICAM-1), and E-selectin resulting in increased leucocyte adhesion. Moreover, they stimulate platelet-derived growth factor (PDGF) pathway and oxidative stress [26]. Beyond their pathogenic role in dermal fibrosis, AECAs have also been linked to complications of SSs, including pulmonary fibrosis and hypertension, and apoptosis of bone marrow EPC [27, 28].

Microarray analyses of EPC from patients with SSc reveal a differential protein expression profile under both basal and hypoxic conditions, with differentiation towards a proinflammatory state. Furthermore, immunohistochemistry of SSc skin samples shows downregulation of TNFS10, TNFAIP3, and HOX-A9 and overexpression of PTGS-2 [29]. Most recently, genomic DNA analysis of eight pairs of monozygotic twins with SSc identified sites that were preferentially hypermethylated or hypomethylated on the X chromosome and corresponded to target genes governing, among other cellular pathways, apoptosis (MTM1), inflammation (ARAF), and oxidative stress (ENOX2) [30]. These latter findings provide some insight into the molecular alterations behind the higher prevalence of morphea and SSc in women.

Vascular abnormalities seem not to be limited to the skin. Patients with SSc have reduced bone marrow vascularity, in spite of normal cell morphology, as measured by microvessel density. Notoriously, peripheral blood mononuclear cells (PMBC) from individuals with SSc release greater amounts of VEGF [31], and its expression is much higher in SSc patients [32, 33] thus suggesting a diminished responsiveness to angiogenic stimuli. Impaired production of TNF-like weak inducer of apoptosis (TWEAK), a newly characterized cytokine, by PMBC may be accountable for aberrant angiogenesis and tissue remodeling in SSc [34]. Lastly, fibroblasts and autoimmunity are also important pathogenic players in morphea and SSc, but in-depth discussion of these topics is beyond the scope of this review.

4. Evaluation

Based on the increasing evidence that vascular changes dominate the early stages of disease development, it is not surprising that there is emerging research looking into ways to rapidly and accurately recognize them. Ultrasonography has gained particular attention as a noninvasive, harmless, and inexpensive diagnostic tool.

Morphea and SSc are characterized by three distinct phases of skin disease: active or edematous; inactive, sclerotic, or fibrosis; and atrophic lesions. Early recognition of the active phase may have both therapeutic and prognostic implications. In a study of 104 morphea lesions, ultrasonography was not inferior to dermatopathologic examination in evaluating active disease. Indeed, when compared to histology, increased cutaneous (dermal or subcutaneous) blood flow and hyperechogenicity of the subcutaneous tissue had both 100% specificity and 100% sensitivity [35]. In keeping with these observations, using fourteen MHz ultrasonography of 16 morphea lesions, hyperechogenicity correlated with the presence of moderate or severe sclerosis on histology. More importantly, ultrasonographic findings were more reliable than clinical-based scores such as the Modified Rodnan Skin Score (mRSS) [36] and have acceptable and reproducible inter- and intraobserver reliability. The inactive and atrophic phases of the disease also exhibit unique sonographic features [37, 38].

Ultrasound can additionally be used to determine the severity of musculoskeletal involvement [39] and endothelial function [40] in SSc and in sclerodermoid GVHD [41]. It has also been shown to be useful in monitoring the response to treatment. For instance, in pediatric patients, the hyperemia and increased echogenicity of active lesions disappeared after successful treatment [42]. In a different series, dermal thickness as measured by ultrasound was decreased in patients treated with phototherapy [43] and topical imiquimod [44]. Due to its depth of penetration, which is a function of frequency, the usefulness of ultrasonography is somewhat limited to the skin and subcutaneous tissue. In this regard MRI is more advantageous and allows for better assessment of deeper structures such as the fascia and underlying muscle [45, 46]. As with ultrasonography, MRI can be resourceful in monitoring disease activity and response to treatment [47].

5. Treatment

The treatment of morphea and skin disease in SSc is challenging, and its efficacy is difficult to assess owing to the absence of validated and standardized outcome measures. Nonetheless, numerous treatment modalities both systemic and topical have been investigated, the majority of which have been abandoned due to lack of response or have not been investigated in larger populations. However, among these interventions, methotrexate (MTX) alone or in combination with systemic steroids and phototherapy have been proven to be beneficial with stronger evidence to support their use.

5.1. Methotrexate. The effectiveness of methotrexate, primarily in conjunction with systemic steroids, has been validated by several retrospective studies. In the recent past, at least six prospective, including double-blind, randomized trials have confirmed the efficacy and safety of this therapeutic regimen. For example, in patients with juvenile morphea, clinical remission for a mean duration of 25 months was achieved with simultaneous use of MTX and prednisone [48]. In another study of pediatric patients with moderate to severe morphea, this combination strategy quickly resulted in clinical improvement, as determined by Modified LS Skin Severity Index, within two months of treatment [49]. Improvement in musculoskeletal involvement has also been observed in a prospective study of adults with deep morphea (mean age 52 years) [47]. When added to MTX and prednisone, imatinib, which inhibits fibroblast activity, halted the progression of skin disease and joint deformity in a 3-year-old patient [50]. MTX likely exerts its antifibrotic effects via inhibition of inflammatory cytokines such as IL-2, IL-4, IL-6, IL-8, and TNF-alpha and adhesion molecules such as ICAM-1 [7, 51, 52].

With regard to the use of MTX in SSc, in 2009 the European League Against Rheumatism/EULAR Scleroderma Trails and Research published recommendations for the management of the multiple manifestations of SSc, including cutaneous involvement. Based on two randomized controlled trials on patients with early diffuse SSc or limited SSc [53, 54], methotrexate was recommended as a first-line treatment for early diffuse SSc (Class A recommendation). Notwithstanding, MTX was superior to placebo in one of these studies [54], whereas the other showed only a trend favoring MTX, but it did not reach statistical significance. Two important considerations can be drawn from these conflicting observations. First, it is conceivable to hypothesize that, relative to morphea, the modest or lack of response to treatment with MTX in SSc is due to the fact that most studies for management of morphea included a combination of MTX and steroids. Second, with widespread involvement, the efficacy of MTX may be reduced or difficult to quantify. Placebo controlled trials assessing the benefits of combined MTX and systemic steroids for diffuse SSc are lacking.

Mycophenolate mofetil is reserved as a second line agent that could be used for treatment of localized and generalized morphea after failed response to MTX and/or phototherapy [55, 56]. Over the past decade, B-cell depletion therapy has gained special attention as a successful intervention for various immune-mediated diseases. Pertaining to its use for sclerodermoid conditions, there are conflicting results in patients with refractory sclerodermoid GVHD either showing improvement [17] or lack of response [57]. A recent case report showed resolution of localized scleroderma with rituximab [58]. Larger case series and prospective studies will help elucidate its potential use as a standard treatment.

5.2. Phototherapy. First documented in 1994 [59], phototherapy for treatment of morphea has since been widely used and studied. By virtue of their longer wavelength and thus deeper penetration, PUVA therapy and UVA1 are the cornerstone of light treatment for localized scleroderma. Its mechanism of action likely involves the combination of various effects such as alteration in cytokine and growth factors expression, modulation of endothelial dysfunction, induction of matrix metalloproteinases that degrade collagen, apoptosis of Langerhans cells and T cells, and inhibition of collagen synthesis [60–63]. The treatment course varies among clinical protocols, but it typically requires approximately 30 sessions before clinical, histological, and ultrasonographic improvement can be appreciated. Furthermore, clinical improvement continues beyond cessation of therapy; thus prolonged treatment is neither needed nor indicated. Phototherapy is effective in all Fitzpatrick skin prototypes and is generally well tolerated, with no serious side effects. The main caveats to the use of UVA1 are the need for prolonged exposure times, diminished effectives after repetitive treatment owing to increased pigmentation, and its availability at specialized centers only. Alternatively, narrowband UVB and broadband UVA can be used with satisfactory results [64–67].

There is a paucity of data on the use of phototherapy for management of diffuse skin involvement in SSc, but PUVA and UVA1 have been reported to be effective. In a study of 18 patients with acrosclerosis, low dose UVA1 resulted in reduction of clinical score from 19.4 to 14.9; this was accompanied by elevation of dermal collagenase [68]. In a larger series of patients with different skin conditions amenable to treatment with UVA1, 12 patients with SSc/CREST had a moderate response (51–75% improvement) as determined by clinical assessment by the same physician before and after treatment [69]. Another study involving 3 patients with systemic scleroderma also reported improvement in the mRSS after UVA1 treatment [70]. Due to the small number of study subjects, evaluation of limited disease with involvement of the hands only, and the subjective (clinical) assessment of response to treatment, the results of these studies cannot be generalized.

On the other hand, provocative data from the basic research literature may be key in providing the foundation for the development of new therapeutic interventions for morphea and SSc. For instance, the tight-skin (Tsk (−/+)) model of SSc shows abnormal fibrillin-1 expression and chronic oxidative damage that may be responsible for impaired angiogenesis [71]. Circulating endothelial cells and EPCs from patients with SSc treated with iloprost, a synthetic analogue of the vasodilatory prostacyclin PGI2, exhibit upregulation of antiapoptotic genes and genes involved in wound healing [72]. Treatment with recombinant human erythropoietin resulted in resolution of a nonhealing digital ulcer and reduction in apoptotic rates of bone marrow endothelial cells [73] in a patient with SSc. In conclusion, the advent of new technology has furthered our understanding of the imbricated mechanisms behind the development of these debilitating and disfiguring conditions. Nonetheless, placebo-controlled trials exploring these newly discovered pathways are much needed to expand our treatment repertoire. This task is rather challenging because, by virtue of its heterogenous presentation, better measures of disease activity and outcomes are necessary to accurately evaluate evidence-based therapies. Fortunately, research in this area is underway.

Conflict of Interests

The authors declare that they have no conflict of interests.

References

[1] R. M. Laxer and F. Zulian, "Localized scleroderma," *Current Opinion in Rheumatology*, vol. 18, no. 6, pp. 606–613, 2006.

[2] L. S. Peterson, A. M. Nelson, and W. P. D. Su, "Classification of morphea (localized scleroderma)," *Mayo Clinic Proceedings*, vol. 70, no. 11, pp. 1068–1076, 1995.

[3] Y. E. Chiu, S. Vora, E. K. Kwon, and M. Maheshwari, "A significant proportion of children with morphea en coup de sabre and Parry-Romberg syndrome have neuroimaging findings," *Pediatric Dermatology*, vol. 29, pp. 738–748, 2012.

[4] T. M. Frech, M. P. Revelo, S. G. Drakos et al., "Vascular leak is a central feature in the pathogenesis of systemic sclerosis," *The Journal of Rheumatology*, vol. 39, pp. 1385–1391, 2012.

[5] M. Hasegawa, S. Sato, T. Nagaoka, M. Fujimoto, and K. Takehara, "Serum levels of tumor necrosis factor and interleukin-13 are elevated in patients with localized scleroderma," *Dermatology*, vol. 207, no. 2, pp. 141–147, 2003.

[6] H. Higley, K. Persichitte, S. Chu, W. Waegell, R. Vancheeswaran, and C. Black, "Immunocytochemical localization and serologic detection of transforming growth factor β1: association with type I procollagen and inflammatory cell markers in diffuse and limited systemic sclerosis, morphea, and Raynaud's phenomenon," *Arthritis and Rheumatism*, vol. 37, no. 2, pp. 278–288, 1994.

[7] H. Ihn, S. Sato, M. Fujimoto, K. Kikuchi, and K. Takehara, "Demonstration of interleukin-2, interleukin-4 and interleukin-6 in sera from patients with localized scleroderma," *Archives of Dermatological Research*, vol. 287, no. 2, pp. 193–197, 1995.

[8] V.-M. Kahari, M. Sandberg, H. Kalimo, T. Vuorio, and E. Vuorio, "Identification of fibroblasts responsible for increased collagen production in localized scleroderma by in situ hybridization," *Journal of Investigative Dermatology*, vol. 90, no. 5, pp. 664–670, 1988.

[9] R. Sgonc, M. S. Gruschwitz, H. Dietrich, H. Recheis, M. E. Gershwin, and G. Wick, "Endothelial cell apoptosis is a primary pathogenetic event underlying skin lesions in avian and human scleroderma," *The Journal of Clinical Investigation*, vol. 98, no. 3, pp. 785–792, 1996.

[10] P. Cipriani, A. Marrelli, V. Liakouli, P. Di Benedetto, and R. Giacomelli, "Cellular players in angiogenesis during the course of systemic sclerosis," *Autoimmunity Reviews*, vol. 10, no. 10, pp. 641–646, 2011.

[11] D. Hamamdzic, R. A. Harley, D. Hazen-Martin, and E. C. LeRoy, "MCMV induces neointima in IFN-γR-/- mice: intimal cell apoptosis and persistent proliferation of myofibroblasts," *BMC Musculoskeletal Disorders*, vol. 2, article 1, 2001.

[12] C. M. Magro, A. N. Crowson, and C. Ferri, "Cytomegalovirus-associated cutaneous vasculopathy and scleroderma sans inclusion body change," *Human Pathology*, vol. 38, no. 1, pp. 42–49, 2007.

[13] C. M. Magro, G. Nuovo, C. Ferri, A. N. Crowson, D. Giuggioli, and M. Sebastiani, "Parvoviral infection of endothelial cells and stromal fibroblasts: a possible pathogenetic role in scleroderma," *Journal of Cutaneous Pathology*, vol. 31, no. 1, pp. 43–50, 2004.

[14] S. S. Koca, A. Isik, I. H. Ozercan, B. Ustundag, B. Evren, and K. Metin, "Effectiveness of etanercept in bleomycin-induced experimental scleroderma," *Rheumatology*, vol. 47, no. 2, pp. 172–175, 2008.

[15] C. Lunardi, M. Dolcino, D. Peterlana et al., "Antibodies against human cytomegalovirus in the pathogenesis of systemic sclerosis: a gene array approach," *PLoS Medicine*, vol. 3, no. 1, article e2, 2006.

[16] R. Pastano, C. Dell'Agnola, C. Bason et al., "Antibodies against human cytomegalovirus late protein UL94 in the pathogenesis of scleroderma-like skin lesions in chronic graft-versus-host disease," *International Immunology*, vol. 24, pp. 583–591, 2012.

[17] V. Ratanatharathorn, L. Ayash, C. Reynolds et al., "Treatment of chronic graft-versus-host disease with anti-CD20 chimeric monoclonal antibody," *Biology of Blood and Marrow Transplantation*, vol. 9, no. 8, pp. 505–511, 2003.

[18] T. C. Barnes, D. G. Spiller, M. E. Anderson, S. W. Edwards, and R. J. Moots, "Endothelial activation and apoptosis mediated by neutrophil-dependent interleukin 6 trans-signalling: a novel target for systemic sclerosis?" *Annals of the Rheumatic Diseases*, vol. 70, no. 2, pp. 366–372, 2011.

[19] R. Sgonc, M. S. Gruschwitz, G. Boeck, N. Sepp, J. Gruber, and G. Wick, "Endothelial cell apoptosis in systemic sclerosis is induced by antibody-dependent cell-mediated cytotoxicity via CD95," *Arthritis and Rheumatism*, vol. 43, pp. 2550–2562, 2000.

[20] J. H. W. Distler, A. Akhmetshina, C. Dees et al., "Induction of apoptosis in circulating angiogenic cells by microparticles," *Arthritis and Rheumatism*, vol. 63, no. 7, pp. 2067–2077, 2011.

[21] S. Guiducci, J. H. W. Distler, A. Jüngel et al., "The relationship between plasma microparticles and disease manifestations in patients with systemic sclerosis," *Arthritis and Rheumatism*, vol. 58, no. 9, pp. 2845–2853, 2008.

[22] J. H. W. Distler, L. C. Huber, S. Gay, O. Distler, and D. S. Pisetsky, "Microparticles as mediators of cellular cross-talk in inflammatory disease," *Autoimmunity*, vol. 39, no. 8, pp. 683–690, 2006.

[23] S. Chabaud, M.-P. Corriveau, T. Grodzicky et al., "Decreased secretion of MMP by non-lesional late-stage scleroderma fibroblasts after selection via activation of the apoptotic fas-pathway," *Journal of Cellular Physiology*, vol. 226, no. 7, pp. 1907–1914, 2011.

[24] G. H. Samuel, S. Lenna, A. M. Bujor, R. Lafyatis, and M. Trojanowska, "Acid sphingomyelinase deficiency contributes to resistance of scleroderma fibroblasts to Fas-mediated apoptosis," *Journal of Dermatological Science*, vol. 67, pp. 166–172, 2012.

[25] C. Mihai and J. W. C. Tervaert, "Anti-endothelial cell antibodies in systemic sclerosis," *Annals of the Rheumatic Diseases*, vol. 69, no. 2, pp. 319–324, 2010.

[26] D. Abraham and O. Distler, "How does endothelial cell injury start? The role of endothelin in systemic sclerosis," *Arthritis Research and Therapy*, vol. 9, supplement 2, article S2, 2007.

[27] H. Dib, M. C. Tamby, G. Bussone et al., "Targets of anti-endothelial cell antibodies in pulmonary hypertension and scleroderma," *European Respiratory Journal*, vol. 39, pp. 1405–1414, 2012.

[28] K. Lewandowska, M. Ciurzynski, E. Gorska et al., "Antiendothelial cells antibodies in patients with systemic sclerosis in relation to pulmonary hypertension and lung fibrosis," *Advances in Experimental Medicine and Biology*, vol. 756, pp. 147–153, 2013.

[29] J. Avouac, N. Cagnard, J. H. Distler et al., "Insights into the pathogenesis of systemic sclerosis based on the gene expression profile of progenitor-derived endothelial cells," *Arthritis and Rheumatism*, vol. 63, no. 11, pp. 3552–3562, 2011.

[30] C. Selmi, C. A. Feghali-Bostwick, A. Lleo et al., "X chromosome gene methylation in peripheral lymphocytes from monozygotic twins discordant for scleroderma," *Clinical & Experimental Immunology*, vol. 169, pp. 253–262, 2012.

[31] M. Bielecki, K. Kowal, A. Lapinska, S. Chwiesko-Minarowska, L. Chyczewski, and O. Kowal-Bielecka, "Peripheral blood mononuclear cells from patients with systemic sclerosis spontaneously secrete increased amounts of vascular endothelial growth factor (VEGF) already in the early stage of the disease," *Advances in Medical Sciences*, vol. 56, no. 2, pp. 255–263, 2011.

[32] V. Carrai, I. Miniati, S. Guiducci et al., "Evidence for reduced angiogenesis in bone marrow in SSc: immunohistochemistry and multiparametric computerized imaging analysis," *Rheumatology*, vol. 51, pp. 1042–1048, 2012.

[33] N. Del Papa, N. Quirici, C. Scavullo et al., "Antiendothelial cell antibodies induce apoptosis of bone marrow endothelial progenitors in systemic sclerosis," *The Journal of Rheumatology*, vol. 37, no. 10, pp. 2053–2063, 2010.

[34] M. Bielecki, K. Kowal, A. Lapinska et al., "Diminished production of TWEAK by the peripheral blood mononuclear cells is associated with vascular involvement in patients with systemic sclerosis," *Folia Histochemica et Cytobiologica*, vol. 47, no. 3, pp. 465–469, 2009.

[35] X. Wortsman, J. Wortsman, I. Sazunic, and L. Carreño, "Activity assessment in morphea using color Doppler ultrasound," *Journal of the American Academy of Dermatology*, vol. 65, no. 5, pp. 942–948, 2011.

[36] K. A. Nezafati, R. L. Cayce, J. S. Susa et al., "14-MHz ultrasonography as an outcome measure in morphea (localized scleroderma)," *Archives of Dermatology*, vol. 147, no. 9, pp. 1112–1115, 2011.

[37] S. C. Li, M. S. Liebling, K. A. Haines, J. E. Weiss, and A. Prann, "Initial evaluation of an ultrasound measure for assessing the activity of skin lesions in juvenile localized scleroderma," *Arthritis Care and Research*, vol. 63, no. 5, pp. 735–742, 2011.

[38] E. Szymańska, M. Maj, M. Majsterek, J. Litniewski, A. Nowicki, and L. Rudnicka, "The usefulness of high frequency ultrasonography in dermatologlcal practice—ultrasound features of selected cutaneous lesions," *Polski Merkuriusz Lekarski*, vol. 31, no. 181, pp. 37–40, 2011.

[39] A. Iagnocco, F. Ceccarelli, C. Vavala et al., "Ultrasound in the assessment of musculoskeletal involvement in systemic sclerosis," *Medical Ultrasonography*, vol. 14, pp. 231–234, 2012.

[40] T. M. Fernandes, B. E. Bica, N. R. Villela et al., "Evaluation of endothelial function in patients with limited systemic sclerosis by use of brachial artery Doppler ultrasound," *Revista Brasileira de Reumatologia*, vol. 52, pp. 561–568, 2012.

[41] A. Osmola-Mankowska, W. Silny, A. Danczak-Pazdrowska et al., "Assessment of chronic sclerodermoid Graft-versus-Host Disease patients, using 20 MHz high-frequency ultrasonography and cutometer methods," *Skin Research and Technology*, vol. 19, no. 1, pp. e417–e422, 2013.

[42] S. C. Li, M. S. Liebling, and K. A. Haines, "Ultrasonography is a sensitive tool for monitoring localized scleroderma," *Rheumatology*, vol. 46, no. 8, pp. 1316–1319, 2007.

[43] R. Buense, I. A. Duarte, and M. Bouer, "Localized scleroderma: assessment of the therapeutic response to phototherapy," *Anais Brasileiros de Dermatologia*, vol. 87, pp. 63–69, 2012.

[44] E. Pope, A. S. Doria, M. Theriault, A. Mohanta, and R. M. Laxer, "Topical imiquimod 5% cream for pediatric plaque morphea: a prospective, multiple-baseline, open-label pilot study," *Dermatology*, vol. 223, no. 4, pp. 363–369, 2011.

[45] S. Schanz, G. Fierlbeck, A. Ulmer et al., "Localized scleroderma: MR findings and clinical features," *Radiology*, vol. 260, no. 3, pp. 817–824, 2011.

[46] S. Schanz, J. Henes, A. Ulmer et al., "Magnetic resonance imaging findings in patients with systemic scleroderma and musculoskeletal symptoms," *European Radiology*, vol. 23, pp. 212–221, 2013.

[47] S. Schanz, J. Henes, A. Ulmer et al., "Response evaluation of musculoskeletal involvement in patients with deep morphea treated with methotrexate and prednisolone: a combined MRI and clinical approach," *American Journal of Roentgenology*, vol. 200, pp. 376–382, 2013.

[48] F. Zulian, C. Vallongo, A. Patrizi et al., "A long-term follow-up study of methotrexate in juvenile localized scleroderma (morphea)," *Journal of the American Academy of Dermatology*, vol. 67, pp. 1151–1156, 2012.

[49] K. S. Torok and T. Arkachaisri, "Methotrexate and corticosteroids in the treatment of localized scleroderma: a standardized prospective longitudinal single-center study," *The Journal of Rheumatology*, vol. 39, no. 2, pp. 286–294, 2012.

[50] Y. Inamo and T. Ochiai, "Successful combination treatment of a patient with progressive Juvenile Localized Scleroderma (Morphea) using Imatinib, Corticosteroids, and Methotrexate," *Pediatric Dermatology*, 2012.

[51] S. Reitamo, A. Remitz, J. Varga et al., "Demonstration of interleukin 8 and autoantibodies to interleukin 8 in the serum of patients with systemic sclerosis and related disorders," *Archives of Dermatology*, vol. 129, no. 2, pp. 189–193, 1993.

[52] S. Visvanathan, J. C. Marini, J. S. Smolen et al., "Changes in biomarkers of inflammation and bone turnover and associations with clinical efficacy following infliximab plus methotrexate therapy in patients with early rheumatoid arthritis," *The Journal of Rheumatology*, vol. 34, no. 7, pp. 1465–1474, 2007.

[53] J. E. Pope, N. Bellamy, J. R. Seibold et al., "A randomized, controlled trial of methotrexate versus placebo in early diffuse scleroderma," *Arthritis and Rheumatism*, vol. 44, pp. 1351–1358, 2001.

[54] F. H. J. van den Hoogen, A. M. T. Boerbooms, A. J. G. Swaak, J. J. Rasker, H. J. J. van Lier, and L. B. A. van de Putte, "Comparison of methotrexate with placebo in the treatment of systemic sclerosis: a 24 week randomized double-blind trial, followed by a 24 week observational trial," *British Journal of Rheumatology*, vol. 35, no. 4, pp. 364–372, 1996.

[55] C. T. Derk, E. Grace, M. Shenin, M. Naik, S. Schulz, and W. Xiong, "A prospective open-label study of mycophenolate mofetil for the treatment of diffuse systemic sclerosis," *Rheumatology*, vol. 48, no. 12, pp. 1595–1599, 2009.

[56] N. Fett and V. P. Werth, "Update on morphea: part II. Outcome measures and treatment," *Journal of the American Academy of Dermatology*, vol. 64, no. 2, pp. 231–242, 2011.

[57] L. George, B. George, D. J. Gottlieb, M. Hertzberg, and P. Fernandez-Peñas, "Lack of efficacy of rituximab in refractory sclerodermatous chronic GVHD," *Bone Marrow Transplantation*, vol. 47, pp. 737–738, 2012.

[58] M. S. Chimenti, M. Teoli, A. D. Stefani, A. Giunta, M. Esposito, and R. Perricone, "Resolution with rituximab of localized scleroderma occurring during etanercept treatment in a patient with rheumatoid arthritis," *European Journal of Dermatology*, vol. 23, no. 2, pp. 273–274, 2013.

[59] M. Kerscher, M. Vokenandt, M. Meurer, P. Lehmann, G. Plewig, and M. Rocken, "Treatment of localised scleroderma with PUVA bath photochemotherapy," *The Lancet*, vol. 343, no. 8907, p. 1233, 1994.

[60] M. El-Mofty, W. Mostafa, S. Esmat et al., "Suggested mechanisms of action of UVA phototherapy in morphea: a molecular study," *Photodermatology Photoimmunology and Photomedicine*, vol. 20, no. 2, pp. 93–100, 2004.

[61] A. Morita, K. Kobayashi, I. Isomura, T. Tsuji, and J. Krutmann, "Ultraviolet A1 (340-400 nm) phototherapy for scleroderma in systemic sclerosis," *Journal of the American Academy of Dermatology*, vol. 43, no. 4, pp. 670–674, 2000.

[62] K. Scharffetter, M. Wlaschek, A. Hogg et al., "UVA irradiation induces collagenase in human dermal fibroblasts in vitro and in vivo," *Archives of Dermatological Research*, vol. 283, no. 8, pp. 506–511, 1991.

[63] B. Stein, H. J. Rahmsdorf, A. Steffen, M. Litfin, and P. Herrlich, "UV-induced DNA damage is an intermediate step in UV-induced expression of human immunodeficiency virus type 1, collagenase, c-fos, and metallothionein," *Molecular and Cellular Biology*, vol. 9, no. 11, pp. 5169–5181, 1989.

[64] M. El-Mofty, W. Mostafa, M. El-Darouty et al., "Different low doses of broad-band UVA in the treatment of morphea and systemic sclerosis. A clinico-pathologic study," *Photodermatology Photoimmunology and Photomedicine*, vol. 20, no. 3, pp. 148–156, 2004.

[65] M. El-Mofty, H. Zaher, M. Bosseila, R. Yousef, and B. Saad, "Low-dose broad-band UVA in morphea using a new method for evaluation," *Photodermatology Photoimmunology and Photomedicine*, vol. 16, no. 2, pp. 43–49, 2000.

[66] A. Kreuter, J. Hyun, M. Stücker, A. Sommer, P. Altmeyer, and T. Gambichler, "A randomized controlled study of low-dose UVA1, medium-dose UVA1, and narrowband UVB phototherapy in the treatment of localized scleroderma," *Journal of the American Academy of Dermatology*, vol. 54, no. 3, pp. 440–447, 2006.

[67] B. A. Zwischenberger and H. T. Jacobe, "A systematic review of morphea treatments and therapeutic algorithm," *Journal of the American Academy of Dermatology*, vol. 65, no. 5, pp. 925–941, 2011.

[68] A. Kreuter, F. Breuckmann, A. Uhle et al., "Low-dose UVA1 phototherapy in systemic sclerosis: effects on acrosclerosis," *Journal of the American Academy of Dermatology*, vol. 50, no. 5, pp. 740–747, 2004.

[69] C. Tuchinda, H. A. Kerr, C. R. Taylor et al., "UVA1 phototherapy for cutaneous diseases: an experience of 92 cases in the United States," *Photodermatology Photoimmunology and Photomedicine*, vol. 22, no. 5, pp. 247–253, 2006.

[70] N. Pereira, F. Santiago, H. Oliveira, and A. Figueiredo, "Low-dose UVA1 phototherapy for scleroderma: what benefit can we expect?" *Journal of the European Academy of Dermatology and Venereology*, vol. 26, no. 5, pp. 619–626, 2012.

[71] H. Xu, M. Zaidi, J. Struve et al., "Abnormal fibrillin-1 expression and chronic oxidative stress mediate endothelial mesenchymal transition in a murine model of systemic sclerosis," *American Journal of Physiology—Cell Physiology*, vol. 300, no. 3, pp. C550–C556, 2011.

[72] E. Tinazzi, M. Dolcino, A. Puccetti et al., "Gene expression profiling in circulating endothelial cells from systemic sclerosis patients shows an altered control of apoptosis and angiogenesis that is modified by iloprost infusion," *Arthritis Research and Therapy*, vol. 12, no. 4, article R131, 2010.

10

Pathophysiological Relationship between Infections and Systemic Vasculitis

Carolina Muñoz-Grajales[1] and Juan C. Pineda[2]

[1]*Rheumatology Department, Pablo Tobón Uribe Hospital, Medellín, Colombia*
[2]*Internal Medicine Department, Fundación Valle del Lili, ICESI University, Cali, Colombia*

Correspondence should be addressed to Juan C. Pineda; jpinedaruiz@gmail.com

Academic Editor: Alexander Szalai

The development of autoimmune disorders requires a combination of genetic, immunological, and environmental factors. Infectious agents, such as viruses and bacteria, can trigger autoimmunity through different mechanisms, and for systemic vasculitis in particular, microbial agents have been suggested to be involved in its pathogenesis. Although the exact mechanisms have not been fully elucidated, different theories have been postulated. This review considers the role of infections in the etiology of primary vasculitis, emphasizing their related immunological events.

1. Introduction

Primary systemic vasculitides are a complex group of disorders that involve multiple organs, often with a severe clinical course. Although uncommon, they require prompt management and adequate handling. Early diagnosis is required to preserve the function of the affected organs and to decrease mortality. Clinical manifestations are varied and nonspecific and may be related to those occurring in other systemic diseases, such as infections or malignancies. Although the origin of primary vasculitis is not fully understood, there is a combination of genetic, immunological, and environmental factors, like infections, which could trigger some of them. In the latest revision of the Chapel Hill Consensus Conference (CHCC), vasculitis associated with hepatitis B (HBV) and hepatitis C (HCV) viruses were included [1]; however, there are many other organisms associated (Table 1). Since Wegener's first description, an association with bacteria [2] has been suspected. There have been attempts to confirm this relationship; however, it remains a subject of debate.

Various mechanisms have been proposed to be involved in the relationship between infection and systemic vasculitis: molecular mimicry, superantigens, cell activation by Toll-like receptors (TLR), and more recently, the anti-idiotypic response by neutrophil extracellular traps in the antineutrophil cytoplasmic antibodies- (ANCA-) associated vasculitis (Table 2) [3–5]. In addition, some infections are accepted as the secondary causes of vasculitis. Bacteria, spirochetes, rickettsia, fungi, viruses, parasites, and protozoa have all been implicated, and various mechanisms have been postulated, including direct vascular invasion, immune complex deposition, and activation of T lymphocytes [6–8]. In this paper, we review the current evidence for the role of infections in the etiology of primary vasculitis. We emphasize immunological events and their relationships to organ damage.

2. Large and Medium-Vessel Vasculitis

For several years, a causal link between Takayasu's arteritis (TA) and tuberculosis (TB) has been proposed due to the granulomatous nature of both diseases. Moreover, the link is supported by the increasing frequency of TA in patients from continents with a high prevalence of TB, such as Asia, Africa, and South America [5]. However, attempts to recover mycobacteria from the tissues of TA patients have been unsuccessful. In 2012, Soto et al. found sequences of the *Mycobacterium tuberculosis* IS 6110 and HupB genes in the aorta of 23 of 33 patients with TA (70% of TA

Table 1: The most important microbial agents presumed to be involved in the development of primary systemic vasculitis.

	Microbial agent	Reference
Type of vasculitis		
Takayasu arteritis	*Mycobacterium tuberculosis*	[5, 9, 10]
Giant cell arteritis	*Burkholderia*	[11]
Polyarteritis nodosa	Hepatitis B virus, hepatitis C virus, and HIV infection	[12]
Immune complex vasculitis		
Antiglomerular basement membrane disease	Increased incidence during influenza epidemics	[13]
Cryoglobulinemic vasculitis	HCV	[14–16]
IgA vasculitis	Many bacteria, viruses, and even protozoa (e.g., *Helicobacter pylori, Staphylococcus aureus,* and *M. pneumonia*)	[17–22]
Hypocomplementemic urticarial vasculitis	Few associations with infections	[23]
ANCA-associated vasculitis		
Microscopic polyangiitis	*Staphylococcus aureus*	[24]
Granulomatosis with polyangiitis	*Staphylococcus aureus, Klebsiella,* and *Escherichia coli* species	[24–36]
Eosinophilic granulomatosis with polyangiitis	—	

tissues compared with 32% of atherosclerotic tissues) [9]. Furthermore, it has been observed that patients with TA have an increased T cell response to the human heat shock protein 60 (hHSP-60) and mycobacteria heat shock protein 65 (mHSP-65) (22 of 26 patients versus 3 of 18 healthy controls). Additionally, an increase in circulating IgG isotype antibodies against these antigens was reported (anti-MHSP-65 in 92% of TA patients versus 11% in controls and anti-hHSP-60 in 84% of TA subjects versus 22% in controls; $P < 0.001$), raising the possibility of molecular mimicry between hHSP-60 and hHSP-65 [10]. Therefore, a previous infection with TB could aid in the development of arteritis because of the reactivity against vascular endothelial peptides with similarity to mycobacterial antigens [37].

In giant cell arteritis (GCA), the presence of certain viruses in the tissues of temporal arteries from affected patients has been suggested. However, a study conducted on 37 samples to detect *Chlamydia pneumoniae*, parvovirus B19, and herpesvirus (excluding serotype 8) showed no differences between the patients with GCA and controls. Nonetheless, Mohammadi et al. found human papilloma virus DNA in 16 of 22 temporal artery samples from patients with GCA vasculitis [50] and Curly et al. reported *Burkholderia* sp. in 9 out of 10 patients [11]. However, a recent microbiome DNA sequencing study in samples from the temporal arteries of patients with GCA showed no increase in the frequency of a particular microorganism [51].

In contrast, polyarteritis nodosa (PAN) is strongly linked to hepatitis B virus (HBV) and also has been linked to hepatitis C virus (HCV), human immunodeficiency virus (HIV), group A *Streptococcus*, human T cell leukemia virus-1, *Cytomegalovirus*, *Epstein-Barr virus*, and parvovirus B19 [12]. Thus, the prevalence of PAN associated with HBV, HCV, and HIV coincides largely with the prevalence of underlying infections [5].

The association between PAN and HBV has been frequently observed (10–54% of patients); in fact, in the last CHCC, this association was grouped in a specific subset of vasculitis called vasculitis associated with probable cause [1]. The vasculitis typically begin within the first 6 months after infection when there is constant viral replication and immune complex deposition composed of viral antigens, more likely HBe antigen, and other specific antibodies [3]. All cases of HBV-PAN are almost always associated with the wild-type HBV infection, characterized by HBe antigenemia and high HBV replication. Whereby, two general mechanisms have been proposed, the first one is a direct injury of the vessel wall by the virus and the second one an endothelial lesion resulting from circulating immune complexes deposition and complement activation, leading to attraction and activation of neutrophils. That could explain the subsequent organ damage [12] but still need further research to confirm this.

3. Small-Vessel Vasculitis

3.1. Immune Complex-Mediated Vasculitis. Regarding basement membrane disease, only a description of infection (influenza outbreak) is thought to be a likely trigger [13]. In contrast, the relationship between HCV and cryoglobulinemia is well known. Although the exact mechanism is unknown, it has been suggested that the virus induces B cell proliferation via the interaction of its envelope E2 protein with CD81 present in hepatocytes and lymphocytes,

Table 2: Theories regarding the role of infection in the development of primary systemic vasculitis. Toll-like receptor (TLR); 3 proteinase (PR3); myeloperoxidase (MPO).

Vasculitis	Mechanism	Microbial agent	Evidence	References
Takayasu's arteritis	Molecular mimicry	*Mycobacterium tuberculosis*	*Mycobacterium tuberculosis* gene sequences IS6110 and HupB in tissues from aorta Increased T cell response to hHSP60 and mHSP65	[9, 10, 37]
MPO-AAV	Neutrophil cell traps	Various	Immunofluorescence analyses revealed MPO located in these extracellular chromatin fibers IgG ANCA induced neutrophil NETs In crescentic glomerulonephritis, lesion associated with AAV has detected NETs Increased levels of MPO-DNA complex in the serum Induced pauci-immune glomerulonephritis and alveolar hemorrhage in rats exposed to PTU/PMA	[38–40]
PR3-AAV	Neutrophil cell traps	Various	Immunofluorescence analyses revealed MPO located in these extracellular chromatin fibers Murine anti-PR3 antibody induced NETs	[38]
	Stimulation of T lymphocytes by *S. aureus* superantigen	*S. aureus*	Persistent activation of circulating T lymphocytes Chronic carriers of *S. aureus* that expressed toxic shock toxin 1 (TSS-1) had increased numbers of relapses	[27, 28, 36]
	Antigens can join to renal basement membranes by charge interaction	*S. aureus*	—	[41]
	Idiotype, anti-idiotype	*S. aureus*	Similarity of some bacterial peptides, including but not limited to *S. aureus*, with complementary PR3 (PR3c)	[42]
	TLR activation	*S. aureus*	During active infection of AAV, TLR9 expression increased significantly compared to uninfected patients Increased expression of TLR9 in monocytes from patients with AAV (*S. aureus* carriers) TLR2 and TLR9 were stimulated *in vitro*, and increased membrane expression of PR3 (PR3m) In patients with AAV-PR3, hypomethylated CpG motifs triggered production of PR3-ANCA by autoreactive LB	[43–45]
	Molecular mimicry	*Klebsiella* and *Escherichia coli* species	Anti-lysosomal-associated membrane protein-2 (hLAMP-2)	[46–49]

thereby generating chronic B lymphocyte stimulation [14–16]. Additionally, although the cause of IgA-mediated vasculitis is unknown, some infectious triggers have been identified. One study reported that 29 of 55 children [17, 18] were isolated with *Helicobacter pylori* (49.3% of Chinese infants with IgA vasculitis compared to 23.4% of controls) [19, 20]. *Staphylococcus aureus* [21] and *Mycoplasma pneumoniae* [22] are additional examples of these associations. Similarly, hypocomplementemic urticarial vasculitis syndrome, an illness that has recently been considered a monogenic form of lupus by some researchers [52], does not have many descriptions related to infection. In a study of 64 patients published in 2009, 70% had no identifiable cause of vasculitis. In only 12% of the cases, infection (primarily of the upper respiratory tract) was considered to be the underlying cause [23].

3.2. ANCA-Associated Vasculitis (AAV). Vasculitis associated with antineutrophil cytoplasmic antibodies (ANCA) includes a group of diseases that cause small-vessel necrosis. These diseases are characterized by the presence of ANCA which vary depending on the vasculitis type and whether they are directed against myeloperoxidase (MPO) or proteinase 3 (PR3) [53, 54]. Some researchers propose that PR-3 ANCA-associated vasculitis patients are more likely to relapse and display predominant extrarenal manifestations and rapid deterioration of renal function compared to patients with MPO-ANCA vasculitis [55–57]. Genetic factors are also different, because PR3-ANCA vasculitis is partnered with HLA-DP and the genes encoding PR3 (PRTN3) and antitrypsin (SERPINA1). In contrast, MPO-ANCA vasculitis is associated with HLA-DQ [58, 59].

Currently, there is only one *in vivo* model for MPO-ANCA vasculitis, but not for the associated PR3. Immunizing MPO-deficient mice produced anti-MPO. The transfer of splenocytes from immunodeficient *Rag2*$^{-/-}$ mice induced necrotizing vasculitis with granulomatous inflammation and pauci-immune glomerulonephritis. Injecting IgG into wild immunodeficient MPO mice also generated a pauci-immune glomerulonephritis [60, 61]. Although immunized mice developed antibodies capable of recognizing PR3 on the surface of neutrophils, the passive transfer of IgG did not lead to vasculitis. Immunizing mice with the human PR3 ANCA produced some of the inflammatory reactions in the lungs, but not glomerulonephritis [62–64]. These differences suggest that although ANCA production is shared between these vasculitides (MPO-ANCA and PR3-ANCA), they have different pathogenic pathways [65] and as discussed below, iPR3-AAV has the most notable microorganism participation in its pathophysiology.

Neutrophil extracellular traps (NETs) have recently been reported to participate in the pathogenesis of various autoimmune diseases, such as AAV (MPO-ANCA and PR3-ANCA vasculitides). Immunofluorescence analyses of NETs induced *in vitro* revealed that both MPO and PR3 are expressed in extracellular chromatin fibers [38, 39]. These authors also found that IgG ANCA induced NETs in the patients with AAV; similarly, it was also observed that murine anti-PR3 could induce NET formation [38]. In serum samples of crescentic glomerulonephritis lesions associated with AAV, increased NETs and DNA-MPO were detected [38]. Furthermore, it has been reported that propylthiouracil (PTU) can generate anti-MPO-ANCA, and some patients may develop ANCA-associated vasculitis. Nakazawa et al. studied the capacity of PTU to induce aberrant or irregular NETs *in vitro*. Typically, NETs are obtained after the *in vitro* stimulation with phorbol myristate acetate (PMA). However, these authors added PTU to PMA, resulting in the production of irregular NETs. These were subsequently inserted into WKY rats and they produced ANCA, which differed from the rats immunized with regular NETs produced by PMA. Pauci-immune glomerulonephritis and alveolar hemorrhage have also been induced in rats exposed to PTU/PMA [40].

For several years, the involvement of *Staphylococcus aureus* infection in the genesis of Wegener granulomatosis (GPA) has been suggested. This theory emerged based on the observation that up to 70% of patients with chronic nasal GPA are carriers of this microorganism [25–30]. Moreover, there is an increased risk of relapse of the limited form in carriers [25, 31], and trimethoprim-sulfamethoxazole prophylaxis reduces the risk of recurrence by up to 60% [32, 33]. Furthermore, a recent retrospective study found that 70% of patients with airway GPA treated with trimethoprim-sulfamethoxazole monotherapy had good clinical responses [34]. Finally, in the microscopic polyangiitis and IgA vasculitis, there are case reports of activation after *S. aureus* infections [24, 35].

Different theories have been developed regarding the relationship between GPA and *S. aureus*. One theory proposes that carriers of the bacteria have low-grade infections in the upper respiratory tract, resulting in the "priming" of neutrophils induced by cell surface PR3 expression, which can be activated by PR3-ANCA. The possibility of polyclonal expansion of B cells, stimulated by the components of the bacterial cell wall, has also been considered. Others have suggested a chronic stimulation of T cells by *S. aureus* superantigens, because they found persistent activation of circulating T lymphocytes in patients with GPA [28, 36, 66, 67].

One study found that, in GPA chronic carrier patients of *S. aureus*, strains expressing toxic shock syndrome toxin 1 (SAT-1) had the increased numbers of relapses (relative risk versus control subjects 13.3; 95% CI: 4.2–42.6) [27]. However, in another study, these same authors reported that although they observed further T lymphocyte expansion in GPA, they found no association with the presence of *S. aureus* or superantigens [7]. Another hypothesis assumes that the antigens of these bacteria can adhere to the renal basement membrane through interaction with the electric charge [41].

More recently, another mechanism based on the similarity of some bacterial peptides was proposed. It includes (but is not limited to) *S. aureus* with the complementary PR3 protein (PR3c) produced in the bacteria by antisense or reverse translation of the *PRTN3* gene, which encodes human PR3, into cDNA that is experimentally incorporated into bacterial DNA [68]. These theories resulted from the observation that seven of 34 patients with PR3-ANCA had antibodies against PR3c (based on ELISA against the PR3c middle region) but had no cross-reactivity with PR3. Therefore, anti-PR3 could be bonded against anti-PR3c, indicating an idiotype anti-idiotype reaction [42].

Because the aforementioned bacterial peptides have similarities with PR3c, GPA carriers of *S. aureus* can theoretically produce antibodies against PR3c through the idiotypic anti-idiotypic reactions equivalent to PR-3 ANCA [42]. In support of this theory, mice immunized with PR3c increased their anti-PR3 antibody production. However, in a subsequent study of 57 Dutch patients with PR3 AAV and 27 healthy controls, no increase in reaction against the middle region of PR3c or any relationship between *S. aureus* was noted [69]. Because IgG subclass affects binding affinity, these contradicting results could be explained by the differences in the profile of IgG subclasses within the populations studied, as suggested by Preston and Falk [70]. Alternatively, perhaps anti-idiotype antibodies may mask or hide the antigen-binding site in the idiotype, preventing binding to the complementary protein used in ELISA assay. This is analogous to observations in a study of anti-idiotype SSA/Ro in patients with systemic lupus erythematosus or Sjögren syndrome [70, 71].

In AAV, TLR expression on monocytes and natural killer cells in peripheral blood [43] was observed to be an important element in the response to infection by innate immunity; therefore, another theory postulates that the activation of neutrophils in patients with AAV is related to TLRs [67]. In a cohort of patients with GPA, the expression of TLR2, TLR4, and TLR9 on granulocytes was not increased in uninfected patients compared to healthy controls, even when the disease was active. However, during active infection, there was a significant increase in the TLR9 expression, compared to uninfected patients; there was also a tendency towards an increased TLR2 and TLR4 expression [44]. Another study found an increased expression of TLR9 in monocytes of *S. aureus* carriers with AAV [43]. In addition, when TLR9 and TLR2 were stimulated *in vitro*, they increased the expression of membrane PR3 (PR3m) [44]. Moreover, it was reported that in patients with PR3-AAV, IL-2 in combination with hypomethylated CpG motifs, which are characteristic of viruses and bacteria, triggered the production of PR3-ANCA by autoreactive B cells [45, 67].

Finally, another important finding, which supports the relationship between AAV and bacterial infection, is the presence of human autoantibodies against protein 2 of the lysosomal membrane (hLAMP-2) in patients with AAV (80% of patients from three European cohorts) [46]. These antibodies activate neutrophils and generate endothelial damage *in vitro* [47] and have homology with the bacterial adhesion FimH protein (a fimbrial adhesin of Gram-negative bacteria). Eight amino acids of an epitope of LAMP-2 (P41–49), which are recognized by the autoantibodies, have a strong homology to several FimH proteins that are common in Gram-negative species, thereby suggesting molecular mimicry between the two proteins [66]. In *in vivo* models, immunization of rats with FimH generates reactive antibodies, LAMP-2, and necrotizing pauci-immune nephritis [47, 48]. However, in other cohorts, an increase in the anti-hLAMP-2 has not been observed [49].

Other organisms, such as *Haemophilus influenzae*, *Streptococcus pneumonia*, and *Klebsiella pneumoniae*, have been found in the lower respiratory tract and have been considered part of the etiology of GPA [72]; however, more evidence is needed. In addition, antibodies against HCV and *Helicobacter pylori* also have been found [73]. Other viruses involved in the onset of AAV include HIV [74] and Epstein-Barr virus (EBV). EBV functionally inactivates a protein expressed primarily in T cells, thus altering the immune response and resulting in systemic vasculitis and lymphocyte proliferation through the mitogenic effect of viral DNA [75, 76]. Cytomegalovirus produces direct cellular damage and induces high plasma levels of immune amplifiers, such as IL-5 and α-lymphotoxin [77].

4. Conclusions

Most infectious agents, including viruses, bacteria, and parasites, can trigger autoimmunity through various mechanisms. Infections are associated with the secondary forms of vasculitis. However, there is growing evidence that microbial agents also play a role in the induction of primary systemic vasculitis. For example, a number of infectious agents have been proposed as potential triggers; however, in most cases, the link remains hypothetical. Different mechanisms and pathogenic hypotheses have been proposed (molecular mimicry, superantigens, cell activation by Toll-like receptors, the anti-idiotypic response, and neutrophil extracellular traps); however, the pathophysiology of the complex relationship between infection and vasculitis remains not fully understood.

Conflict of Interests

The authors declare no conflict of interests.

References

[1] J. C. Jennette, R. J. Falk, P. A. Bacon et al., "2012 Revised International Chapel Hill consensus conference nomenclature of vasculitides," *Arthritis and Rheumatism*, vol. 65, no. 1, pp. 1–11, 2013.

[2] F. Wegener, "Über generalisierte, septische Gefässerkrankungen," *Verhandlungen der Deutschen Gesellschaft für Pathologie*, vol. 26, pp. 202–210, 1936.

[3] C. C. Belizna, M. A. Hamidou, H. Levesque, L. Guillevin, and Y. Shoenfeld, "Infection and vasculitis," *Rheumatology*, vol. 48, no. 5, pp. 475–482, 2009.

[4] R. Root-Bernstein and D. Fairweather, "Complexities in the relationship between infection and autoimmunity," *Current Allergy and Asthma Reports*, vol. 14, no. 1, article 407, 2014.

[5] M. M. van Timmeren, P. Heeringa, and C. G. M. Kallenberg, "Infectious triggers for vasculitis," *Current Opinion in Rheumatology*, vol. 26, no. 4, pp. 416–423, 2014.

[6] A. J. dal Canto and H. W. Virgin IV, "Animal models of infection-mediated vasculitis," *Current Opinion in Rheumatology*, vol. 11, no. 1, pp. 17–23, 1999.

[7] E. R. Popa, C. A. Stegeman, N. A. Bos, C. G. M. Kallenberg, and J. W. C. Tervaert, "Staphylococcal superantigens and T cell expansions in Wegener's granulomatosis," *Clinical & Experimental Immunology*, vol. 132, no. 3, pp. 496–504, 2003.

[8] O. Oyoo and L. R. Espinoza, "Infection-related vasculitis," *Current Rheumatology Reports*, vol. 7, no. 4, pp. 281–287, 2005.

[9] M. E. Soto, M. Del Carmen Ávila-Casado, C. Huesca-Gómez et al., "Detection of *IS6110* and *HupB* gene sequences of *Mycobacterium tuberculosis* and bovis in the aortic tissue of patients with Takayasu's arteritis," *BMC Infectious Diseases*, vol. 12, article 194, 2012.

[10] S. K. Chauhan, N. K. Tripathy, N. Sinha, M. Singh, and S. Nityanand, "Cellular and humoral immune responses to mycobacterial heat shock protein-65 and its human homologue in Takayasu's arteritis," *Clinical and Experimental Immunology*, vol. 138, no. 3, pp. 547–553, 2004.

[11] L. K. Curly, J. K. Bradley, J. Hernandez-Rodriguez, M. Corbera-Bellalta, M. C. Cid, and H. P. Schweizer, "Identification of a Burkholderia-like strain from temporal arteries of subjects with giant cell arteritis," *Arthritis & Rheumatism*, vol. 64, supplement 10, p. S373, 2012.

[12] C. Pagnoux, P. Cohen, and L. Guillevin, "Vasculitides secondary to infections," *Clinical and Experimental Rheumatology*, vol. 24, no. 2, pp. S71–S81, 2006.

[13] A. J. Proskey, L. Weatherbee, R. E. Easterling, J. A. Greene Jr., and J. M. Weller, "Goodpasture's syndrome. A report of five cases and review of the literature," *The American Journal of Medicine*, vol. 48, no. 2, pp. 162–173, 1970.

[14] P. Pileri, Y. Uematsu, S. Campagnoli et al., "Binding of hepatitis C virus to CD81," *Science*, vol. 282, no. 5390, pp. 938–941, 1998.

[15] D. Rosa, G. Saletti, E. De Gregorio et al., "Activation of naïve B lymphocytes via CD81, a pathogenetic mechanism for hepatitis C virus-associated B lymphocyte disorders," *Proceedings of the National Academy of Sciences of the United States of America*, vol. 102, no. 51, pp. 18544–18549, 2005.

[16] E. D. Charles, R. M. Green, S. Marukian et al., "Clonal expansion of immunoglobulin $M^{+}CD27^{+}$ B cells in HCV-associated mixed cryoglobulinemia," *Blood*, vol. 111, no. 3, pp. 1344–1356, 2008.

[17] C. S. Alfredo, N. A. Nunes, C. A. Len, C. M. P. Barbosa, M. T. R. A. Terreri, and M. O. E. Hilário, "Henoch-Schönlein purpura: recurrence and chronicity," *Jornal de Pediatria*, vol. 83, no. 2, pp. 177–180, 2007.

[18] D. Rigante, L. Castellazzi, A. Bosco, and S. Esposito, "Is there a crossroad between infections, genetics, and Henoch-Schönlein purpura?" *Autoimmunity Reviews*, vol. 12, no. 10, pp. 1016–1021, 2013.

[19] L.-J. Xiong, Y. Tong, Z.-L. Wang, and M. Mao, "Is helicobacter pylori infection associated with Henoch-Schonlein purpura in Chinese children? A meta-analysis," *World Journal of Pediatrics*, vol. 8, no. 4, pp. 301–308, 2012.

[20] T. Ulas, I. Tursun, M. S. Dal, M. A. Eren, and H. Buyukhatipoglu, "Rapid improvement of Henoch-Schonlein purpura associated with the treatment of *Helicobacter pylori* infection," *Journal of Research in Medical Sciences*, vol. 17, no. 11, pp. 1086–1088, 2012.

[21] S. Mandai, M. Aoyagi, K. Nagahama et al., "Post-staphylococcal infection Henoch-Schönlein purpura nephritis: a case report and review of the literature," *Renal Failure*, vol. 35, no. 6, pp. 869–874, 2013.

[22] P. Yiallouros, M. Moustaki, A. Voutsioti, F. Sharifi, and T. Karpathios, "Association of *Mycoplasma pneumoniae* infection with Henoch-Schonlein purpura," *Prague Medical Report*, vol. 114, no. 3, pp. 177–179, 2013.

[23] K. Kulthanan, M. Cheepsomsong, and S. Jiamton, "Urticarial vasculitis: etiologies and clinical course," *Asian Pacific Journal of Allergy and Immunology*, vol. 27, no. 2-3, pp. 95–102, 2009.

[24] R. Kasmani, K. Okoli, K. Naraharisetty, W. Gunning, J. I. Shapiro, and S. Ratnam, "Microscopic polyangiitis triggered by recurrent methicillin-resistant *Staphylococcus aureus* bacteremia," *International Urology and Nephrology*, vol. 42, no. 3, pp. 821–824, 2010.

[25] C. A. Stegeman, J. W. Cohen Tervaert, W. J. Sluiter, W. L. Manson, P. E. De Jong, and C. G. M. Kallenberg, "Association of chronic nasal carriage of *Staphylococcus aureus* and higher relapse rates in Wegener granulomatosis," *Annals of Internal Medicine*, vol. 120, no. 1, pp. 12–17, 1994.

[26] M. Laudien, S. D. Gadola, R. Podschun et al., "Nasal carriage of *Staphylococcus aureus* and endonasal activity in Wegener's granulomatosis as compared to rheumatoid arthritis and chronic rhinosinusitis with nasal polyps," *Clinical and Experimental Rheumatology*, vol. 28, no. 1, supplement 57, pp. S51–S55, 2010.

[27] E. R. Popa, C. A. Stegeman, W. H. Abdulahad et al., "Staphylococcal toxic-shock-syndrome-toxin-1 as a risk factor for disease relapse in Wegener's granulomatosis," *Rheumatology*, vol. 46, no. 6, pp. 1029–1033, 2007.

[28] E. R. Popa, C. A. Stegeman, C. G. M. Kallenberg, and J. W. C. Tervaert, "*Staphylococcus aureus* and Wegener's granulomatosis," *Arthritis Research*, vol. 4, no. 2, pp. 77–79, 2002.

[29] K. Zycinska, K. A. Wardyn, T. M. Zielonka, U. Demkow, and M. S. Traburzynski, "Chronic crusting, nasal carriage of *Staphylococcus aureus* and relapse rate in pulmonary Wegener's granulomatosis," *Journal of Physiology and Pharmacology*, vol. 59, supplement 6, pp. 825–831, 2008.

[30] J. van Putten, E. van Haren, and J. Lammers, "Association between Wegener's granulomatosis and *Staphylococcus aureus* infection?" *The European Respiratory Journal*, vol. 9, no. 9, pp. 1955–1957, 1996.

[31] K. Zycinska, K. A. Wardyn, T. M. Zielonka, U. Demkow, and M. S. Traburzynski, "Chronic crusting, nasal carriage of *Staphylococcus aureus* and relapse rate in pulmonary Wegener's granulomatosis," *Journal of Physiology and Pharmacology*, vol. 59, supplement 6, pp. 825–831, 2008.

[32] K. Zycinska, K. A. Wardyn, T. M. Zielonka, R. Krupa, and W. Lukas, "Co-trimoxazole and prevention of relapses of PR3-ANCA positive vasculitis with pulmonary involvement," *European Journal of Medical Research*, vol. 14, supplement 4, pp. 265–267, 2009.

[33] C. A. Stegeman, J. W. Tervaert, P. E. de Jong, and C. G. Kallenberg, "Trimethoprim-sulfamethoxazole (co-trimoxazole) for the prevention of relapses of Wegener's granulomatosis. Dutch Co-Trimoxazole Wegener Study Group," *The New England Journal of Medicine*, vol. 335, no. 1, pp. 16–20, 1996.

[34] J. Tuin, J. Sanders, and C. Stegeman, "Co-trimoxazole monotherapy as induction therapy for localized granulomatosis with polyangiitis," *La Presse Médicale*, vol. 42, no. 4, p. 771, 2013.

[35] J. J. Gao, J. M. Wei, Y. H. Gao, S. Li, and Y. Na, "Central venous catheter infection-induced Henoch-Schönlein purpura in a patient on hemodialysis," *Renal Failure*, vol. 36, no. 7, pp. 1145–1147, 2014.

[36] E. R. Popa, C. A. Stegeman, N. A. Bos, C. G. M. Kallenberg, and J. W. Cohen Tervaert, "Staphylococcal superantigens and T cell expansions in Wegener's granulomatosis," *Clinical and Experimental Immunology*, vol. 132, no. 3, pp. 496–504, 2003.

[37] D. Castillo-Martínez and L. M. Amezcua-Guerra, "Self-reactivity against stress-induced cell molecules: the missing link between Takayasu's arteritis and tuberculosis?" *Medical Hypotheses*, vol. 78, no. 4, pp. 485–488, 2012.

[38] K. Kessenbrock, M. Krumbholz, U. Schönermarck et al., "Netting neutrophils in autoimmune small-vessel vasculitis," *Nature Medicine*, vol. 15, no. 6, pp. 623–625, 2009.

[39] V. Brinkmann, U. Reichard, C. Goosmann et al., "Neutrophil extracellular traps kill bacteria," *Science*, vol. 303, no. 5663, pp. 1532–1535, 2004.

[40] D. Nakazawa, U. Tomaru, and A. Ishizu, "Possible implication of disordered neutrophil extracellular traps in the pathogenesis of MPO-ANCA-associated vasculitis," *Clinical and Experimental Nephrology*, vol. 17, no. 5, pp. 631–633, 2013.

[41] R. H. Brons, H. I. Bakker, R. T. Van Wijk et al., "Staphylococcal acid phosphatase binds to endothelial cells via charge interaction; a pathogenic role in Wegener's granulomatosis?" *Clinical and Experimental Immunology*, vol. 119, no. 3, pp. 566–573, 2000.

[42] W. F. Pendergraft III, G. A. Preston, R. R. Shah et al., "Autoimmunity is triggered by cPR-3(105–201), a protein complementary to human autoantigen proteinase-3," *Nature Medicine*, vol. 10, no. 1, pp. 72–79, 2004.

[43] H. Tadema, W. H. Abdulahad, C. A. Stegeman, C. G. M. Kallenberg, and P. Heeringa, "Increased expression of toll-like receptors by monocytes and natural killer cells in anca-associated vasculitis," *PLoS ONE*, vol. 6, no. 9, Article ID e24315, 2011.

[44] J. U. Holle, M. Windmöller, C. Lange, W. L. Gross, K. Herlyn, and E. Csernok, "Toll-like receptor TLR2 and TLR9 ligation triggers neutrophil activation in granulomatosis with polyangiitis," *Rheumatology*, vol. 52, no. 7, pp. 1183–1189, 2013.

[45] H. Tadema, W. H. Abdulahad, N. Lepse, C. A. Stegeman, C. G. M. Kallenberg, and P. Heeringa, "Bacterial DNA motifs trigger ANCA production in ANCA-associated vasculitis in remission," *Rheumatology*, vol. 50, no. 4, pp. 689–696, 2011.

[46] R. Kain, H. Tadema, E. F. McKinney et al., "High prevalence of autoantibodies to hLAMP-2 in anti-neutrophil cytoplasmic antibody-associated vasculitis," *Journal of the American Society of Nephrology*, vol. 23, no. 3, pp. 556–566, 2012.

[47] R. Kain, M. Exner, R. Brandes et al., "Molecular mimicry in pauci-immune focal necrotizing glomerulonephritis," *Nature Medicine*, vol. 14, no. 10, pp. 1088–1096, 2008.

[48] R. Kain, D. A. Firmin, and A. J. Rees, "Pathogenesis of small vessel vasculitis associated with autoantibodies to neutrophil cytoplasmic antigens: new insights from animal models," *Current Opinion in Rheumatology*, vol. 22, no. 1, pp. 15–20, 2010.

[49] A. J. Roth, M. C. Brown, R. N. Smith et al., "Anti-LAMP-2 antibodies are not prevalent in patients with antineutrophil cytoplasmic autoantibody glomerulonephritis," *Journal of the American Society of Nephrology*, vol. 23, no. 3, pp. 545–555, 2012.

[50] A. Mohammadi, J. D. Pfeifer, and J. S. Lewis, "Association between human papillomavirus DNA and temporal arteritis," *BMC Musculoskeletal Disorders*, vol. 13, article 132, 2012.

[51] A. S. Bhatt, V. E. Manzo, C. S. Pedamallu et al., "Brief REPORT: in search of a candidate pathogen for giant cell arteritis: sequencing-based characterization of the giant cell arteritis microbiome," *Arthritis & Rheumatology*, vol. 66, no. 7, pp. 1939–1944, 2014.

[52] J. E. Maldonado and A. Iglesias-Gamarra, "Vasculitis urticarial hipocomplementémica: aclaración histórica," *Revista Colombiana de Reumatología*, vol. 21, no. 2, pp. 84–90, 2014.

[53] J. C. Jennette and R. J. Falk, "Antineutrophil cytoplasmic autoantibodies and associated diseases: a review," *American Journal of Kidney Diseases*, vol. 15, no. 6, pp. 517–529, 1990.

[54] J. C. Jennette and R. J. Falk, "Small-vessel vasculitis," *The New England Journal of Medicine*, vol. 337, no. 21, pp. 1512–1523, 1997.

[55] C. F. M. Franssen, C. A. Stegeman, C. G. M. Kallenberg et al., "Antiproteinase 3- and antimyeloperoxidase-associated vasculitis," *Kidney International*, vol. 57, no. 6, pp. 2195–2206, 2000.

[56] C. Geffriaud-Ricouard, L. H. Noël, D. Chauveau, S. Houhou, J. P. Grünfeld, and P. Lesavre, "Clinical spectrum associated with ANCA of defined antigen specificities in 98 selected patients," *Clinical Nephrology*, vol. 39, no. 3, pp. 125–136, 1993.

[57] C. Franssen, R. Gans, C. Kallenberg, C. Hageluken, and S. Hoorntje, "Disease spectrum of patients with antineutrophil cytoplasmic autoantibodies of defined specificity: distinct differences between patients with anti-proteinase 3 and anti-myeloperoxidase autoantibodies," *Journal of Internal Medicine*, vol. 244, no. 3, pp. 209–216, 1998.

[58] P. A. Lyons, T. F. Rayner, S. Trivedi et al., "Genetically distinct subsets within ANCA-associated vasculitis," *The New England Journal of Medicine*, vol. 367, no. 3, pp. 214–223, 2012.

[59] C. G. M. Kallenberg, C. A. Stegeman, W. H. Abdulahad, and P. Heeringa, "Pathogenesis of ANCA-associated vasculitis: new possibilities for intervention," *American Journal of Kidney Diseases*, vol. 62, no. 6, pp. 1176–1187, 2013.

[60] M. A. Little, C. L. Smyth, R. Yadav et al., "Antineutrophil cytoplasm antibodies directed against myeloperoxidase augment leukocyte-microvascular interactions in vivo," *Blood*, vol. 106, no. 6, pp. 2050–2058, 2005.

[61] H. Xiao, P. Heeringa, P. Hu et al., "Antineutrophil cytoplasmic autoantibodies specific for myeloperoxidase cause glomerulonephritis and vasculitis in mice," *The Journal of Clinical Investigation*, vol. 110, no. 7, pp. 955–963, 2002.

[62] Y. Tomer, B. Gilburd, M. Blank et al., "Characterization of biologically active antineutrophil cytoplasmic antibodies induced in mice: pathogenetic role in experimental vasculitis," *Arthritis & Rheumatism*, vol. 38, no. 10, pp. 1375–1381, 1995.

[63] H. Pfister, M. Ollert, L. F. Fröhlich et al., "Antineutrophil cytoplasmic autoantibodies against the murine homolog of proteinase 3 (Wegener autoantigen) are pathogenic in vivo," *Blood*, vol. 104, no. 5, pp. 1411–1418, 2004.

[64] Y. M. van der Geld, T. Hellmark, D. Selga et al., "Rats and mice immunised with chimeric human/mouse proteinase 3 produce autoantibodies to mouse Pr3 and rat granulocytes," *Annals of the Rheumatic Diseases*, vol. 66, no. 12, pp. 1679–1682, 2007.

[65] C. G. M. Kallenberg, "Pathogenesis of PR3-ANCA associated vasculitis," *Journal of Autoimmunity*, vol. 30, no. 1-2, pp. 29–36, 2008.

[66] J. Alam, Y. C. Kim, and Y. Choi, "Potential role of bacterial infection in autoimmune diseases: a new aspect of molecular mimicry," *Immune Network*, vol. 14, no. 1, pp. 7–13, 2014.

[67] H. Tadema, P. Heeringa, and C. G. M. Kallenberg, "Bacterial infections in Wegener's granulomatosis: mechanisms potentially involved in autoimmune pathogenesis," *Current Opinion in Rheumatology*, vol. 23, no. 4, pp. 366–371, 2011.

[68] S. Borgmann, "Infectious trigger of anca-associated vasculitides and other autoimmune diseases," *Journal of Bacteriology & Parasitology*, vol. 3, no. 8, 2012.

[69] H. Tadema, C. G. M. Kallenberg, C. A. Stegeman, and P. Heeringa, "Reactivity against complementary proteinase-3 is not increased in patients with PR3-ANCA-associated vasculitis," *PLoS ONE*, vol. 6, no. 3, Article ID e17972, 2011.

[70] G. Preston and R. Falk, "Autoimmunity: does autoantigen complementarity underlie PR3-ANCA AAV?" *Nature Reviews Rheumatology*, vol. 7, no. 8, pp. 439–440, 2011.

[71] J. G. Routsias, E. Touloupi, E. Dotsika et al., "Unmasking the anti-La/SSB response in sera from patients with Sjogren's Syndrome by specific blocking of anti-idiotypic antibodies to La/SSB antigenic determinants," *Molecular Medicine*, vol. 8, no. 6, pp. 293–305, 2002.

[72] A. G. Richter, R. A. Stockley, L. Harper, and D. R. Thickett, "Pulmonary infection in Wegener granulomatosis and idiopathic pulmonary fibrosis," *Thorax*, vol. 64, no. 8, pp. 692–697, 2009.

[73] M. Lidar, N. Lipschitz, P. Langevitz et al., "Infectious serologies and autoantibodies in wegener's granulomatosis and other vasculitides: novel associations disclosed using the rad BioPlex

2200," *Annals of the New York Academy of Sciences*, vol. 1173, pp. 649–657, 2009.

[74] N. Patel, N. Patel, T. Khan, N. Patel, and L. R. Espinoza, "HIV infection and clinical spectrum of associated vasculitides," *Current Rheumatology Reports*, vol. 13, no. 6, pp. 506–512, 2011.

[75] M. Mirsaeidi, F. Syed, and E. S. Jaffe, "Antineutrophil cytoplasmic autoantibody-associated systemic vasculitis is associated with epstein-barr virus in the setting of HIV infection," *Infectious Diseases in Clinical Practice*, vol. 21, no. 1, pp. 50–53, 2013.

[76] P. Xu, S. Lin, L. Wei, and W. Shang, "Antineutrophil cytoplasmic antibody-associated vasculitis associated with Epstein-Barr virus infection: a case report and review of the literature," *Infection*, vol. 42, no. 3, pp. 591–594, 2014.

[77] S. Varani, A. Mastroianni, G. Frascaroli et al., "Generalized Wegener's granulomatosis in an immunocompetent adult after cytomegalovirus mononucleosis and bacterial urinary tract infection," *Arthritis and Rheumatism*, vol. 60, no. 5, pp. 1558–1562, 2009.

11

Immunological Parameters Associated With Vitiligo Treatments: A Literature Review Based on Clinical Studies

Ana Cláudia Guimarães Abreu,[1] Gabriela Guy Duarte,[1] Juliana Yasmin Pains Miranda,[1] Daniel Gontijo Ramos,[2,3] Camila Gontijo Ramos,[1,3] and Mariana Gontijo Ramos[1,3]

[1] *Faculdade de Ciências Humanas, Sociais e da Saúde, Universidade Fumec, 30310-190 Belo Horizonte, MG, Brazil*
[2] *Departamento de Dermatologia, Santa Casa de Belo Horizonte, 30150-221 Belo Horizonte, MG, Brazil*
[3] *Clínica de Dermatologia, Edifício Life Center, 30110-921 Belo Horizonte, MG, Brazil*

Correspondence should be addressed to Mariana Gontijo Ramos; marianagontijoramos@gmail.com

Academic Editor: Corrado Betterle

Vitiligo, a depigmentary disorder, caused by the loss of melanocytes, affects approximately 1% of the world population, irrespective of skin type, with a serious psychological impact on the patient quality of life. So far, the origin of vitiligo has not been traced and the pathogenesis is complex, involving the interplay of a multitude of variables. Although there is no treatment that ensures the complete cure of the disorder, there are some pharmacological, phototherapy, and surgical therapies available. A series of variables can affect treatment outcome, such as individual characteristics, emotional issues, type of vitiligo, stability of the lesions, and immunological status. The present literature review identified the main immunological parameters associated with treatments for vitiligo. Cytotoxic CD8+ T lymphocytes are the main cell type involved in treatment success, as fewer cells in skin lesions are associated with better results. Other parameters such as cytokines and regulatory T cells may also be involved. Further clinical scientific studies are needed to elucidate the complex mechanisms underlying vitiligo and its treatments, in order to expand the range of therapeutic approaches for each individual case.

1. Introduction

Vitiligo is an acquired, usually asymptomatic pigmentary disorder that results in the loss of functional melanocytes and is often associated with other autoimmune diseases. At the onset of the disease white patches of different sizes appear on different parts of the body [1, 2]. Vitiligo affects approximately 1% of the world population of all skin types, usually before the age of 20 [3]. Its psychological impact on the quality of life can be disastrous, as dissatisfaction with body image can smother self-esteem and develop a depressive state, especially among dark or tan-skinned patients [4]. The course of the disease is unpredictable, with peaks of anxiety, which makes the patient feel an urge to try different types of treatments. The fact that it can be rather hard to hide the white patches from the eyes of other people makes it difficult for the patient to cope with the disease on a daily basis [5, 6]. Vitiligo can be clinically classified as follows: Nonsegmental or generalized vitiligo is a group that includes acrofacial, vulgaris, universalis, and mixed forms. Localized vitiligo can affect one, two, or multiple segments and includes focal, segmental, and mucosal forms. There are also mixed and undetermined forms of vitiligo [7, 8].

2. Pathogenesis of Vitiligo

Vitiligo is an intriguing disorder whose cause has been an extensive topic of debate. The exact origin of vitiligo is still unclear, and the pathogenesis is complex and involves the interplay of a series of variables [9–11]. There is a multifactorial genetic component predisposing certain individuals to vitiligo and family history is a variable found in approximately one-third of the people with the disease [3, 7]. There is also strong genetic evidence of a link between vitiligo and other autoimmune diseases [12].

According to the neural theory, segmental vitiligo follows the same path as dermatome, and dysfunction of the sympathetic nervous system can curb melanin production and lead to depigmentation [8].

The intrinsic theory suggests that defects in vitiligo melanocytes lead to their death. These include morphologic defects, decreased adhesive properties, and deficient melanocyte growth factors [13, 14]. Increased oxidative stress has also proved to be an important cause for melanocytes destruction [15, 16].

The theory of autoimmune mediated destruction of melanocytes is well accepted and seems to have currently become the leading hypothesis in vitiligo pathogenesis. The immune reaction can be mediated by cellular immunity, humoral antibody-mediated immunity, and the action of cytokines [8].

The action of antibodies against different melanocyte-associated antigens was confirmed in vitiligo. The main antigen recognized by these antibodies is tyrosinase, but antibodies against tyrosine hydroxylase, pigment cell surface antigens, and antithyroid antigens have also been found [17, 18].

Cell-mediated immunity in vitiligo is demonstrated by the presence of inflammatory infiltrates in perilesional vitiligo skin. Decreased CD4+ to CD8+ lymphocytes ratio in vitiligo-stricken skin compared to healthy skin and CD8 T cells directed against melanocytic antigens have been found both in perilesional skin and in the blood of vitiligo patients [19–21]. This shows that the elimination of melanocytes by cytotoxic T cells is a mechanism leading to depigmentation in vitiligo.

Cytokines also seem to play an important role in vitiligo pathogenesis. There is an increase in the expression of tumor necrosis alpha (TNF-α) and interferon-gama (IFN-γ), suggesting that vitiligo is mediated by a T helper cell-1 (Th1) response [22].

The role of regulatory T cells in vitiligo pathogenesis has been a recent topic of research, and there is evidence that Treg is jeopardized in vitiligo patients. However, there is some contradicting data and this subject demands further investigation [8].

Given the importance of the immune system in depigmentation lesions in vitiligo, a series of treatments meant for altering or decreasing immunological reactions has been developed.

3. Vitiligo Treatment

There are no treatments ensuring the complete cure of vitiligo. The main goal of the current treatments is either to control the autoimmune destruction of melanocytes or stimulate their growth on affected areas. Treatment can encompass pharmacological, physical, and surgical approaches or still a combination of different procedures [7].

Pharmacological treatment consists of a topical and systemic corticosteroid therapy, topical calcineurin inhibitors such as tacrolimus and pimecrolimus, pseudocatalase, melagenina (human placental extract), and vitamin-D derivatives [3, 7].

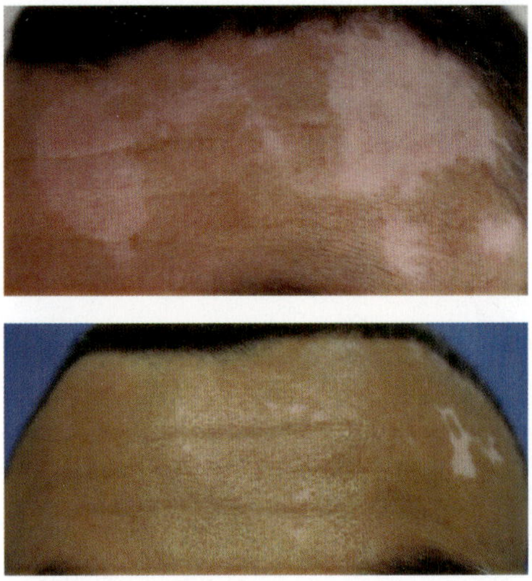

Figure 1: Repigmentation observed after melanocyte transplantation for the treatment of stable vitiligo.

Light therapy includes sunlight, PUVA, narrowband UVB (NB-UVB), and excimer laser. These treatments are frequently combined with topical treatment and transplantation processes [23].

Surgical treatment can be an option and is usually recommended for patients with stable vitiligo (with no change in lesions numbers or morphology), for which other treatments had no significant results. There are various techniques, but the most usual technique consists of transplanting a pigmented skin graft from a donor onto the patient's affected areas. Surgical treatments include suction blister grafts, punch grafts, minigrafts, and split thickness skin grafts [24, 25]. Melanocytes and keratinocytes transplantation is also a surgical intervention by which cell suspension is transferred from a donor's pigmented skin onto a previously prepared recipient, usually by means of dermabrasion. Cultured and noncultured cells can be used [26–28]. Noncultured melanocytes-keratinocytes cellular grafting yields significant pigmentation results in patients with stable forms of vitiligo, as seen from data previously collected by our group (Figure 1) [29].

Although there are several options for the treatment of vitiligo, the results are different for each patient and hardly ever satisfying, as these people can be affected by a series of unknown factors. Knowledge of the immune parameters associated with vitiligo pathogenesis is therefore vital in predicting and suggesting the right type of treatment for each patient.

4. Immunological Parameters Associated with Vitiligo Treatments

Different treatments for vitiligo can lead to good repigmentation and great satisfaction for some patients. However, they may not work so well for others. Treatment outcome will depend on some rather complex mechanisms, such as

Table 1: Summary of immunological parameters associated with vitiligo treatments reported in the literature.

Author	Type of vitiligo	Treatment	Main findings in immunological parameters	Reference
Rao et al.	Generalized	Surgical by suction blister epidermal grafting	Patients with active vitiligo and poor treatment response had increased levels of CD8+ and CD45RO+ cells in skin lesions	[30]
Abdallah et al.	Generalized	Surgical by autologous minigrafting	Patients unresponsive to treatment had increased cytotoxic T lymphocyte in skin lesions	[31]
Zhou et al.	Localized and generalized	Surgical by autologous melanocyte transplantation	Patients with poor repigmentation response had higher levels of CD8+ T cells in perilesional skin and increased levels of proinflammatory cytokines in epidermis fluid	[32]
Reyes et al.	Generalized	PUVA and *Polypodium leucotomos*	Abnormal activation and decrease in CD8+CD45RO+ blood lymphocytes	[33]
Antelo et al.	Generalized	PUVA	Reduction of CD8+CLA+ lymphocytes in peripheral blood	[34]
Shi et al.	Vitiligo with qi-stagnancy and blood-stasis	Chinese herbs Zengse pill combined with cobalamin and psoralea tincture	Increased CD4/CD8 ration and reduced CD8+ in peripheral blood	[35]
Tembhre et al.	Generalized	NB-UVB	Increased serum IL-10, IL-13, and IL-17 and decreased TGF-β in active vitiligo patients. NB-UVB may be able to modulate T helper and Treg cytokines.	[36]
Moftah et al.	Generalized	NB-UVB	NB-UVB treatment decreased peripheral blood Treg cells.	[37]

individual characteristics, emotional issues, type of vitiligo, stability of the lesions, and immunological status.

Although there are many studies showing the importance of the immune reaction to the pathogenesis of vitiligo, few of them were conducted in vivo in human patients submitted to treatments.

The purpose of the present literature review is to investigate and analyze clinical studies about the association of immunological parameters with treatments for vitiligo. Data collected from Pubmed database suggested that there is a growing interest in this subject, as most of the studies have been published quite recently, after 2010. It was also observed that research groups are mainly from Asian countries, such as India and China. The main findings of the studies are summarized in Table 1.

Most of the patients enrolled in the studies suffered from generalized vitiligo and were submitted to different types of treatments, such as NB-UVB, PUVA alone or combined with *Polypodium leucotomos,* alternative treatment with Chinese herbs or minigrafts, surgical treatment, or autologous melanocytes transplantation.

The importance of the patient's immunological status for the outcome of vitiligo treatments was observed in all studies.

Cellular immunity seems to play a vital role in the outcome of vitiligo treatments, as CD8+ T cells are involved in the autoimmune destruction of melanocytes resulting in skin depigmentation. In 2012, Rao et al. reported that patients with active vitiligo, when compared to patients with stable vitiligo, presented increased numbers of CD8+ and CD45RO+ cells (effector lymphocytes) on perilesional skin and had the worst response to the treatment with melanocyte transplantation [30]. A similar result showing increased cytotoxic T lymphocytes in vitiligo skin lesions and poor response to minigraft transplantation was demonstrated by Abdallah et al. [31].

Zhou et al. treated patients with melanocyte transplantation and observed an increased number of CD8+ lymphocytes in the perilesional skin of patients with poor repigmentation results. They also demonstrated that dermal mesenchymal stem cells (DMSC) had an inhibitory effect against CD8+ T cells skin-homing, inhibited cell proliferation, induced apoptosis, and regulated the production of cytokines and chemokines by CD8+ lymphocytes [32]. A decrease in peripheral blood CD8+ lymphocytes can be associated with the increased homing of these cells to vitiligo-affected skin sites; once in the active disease the lymphocytes migrate to the skin, due to cutaneous lymphocyte-associated antigen (CLA) molecule expression [33, 34].

Alternative treatments, which can be administered alone or in combination with other procedures, are sometimes an option for patients who are unresponsive to regular treatments. Oral administration of Chinese herbs (Zengse pill) combined with oral cobalamin and topic psoralea tincture induced significant repigmentation and increased blood CD4+/CD8+ ratio, regulating the immunity of the organism [35].

Treatment with PUVA alone has proved inefficient and incapable of altering immunologic parameters in patients [34]. However, a combination of PUVA and *Polypodium leucotomos* succeeded in inducing repigmentation and curbed the proliferation of lymphocytes in patients with generalized vitiligo [33].

Regulatory T cells (Treg) are lymphocytes specialized in self-tolerance and in preserving immune system homeostasis.

These cells are responsible for the production of modulatory cytokines. There have been advances in the research on Treg cells in the pathogenesis of vitiligo and on successful treatments. Regulatory cytokines produced by Treg cells, such as interleukin-10 and tumor growth factor beta (TGF-β), are suggested to be related to the stability of the disease. In 2013, Tembhre et al. found increased cytokine levels in patients with stable vitiligo, and treatment with NB-UVB was capable of elevating TGF-β levels, suggesting that Treg cytokines played an important role in repigmentation [36]. However, no evidence of a correlation between Treg and duration or activity of vitiligo was found by Moftah et al. in 2014, indicating that more studies are needed to further elucidate these mechanisms [37].

Other cytokines are probably involved in vitiligo pathogenesis and treatment. Higher levels of the proinflammatory cytokines Interleukin-1α, Interleukin-1β, and interleukin-12, measured in epidermis fluid, were present in patients whose response to melanocyte transplantation was unsatisfactory [32]. Patients with active vitiligo also showed an increase in blood proinflammatory cytokines [36]. These data suggest that an increased inflammatory response mediated by Th1 cytokines is associated with disease activity and consequently poor skin repigmentation.

It is common knowledge that stable vitiligo can help predict response to different treatments, mainly surgical procedures for the replacement of melanocytes in depigmented skin sites. The course of the disease is difficult to predict, as it can either stay stable for years and then become active again or regress spontaneously. Literature review indicates that more stable lesions present lower numbers of cytotoxic T cells and inflammatory cytokines, leading to a better prognosis [30, 36].

Regarding the type of vitiligo, it is possible to conclude that patients with the generalized form of the disease will have the worst response to different treatments, compared to those with segmental vitiligo. An explanation for this observation is the fact that generalized vitiligo patients have more lesions in many body areas and thus need more aggressive and long lasting treatments.

5. Conclusions

Literature review shows that immunological parameters, mainly cytotoxic T lymphocytes, cytokines, and regulatory T cells, can influence the outcome of different treatments for vitiligo. Lower levels of CD8+ cells in skin lesions are usually associated with better repigmentation results. However, further scientific studies and efforts are needed, especially through clinical studies, to elucidate the complex mechanisms underlying vitiligo and its treatments, leading to better therapeutic choices for each individual case.

Conflict of Interests

The authors declare that there is no conflict of interests regarding the publication of this paper.

References

[1] J. S. Bellet and N. S. Prose, "Vitiligo in children: a review of classification, hypotheses of pathogenesis and treatment," *Anais Brasileiros de Dermatologia*, vol. 80, no. 6, pp. 631–636, 2005.

[2] R. Czajkowski and K. Męcińska-Jundziłł, "Current aspects of vitiligo genetics," *Dermatology and Allergology*, vol. 31, no. 4, pp. 247–255, 2014.

[3] M. E. Whiton, M. Pinart, J. Batchelor et al., "Interventions for vitiligo," *Cochrane Database of Systematic Reviews*, no. 1, Article ID CD003263, 2015.

[4] K. Ezzedine, V. Eleftheriadou, M. Whitton, and N. van Geel, "Vitiligo," *The Lancet*, vol. 386, no. 9988, pp. 74–84, 2015.

[5] G. Schmid-Ott, H.-W. Künsebeck, E. Jecht et al., "Stigmatization experience, coping and sense of coherence in vitiligo patients," *Journal of the European Academy of Dermatology & Venereology*, vol. 21, no. 4, pp. 456–461, 2007.

[6] C. Krüger and K. Schallreuter, "Stigmatisation, avoidance behaviour and difficulties in coping are common among adult patients with vitiligo," *Acta Dermato Venereologica*, vol. 95, no. 5, pp. 553–558, 2015.

[7] A. R. Faria, M. T. Mira, R. G. Tarlé, C. C. Silva de Castro, and G. Dellatorre, "Vitiligo—part 2—classification, histopathology and treatment," *Anais Brasileiros de Dermatologia*, vol. 89, no. 5, pp. 784–790, 2014.

[8] G. F. Mohammed, A. H. A. Gomaa, and M. S. Al-Dhubaibi, "Highlights in pathogenesis of vitiligo," *World Journal of Clinical Cases*, vol. 3, no. 3, pp. 221–230, 2015.

[9] K. U. Schallreuter, P. Bahadoran, M. Picardo et al., "Vitiligo pathogenesis: autoimmune disease, genetic defect, excessive reactive oxygen species, calcium imbalance, or what else?" *Experimental Dermatology*, vol. 17, no. 2, pp. 139–140, 2008.

[10] J. M. Richmond, M. L. Frisoli, and J. E. Harris, "Innate immune mechanisms in vitiligo: danger from within," *Current Opinion in Immunology*, vol. 25, no. 6, pp. 676–682, 2013.

[11] K. Ezzedine, A. Mahé, N. van Geel et al., "Hypochromic vitiligo: delineation of a new entity," *British Journal of Dermatology*, vol. 173, no. 3, pp. 716–721, 2015.

[12] R. A. Spritz, "Modern vitiligo genetics sheds new light on an ancient disease," *Journal of Dermatology*, vol. 40, no. 5, pp. 310–318, 2013.

[13] R. Speeckaert, M. M. Speeckaert, and N. van Geel, "Why treatments do(n't) work in vitiligo: an autoinflammatory perspective," *Autoimmunity Reviews*, vol. 14, no. 4, pp. 332–340, 2015.

[14] M. Picardo and E. Bastonini, "A new view of vitiligo: looking at normal-appearing skin," *Journal of Investigative Dermatology*, vol. 135, no. 7, pp. 1713–1714, 2015.

[15] S. Li, G. Zhu, Y. Yang et al., "Oxidative stress-induced chemokine production mediates $CD8^+$ T cell skin trafficking in vitiligo," *Journal of Investigative Dermatology Symposium Proceedings*, vol. 17, no. 1, pp. 32–33, 2015.

[16] G. Güntaş, B. Engin, Ö. B. Ekmekçi et al., "Evaluation of advanced oxidation protein products, prooxidant-antioxidant balance, and total antioxidant capacity in untreated vitiligo patients," *Annals of Dermatology*, vol. 27, no. 2, pp. 178–183, 2015.

[17] E. H. Kemp, S. Emhemad, S. Akhtar, P. F. Watson, D. J. Gawkrodger, and A. P. Weetman, "Autoantibodies against tyrosine hydroxylase in patients with non-segmental (generalised) vitiligo," *Experimental Dermatology*, vol. 20, no. 1, pp. 35–40, 2011.

[18] V. Ingordo, C. Gentile, S. S. Iannazzone, F. Cusano, and L. Naldi, "Vitiligo and autoimmunity: an epidemiological study in a representative sample of young Italian males," *Journal of the European Academy of Dermatology and Venereology*, vol. 25, no. 1, pp. 105–109, 2011.

[19] N. A. C. van Geel, I. G. Mollet, S. De Schepper et al., "First histopathological and immunophenotypic analysis of early dynamic events in a patient with segmental vitiligo associated with halo nevi," *Pigment Cell and Melanoma Research*, vol. 23, no. 3, pp. 375–384, 2010.

[20] R. M. Luiten, J. G. van den Boorn, D. Konijnenberg et al., "Autoimmune destruction of skin melanocytes by perilesional T cells from vitiligo patients," *Journal of Investigative Dermatology*, vol. 129, no. 9, pp. 2220–2232, 2009.

[21] N. Oiso, T. Suzuki, K. Fukai, I. Katayama, and A. Kawada, "Non-segmental vitiligo and autoimmune mechanism," *Dermatology Research and Practice*, vol. 2011, Article ID 518090, 7 pages, 2011.

[22] Z. A. Taher, G. Lauzon, S. Maguiness, and M. T. Dytoc, "Analysis of interleukin-10 levels in lesions of vitiligo following treatment with topical tacrolimus," *British Journal of Dermatology*, vol. 161, no. 3, pp. 654–659, 2009.

[23] Y. H. Jang, S.-E. Jung, J. Shin, and H. Y. Kang, "Triple combination of systemic corticosteroids, excimer laser, and topical tacrolimus in the treatment of recently developed localized vitiligo," *Annals of Dermatology*, vol. 27, no. 1, pp. 104–107, 2015.

[24] A. Budania, D. Parsad, A. J. Kanwar, and S. Dogra, "Comparison between autologous noncultured epidermal cell suspension and suction blister epidermal grafting in stable vitiligo: a randomized study," *British Journal of Dermatology*, vol. 167, no. 6, pp. 1295–1301, 2012.

[25] V. M. Sheth, S. D. Currimbhoy, H. J. Feetham et al., "Efficacy of narrowband ultraviolet B versus excimer radiation in repigmenting vitiligo after minigrafting on the distal arms," *Journal of the American Academy of Dermatology*, vol. 67, no. 2, pp. 318–320, 2012.

[26] S. V. Mulekar, A. Al Issa, and A. Al Eisa, "Treatment of vitiligo on difficult-to-treat sites using autologous noncultured cellular grafting," *Dermatologic Surgery*, vol. 35, no. 1, pp. 66–71, 2009.

[27] S. V. Mulekar, A. Al Eisa, M. B. Delvi, A. Al Issa, and A. H. Al Saeed, "Childhood vitiligo: a long-term study of localized vitiligo treated by noncultured cellular grafting," *Pediatric Dermatology*, vol. 27, no. 2, pp. 132–136, 2010.

[28] L. Komen, C. Vrijman, E. P. Tjin et al., "Autologous cell suspension transplantation using a cell extraction device in segmental vitiligo and piebaldism patients: a randomized controlled pilot study," *Journal of the American Academy of Dermatology*, vol. 73, no. 1, pp. 170–172, 2015.

[29] M. G. Ramos, D. G. Ramos, G. Gontijo, C. G. Ramos, T. N. Rocha, and R. H. Rocha, "Non-cultured melanocyte/keratinocyte transplantation for the treatment of stable vitiligo on the face: report of two cases," *Anais Brasileiros de Dermatologia*, vol. 88, no. 5, pp. 811–813, 2013.

[30] A. Rao, S. Gupta, A. K. Dinda et al., "Study of clinical, biochemical and immunological factors determining stability of disease in patients with generalized vitiligo undergoing melanocyte transplantation," *British Journal of Dermatology*, vol. 166, no. 6, pp. 1230–1236, 2012.

[31] M. Abdallah, M. B. Abdel-Naser, M. H. Moussa, C. Assaf, and C. E. Orfanos, "Sequential immunohistochemical study of depigmenting and repigmenting minigrafts in vitiligo," *European Journal of Dermatology*, vol. 13, no. 6, pp. 548–552, 2003.

[32] M.-N. Zhou, Z.-Q. Zhang, J.-L. Wu et al., "Dermal mesenchymal stem cells (DMSCs) inhibit skin-homing CD8+ T cell activity, a determining factor of vitiligo patients' autologous melanocytes transplantation efficiency," *PLoS ONE*, vol. 8, no. 4, Article ID e60254, 10 pages, 2013.

[33] E. Reyes, P. Jaén, E. D. L. Heras et al., "Systemic immunomodulatory effects of *Polypodium leucotomos* as an adjuvant to PUVA therapy in generalized vitiligo: a pilot study," *Journal of Dermatological Science*, vol. 41, no. 3, pp. 213–216, 2006.

[34] D. P. Antelo, A. L. Filgueira, and J. M. T. Cunha, "Reduction of skin-homing cytotoxic T cells ($CD8^+$–CLA^+) in patients with vitiligo," *Photodermatology Photoimmunology and Photomedicine*, vol. 27, no. 1, pp. 40–44, 2011.

[35] N. Shi, Y. J. Chen, J. Wang, and H. Ni, "Clinical observation on the effect of Zengse Pill in treating patients with vitiligo of qi-stagnancy and blood-stasis syndrome type," *Chinese Journal of Integrative Medicine*, vol. 14, no. 4, pp. 303–306, 2008.

[36] M. K. Tembhre, V. K. Sharma, A. Sharma, P. Chattopadhyay, and S. Gupta, "T helper and regulatory T cell cytokine profile in active, stable and narrow band ultraviolet B treated generalized vitiligo," *Clinica Chimica Acta*, vol. 424, pp. 27–32, 2013.

[37] N. H. Moftah, R. A. H. El-Barbary, M. A. Ismail, and N. A. M. Ali, "Effect of narrow band-ultraviolet B on $CD4^+CD25^{high}$ $FoxP3^+$T-lymphocytes in the peripheral blood of vitiligo patients," *Photodermatology Photoimmunology and Photomedicine*, vol. 30, no. 5, pp. 254–261, 2014.

12

Occurrence of Autoimmune Diseases Related to the Vaccine against Yellow Fever

Ana Cristina Vanderley Oliveira,[1,2] Licia Maria Henrique da Mota,[1] Leopoldo Luiz dos Santos-Neto,[1] Jozélio Freire De Carvalho,[3] Iramaya Rodrigues Caldas,[4] Olindo Assis Martins Filho,[5] and Pedro Luis Tauil[1]

[1] *Faculdade de Medicina, Universidade de Brasília, Brasília, DF, Brazil*
[2] *CRDF, SHLN Bloco L Centro Cínico Norte II, 70910-900 Brasília, DF, Brazil*
[3] *Hospital Universitário Professor Edgard Santos da Universidade Federal da Bahia, 70390-700 Salvador, BA, Brazil*
[4] *Coordenação de Pesquisa da Fundação Oswaldo Cruz (FIOCRUZ), 41810-080 Brasília, DF, Brazil*
[5] *Laboratório de Biomarcadores de Diagnóstico e Monitoração do Centro de Pesquisas René Rachou, FIOCRUZ, 21040-900 Belo Horizonte, MG, Brazil*

Correspondence should be addressed to Ana Cristina Vanderley Oliveira; acvanderley@gmail.com

Academic Editor: Ricard Cervera

Yellow fever is an infectious disease, endemic in South America and Africa. This is a potentially serious illness, with lethality between 5 and 40% of cases. The most effective preventive vaccine is constituted by the attenuated virus strain 17D, developed in 1937. It is considered safe and effective, conferring protection in more than 90% in 10 years. Adverse effects are known as mild reactions (allergies, transaminases transient elevation, fever, headache) and severe (visceral and neurotropic disease related to vaccine). However, little is known about its potential to induce autoimmune responses. This systematic review aims to identify the occurrence of autoinflammatory diseases related to 17D vaccine administration. Six studies were identified describing 13 possible cases. The diseases were Guillain-Barré syndrome, multiple sclerosis, multiple points evanescent syndrome, acute disseminated encephalomyelitis, autoimmune hepatitis, and Kawasaki disease. The data suggest that 17D vaccination may play a role in the mechanism of loss of self-tolerance.

1. Introduction

Yellow fever is an infectious disease endemic in South America and Africa. The presence of viral reservoirs and the large number of viral vectors are prerequisites for the outbreaks of yellow fever observed in these areas [1]. The virus is transmitted by the bite of blood-sucking insects of the family Culicidae, in particular the genera *Aedes* and *Haemagogus* [2].

The yellow fever virus is a single-stranded RNA virus that belongs to the family Flaviviridae [1, 2]. The virus most likely originated in Africa and was brought to America during the slave trade [1, 3].

Epidemiologically, yellow fever exists in two forms, rural and urban, which are similar in their clinical and pathophysiological characteristics [2]. The disease lethality is estimated between 5 and 40%. In more severe cases, yellow fever evolves with sepsis, ictero-, and hepatorenal hemorrhagic syndromes, myocardial injury, and shock [1, 2]. According to the World Health Organization (WHO), more than 50% of people without treatment will die from the disease [4]. Some series report 94,8% of lethality at severe disease [5].

The clinical manifestations range from oligosymptomatic forms to severe and fatal cases [1, 2]. Only one in seven infected individuals develops symptoms [6]. The extremes of age are related to the severity and lethality of infection [7].

The incubation period is 3–6 days [8]. In the milder forms, infected individuals may develop nonspecific malaise, myalgia, nausea and vomiting, fever, and headaches. In this presentation, severe hemorrhage, hematemesis, epistaxis, ecchymosis, jaundice, dehydration, and oligo/anuria complete the picture [1, 2, 7]. Infection with the yellow fever virus is distinguished from other flaviviruses by liver damage and jaundice. Late manifestations, such as mental confusion, seizures, and coma, can occur. Death occurs between 7 and 10 days after the onset of symptoms [1].

The best method to prevent yellow fever is vaccination [2, 8]. The 17D vaccine, made with live attenuated virus, has been used since 1937 and is considered one of the safest and most effective vaccines ever produced [2, 9]. The vaccine induces neutralizing antibodies in 90% of recipients after 10 days and in 99% of recipients after 30 days [6]. Today, the vaccines for yellow fever are derived from two substrains, 17D and 17D-204 [8]. The vaccines are produced by four centers: Institut Pasteur in Dakar, Senegal; Bio-Manguinhos Wire Cruz, Rio de Janeiro, Brazil; Sanofi Pasteur, US; and Sanofi Pasteur, France [1]. The WHO recommended that the vaccine be administered every 10 years until 2013. However, some authors believe that the vaccine's protection can extend throughout an individual's lifetime [2, 3]. Thus, based on the existing data, the WHO changed the recommendation: there is no need for revaccination for the immune-competent individuals [10]. It is estimated that over 500 million doses have been applied [9].

However, the yellow fever vaccine is not free of adverse effects [2, 8]. In general the adverse effects are mild and well tolerated, including pain in the injection site, headache, myalgia, fever, and lower back pain. These symptoms occur between the second and 11th day after the application [8]. Among the serious adverse events, a multisystem disease (YEL-AVD) and a neurological disease (YEL-AND) are associated with the yellow fever vaccination. Both are a consequence of infection by the vaccine virus [2, 8, 9]. YEL-AVD exhibits a clinical picture similar to wild yellow fever, whereas YEL-AND encompasses neurological manifestations, such as encephalitis and meningitis. Some autoimmune manifestations, such as Guillain-Barré or ADEM (acute disseminated encephalomyelitis), are also described [8, 11].

The development of autoimmune manifestations has been linked to vaccination and to infection by wild-type microorganisms [12]. Infections are potentially relevant events in the development of autoimmune diseases, as they have the ability to hyperstimulate the immune system. Antigens similar to human cells and tissues may stimulate autoantibody production because of the molecular mimicry in genetically predisposed individuals [9].

As the infection mechanisms due to the vaccine virus and wild microorganisms are the same, it is theoretically possible for autoimmunity to occur after vaccination [12, 13]. Another factor to be considered is the potential induction of autoimmunity by vaccine adjuvants [13].

In this study, we performed the first systematic review to identify the occurrence of autoimmune diseases related to the vaccine against yellow fever.

2. Methods

The search for articles was performed on September 9, 2012, in the following databases: PubMed, MEDLINE, LILACS, and SCiELO.

We used the words or phrases "yellow fever vaccine" or "yellow fever vaccination" in combination with "autoimmune," "autoimmunity," "immune response," "adverse effects," and "adverse events."

We included only studies published between 1937, the year the 17D vaccine was introduced, and September 9, 2012. We limited the included studies to those performed on humans and on the 17D vaccine (17D, 17DD, or 17D 204). The adverse event must have occurred within 30 days of the vaccination. Only articles written in English, Portuguese, or Spanish were considered.

After the initial screening, duplicate articles and those which were not case series were excluded.

The remaining abstracts were read, and those that cited the occurrence of some autoimmune disease were selected for reading. For purposes of this review, autoimmune diseases are considered to be any autoimmune disorders that are characterized by the production of autoantibodies. These must react with host tissues or immune effector cells that are reactive to endogenous peptides.

We found 602 articles. After applying the inclusion criteria, 463 articles remained and were screened by title. Of those remaining, we selected case series and case reports, totaling 132 articles, of which 82 were duplicates. Thus, 50 articles were selected for an analysis of the abstracts. Selected articles should cite at least one occurrence of autoimmune disease related to the 17D vaccine. At the end of our selection, we were left with 6 articles.

The quality of the selected articles was assessed by the McHarm tool, developed by McMaster University, Canada [14].

3. Results

There were 13 cases time-related to the development of autoimmune diseases (Table 1). Eight men (61.5%) and 5 women (38.5%) comprised the sample. Their ages ranged between 12 and 68 years, with a mean age of 42.31 years and a standard deviation of 20.43 years. The hepatitis A vaccine was applied in 8 of the cases described in this work. The time between the application of the vaccine and the clinical manifestations ranged between 7 and 27 days, with an average of 13.92 days.

In 1967, Miller et al. reported a series of 9 cases related to vaccination and multiple sclerosis. One case concerns a woman, aged 22 years, vaccinated against yellow fever in 1942. Six weeks prior to her yellow fever vaccine, she had been immunized with tetanus, typhoid vaccine, and smallpox without adverse effects. Hours after receiving the vaccine against yellow fever, she developed progressive loss of vision in both eyes, with recovery in a few weeks. One year after receiving the yellow fever vaccine, retrobulbar neuritis presented in the right eye. Over 12 episodes of retrobulbar neuritis between 1944 and 1951 were reported by

Table 1: Cases of autoimmune diseases after yellow fever vaccination.

	Author	Disease	Age (years)	Gender	Time between vaccine and symptoms (days)	Symptoms	McHarm (quality)	Other vaccines
1	McMahon et al. [11]	GBS	49	M	10	Headache, diplopia	Good	Meningitis, dT, typhoid fever, Salk
2	McMahon et al. [11]	GBS	37	M	16	Headache, blurred vision	Good	Hep B, meningitis, dT
3	McMahon et al. [11]	GBS	17	F	7	Difficulty breathing	Good	Typhoid, Hep A, dT
4	McMahon et al. [11]	GBS	56	M	27	Paresis	Good	Hep A, Hep B, typhoid fever, meningitis
5	McMahon et al. [11]	GBS	63	F	16	Headache, unsteady gait	Good	Hep A
6	McMahon et al. [11]	GBS	68	F	8	Paresis	Good	dT, Hep A, typhoid
8	McMahon et al. [11]	ADEM	18	M	20	Eye pain, paresis, blurred vision	Good	dT, MMR
9	McMahon et al. [11]	ADEM	61	M	7	Unsteady gait	Good	dT, hepatitis A
10	Miller et al. [15]	MS	22	M	"Few hours"	Visual loss, paresis	Bad	Typhoid, tetanus, chickenpox
11	Perumalswami et al. [16]	AIH	31	F	11	Liver failure	Intermediate	Hep A
12	Schmöeller et al. [17]	KD	12	M	20	Conjunctivitis, fever, coronary aneurism	Bad	None
13	Stangos et al. [18]	MEWDS	50	F	10	Temporary visual loss	Intermediate	Hepatitis A
14	Vital et al. [19]	MS?	66	M	15	Facial paralysis	Bad	None

GBS: Guillain-Barré syndrome; ADMS: acute demyelinating multiple sclerosis; AIH: autoimmune hepatitis; KD: Kawasaki disease; MEWDS: multiple evanescent white dot syndrome; dT: dyphteria and tetanus; Hep B: hepatitis B; Hep A: hepatitis A; MMR: Measles-Mumps-Rubella.

the authors. The patient exhibited unilateral or bilateral paresis and emotional lability. Fifteen years after the vaccination, an examination revealed sequelae such as atrophy of the left optic nerve, residual intention tremor, and ataxia. The remaining cases cited by Miller involved vaccinations against other diseases [15].

In 2009, Schmöeller and colleagues described an atypical case after yellow fever vaccination that occurred in Rio Grande do Sul, Brazil. A male child, aged 12 years, developed the typical manifestations of Kawasaki disease. Kawasaki disease is a vasculitis of medium-caliber vessels with involvement of cardiac vessels and possible autoimmune etiology. Twenty days after the vaccination, the patient developed fever, fatigue, and myalgia, followed by conjunctivitis and cervical lymphadenopathy. Investigations revealed leukocytosis (17×10^9 cells/L), eosinophilia (1.5×10^9 cells/L), and moderate anemia. The erythrocyte sedimentation rate was 112 mm/h. Tests for cytomegalovirus, Epstein-Barr virus, and toxoplasmosis were negative. Echocardiography revealed coronary dilation. Treatment was started after the diagnosis, and the patient was medicated with immunoglobulin (2 g/kg, one day) plus aspirin. There was improvement for 2 weeks followed by arthralgia and recrudescence of conjunctivitis. The team opted to start prednisone therapy at 10 mg/kg, and symptom remission was observed. One month later, the child exhibited improved echocardiographic parameters and good recovery. The child remained asymptomatic and continued low-dose-aspirin therapy according to the authors of the publication [17].

Stangos and colleagues described a case of multiple evanescent white dot syndrome (MEWDS) after simultaneous vaccination against hepatitis A and yellow fever. This disease is benign, is characterized by white spots in the retinal pigment epithelium, and manifests clinically by unilateral involvement with painless loss of visual field scotomas and fotopsias. The disease mainly affects females, as in the case described. This patient was a woman of 50 years who developed visual loss in photopsia and painless paracentral scotoma in the left eye 10 days after vaccination. Examination revealed a visual acuity of 20/40, and fundoscopy revealed papillitis, macular granularity, and multiple white spots. Fluorescein angiography of the affected eye revealed numerous hypofluorescent injuries gradually radiating from the optic nerve. These findings, associated with the exclusion of sarcoidosis, tuberculosis, and syphilis, led researchers to diagnose MEWDS. The patient exhibited spontaneous clinical remission after 6 weeks, with normalization of her examinations. The authors believe that her older age might have favored the development of MEWDS [18].

Vital et al. analyzed the case of a 66-year-old patient vaccinated against yellow fever who developed progressive motor and sensory neuropathy associated with bilateral facial paralysis 15 days after vaccination. CSF analysis revealed a protein concentration of 3 g/L and 5 lymphocytes. Six weeks after the onset of symptoms, the patient underwent a tracheotomy. The patient required rehabilitation for 9 months. In the paper, there is no detailed description of the type of rehabilitation or the drugs that were used. Biopsy samples were necessary and were taken from the superficial peroneal nerve and peroneal muscle. Histological analysis revealed destruction of the myelin sheath and associated macrophages [19].

There are also reports of a 31-year-old patient, previously healthy, who developed autoimmune hepatitis 11 days after vaccination against hepatitis A and yellow fever. Perumalswami and colleagues described the clinical findings, which began with fever, dark urine, nausea, and vomiting. On physical examination, the patient exhibited jaundice and hepatomegaly. Laboratory tests reported values of 12 g/dL hemoglobin, 575 U/L ALT, 1276 U/L AST, and 162 U/L alkaline phosphatase. Serology for Epstein-Barr virus, leptospira, and hepatitides A, B, C, and E were negative. The following autoantibodies were measured and showed no reactions: antinuclear antibodies (ANA), liver-kidney microsomal (LKM) antibody, antimitochondrial antibodies, and anti-smooth muscle antibodies. A slight increase in IgG that reached 18.7 g/L was observed (VR $<$ 17.28 g/L). PCR for viral RNA of the yellow fever virus was negative. The patient's clinical and laboratory findings improved over 3 weeks. New analysis indicated further increases in transaminases and bilirubin. The presumptive diagnosis of autoimmune hepatitis was made based on the criteria of the International Autoimmune Hepatitis Group (International Autoimmune Hepatitis Group (IAIGH)). Liver biopsy revealed lymphoplasmocytes periportal infiltrates, parenchymal necrosis, and lobular inflammation. The patient was treated with 40 mg of prednisone and 50 mg of azathioprine per day. After 3 months, the transaminases had normalized. After 1 year, a biopsy indicated a significant reduction in periportal inflammation. Previously necrotic areas were replaced by fibrous septa [16].

By analyzing data from 1990 in the 2005 American surveillance system, "Vaccine Adverse Event Reporting System (VAERS)," McMahon and colleagues sought to identify neurological syndromes associated with vaccination against yellow fever. Acute disseminated encephalomyelitis (ADEM) is defined by the presence of disseminated demyelination on imaging, as supported by the clinical presentation. Guillain-Barré syndrome (GBS) is defined by the presence of peripheral neuropathy and electrodiagnostic findings consistent with acute axonal demyelination. For the purpose of their analysis, encephalitis had to be caused after vaccination. Therefore, it is necessary to confirm the presence of the virus or specific IgM in the CSF. GBS and ADEM are considered autoimmune events. The authors considered a range of 30 days to classify the events as related to the yellow fever vaccine. We identified 3 cases of suspected ADEM in patients between 18 and 61 years of age. The clinical symptoms began between 7 and 20 days after vaccination. One of these patients exhibited retrobulbar optic neuritis with bilateral eye pain, blurred vision, numbness in the upper limb, lower limb paresis, and difficulty urinating. The patient developed persistent paresthesia but with almost total recovery of the other symptoms. The others, aged 19 and 61 years, progressed to paresis and difficulty walking. The oldest did not fully recover and was later referred to a recovery center. The youngest, although he exhibited associated urinary dysfunction, showed improvement and was able to walk without assistance. This last patient, diagnosed with ADEM, was not considered by our criteria to exhibit positive CSF IgM, indicating that the vaccine virus did not penetrate into the central nervous system. This consideration was not made by the authors. Six patients, aged 17 to 68 years, developed suspected Guillain-Barré between 7 and 27 days after immunization. IgM CSF was evaluated in only one case and produced a negative result. Three patients required immunoglobulin, one patient required plasmapheresis, and another patient required two high doses of metilprednisolone. Of the six patients, one had diplopia at discharge, whereas the others exhibited minimal sequelae. None of the patients diagnosed with Guillain-Barré or ADEM in this publication had received the yellow fever vaccine alone [11].

Although it has been retracted because the author of the revision considered the disease secondary to an infection with the vaccine virus, Merlo et al. describe one possible case in 1993. The author published the first time-related description of vaccine associated encephalitis due to 17D in an adult. The patient was a 29-year-old individual immunized for the first time against yellow fever. The patient received vaccinations against diphtheria and tetanus on the same day as the yellow fever vaccine. At the third day, the patient had fever and headache and vomited. Nineteen days after, his clinical findings consisted of blurred vision, headache, dizziness, and ataxia. The sequela was persistent mild ataxia. Serological investigation for neurotropic viruses and bacteria was negative. The yellow fever neutralizing antibody was found in serum after 60 days (titer 1:80). Specific IgM or viral RNA in the CSF were not measured, and, thus, it was not possible to determine whether the symptoms were due to infection with the vaccine virus or to the occurrence of a secondary autoimmune response [20].

4. Discussion

Several studies in the literature have reported the association of vaccination with the development of autoimmune diseases [12]. Autoimmune events after vaccination are rare; therefore, the number of subjects studied would need to be quite high to identify the appropriate number of cases. Accordingly, the human and material cost becomes high in cohort studies. Additionally, it is difficult to control all of the factors that can alter the results of the study, such as environmental factors, genetic factors, or infections. The unpredictability of autoimmunity and the lack of previous studies make the study design even more complex. Even though one might identify the presence of an eventual relationship between the 17D vaccine and autoimmunity, new studies are needed to establish a relation cause and effect.

Although there are few case reports, a series of cases presents other limitations. The identification of cases was conducted passively, leading to underreporting. The amount of information collected and the data quality may be different in each study. Some of the reasons are the lack of resources, delayed diagnosis, or differences between examiners. Although the vaccines are derived from the same original strain, they are produced by four distinct centers, and differences in handling and preservatives may occur. Such differences can be responsible for the development of autoimmune events. Thus, the comparison between cases involving vaccines of different manufacturers can lead to less reliable results. However, given the lack of studies on the topic, a series of cases remains an important tool.

Our study was heavily weighted by McMahon data, which were extracted from VAERS. It is a system of passive reporting and it was not designed for the establishment of cause and effect relationship. Some of its limitations are variability of data quality, underreporting, lacking of denominator information, and reporter bias. However, this system identifies adverse effects related to vaccines that must be further studied. Since there is a little amount of scientific literatures to establish or refute causal relationships for many adverse effects, VAERS is an important tool to be considered because it may highlight the red flags about vaccines [21].

Several MS cases have been reported around the time of vaccination, notably with hepatitis B [12, 13, 22]. The possible mechanisms involved include molecular mimicry between proteins of hepatitis B virus and myelin, the general immune stimulation by antigens or even toxic contaminants of the vaccine [22]. Among the myelin antigens, the major target of multiple sclerosis (MS) and experimental autoimmune encephalomyelitis (EAE) is the myelin basic protein (MBP). The humoral immunity against myelin oligodendrocyte glycoprotein (MOG) is related to myelin damage. The MBP and MOG share homologies with the antigen of hepatitis B, HBsAg. Using synthetized peptides that mimic MBP and MOG, Bogdanos et al. studied 234 serum samples and identified double reactivity between HBsAg and MOG after hepatitis B immunization. At 3 months postvaccination reactivity to at least one of the MOG mimics was present in 53% of the cases. The data suggest that HBsAg share important homologies with myelin antigens and that the antiviral response can induce cross-reactive anti-self immune responses that reduce after time. The author indicates that the tolerance mechanisms may be responsible for this decrease [23]. The number of cases reported following immunization against yellow fever is considerably lower compared to hepatitis B. However, among autoimmune events reported following yellow fever vaccine, myelin is the target in more than 80% of the cases described. Therefore, it is plausible that the mechanisms suggested for hepatitis B may also apply to the yellow fever vaccine.

In evaluating the studies, some limitations should be considered. Some studies have reported the specific type of yellow fever vaccine. However, since 1937, the 17D vaccine has been used. This can be derived from two different 17D substrains, DD-17 and D-17 204, which differ by the number of passages in murine tissues and chickens [8]. Despite the existence of two subtypes of the vaccine in addition to the original 17D vaccine, the absence of this information does not invalidate the studies presented.

The type of surveillance used in our study, often passive, underestimates the actual number of cases. Furthermore, different countries have different ways of collecting data and different methods of diagnosis, which may affect the outcome. In some cases included in this series of cases, there was no detailed information on the diagnostic procedures performed or the possible exclusion of other differential diagnoses.

The time between the onset of symptoms and the immunization can also interfere with the data analysis. Most of the studies regarding adverse events related to yellow fever vaccine consider a 30-day period for analysis. Autoimmune events may occur over periods longer than 30 days and are not considered related to the vaccine. The development of autoimmune events and autoimmune diseases is rare. Because they are nonspecific, they can be very difficult to be diagnosed. Thus, it is possible that there is a subnotification. On the other hand, symptoms caused by other variables, such as other virus infections or bad alimentation, must be interpreted as 17D adverse events if they occur within 30 days.

Many studies included in this series of cases describe adverse events after administering more than one vaccine at a time. In this situation, it is not possible to attribute the adverse effects solely to the vaccine against yellow fever. The case of multiple evanescent white dot syndrome (MEWDS) described by Stangos et al. occurred after simultaneous vaccination against hepatitis A and yellow fever [18]. However, a case of MEWDS has been reported by Fine in a male patient of 30 years, 13 days before vaccination against hepatitis A alone [24]. Thus, there is no way to exclude the participation of any of the vaccines. The disease may have developed by chance or was caused by one or both vaccines. Perumalswami and colleagues also describe autoimmune hepatitis in this case after simultaneous vaccination against hepatitis A and yellow fever [16].

There is no description of synergism between vaccines in the induction or promotion of self-reactive events. Vaccination against multiple agents has been reported to be well tolerated but should be avoided in those more susceptible to autoimmune events (e.g., those with a family history or previous occurrence of other autoimmune diseases) [16].

Exacerbation of preexisting autoimmune diseases was not identified in this series of cases. Our group identified 70 patients with rheumatic diseases who were inadvertently vaccinated against yellow fever [25]. In this study, only mild adverse effects were observed (mild skin rash, headache, myalgia, and transient elevation of liver enzymes) at a frequency similar to that reported in the population without a diagnosis of autoimmune diseases. Among patients evaluated by Mota et al., there were cases of rheumatoid arthritis, systemic lupus erythematosus, systemic sclerosis, and spondyloarthritis, and no cases of reactivation or flare of the underlying disease in the immediate period after the yellow fever vaccination were observed. The lack of studies evaluating the activity of autoimmune diseases is due to the inability to perform controlled studies due to increased risk of YEL-AVD in this group of individuals. Because the vaccine is made from the live virus, it is contraindicated in immunocompromised individuals [8, 9, 26].

The use of adjuvants in vaccines was also related to the appearance of autoantibodies and constitutional symptoms [27, 28]. The antiphospholipid syndrome can be induced by tetanus vaccine in murines [29]. Anticardiolipin autoantibodies can be elevated after influenza immunization in patients with lupus [30]. The adjuvant's use in the manufacture of vaccines increases the immune response and its duration against the antigen, promoting physical protection against the pathogen and facilitating its translocation to lymph nodes [27]. In 2001, Schoenfeld and Agmon-Levin described a syndrome known as autoimmune/inflammatory syndrome induced by adjuvants (ASIA). This syndrome includes 4 conditions with common features and exposure to a component with adjuvant effect: macrophagic myofasciitis syndrome, Gulf War syndrome, Siliconosis, and the adjuvant disease. Some criteria were suggested. The major criteria are exposure to an external stimuli, typical clinical manifestations (myalgia, myositis, muscle weakness, arthralgia/arthritis, chronic fatigue, sleep disturbances, neurological manifestations, cognitive impairment, memory loss, and pyrexia), improvement while removing the agent, and typical biopsy. The minor criteria are the appearance of antibodies or autoantibodies related to the suspected adjuvant, other clinical manifestations, specific HLA, and evolvement of autoimmune disease [27]. The syndrome is very rare although the exposure to antigens is very common, which suggests other risk factors such as genetic features or coexposure [31].

Although the 17D yellow fever vaccine has its limitations, such as the risk for immunocompromised persons, it is the safest and most effective arboviral vaccine [32]. The development of an inactivated vaccine would be a solution for the immunosuppressed ones. The virus inactivation made by pressure could reduce the use of external agents. Thus, the yellow fever vaccine could be more secure [32]. However, killed vaccines may have disadvantages as risk of incomplete inactivation, change in immunogenic properties of the virus, and the use of multiple doses [32, 33].

Among the abstracts selected for reading, there was greater interest in the occurrence of YEL-AVD; 27 cases were identified in all. It is believed that the occurrence of serious adverse effects is related to the host. Therefore, it is possible that autoimmune phenomena may be related to host characteristics as well [34, 35].

5. Conclusion

Although we have to consider the limitations of the data presented, due to the scarcity of information on the subject and quality of available studies, this is the first systematic review to evaluate events specifically related to autoimmunity developing after vaccination against yellow fever.

While it is plausible to consider the possibility of autoimmune events after yellow fever vaccine, considering the massive coverage in endemic regions, a systematic review of the literature reveals that there are few reports of such autoimmunity. The data set found may suggest that the increase in risk of autoimmunity when the yellow fever vaccine is applied is unlikely.

Abbreviations

WHO: World Health Organization
YEL-AVD: Yellow fever vaccine associated viscerotropic disease
YEL-AND: Yellow fever vaccine associated neurotropic disease
ADEM: Acute disseminated encephalomyelitis
MEWDS: Multiple evanescent white dot syndrome
GBS: Guillain-Barré syndrome.

Conflict of Interests

The authors declare that there is no conflict of interests regarding the publication of this paper.

References

[1] C. L. Gardner and K. D. Ryman, "Yellow fever: a reemerging threat," *Clinics in Laboratory Medicine*, vol. 30, no. 1, pp. 237–260, 2010.

[2] P. F. Vasconcelos, "Yellow fever," *Revista da Sociedade Brasileira de Medicina Tropical*, vol. 36, no. 2, pp. 275–293, 2003.

[3] J. E. Staples and T. P. Monath, "Yellow fever: 100 Years of discovery," *Journal of the American Medical Association*, vol. 300, no. 8, pp. 960–962, 2008.

[4] W. H. Organization, Yellow fever, Fact Sheet no. 100, 2011, http://www.who.int/mediacentre/factsheets/fs100/en/.

[5] A. C. Lopes, *Tratado de Clínica Médica*, 2nd edition, 2009.

[6] C. Domingo and M. Niedrig, "Safety of 17D derived yellow fever vaccines," *Expert Opinion on Drug Safety*, vol. 8, no. 2, pp. 211–221, 2009.

[7] E. D. Barnett, "Yellow fever: epidemiology and prevention," *Clinical Infectious Diseases*, vol. 44, no. 6, pp. 850–856, 2007.

[8] A. D. Barrett and D. E. Teuwen, "Yellow fever vaccine-how does it work and why do rare cases of serious adverse events take place?" *Current Opinion in Immunology*, vol. 21, no. 3, pp. 308–313, 2009.

[9] E. B. Hayes, "Is it time for a new yellow fever vaccine?" *Vaccine*, vol. 28, no. 51, pp. 8073–8076, 2010.

[10] M. P. Grobusch, A. Goorhuis, R. W. Wieten et al., "Yellow fever revaccination guidelines change—a decision too feverish?" *Clinical Microbiology and Infection*, vol. 19, no. 10, pp. 885–886, 2013.

[11] A. W. McMahon, R. B. Eidex, A. A. Marfin et al., "Neurologic disease associated with 17D-204 yellow fever vaccination: a report of 15 cases," *Vaccine*, vol. 25, no. 10, pp. 1727–1734, 2007.

[12] M. Tishler and Y. Shoenfeld, "Vaccination may be associated with autoimmune diseases," *The Israel Medical Association Journal*, vol. 6, no. 7, pp. 430–432, 2004.

[13] H. Orbach, N. Agmon-Levin, and G. Zandman-Goddard, "Vaccines and autoimmune diseases of the adult," *Discovery Medicine*, vol. 9, no. 45, pp. 90–97, 2010.

[14] P. Santaguida and P. Raina, "McMaster Quality Assessment Scale of Harms (McHarm) for primary studies," http://hiru.mcmaster.ca/epc/mcharm.pdf.

[15] H. Miller, W. Cendrowski, and K. Shapira, "Multiple sclerosis and vaccination," *British Medical Journal*, vol. 2, no. 546, pp. 210–213, 1967.

[16] P. Perumalswami, L. Peng, and J. A. Odin, "Vaccination as a triggering event for autoimmune hepatitis," *Seminars in Liver Disease*, vol. 29, no. 3, pp. 331–334, 2009.

[17] D. Schmöeller, M. W. Keiserman, H. L. Staub, F. P. Velho, and M. De Fátima Grohe, "Yellow fever vaccination and kawasaki disease," *Pediatric Infectious Disease Journal*, vol. 28, no. 11, pp. 1037–1038, 2009.

[18] A. Stangos, M. Zaninetti, I. Petropoulos, E. Baglivo, and C. Pournaras, "Multiple evanescent white dot syndrome following simultaneous hepatitis-A and yellow fever vaccination," *Ocular Immunology and Inflammation*, vol. 14, no. 5, pp. 301–304, 2006.

[19] C. Vital, A. Vital, G. Gbikpi-Benissan et al., "Postvaccinal inflammatory neuropathy: peripheral nerve biopsy in 3 cases," *Journal of the Peripheral Nervous System*, vol. 7, no. 3, pp. 163–167, 2002.

[20] C. Merlo, R. Steffen, T. Landis, T. Tsai, and N. Karabatsos, "Possible association of encephalitis and 17D yellow fever vaccination in a 29-year-old traveller," *Vaccine*, vol. 11, no. 6, p. 691, 1993.

[21] A. M. Loughlin, C. D. Marchant, W. Adams et al., "Causality assessment of adverse events reported to the vaccine adverse event reporting system (VAERS)," *Vaccine*, vol. 30, no. 50, pp. 7253–7259, 2012.

[22] O. Gout, "Vaccinations and multiple sclerosis," *Neurological Sciences*, vol. 22, no. 2, pp. 151–154, 2001.

[23] D. P. Bogdanos, H. Smith, Y. Ma, H. Baum, G. Mieli-Vergani, and D. Vergani, "A study of molecular mimicry and immunological cross-reactivity between hepatitis B surface antigen and myelin mimics," *Clinical and Developmental Immunology*, vol. 12, no. 3, pp. 217–224, 2005.

[24] L. Fine, A. Fine, and E. T. Cunningham Jr., "Multiple evanescent white dot syndrome following hepatitis A vaccination," *Archives of Ophthalmology*, vol. 119, no. 12, pp. 1856–1858, 2001.

[25] L. M. Mota, A. C. V. Oliveira, R. A. C. Lima, L. L. Dos Santos-Neto, and P. L. Tauil, "Vaccination against yellow fever among patients on immunosuppressors with diagnoses of rheumatic diseases," *Revista da Sociedade Brasileira de Medicina Tropical*, vol. 42, no. 1, pp. 23–27, 2009.

[26] M. Löbermann, D. Boršo, I. Hilgendorf, C. Fritzsche, U. K. Zettl, and E. C. Reisinger, "Immunization in the adult immunocompromised host," *Autoimmunity Reviews*, vol. 11, no. 3, pp. 212–218, 2012.

[27] Y. Shoenfeld and N. Agmon-Levin, ""ASIA"—autoimmune/inflammatory syndrome induced by adjuvants," *Journal of Autoimmunity*, vol. 36, no. 1, pp. 4–8, 2011.

[28] A. Lerner, "Aluminum as an adjuvant in Crohn's disease induction," *Lupus*, vol. 21, no. 2, pp. 231–238, 2012.

[29] L. Dimitrijević, I. Živković, M. Stojanović, V. Petrušić, and S. Živančević-Simonović, "Vaccine model of antiphospholipid syndrome induced by tetanus vaccine," *Lupus*, vol. 21, no. 2, pp. 195–202, 2012.

[30] E. S. Vista, S. R. Crowe, L. F. Thompson et al., "Influenza vaccination can induce new-onset anticardiolipins but not $\beta 2$-glycoprotein-I antibodies among patients with systemic lupus erythematosus," *Lupus*, vol. 21, no. 2, pp. 168–174, 2012.

[31] N. Agmon-Levin, G. Hughes, and Y. Shoenfeld, "The spectrum of ASIA: 'autoimmune (auto-inflammatory) syndrome induced by adjuvants'," *Lupus*, vol. 21, no. 2, pp. 118–120, 2012.

[32] L. P. Gaspar, Y. S. Mendes, A. M. Y. Yamamura et al., "Pressure-inactivated yellow fever 17DD virus: implications for vaccine development," *Journal of Virological Methods*, vol. 150, no. 1-2, pp. 57–62, 2008.

[33] T. P. Monath, E. Fowler, C. T. Johnson et al., "An inactivated cell-culture vaccine against yellow fever," *The New England Journal of Medicine*, vol. 364, no. 14, pp. 1326–1333, 2011.

[34] M. L. Silva, L. R. Espírito-Santo, M. A. Martins et al., "Clinical and immunological insights on severe, adverse neurotropic and viscerotropic disease following 17D yellow fever vaccination," *Clinical and Vaccine Immunology*, vol. 17, no. 1, pp. 118–126, 2010.

[35] C. Vellozzi, T. Mitchell, E. Miller et al., "Yellow fever vaccine-associated viscerotropic disease (YEL-AVD) and corticosteroid therapy: eleven United States cases, 1996–2004," *The American Journal of Tropical Medicine and Hygiene*, vol. 75, no. 2, pp. 333–336, 2006.

13

Evaluation of SLE Susceptibility Genes in Malaysians

Julio E. Molineros,[1] Kek Heng Chua,[2] Celi Sun,[1] Lay Hoong Lian,[3] Prasenjeet Motghare,[1] Xana Kim-Howard,[1] and Swapan K. Nath[1]

[1] *Arthritis and Clinical Immunology Research Program, Oklahoma Medical Research Foundation, 1025 NE 13th Street, Oklahoma City, OK 73104, USA*
[2] *Department of Biomedical Science, Faculty of Medicine, University of Malaya, 50603 Kuala Lumpur, Malaysia*
[3] *Department of Molecular Medicine, Faculty of Medicine, University of Malaya, 50603 Kuala Lumpur, Malaysia*

Correspondence should be addressed to Swapan K. Nath; swapan-nath@omrf.org

Academic Editor: Juan-Manuel Anaya

Systemic Lupus Erythematosus (SLE) is a clinically heterogeneous autoimmune disease with strong genetic and environmental components. Our objective was to replicate 25 recently identified SLE susceptibility genes in two distinct populations (Chinese (CH) and Malays (MA)) from Malaysia. We genotyped 347 SLE cases and 356 controls (CH and MA) using the ImmunoChip array and performed an admixture corrected case-control association analysis. Associated genes were grouped into five immune-related pathways. While CH were largely homogenous, MA had three ancestry components (average 82.3% Asian, 14.5% European, and 3.2% African). Ancestry proportions were significantly different between cases and controls in MA. We identified 22 genes with at least one associated SNP ($P < 0.05$). The strongest signal was at HLA-DRA ($P_{\text{Meta}} = 9.96 \times 10^{-9}$; $P_{\text{CH}} = 6.57 \times 10^{-8}$, $P_{\text{MA}} = 6.73 \times 10^{-3}$); the strongest non-HLA signal occurred at *STAT4* ($P_{\text{Meta}} = 1.67 \times 10^{-7}$; $P_{\text{CH}} = 2.88 \times 10^{-6}$, $P_{\text{MA}} = 2.99 \times 10^{-3}$). Most of these genes were associated with B- and T-cell function and signaling pathways. Our exploratory study using high-density fine-mapping suggests that most of the established SLE genes are also associated in the major ethnicities of Malaysia. However, these novel SNPs showed stronger association in these Asian populations than with the SNPs reported in previous studies.

1. Introduction

Systemic Lupus Erythematosus (SLE) is a heterogeneous autoimmune disease, in terms of both clinical presentation and incidence and severity across ethnically diverse populations. Asians are among those with a greater risk of SLE and have more severe disease presentations such as lupus nephritis [1]. SLE has strong and complex genetic components. While several genomewide association studies (GWAS) have been reported for European SLE populations, few Asian GWAS have been performed [2–4]. Among European identified SLE loci were HLA loci *HLA-DRA* [5] and *ATG5* [5], immune signal transduction loci *BANK1* [6], *BLK* [5], *LYN* [5], TLR, and IFN pathway related loci *IFIH1* [7], *STAT4* [8], *TNFAIP3* [9], *IRF7* [5], *IRF8* [7], as well as *NCF2* [7], *IL10* [10], *PHRF1* [5], *CD44* [11], *ICAM1_ICAM4* [7], *TYK2* [7], and *UBE2L3* [5]. Loci identified through Asian GWAS include *ETS1* [12], *SLC15A4* [12], *IKZF1* [12], *RASGRP3* [12], *TNFSF4* [12], and *TNIP1* [10].

Malaysia has a population of around 28 million with three major ethnic groups (Malays (60.3%), Chinese (22.9%), and Indians (7.1%)). SLE patients and controls from Malaysia offer a unique opportunity to explore the effect of different ancestral backgrounds [13] on SLE genetic architecture. We explored association of SLE-associated loci identified through GWAS in two majority populations, Chinese and Malays. Given that these cohorts may be admixed, we expect that ancestry proportion may influence SLE association. Although previous studies [13–18] reported genetic associations with some candidate genes in Malaysians. To our knowledge, this is the first study which assessed SLE susceptibility genes using large scale targeted fine-mapping on Malaysian populations.

Our objective was to replicate and fine-map genetic association in 25 previously reported SLE susceptibility loci and to assess population structure and individuals admixture in the two ethnically distinct Malaysian cohorts.

2. Materials and Methods

2.1. Subjects and Genotyping. We genotyped 347 cases and 356 controls from the two major Malaysian ethnic groups (Malays (MA) and Chinese (CH)) using the Illumina custom designed ImmunoChip array [19] as part of a separate ongoing genetic association project. The ImmunoChip is a dense fine-mapping genotype array that contains ~196,000 SNPs from 184 genes associated with at least one of 12 autoimmune diseases, including SLE. Genotyping was conducted through the Genotyping Core Facility of the Oklahoma Medical Research Foundation (OMRF), Oklahoma City, USA. Subjects were recruited in compliance with the Internal Review Boards of OMRF and the University of Malaya Medical Centre. All SLE cases fulfilled the ACR criteria for SLE classification [20, 21]. Controls were matched by ethnicity and gender. Our CH cohort included 288 cases and 292 controls (187 males and 393 females); MA included 59 cases and 64 controls (48 males and 75 females) (Supplementary Table 1 in Supplementary Material available online at http://dx.doi.org/10.1155/2014/305436).

2.2. Quality Control. Individuals were removed from analysis if they were genetically related to other study subjects ($r > 0.25$), as estimated through the relatedness coefficient implemented in GCTA, or if they were outliers (mean ± 2 standard deviations) determined by principal component analysis. SNPs were excluded according to the following criteria: poor genotyping clustering, missing genotype rate greater than 90%, Hardy-Weinberg disequilibrium $P < 0.001$ in controls, or minor allele frequency below 0.5% (Supplementary Figure 1). SNP positions were aligned with HG19. The analysis set contained 6,991 SNPs from 25 previously reported genes genotyped on 580 CH and 123 MA unrelated individuals.

2.3. Population Structure. In order to estimate population structure of our cohorts, we selected 14,134 SNPs with very low intermarker linkage disequilibrium (LD, $r^2 < 0.2$). This SNP set was enriched by variants with pairwise allele frequency difference >20%. We merged our cohorts with individuals from the 1000 Genomes Project (103 CEU, 100 CHB + 100 JPT, and 101 YRI). We estimated the first ten principal components using GCTA [22], as well as the mean and standard deviation for the first three principal components within each cohort (Figure 1). The same dataset was used to estimate individual admixture proportions in ADMIXTURE [23]. We estimated models of admixture using 1 to 7 ancestry components and determined the optimal admixture model by minimizing the cross-validation error using the Bayesian information criterion and the Akaike information criterion. Mean ancestry between cases and controls was compared with a two-tailed t-test.

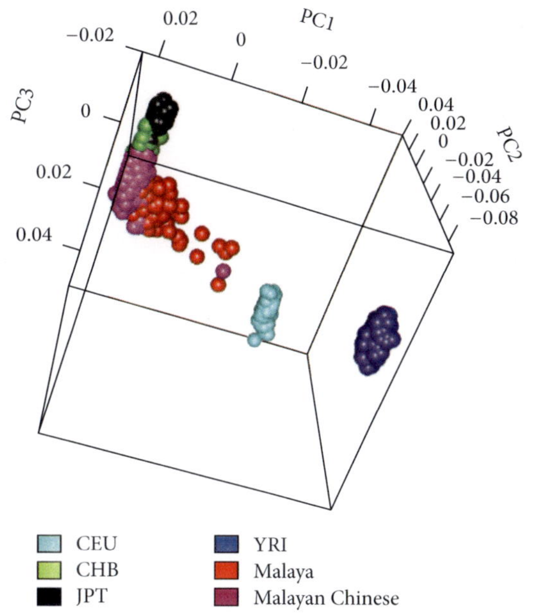

Figure 1: Principal components analysis of Chinese and Malay cohorts. Notably the Malaysian Chinese were a more homogeneous population than the Malays (CEU: North Europeans from CEPH; CHB: Beijing Chinese; JPT: Japanese; YRI: Yorubans from Nigeria).

2.4. Association Analysis. We performed individual SNP case-control association analysis using a chi-square statistic in PLINK [24]. Given the sample size of our cohorts and that this is a replication study, association was considered significant if $P < 0.05$ (alpha = 0.05). We guarded against type 1 error by performing permutation tests (100,000 permutations). Possible influence of admixture was corrected using a logistic regression model in PLINK [24] with the Asian ancestry proportion as a covariate. We used meta-analysis (Fisher's combined P value, four degrees of freedom) to combine association P values from both cohorts. For SNPs which were not significant in either cohort or when odds ratios were not in the same direction, no P_{Meta} was calculated. All associated SNPs passed the permutation test (results not shown).

The best SNP was selected for each region starting with the most significant combined P. We performed epistasis analysis using PLINK [24] and GAIA [25] in order to identify possible gene-gene interactions. We performed a conditional analysis using a logistic regression model (PLINK) for all significant SNPs from *STAT4* and *HLA-DRA* regions. We used the strongest associated SNP from each loci as the initial conditioned SNP to identify additional independent variants.

In order to check for additional sources of stratification, we used mixed models as implemented on EMMAX [26] (Supplementary Table 2).

RegulomeDB [27] and HaploReg [28] were used to identify functional elements overlapping with the selected SNPs.

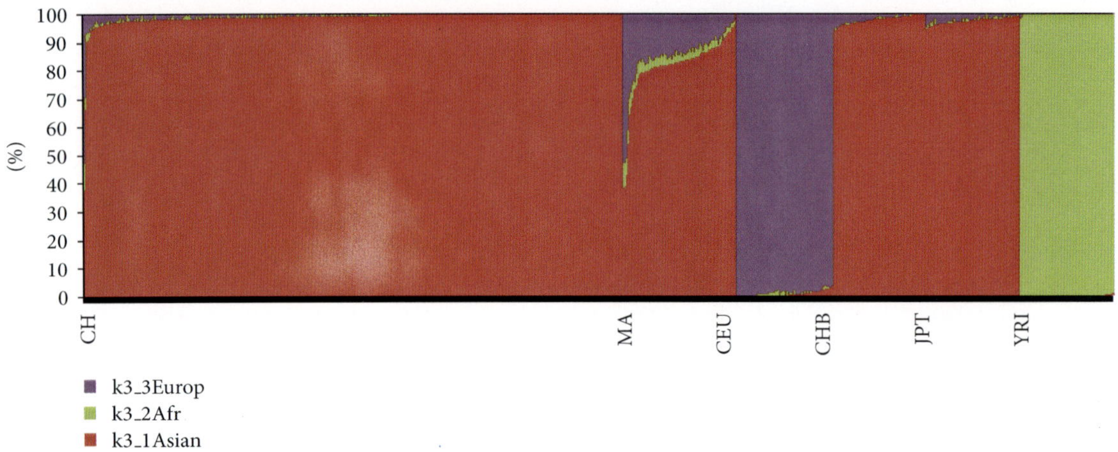

FIGURE 2: Admixture proportions of Chinese and Malays. Malaysian Chinese had less evidence of admixture from Europeans and Africans than Malaysian Malays (CH: Malaysian Chinese; MA: Malaysian Malays; CEU: North Europeans from CEPH; CHB: Beijing Chinese; JPT: Japanese; YRI: Yorubans from Nigeria).

2.5. Pathway Analysis. We chose to study five main pathways which contained the majority of the 25 target genes. All of these pathways are reported to be involved in SLE pathogenesis [29]. In order to determine if there were overrepresented pathways in these two cohorts we performed a gene set enrichment analysis (GSEA) weighted by the strength of the meta-analysis association using i-GSEA4GWAS [30]. The objective of this mode of GSEA was to identify the possible biological mechanisms that involve associated loci, and to identify candidate causal SNPs that affect the normal function in these pathways. Since we used a small set of loci we looked for pathways that contained at least two reported genes.

2.6. Power Analysis. We estimated the required sample size for detection of additional association signals in our cohorts using the method developed by Hoggart et al. [31] for alpha = 0.05. This method takes into account the effect of admixture on the probability of identifying an associated variant in a mixed population. The parameters included populations with similar characteristics as CH and MA (admixture proportions of 10% for CH and 20% for MA) and a power of detection of 80%.

3. Results

3.1. Population Structure. Based on the proportions of the 1000 Genomes Project populations we estimated optimal population structure for Asian, African, and European ancestries. CH were very homogenous compared to the MA. As expected, mean Asian ancestral proportion was the highest in both populations ($ASN_{CH} = 99.0 \pm 3.2$; $ASN_{MA} = 82.3 \pm 10.6$), followed by European ancestry ($EUR_{CH} = 0.7 \pm 2.7$; $EUR_{MA} = 14.5 \pm 9.4$) and then African ancestry ($AFR_{CH} = 0.3 \pm 0.7$; $AFR_{MA} = 3.2 \pm 1.6$) (Figure 2). There was a significant mean ancestry difference between cases and controls in MA (case/control: 84.5/80.3: $P_{ASN} = 0.02$; 3/3.3: 12.5/16.4: $P_{AFR} = 0.27$; $P_{EUR} = 0.02$) but not in CH.

3.2. Association Analysis. We identified associated SNPs in 20 previously reported genes in either cohort. However, not all associated SNPs were significant in both cohorts. In CH published non-HLA loci SNPs showed significant association with SLE (Supplementary Table 3), including *ETS1* (rs1128334, $P_{CH} = 2.4 \times 10^{-3}$), *IRF8* (rs2280381, $P_{CH} = 1.38 \times 10^{-2}$), *TNFAIP3* (rs5029939, $P_{CH} = 1.62 \times 10^{-2}$), *STAT4* (rs3821236, $P_{CH} = 1.86 \times 10^{-2}$), and *RASGRP3* (rs13385731, $P_{CH} = 3.63 \times 10^{-2}$). In MA, *IKZF1* (rs4917014, $P_{MA} = 1.06 \times 10^{-2}$), *RASGRP3* (rs13385731, $P_{MA} = 2.14 \times 10^{-2}$), *KIAA1542* (rs4963128, $P_{MA} = 2.25 \times 10^{-2}$), *TNIP1* (rs10036748, $P_{MA} = 2.55 \times 10^{-2}$), and *IL21R* (rs3093301, $P_{MA} = 3.28 \times 10^{-2}$) were significantly associated with SLE. For the HLA locus, we replicated association for rs9271366 (*HLA-DRB1_HLA-DQA1* $P_{Meta} = 1.33 \times 10^{-6}$, $P_{CH} = 2.62 \times 10^{-6}$; $P_{MA} = 2.92 \times 10^{-2}$), consistent with the previous report on Malays and Chinese [13].

For all genes SNPs with the strongest association in this study differed from those previously reported. We identified 22 previously reported genes with at least one associated variant; the most significantly associated SNP for each gene was based on Fisher's combined *P* value. The strongest association was in the HLA region in the vicinity of *HLA-DRA* (rs6911777, $P_{Meta} = 9.96 \times 10^{-9}$, $P_{CH} = 6.58 \times 10^{-8}$, and $P_{MA} = 6.73 \times 10^{-3}$). The strongest non-HLA association was observed at *STAT4* (rs7568275, $P_{Meta} = 1.68 \times 10^{-7}$, $P_{CH} = 2.88 \times 10^{-6}$, and $P_{MA} = 2.99 \times 10^{-3}$). Also Asian identified *TNFSF4* (rs10798269, $P_{Meta} = 5.98 \times 10^{-3}$, $P_{CH} = 3.87 \times 10^{-2}$, and $P_{MA} = 1.88 \times 10^{-2}$) and *SLC15A4* (rs6486738, $P_{Meta} = 4.88 \times 10^{-2}$, $P_{CH} = 0.122$, and $P_{MA} = 6.9 \times 10^{-2}$) were replicated. We identified variants in LD with published variants *RASGRP3* (rs13425999, $r^2 = 0.95$, $P_{Meta} = 6.82 \times 10^{-3}$, $P_{CH} = 3.30 \times 10^{-2}$, and $P_{MA} = 2.79 \times 10^{-2}$), *TNIP1* (rs3792782,

Table 1: SLE susceptibility genes in Malay (MA) and Chinese (CH).

Gene	Cytogenetic band	SNP	Base position	A1/A2	Chinese				Malay				Meta-analysis P value*
					F_A	F_U	P value	OR 95% CI	F_A	F_U	P value	OR 95% CI	
TNFSF4-LOC730070	1q25	rs10798269	173,309,713	A/G	0.342	0.401	3.87×10^{-2}	0.78 (0.61–0.99)	0.314	0.460	1.88×10^{-2}	0.54 (0.32–0.9)	5.98×10^{-3}
NCF2	1q25	rs13306575	183,532,437	T/C	0.080	0.043	8.11×10^{-3}	1.95 (1.18–3.22)	0.119	0.070	1.93×10^{-1}	1.78 (0.74–4.28)	1.17×10^{-2}
MAPKAPK2-IL10	1q31-32	rs2232360	207,040,659	A/G	0.328	0.351	3.98×10^{-1}	0.9 (0.71–1.15)	0.576	0.397	5.06×10^{-3}	2.07 (1.24–3.45)	—
RASGRP3	2p25.1-24.1	rs13425999	33,702,203	T/C	0.129	0.174	3.03×10^{-2}	0.7 (0.51–0.97)	0.102	0.203	2.79×10^{-2}	0.44 (0.21–0.93)	6.82×10^{-3}
IFIH1	2q24	rs13023380	163,154,363	A/G	0.010	0.002	5.56×10^{-2}	6.14 (0.74–51.13)	0.025	0.103	1.42×10^{-2}	0.23 (0.06–0.82)	—
STAT4	2q32.2-32.3	rs7568275	191,966,452	G/C	0.453	0.317	2.88×10^{-6}	1.78 (1.4–2.27)	0.422	0.236	2.99×10^{-3}	2.36 (1.33–4.19)	1.68×10^{-7}
BANK1	4q24	rs17031870	102,940,788	G/A	0.092	0.058	2.89×10^{-2}	1.64 (1.05–2.56)	0.237	0.143	5.95×10^{-2}	1.87 (0.97–3.59)	1.26×10^{-2}
TNIP1	5q32-33.1	rs3792782	150,456,677	C/T	0.214	0.247	1.81×10^{-1}	0.83 (0.63–1.09)	0.305	0.453	1.70×10^{-2}	0.53 (0.31–0.89)	2.09×10^{-2}
HLA-DRA	6p21.3	rs6911777	32,409,996	C/T	0.264	0.137	6.57×10^{-8}	2.26 (1.67–3.05)	0.161	0.055	6.73×10^{-3}	3.32 (1.34–8.21)	9.96×10^{-9}
PRDM1-ATG5	6q21	rs9398065	106,546,034	C/G	0.075	0.039	9.52×10^{-3}	1.97 (1.17–3.31)	0.119	0.039	1.95×10^{-2}	3.31 (1.15–9.5)	1.78×10^{-3}
TNFAIP3	6q23	rs5029928	138,189,942	T/C	0.083	0.046	1.02×10^{-2}	1.88 (1.15–3.05)	0.059	0.031	2.87×10^{-1}	1.96 (0.56–6.86)	2.00×10^{-2}
C7orf721-IKZF1	7p13-11.1	rs11185603	50,306,810	G/C	0.236	0.282	7.61×10^{-2}	0.79 (0.61–1.03)	0.144	0.302	3.25×10^{-3}	0.39 (0.21–0.74)	2.30×10^{-3}
BLK	8p23-22	rs11782375	11,294,934	C/T	0.277	0.380	1.88×10^{-4}	0.62 (0.49–0.8)	0.297	0.375	1.94×10^{-1}	0.7 (0.41–1.2)	4.09×10^{-4}
LYN	8q13	rs7828258	56,867,945	T/C	0.223	0.242	4.38×10^{-1}	0.9 (0.68–1.18)	0.136	0.281	5.18×10^{-3}	0.4 (0.21–0.77)	1.61×10^{-2}
KIAA1542-PHRF1	11p15.5	rs4963128	589,564	T/C	0.083	0.070	4.01×10^{-1}	1.2 (0.78–1.86)	0.059	0.156	1.51×10^{-2}	0.34 (0.14–0.84)	—
IRF7	11p15.5	rs7943546	612,148	C/T	0.024	0.033	3.99×10^{-1}	0.74 (0.37–1.49)	0.025	0.055	2.46×10^{-1}	0.45 (0.11–1.79)	3.26×10^{-1}
PDHX-CD44	11p13	rs12362140	35,142,019	A/C	0.007	0.027	7.46×10^{-3}	0.25 (0.08–0.75)	0.085	0.148	1.22×10^{-1}	0.53 (0.24–1.2)	7.27×10^{-3}
ETS1	11q23.3	rs76404385	128,333,055	T/C	0.202	0.138	3.41×10^{-3}	1.59 (1.16–2.17)	0.178	0.063	5.02×10^{-3}	3.25 (1.38–7.65)	2.05×10^{-4}
SLC15A4	12q24.32	rs6486738	129,432,715	G/C	0.295	0.337	1.22×10^{-1}	0.82 (0.64–1.05)	0.203	0.305	6.90×10^{-2}	0.58 (0.32–1.05)	4.88×10^{-2}
IL21R	16p11	rs8060368	27,412,414	T/C	0.012	0.039	3.59×10^{-3}	0.3 (0.13–0.71)	0.170	0.109	1.72×10^{-1}	1.66 (0.8–3.46)	—
ITGAM	16p11.2	rs12444713	31,378,235	A/G	0.284	0.369	2.48×10^{-3}	0.68 (0.53–0.87)	0.5	0.52	7.10×10^{-1}	1.1 (0.67–1.82)	—
ORF8-LOC100131952	16q24.1	rs34912238	86,001,903	T/C	0.039	0.077	6.25×10^{-3}	0.49 (0.29–0.82)	0.076	0.031	1.15×10^{-1}	2.56 (0.77–8.55)	—
ICAM1-ICAM4	19p13.2	rs5498	10,395,683	G/A	0.250	0.267	5.06×10^{-1}	0.91 (0.7–1.19)	0.314	0.242	2.11×10^{-1}	1.43 (0.82–2.51)	—
TYK2	19p13.2	rs12975591	10,627,814	G/A	0.415	0.454	1.84×10^{-1}	0.85 (0.67–1.08)	0.232	0.121	2.62×10^{-2}	2.19 (1.09–4.41)	—
UBE2L3	22q11.21	rs2236642	21,989,621	T/C	0.089	0.127	3.61×10^{-2}	0.67 (0.46–0.98)	0.144	0.172	5.51×10^{-1}	0.81 (0.41–1.62)	9.77×10^{-2}

*When ORs from CH and MA are in different directions, we did not perform the meta-analysis.
— indicated SNPs where no meta-analysis was performed.
OR: odds ratio. Minor allele frequencies are given for the minor allele A1. F_A: minor allele frequency for cases; F_U: minor allele frequency for controls.

$r^2 = 0.74$, $P_{Meta} = 2.09 \times 10^{-2}$, $P_{CH} = 0.181$, and $P_{MA} = 1.7 \times 10^{-2}$), *C7orf72-IKZF1* (rs11185603, $r^2 = 1$, $P_{Meta} = 2.3 \times 10^{-3}$, $P_{CH} = 7.61 \times 10^{-2}$, and $P_{MA} = 3.25 \times 10^{-3}$). Even though these variants have a stronger association signal, they can be explained by their published counterparts.

We also identified a variant in *ETS1* (rs76404385, $P_{Meta} = 2.05 \times 10^{-4}$, $P_{CH} = 3.41 \times 10^{-3}$, and $P_{MA} = 5.02 \times 10^{-3}$) that was completely independent of published variant (rs1128334 $r^2 = 0$). European GWAS identified loci *IL10* (rs2232360, $P_{CH} = 0.398$, and $P_{MA} = 5.06 \times 10^{-3}$), *BANK1* (rs17031870, $P_{Meta} = 1.26\times10^{-2}$, $P_{CH} = 2.89\times10^{-2}$, and $P_{MA} = 5.95\times10^{-2}$), *PRDM1-ATG5* (rs9398065, $P_{Meta} = 1.78 \times 10^{-3}$, $P_{CH} = 9.52 \times 10^{-3}$, and $P_{MA} = 1.95 \times 10^{-2}$), *BLK-FAM167A* (rs11782375, $P_{Meta} = 4.09 \times 10^{-4}$, $P_{CH} = 1.88 \times 10^{-4}$, and $P_{MA} = 0.194$), *LYN* (rs7828258, $P_{Meta} = 1.61 \times 10^{-2}$, $P_{CH} = 4.38 \times 10^{-1}$, and $P_{MA} = 5.18 \times 10^{-3}$), *PDHX-CD44* (rs12362140, $P_{Meta} = 7.27 \times 10^{-3}$, $P_{CH} = 7.46 \times 10^{-3}$, and $P_{MA} = 0.122$), *ITGAM* (rs12444713, $P_{CH} = 2.48 \times 10^{-3}$, and $P_{MA} = 0.71$), *NCF2* (rs13306575, $P_{Meta} = 1.17 \times 10^{-2}$, $P_{CH} = 8.11 \times 10^{-3}$, and $P_{MA} = 0.193$), *IFIH1* (rs13023380, $P_{CH} = 5.56 \times 10^{-2}$, and $P_{MA} = 1.42 \times 10^{-2}$), *TNFAIP3* (rs5029928, $P_{Meta} = 2 \times 10^{-2}$, $P_{CH} = 1.02 \times 10^{-2}$, and $P_{MA} = 0.287$), *PHRF1* (rs4963128, $P_{CH} = 0.4$, and $P_{MA} = 1.51 \times 10^{-2}$), *IL21R* (rs8060368, $P_{CH} = 3.59 \times 10^{-3}$, $P_{MA} = 0.172$), *IRF8* (rs34912238, $P_{CH} = 6.25 \times 10^{-3}$, and $P_{MA} = 0.115$), and *ICAM1-ICAM4-TYK2* region (rs12975591, $P_{CH} = 0.184$, and $P_{MA} = 3.06 \times 10^{-2}$) also had a strong combined association with SLE (Table 1).

Notably, the scales of the odds ratio for rs7568275 (*STAT4*: $OR_{CH} = 1.78$, $OR_{MA} = 2.36$), rs9398065 (*PRDM1-ATG5*: $OR_{CH} = 1.97$, $OR_{MA} = 3.31$), rs5029928 (*TNFAIP3*: $OR_{CH} = 1.88$, $OR_{MA} = 1.96$), and rs76404385 (*ETS1*: $OR_{CH} = 1.59$, $OR_{MA} = 3.25$) were very close to *HLA-DRA* levels of OR (rs6911777 $OR_{CH} = 2.26$, $OR_{MA} = 3.32$).

Among the aforementioned 22 SNPs, we identified that rs11782375 (*FAM167A_BLK*) overlaps with an eQTL that potentially affects gene expression [32]. Additionally, rs13425999 (*RASGRP3*), rs5029928 (*TNFAIP3*), and rs11185603 (*IKZF1*) were identified as likely to affect binding by RegulomeDB [27]. These three SNPs contained enhancer and promoter histone marks in multiple cell types (in particular lymphoblastoid cell type GM12787) and also colocated with DNAse binding sites.

We used conditional analysis to identify multiple independent SNPs for each gene. In particular, *STAT4* had rs6740131 ($P_{CH} = 2.89 \times 10^{-4}$, $P_{CH} = 5.76 \times 10^{-3}$ after conditioning) as an additional independent SNP in CH. In the case of HLA, there were two additional independent SNPs in CH (rs2239806, $P_{CH} = 9.3 \times 10^{-5}$, and $P_{CH} = 2.47 \times 10^{-6}$ after conditioning and rs532098, $P_{CH} = 7.44 \times 10^{-5}$, and $P_{CH} = 7.05 \times 10^{-5}$ after conditioning).

3.3. Pathway Related Loci. We identified five important pathways involved in SLE pathogenesis which contained at least one of the 25 genes examined in our study. Both B- and T-cell function and signaling pathways had the greatest number of associated variants (Table 2). Neutrophil/monocyte function and signaling had four significantly associated SNPs, whereas TLR and type I IFN signaling pathways each included five genes with significantly associated SNPs. NFκB signaling also contained SNPs significantly associated with SLE. We did not observe any significantly associated SNPs in DNA degradation apoptosis and clearance of cellular debris pathways.

The only significantly enriched pathway was hsa04514 [cell adhesion molecules (CAMs)]. We derived four causal SNPs that potentially explain enrichment of this pathway, where rs2071554 (nonsynonymous, coding (deleterious) in *HLA-DOB*) and rs1129740 (nonsynonymous, coding in *HLA-DQA1*) are candidate causal SNPs through their RECEPTOR_ACTIVITY/TRANSMEMBRANE_RECEPTOR_ACTIVITY; rs8084 (essential splice site and intronic in *HLA-DQB*) and rs7192 (nonsynonymous, coding in *HLA-DRA*) were candidate causal SNPs through TRANSMEMBRANE_RECEPTOR_ACTIVITY.

3.4. Gene-Gene Interactions. We did not identify any gene-gene interaction between significant SNPs in either cohort.

3.5. Admixture Correction. We determined potential effects of admixture on associated variants within these pathways by adjusting case-control association analysis with admixture proportions. After admixture correction, only two MA SNPs were no longer significantly associated ($P > 0.05$). All CH SNPs passed the association threshold ($P < 0.05$).

4. Discussion

In this fine-mapping study we examined two understudied Malaysian populations to replicate previously known SLE genetic associations and to localize the most associated SNP within known SLE genes. Since SLE heterogeneity may be amplified in admixed populations, we adjusted association for admixture (Asian and European). We also categorized associated variants by pathways involvement and identified particular pathways with accumulation of reported associated variants in our Malaysian populations.

We found no effect of admixture on CH, which was not surprising since they are considered a homogenous population. In fact, the ancestry proportions of European and African were very small, and the minor allele frequencies for the top 25 genes were remarkably similar (Figure 3). Correlation between allele frequencies of CH versus CHB ($P = 0.94$) was higher than MA versus CHB ($P = 0.65$) further supporting our conclusion of the similarity between CH and CHB.

We replicated SLE association in *RASGP3* [12], *STAT4* [8], *TNIP1* [10], *IKZF1* [7], *IL21R* [33], *ETS1* [12], and *IRF8* [7]. It is not surprising that we did not identify more previously reported loci since the majority of loci were identified from studies of European and European American populations. Given the differences in LD structure between European and Asian populations, we identified new SNPs associated with SLE which could be either causal or in LD with the true causal SNPs within gene.

Associated variants were framed within their possible functional roles in immune-related pathways. The most

Table 2: Replicated genes and five immune-related pathways. Cells marked with an X represent presence of SNPs associated with SLE in those genes in either cohort. *Marks genes present in the pathway.

Gene	B-cell function and signaling	Neutrophil and monocyte function and signaling	NFκB signaling	T-cell function and signaling	TLR and type I IFN signaling
ATG5			*		
BANK1	X*				
BLK	X*				
CD44				X*	
ETS1	X*			X*	
HLA-DR2	X*			X*	
HLA-DR3	X*			X*	
ICAMs		X*			
IFIH1					X*
IKZF1	X*			X*	
IL10	X*	X*		X*	
IL21	X*			X*	
IRF7					*
IRF8	X*	X*			X*
ITGAM		X*			
LYN	X*				
NCF2	X*				
PHRF1					X*
PRDM1	X*			X*	X*
RASGRP3	X*				
SLC15A4			X*		
STAT4				X*	X*
TNFAIP3			X*		
TNFSF4				X*	
TNIP1			X*		
TYK2				*	
UBE2L3			*		
Total	13	4	3	10	5

important SLE-associated pathways in these populations were related to the B- and T-cell function and signaling pathways. We also introduced a causality model for gene set enrichment based on HLA SNPs in the cell adhesion molecules pathway (hsa04514). We identified four SNPs with potential functional effects through an eQTL and histone marks.

Although these results are encouraging, our study is limited due to the small sample size of our cohorts. Given the admixture proportions of these cohorts, we have estimated that we would require at least 1000 cases and controls to identify novel genomewide significant variants ($P < 5 \times 10^{-8}$) with moderate effects (OR > 1.5) for MA and almost double that for CH. Future large scale admixture mapping with the MA will be especially useful to identify novel SLE susceptibility genes. On the other hand, the CH population can be useful for straightforward association mapping for identifying novel genes or localizing the most likely causal variants.

In conclusion, our high-density fine-mapping on SLE targeted genes is one of the first such undertakings in Malaysian populations. Based on our rigorous analysis, we were able to replicate European and Asian SLE-associated loci in both Malaysian Malays and Malaysian Chinese and were able to identify additional variants that might serve as better tag SNPs for causal variants within these cohorts.

Conflict of Interests

The authors declare that there is no conflict of interests regarding the publication of this paper.

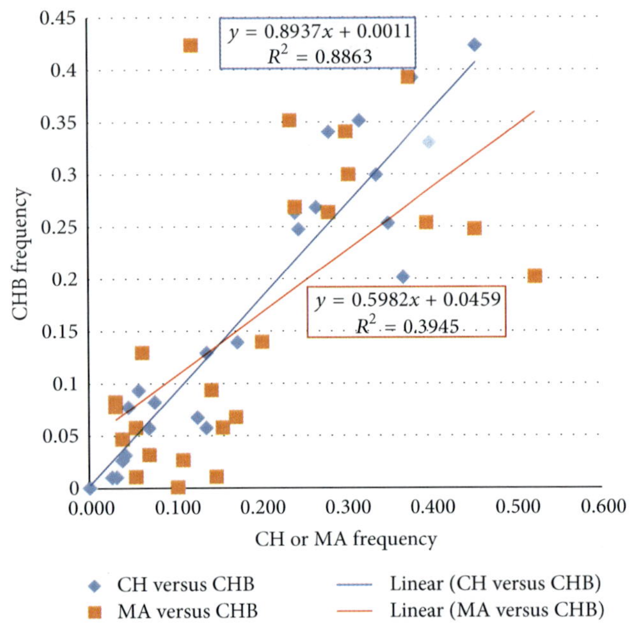

FIGURE 3: Comparison of allele frequencies of the top 25 SNPs from CH versus HapMap Chinese from Beijing (CHB) and MA versus CHB.

Acknowledgments

We are grateful to the affected and unaffected individuals who participated in this study. This work was supported by grants from the US National Institutes of Health (R01AR060366, R21AI094377, and R21AI103399).

References

[1] M. Y. Mok and W. L. Li, "Do Asian patients have worse lupus?" *Lupus*, vol. 19, no. 12, pp. 1384–1390, 2010.

[2] J. M. Kelley, J. C. Edberg, and R. P. Kimberly, "Pathways: strategies for susceptibility genes in SLE," *Autoimmunity Reviews*, vol. 9, no. 7, pp. 473–476, 2010.

[3] Y. Deng and B. P. Tsao, "Genetic susceptibility to systemic lupus erythematosus in the genomic era," *Nature Reviews Rheumatology*, vol. 6, no. 12, pp. 683–692, 2010.

[4] A. L. Sestak, B. G. Fürnrohr, J. B. Harley, J. T. Merrill, and B. Namjou, "The genetics of systemic lupus erythematosus and implications for targeted therapy," *Annals of the Rheumatic Diseases*, vol. 70, supplement 1, pp. i37–i43, 2011.

[5] J. B. Harley, M. E. Alarcón-Riquelme, L. A. Criswell et al., "Genome-wide association scan in women with systemic lupus erythematosus identifies susceptibility variants in ITGAM, PXK, KIAA1542 and other loci," *Nature Genetics*, vol. 40, no. 2, pp. 204–210, 2008.

[6] S. V. Kozyrev, A. Abelson, J. Wojcik et al., "Corrigendum: functional variants in the B-cell gene BANK1 are associated with systemic lupus erythematosus," *Nature Genetics*, vol. 40, pp. 211–216, 2008.

[7] D. S. C. Graham, D. L. Morris, T. R. Bhangale et al., "Association of NCF2, IKZF1, IRF8, IFIH1, and TYK2 with systemic lupus erythematosus," *PLoS Genetics*, vol. 7, no. 10, Article ID e1002341, 2011.

[8] E. F. Remmers, R. M. Plenge, A. T. Lee et al., "STAT4 and the risk of rheumatoid arthritis and systemic lupus erythematosus," *The New England Journal of Medicine*, vol. 357, no. 10, pp. 977–986, 2007.

[9] R. R. Graham, C. Cotsapas, L. Davies et al., "Genetic variants near TNFAIP3 on 6q23 are associated with systemic lupus erythematosus," *Nature Genetics*, vol. 40, no. 9, pp. 1059–1061, 2008.

[10] V. Gateva, J. K. Sandling, G. Hom et al., "A large-scale replication study identifies TNIP1, PRDM1, JAZF1, UHRF1BP1 and IL10 as risk loci for systemic lupus erythematosus," *Nature Genetics*, vol. 41, no. 11, pp. 1228–1233, 2009.

[11] C. J. Lessard, I. Adrianto, J. A. Kelly et al., "Identification of a systemic lupus erythematosus susceptibility locus at 11p13 between PDHX and CD44 in a multiethnic study," *American Journal of Human Genetics*, vol. 88, no. 1, pp. 83–91, 2011.

[12] J. W. Han, H. F. Zheng, Y. Cui et al., "Genome-wide association study in a Chinese Han population identifies nine new susceptibility loci for systemic lupus erythematosus," *Nature Genetics*, vol. 41, pp. 1234–1237, 2009.

[13] H. C. Chai, M. E. Phipps, I. Othman, L. P. Tan, and K. H. Chua, "HLA variants rs9271366 and rs9275328 are associated with systemic lupus erythematosus susceptibility in Malays and Chinese," *Lupus*, vol. 22, pp. 198–204, 2013.

[14] H. C. Chai, M. E. Phipps, and K. H. Chua, "Genetic risk factors of systemic lupus erythematosus in the malaysian population: a minireview," *Clinical and Developmental Immunology*, vol. 2012, Article ID 963730, 9 pages, 2012.

[15] K. Chua, T. Lau, Z. Tee, S. Tan, and L. Liana, "Genetic polymorphisms of the interleukin-1 beta (IL-1β) −511 and +3954 single nucleotide polymorphisms (SNPs) in Malaysian systemic lupus erythematosus (SLE) patients," *Journal of Health Science*, vol. 55, no. 4, pp. 657–662, 2009.

[16] M. R. Azizah, S. S. Ainol, S. H. Kuak, N. C. T. Kong, Y. Normaznah, and M. N. Rahim, "The association of the HLA class II antigens with clinical and autoantibody expression in Malaysian Chinese patients with systemic lupus erythematosus," *Asian Pacific Journal of Allergy and Immunology*, vol. 19, no. 2, pp. 93–100, 2001.

[17] M. R. Azizah, S. S. Ainol, N. C. Kong, Y. Normaznah, and M. N. Rahim, "HLA antigens in Malay patients with systemic lupus erythematosus: association with clinical and autoantibody expression," *The Korean Journal of Internal Medicine*, vol. 16, no. 2, pp. 123–131, 2001.

[18] M. R. Azizah, S. H. Kuak, S. S. Ainol, M. N. Rahim, Y. Normaznah, and K. Norella, "Association of the tumor necrosis factor alpha gene polymorphism with susceptibility and clinical-immunological findings of systemic lupus erythematosus," *Asian Pacific Journal of Allergy and Immunology*, vol. 22, no. 2-3, pp. 159–163, 2004.

[19] A. Cortes and M. A. Brown, "Promise and pitfalls of the Immunochip," *Arthritis Research & Therapy*, vol. 13, no. 1, p. 101, 2011.

[20] E. M. Tan, A. S. Cohen, and J. F. Fries, "The 1982 revised criteria for the classification of systemic lupus erythrematosus," *Arthritis and Rheumatism*, vol. 25, no. 11, pp. 1271–1277, 1982.

[21] M. C. Hochberg, "Updating the American College of Rheumatology revised criteria for the classification of systemic lupus erythematosus," *Arthritis and Rheumatism*, vol. 40, no. 9, p. 1725, 1997.

[22] J. Yang, S. H. Lee, M. E. Goddard, and P. M. Visscher, "GCTA: a tool for genome-wide complex trait analysis," *American Journal of Human Genetics*, vol. 88, no. 1, pp. 76–82, 2011.

[23] D. H. Alexander, J. Novembre, and K. Lange, "Fast model-based estimation of ancestry in unrelated individuals," *Genome Research*, vol. 19, no. 9, pp. 1655–1664, 2009.

[24] S. Purcell, B. Neale, K. Todd-Brown et al., "PLINK: a tool set for whole-genome association and population-based linkage analyses," *American Journal of Human Genetics*, vol. 81, no. 3, pp. 559–575, 2007.

[25] S. Macgregor and I. A. Khan, "GAIA: an easy-to-use web-based application for interaction analysis of case-control data," *BMC Medical Genetics*, vol. 7, article 34, 2006.

[26] H. M. Kang, J. H. Sul, S. K. Service et al., "Variance component model to account for sample structure in genome-wide association studies," *Nature Genetics*, vol. 42, no. 4, pp. 348–354, 2010.

[27] A. P. Boyle, E. L. Hong, M. Hariharan et al., "Annotation of functional variation in personal genomes using RegulomeDB," *Genome Research*, vol. 22, pp. 1790–1797, 2012.

[28] L. D. Ward and M. Kellis, "HaploReg: a resource for exploring chromatin states, conservation, and regulatory motif alterations within sets of genetically linked variants," *Nucleic Acids Research*, vol. 40, pp. D930–D934, 2012.

[29] O. J. Rullo and B. P. Tsao, "Recent insights into the genetic basis of systemic lupus erythematosus," *Annals of the Rheumatic Diseases*, vol. 72, supplement 2, pp. ii56–ii61, 2013.

[30] K. Zhang, S. Cui, S. Chang, L. Zhang, and J. Wang, "i-GSEA4GWAS: a web server for identification of pathways/gene sets associated with traits by applying an improved gene set enrichment analysis to genome-wide association study," *Nucleic Acids Research*, vol. 38, no. 2, pp. W90–W95, 2010.

[31] C. J. Hoggart, M. D. Shriver, R. A. Kittles, D. G. Clayton, and P. M. McKeigue, "Design and analysis of admixture mapping studies," *American Journal of Human Genetics*, vol. 74, no. 5, pp. 965–978, 2004.

[32] B. E. Stranger, A. C. Nica, M. S. Forrest et al., "Population genomics of human gene expression," *Nature Genetics*, vol. 39, no. 10, pp. 1217–1224, 2007.

[33] R. Webb, J. T. Merrill, J. A. Kelly et al., "A polymorphism within IL21R confers risk for systemic lupus erythematosus," *Arthritis and Rheumatism*, vol. 60, no. 8, pp. 2402–2407, 2009.

14

Anti-Transglutaminase 6 Antibodies in Children and Young Adults with Cerebral Palsy

Reidun Stenberg,[1] Marios Hadjivassiliou,[2] Pascale Aeschlimann,[3] Nigel Hoggard,[2] and Daniel Aeschlimann[3]

[1] *Department of Pediatrics, Centre for Rehabilitation Research and Department of Clinical Medicine, School of Health and Medical Sciences, Örebro University, 70185 Örebro, Sweden*
[2] *Department of Neurology and Department of Neuroradiology, The Royal Hallamshire Hospital, Sheffield S10 2JF, UK*
[3] *Matrix Biology & Tissue Repair Research Unit, College of Biomedical and Life Sciences, School of Dentistry, Cardiff University, Cardiff CF14 4XY, UK*

Correspondence should be addressed to Reidun Stenberg; reidun.stenberg@orebroll.se

Academic Editor: Kalle Kurppa

Objectives. We have previously reported a high prevalence of gluten-related serological markers (GRSM) in children and young adults with cerebral palsy (CP). The majority had no enteropathy to suggest coeliac disease (CD). Antibodies against transglutaminase 6 (anti-TG6) represent a new marker associated with gluten-related neurological dysfunction. The aim of this study was to investigate the prevalence of anti-TG6 antibodies in this group of individuals with an early neurological injury resulting in CP. *Materials and Methods.* Sera from 96 patients with CP and 36 controls were analysed for IgA/IgG class anti-TG6 by ELISA. *Results.* Anti-TG6 antibodies were found in 12/96 (13%) of patients with CP compared to 2/36 (6%) in controls. The tetraplegic subgroup of CP had a significantly higher prevalence of anti-TG6 antibodies 6/17 (35%) compared to the other subgroups and controls. There was no correlation of anti-TG6 autoantibodies with seropositivity to food proteins including gliadin. *Conclusions.* An early brain insult and associated inflammation may predispose to future development of TG6 autoimmunity.

1. Introduction

Patients with cerebral palsy (CP) are characterized by abnormal muscle tone, coordination problems, and delay in motor development leading to difficulties in gait, balance, and involuntary movements. Muscle spasticity is very common. Associated conditions include epilepsy, dysarthria, cognitive impairment, and feeding problems, which may result in difficulties in weight gain and growth [1, 2] particularly for the most severely affected CP groups (tetraplegic and dyskinetic subgroups). The aetiology of the brain damage causing CP is among others mainly hypoxia due to asphyxia leading to ischemic brain injury. Another cause could be intrauterine infection [3–5].

Since coeliac disease (CD) is a common cause of poor growth, we previously analysed our cohort of CP patients for IgA and IgG-antibodies against gliadin and transglutaminase 2 (TG2) and found a high prevalence of seropositive patients. The highest prevalence was for IgG-AGA 36 and 61%, respectively [6, 7] which is of low diagnostic value for CD [8]. The majority of these patients also did not have enteropathy on routine histological or extended immunohistochemical examination of small bowel biopsies [6, 9, 10]. However, a number of patients tested positive for TG2 IgA (7/99) and/or had circulating antibodies to deamidated gliadin peptides (DGP; 7/40 tested), accepted markers in CD diagnosis [6, 10]. The seropositive CP patients had a significantly lower weight, height, and body mass index (BMI) and they were also more severely handicapped, according to gross motor function classification (GMFCS) [11].

Increasing numbers of studies have reported that gluten-related disorders include extraintestinal manifestations, for example, involving skin (dermatitis herpetiformis) and brain (gluten Ataxia) [12–15]. Such manifestations may occur in the absence of overt gastrointestinal involvement and patients may be seronegative for anti-TG2 IgA autoantibodies, the commonly used diagnostic marker for CD [16].

TG2 is the autoantigen in CD, whilst TG3 is the autoantigen in dermatitis herpetiformis, a blistering skin disease with gluten-induced granular IgA-deposits in the papillary dermis [12]. Another enzyme in the transglutaminase family that is primarily expressed in the central nervous system is transglutaminase 6 (TG6) [17]. We have demonstrated the presence of circulating anti-TG6 antibodies in adults with gluten Ataxia, independent of intestinal involvement [16]. This may suggest a bias of the immune response towards different TG isozymes in extraintestinal manifestations (i.e., TG6 in gluten Ataxia and TG3 in dermatitis herpetiformis).

The aim of this study was to investigate the prevalence of antibodies against TG6 in patients with CP.

2. Material and Methods

2.1. Participants

2.1.1. CP-Group. The study recruited 99 children and young adults with CP living in the Swedish county council of Värmland and Örebro. In Sweden children and young adults with CP are treated at specialized rehabilitation centers where they can obtain specific support such as medical care, physiotherapy, speech, occupational, and psychological therapy until they have finished school. In some cases they are 24 years of age before they are referred to the adult clinic.

There were 46 girls and 53 boys. At the time of enrolment the age ranged from 18 months to 24 years (median age 11 years). There was no comorbidity for CD such as diabetes mellitus or dermatitis herpetiformis at the time of inclusion. The diagnosis of CP subgroups was based on studies by Mutch et al. [18, 19]. A functional assessment of each child was made on the basis of the Gross Motor Function Classification System (GMFCS), graded I–V, where GMFCS V represent the most severe disability [11]. Medical data of the CP-group were reviewed retrospectively in medical files (RS). Thirteen children had percutaneous gastrostomy (PEG) but also received some gluten containing food orally. Eleven children had treatment for gastroesophageal reflux disease (GERD).

2.1.2. Controls. 36 children, aged 2–18 years (19 boys and 17 girls), were included in the serological analysis as controls. These children had been investigated with laboratory analyses for allergy but were found negative. No further clinical information about the children was available.

2.2. Serology. Data on IgG and IgA AGA and TG2, DGP antibodies and HLA testing were available from our previous studies [6, 10] as well as the data of antibodies against dietary proteins [7].

None in the CP-group had IgA deficiency (<0.07 g/L).

2.3. TG6 Antibody ELISA. Detection of antibodies to TG6 by ELISA followed our previously published protocol with minor modifications [16]. Briefly, full-length human TG6 produced in SF9 cells was obtained from Zedira (Darmstadt, Germany). Results with this antigen were comparable to those obtained with recombinant TG6 produced in house in *E. coli* (data not shown) [16]. TG6 was diluted to 2 μg/mL in 20 mM Tris/HCl, 300 mM NaCl, pH 7.6 immediately prior to use and applied to high-capacity protein binding 96-well plates (Immulon 2HB; Thermo Electron, Waltham, MA, USA) overnight at 4°C. All subsequent incubations were conducted at room temperature. Nonspecific binding was blocked by incubation with 3% BSA (immunoassay grade, Sigma 05477) in TBS (20 mM Tris/HCl, pH 7.4, 150 mM NaCl) for 1 h. Patient sera were diluted 1 : 100 in 1% BSA in TBS and any protein aggregates present removed by centrifugation at 10,000 ×g for 5 min prior to being applied to coated plates. All binding steps were carried out for 90 min and followed by five rinses with TBS/0.01% Tween 20. Antibody binding was detected by incubation with peroxidase-conjugated affinity purified anti-human IgA (Jackson ImmunoResearch, West Grove, PA, USA; 109-035-011, diluted 1 : 1000 in 1% BSA/TBS) or anti-human IgG (Dako, Carpinteria, CA, USA; P0214, diluted 1 : 250 in 1% BSA/TBS). The reaction was finally developed for 2 h using 5 mM 5-amino-2-hydroxybenzoic acid/NaOH, pH 6.0, 0.005% H_2O_2, as a peroxidase substrate solution and stopped by addition of an equal volume of 1 M NaOH to each well. After 15 minutes, the absorbance at 490 nm was measured.

All serum samples were analysed in duplicate on wells containing antigen or only BSA, included on the same plate. The BSA only background was subtracted from values for antigen. Units were calculated from a series of standards (0, 1, 3, 10, and 100 U/mL; 1st generation assay) (Zedira) run in parallel. Results are given as the mean of two independent determinations. A measurement >14 U/mL for IgA or >34 U/mL for IgG was considered positive. Thresholds were set as the 98th percentile on a blood donor collective. As anti-BSA antibodies may be prevalent in this patient cohort which has enhanced immunity to dietary components [7] and this may potentially impact on the analysis, we have evaluated all samples also in a commercial assay without background subtraction (Zedira). There was good agreement between the results of the two ELISA methods (supplementary figure).

2.4. Ethics. The study was approved by Regional Ethical Review Board in Uppsala. Participants or parents, as appropriate, gave written informed consent.

2.5. Statistical Analyses. All data were analyzed using the Statistical Package for the Social sciences (SPSS) program, version 15. Differences between groups were evaluated with Pearson's χ^2 test in cross tabulations and when appropriate Fisher's Exact Test. An independent t-test was used for body mass index (BMI) (standard deviation, SD), height (SD), and weight (SD), using 2-tailed significance.

$P < 0.05$ was considered significant.

3. Results

3.1. Serological Analysis for Anti-TG6 Autoantibodies. Sera from 96 patients with CP and 36 controls (children from same geographical area) were available for analysis of autoantibodies against TG6. We found elevated levels of anti-TG6 antibodies (IgG and/or IgA) in 12/96 (13%) in the CP-group and 2/36 (6%) in the control group ($P = 0.35$). (Figure 1) However, a positive test for TG6 antibodies was significantly more frequent in the tetraplegic subgroup of CP, 6/17 (35%) compared to the control group 6% ($P = 0.01$). We also found statistical significance when the tetraplegic subgroup was compared to the other CP subgroups ($P = 0.006$) (Figure 2). IgA anti-TG6 antibodies were found in 7/96 (7%) compared to 1/36 (3%) in the control group. ($P = 0.45$) IgG anti-TG6 antibodies were found in 6/96 (6%) compared to 1/36 (3%) in the control group ($P = 0.67$). One child had elevated levels of both IgA and IgG to TG6.

This CP cohort has been tested for CD as reported previously. [6, 10] There was an association between anti-TG6 antibodies and IgA antibodies to TG2 ($P = 0.04$) but not for any of the other gluten-related serological markers analysed (anti-TG2 IgG or AGA IgA/IgG) (Table 1(b)). Five of the twelve patients with CP that tested positive for anti-TG6 antibodies were negative for all gluten-related serological markers. Also, there was no correlation between anti-TG6 antibody titres and the presence of other indicators of CD (Table 1(b)). Eleven of the twelve individuals with TG6 positivity had previously been tested for the coeliac HLA type (DQB1 typing) and 6/11 were positive for HLA-DQ2 and/or HLA-DQ8, and a further 2 carried one-half of the DQ2 heterodimer (DQ7, $\alpha5$ subunit) which is known to confer susceptibility to CD [21]. A further patient carries the rare HLA-DQ9 which may also confer susceptibility according to recent evidence [22].

3.2. Clinical Data of Patients Testing Positive for Anti-TG6 Antibodies. The clinical data of the 12 CP patients positive for anti-TG6 antibodies are summarized in Table 1(a). The median age was significantly higher in the TG6 positive group, 14.4 years compared to 10.7 years in the TG6 negative group ($P = 0.021$).

The majority was born at term (8/12) and had asphyxia. Five had epilepsy-requiring medication. There was no significant difference in weight ($P = 0.318$) or BMI ($P = 0.987$) between TG6 antibody positive and negative patients. There was, however, a significant difference in height between the 2 groups. The children and young adults with CP positive for anti-TG6 were shorter ($P = 0.021$). As height correlates to the degree of disability this may reflect a more severe disability, consistent with a higher prevalence of anti-TG6 antibodies in the tetraplegic subgroup [1].

Seven of these patients had previously been investigated on clinical grounds using MRI or CT and the results were reviewed as part of this study (NH). Brain malformation was seen in one child and traumatic injury in another two. Developmental malformations or defects as a consequence of ischemia were seen in 3 cases. In one child with Ataxia no significant abnormalities were found (Table 1(a)). As

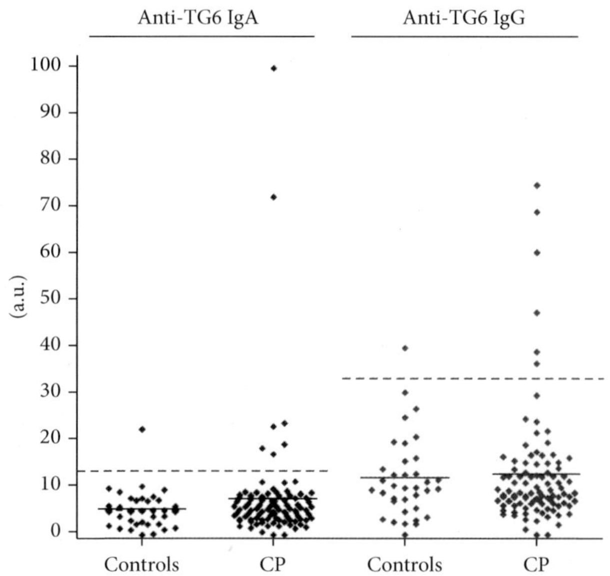

FIGURE 1: Analysis of serum for antibodies against transglutaminase type 6 (TG6) by ELISA. Relative concentration of antibodies in children ($n = 96$) with cerebral palsy (CP) and controls ($n = 36$) is given in arbitrary units. Bolded line represents the mean titre of the group and dotted line the threshold for a positive test.

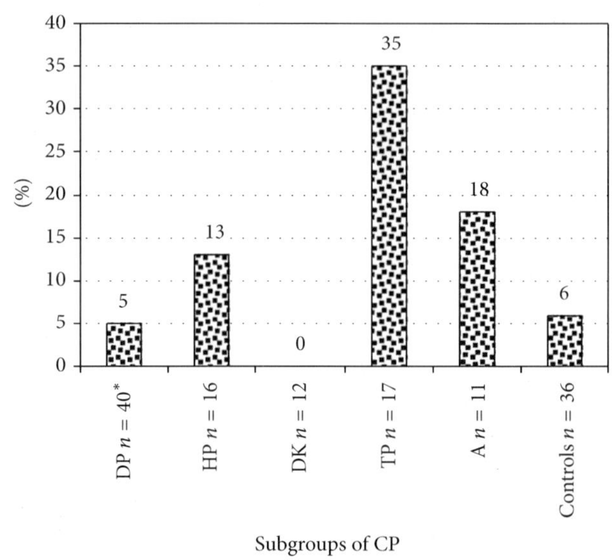

FIGURE 2: Percentage of patients testing positive for IgA/IgG antibodies to TG6 in different CP subgroups and in a control group. The tetraplegic subgroup compared to the other CP subgroups ($P = 0.006$) and to controls ($P = 0.01$); $^{*}n = 3$ missing for TG6 antibody analysis. HP: CP-Hemiplegia, DP: CP-Diplegia, TP: CP-Tetraplegia, DK: CP-Dyskinesia, and A: CP-Ataxia.

gastrointestinal dysfunction typically seen in the most severe forms of CP may impact on gut permeability and lead to enhanced immunity to food-derived antigens, we further evaluated whether a correlation existed between TG6 autoantibodies and indicators of feeding difficulties. There was no significant difference for either the group that had treated

Table 1: (a) Clinical data of children with cerebral palsy and autoantibodies to TG6. (b) Summary of gastrointestinal data and laboratory results previously performed [6, 10] for those CP children testing positive for autoantibodies to TG6.

(a)

Patients sex/age (—/yr)	IQ N = normal MR = mental retardation	Diagnosis/subdiagnosis of CP	GMFCS	CP etiology	Neonatal data W = gestational age when born	Brain MRI/CT/US	Epilepsy and treatment
F/17	N	AU/ A	I	Unknown	PN	MRI, normal	—
M/18	MR	TP	V	Asphyxia	PN Asphyxia at birth	US, wide ventricles, small subependymal bleeding	—
M/4	MR	TP	IV-V	Traumatic injury 3 months of age	PN	CT, focal infarct, cortical, subcortical, and basal ganglia damage	Lamotrigine
M/12	N	A	II	Hydrops fetalis	Hydrops fetalis CS; W 28	MRI, cortical and subcortical damage	—
F/18	MR	TP	V	Asphyxia	CS; W 40	CT, focal infarct	—
F/18	N	HF/HP	II	Left cerebral infarction at 1 years of age	PN	MRI and CT, cortical and subcortical damage, and hydrocephalus	—
M/20	MR	TP	V	Asphyxia	CS; W 40	NA	—
F/7	N	HP	I	Asphyxia	CS; W 32	NA	—
F/14	MR	DP	III	Asphyxia	W 26. Asphyxia at birth	NA	Carbamazepine
F/17	MR	HC/ HP	II	Brain malformation at birth	PN	MRI, brain malformation	Valproate
M/20	MR	TP	V	Asphyxia		NA	Valproate
M/9	MR	TP	V	Traumatic injury 1 years of age	PN	CT, focal infarct	Valproate, lamotrigine, and vigabatrin

(b)

Patients sex/age (—/yr)	IgA anti-TG6 cutoff value >14 U/mL	IgG anti-TG6 cutoff value >34 U/mL	IgA AGA	IgG AGA	IgA TG2	IgG TG2	HLA DQ-type	IgA/IgG DGP cutoff >20 U/mL	Small bowel biopsies	GI symptoms
F/17	17.3	—	—	Pos.	—	—	7.8	—	Positive DR staining grade 1	NA
M/18	18.5	—	Pos.	—	Pos.	NA	6.8	—	Positive DR staining grade 2	—
M/4	19.4	—	—	—	—	—	5	NA	NA	—
M/12	23.9	—	—	Pos.	—	Pos.	6	—	NA	Oral dysfunction
F/18	23.1	—	—	Pos.	Pos.	Pos.	2.5	26	IgA deposits and $\alpha\beta/\gamma\delta$ IEL's, DR staining grade 2	C
F/18	72.4	—	—	—	—	—	7	NA	NA	Unspecific abdominal pain
M/20	>100	39.2	—	—	—	—	2.9	NA	NA	GERD, C, D
F/7	—	36.7	—	—	—	—	6.9	NA	NA	—
F/14	—	47.6	—	Pos.	Pos.	Pos.	6.7	32	NA	GERD
F/17	—	60.5	—	—	—	—	2	—	NA	—
M/20	—	69.1	Pos.	—	—	—	NA	—	NA	GERD, PEG, C
M/9	—	74.8	—	Pos.	—	Pos.	6.8	—	NA	PEG, C

Abbreviations: A: Ataxia; HP: Hemiplegia; TP: Tetraplegia; DP: Diplegia; AU: Autism; HC: Hydrocephalus; HF: Heart Failure; GERD: gastroesophageal reflux disease; PN: partus normalis and born term; CS: Caesarean section; C: Constipation; N: normal; MRI: magnetic resonance imaging; CT: computer tomography; US: Ultrasound; PEG: percutaneous endoscopic gastrostomy; GMFCS: Gross Motor Function Classification System, graded I–V; D: Diarrhoea; NA: not applicable; Pos: positive; IEL: intraepithelial lymphocytes.

TABLE 2: Correlation between indicators of feeding problems and immunity to TG6 and to AGA analysed previously ($n = 99$)* [6].

	AGA positive 41/99* (41%)	AGA negative 58/99* (59%)	P value	TG6 antibody positive 12/96 (12.5%)	TG6 antibody negative 84/96 (87.5%)	P value
Weight	−1.960 SD	−1.00 SD	$P = 0.016$	−1.917 SD	−1.304 SD	$P = 0.318$
BMI	−1.175 SD	−0.136 SD	$P = 0.006$	−0.528 SD	−0.537 SD	$P = 0.987$
PEG $n = 13$	10/13	3/13	$P = 0.005$	2/13	11/13	$P = 0.664$
GERD $n = 11$	6/11	5/11	$P = 0.348$	3/10♦	7/10♦	$P = 0.111$

*90 children age < 18 year were published in the referred paper. Here we have calculated with the whole cohort, $n = 99$, since we have the data available.
♦1 missing for analysis of TG6-antibodies.
SD: weight ± standard deviation (SD), also referred to as weight z-scores, standardized to the Swedish general population by age and sex and based on 3,650 healthy children [20]. GERD: gastroesophageal reflux disease; PEG: percutan endoscopic gastrostomy; AGA: IgA and IgG gliadin antibodies TG6: transglutaminase 6.

GERD or assisted feeding (PEG) with regard to TG6 antibody positivity (Table 2). In contrast, anti-gliadin antibodies previously identified [6] showed a strong association with PEG and also correlated with patient weight and BMI (Table 2).

4. Discussions

The rational for the study was that anti-TG6 antibodies have been described in the context of neurological manifestations in gluten-related disorders and may identify gluten sensitivity in patients serologically negative for anti-TG2 antibodies [23].

There was a significantly higher prevalence of TG6 antibodies in the subgroup of patients with the most severe form of CP but not in the CP group as a whole. Furthermore, a positive correlation of TG6 antibodies with TG2 IgA antibodies but not to other antibodies tested is in keeping with a shared/overlapping mechanistic origin of these autoantibodies as has been suggested [24].

CP is a heterogeneous condition and is likely to have a number of different causes. The most common cause is an ischemic event in the immature brain. Bax et al. showed that magnetic resonance imaging (MRI) abnormalities were detectable in 88% of 351 children with CP [3]. The major findings seen on MRI in the tetraplegic subgroup was white matter damage of immaturity, including periventricular leukomalacia (PVL) (35.1%) and to a lesser extent cortical lesions. The finding of PVL was previously thought to be a typical damage seen in premature-born children. However, this neuroimaging study [3] has shown that white matter damage can be a common finding also among term infants and that in such cases the white matter loss tends to be more extensive. The localisation and severity of the brain lesions depend on the timing of the event in the immature brain and differ between the subgroups of cerebral palsy [3] and so also the clinical outcome of the lesion.

The weight is in general lower in the children with CP compared to normal children and some children with CP require food intake in an alternative way, that is, by a percutaneous gastrostomy (PEG), to gain weight due to their oral and gastrointestinal dysfunction. The most severe forms of CP are in the subgroups of Dyskinesia (DK) and Tetraplegia (TP). These patients also suffer most from gastrointestinal disturbances and have the lowest weight gain of the CP subgroups. In our recently published study from the same cohort of patients, we found mainly IgG-antibodies not only to gluten but also to other food proteins (lactoglobulin and casein) in the DK and TP subgroups of CP who also had the lowest weight [7]. It is likely that these patients have increased intestinal permeability allowing entrance of undigested proteins across the gut barrier into the circulation [25] and therefore have enhanced immunity to food-derived antigens. Such immune reactivity to dietary constituents has also been reported in studies of underweight children from underdeveloped countries [25, 26]. However, we could not find a significant association between lower body weights or the use of PEG and the presence of anti-TG6 autoantibodies; in contrast, AGA antibodies significantly correlated with low weight and assisted feeding (PEG).

There was a significantly higher prevalence of TG6 autoantibodies in the tetraplegic subgroup of patients compared to controls and the other subgroups. In fact there was no antibody response to TG6 in the other subgroup of CP with severe deficiencies, the dyskinetic group. The reason for that is not clear. One possibility could be that the type of brain damage in the tetraplegic subgroup (extensive white matter involvement) may predispose to future development of an immune reaction against TG6. Indeed white matter abnormalities on brain MR imaging are a common finding in patients with CD and headaches [8, 27–30]. The hypothesis of a primary brain insult leading to sensitisation to gluten is supported by a recent study demonstrating increased prevalence of CD in patients with previous head injury [31].

TGs are a family of structurally and functionally related cross-linking enzymes. In mice, TG6 expression is associated with neurogenesis in CNS development and in the mature brain, in neurons in regions associated with motor function including the cerebral cortex and cerebellum [17]. Antibodies isolated from CD patients frequently react with human and mouse neurons. Such antibodies are not the predominant anti-TG2 IgA but either directed to TG6 or cross-reactive between the closely related isozymes, TG2, TG3 and TG6 [32]. Intraventricular injection of such patient-derived

TG-specific immunoglobulins in mice induced Ataxia-like deficits [32]. These data not only indicate that autoantibodies to TG6 could be a marker of brain lesions but that such antibodies may play a part in pathogenesis. The role of TG6 in cerebellar functioning has recently been further highlighted by the identification of mutations in the human gene encoding TG6, causing autosomal dominant spinocerebellar Ataxia [33, 34].

5. Conclusion

This study group of children with CP does not have a higher prevalence of celiac disease than expected in the regional population but they do have more frequent immunoreactivity to gluten and other dietary food components compared to matched controls [6, 7]. Here, we report significantly increased prevalence of anti-TG6 autoantibodies in the tetraplegic subgroup of patients with CP. This antibody response seems not to be correlated with low body weight and the associated immune response to food constituents. The aetiology of anti-TG6 antibodies in this CP subgroup remains unclear, but the results could support the hypothesis of a primary brain insult leading to TG6 autoimmunity.

Abbreviations

A:	CP-Ataxia
AU:	Autism
CP:	Cerebral palsy
CT:	Computer tomography
DP:	CP-Diplegia
DK:	CP-Dyskinesia
GMFCS:	Gross Motor Function Classification System, graded I–V
GERD:	Gastroesophageal reflux
GRSM:	Gluten-related serological markers (IgG/IgA-TG2, IgG/IgA-AGA)
HP:	CP-Hemiplegia
MRI:	Magnetic resonance imaging
PEG:	Percutaneous endoscopic gastrostomy
TP:	CP-Tetraplegia
US:	Ultrasound.

Conflict of Interests

The authors report no potential conflict of interests or commercial or other financial relationships. D. Aeschlimann serves as a scientific advisor/collaborator to Zedira (without financial incentives) but receives royalties from Zedira for patents.

Acknowledgments

The authors acknowledge the participating children and young adults with cerebral palsy from Habilitation Centre in Örebro County Council and Värmland County Council in Sweden and their parents. The work was supported by Grants from the Research Committee of Örebro County Council and from Norrbacka-Eugeniastiftelsen, Sweden, to Reidun Stenberg and Grants from the Sheffield Hospitals Charitable Trust (no. 7877), Coeliac UK, and BRET (Bardhan Research and Education Trust of Rotherham), UK, to Daniel Aeschlimann and Marios Hadjivassiliou.

References

[1] K. Himmelmann, E. Beckung, G. Hagberg, and P. Uvebrant, "Bilateral spastic cerebral palsy—prevalence through four decades, motor function and growth," *European Journal of Paediatric Neurology*, vol. 11, no. 4, pp. 215–222, 2007.

[2] M. O. Dahlseng, A.-K. Finbråten, P. B. Júlíusson, J. Skranes, G. Andersen, and T. Vik, "Feeding problems, growth and nutritional status in children with cerebral palsy," *Acta Paediatrica*, vol. 101, no. 1, pp. 92–98, 2012.

[3] M. Bax, C. Tydeman, and O. Flodmark, "Clinical and MRI correlates of cerebral palsy: the European cerebral palsy study," *Journal of the American Medical Association*, vol. 296, no. 13, pp. 1602–1608, 2006.

[4] Y. W. Wu, G. J. Escobar, J. K. Grether, L. A. Croen, J. D. Greene, and T. B. Newman, "Chorioamnionitis and cerebral palsy in term and near-term infants," *Journal of the American Medical Association*, vol. 290, no. 20, pp. 2677–2684, 2003.

[5] A. T. Pakula, K. Van Naarden Braun, and M. Yeargin-Allsopp, "Cerebral palsy: classification and epidemiology," *Physical Medicine and Rehabilitation Clinics of North America*, vol. 20, no. 3, pp. 425–452, 2009.

[6] R. Stenberg, C. Dahle, E. Lindberg, and J. Schollin, "Increased prevalence of anti-gliadin antibodies and anti-tissue transglutaminase antibodies in children with cerebral palsy," *Journal of Pediatric Gastroenterology and Nutrition*, vol. 49, no. 4, pp. 424–429, 2009.

[7] R. Stenberg, C. Dahle, A. Magnuson, and D. Hellberg, "Increased prevalence of antibodies against dietary proteins in children and young adults with cerebral palsy," *Journal of Pediatric Gastroenterology and Nutrition*, vol. 56, no. 2, pp. 233–238, 2013.

[8] U. Volta, F. Tovoli, R. Cicola et al., "Serological tests in gluten sensitivity (nonceliac gluten intolerance)," *Journal of Clinical Gastroenterology*, vol. 46, no. 8, pp. 680–685, 2012.

[9] R. Stenberg and J. Schollin, "Is there a connection between severe cerebral palsy and increased gluten sensitivity?" *Acta Paediatrica*, vol. 96, no. 1, pp. 132–134, 2007.

[10] R. Stenberg, K. Kaukinen, M. Bengtsson, E. Lindberg, and C. Dahle, "Early developing celiac disease in children with cerebral palsy," *Journal of Pediatric Gastroenterology and Nutrition*, vol. 53, no. 6, pp. 674–678, 2011.

[11] R. Palisano, P. Rosenbaum, S. Walter, D. Russell, E. Wood, and B. Galuppi, "Development and reliability of a system to classify gross motor function in children with cerebral palsy," *Developmental Medicine and Child Neurology*, vol. 39, no. 4, pp. 214–223, 1997.

[12] M. Sárdy, S. Kárpáti, B. Merkl, M. Paulsson, and N. Smyth, "Epidermal transglutaminase (TGase 3) is the autoantigen of dermatitis herpetiformis," *Journal of Experimental Medicine*, vol. 195, no. 6, pp. 747–757, 2002.

[13] M. Hadjivassiliou, S. Boscolo, G. A. B. Davies-Jones et al., "The humoral response in the pathogenesis of gluten ataxia," *Neurology*, vol. 58, no. 8, pp. 1221–1226, 2002.

[14] M. Hadjivassiliou, M. Mäki, D. S. Sanders et al., "Autoantibody targeting of brain and intestinal transglutaminase in gluten ataxia," *Neurology*, vol. 66, no. 3, pp. 373–377, 2006.

[15] M. Hadjivassiliou, D. S. Sanders, R. A. Grünewald, N. Woodroofe, S. Boscolo, and D. Aeschlimann, "Gluten sensitivity: from gut to brain," *The Lancet Neurology*, vol. 9, no. 3, pp. 318–330, 2010.

[16] M. Hadjivassiliou, P. Aeschlimann, A. Strigun, D. S. Sanders, N. Woodroofe, and D. Aeschlimann, "Autoantibodies in gluten ataxia recognize a novel neuronal transglutaminase," *Annals of Neurology*, vol. 64, no. 3, pp. 332–343, 2008.

[17] H. Thomas, K. Beck, M. Adamczyk et al., "Transglutaminase 6: a protein associated with central nervous system development and motor function," *Amino Acids*, vol. 44, no. 1, pp. 161–177, 2013.

[18] L. Mutch, E. Alberman, B. Hagberg, K. Kodama, and M. V. Perat, "Cerebral palsy epidemiology: where are we now and where are we going?" *Developmental Medicine and Child Neurology*, vol. 34, no. 6, pp. 547–551, 1992.

[19] B. Hagberg, G. Hagberg, and I. Olow, "The changing panorama of cerebral palsy in Sweden 1954-1970. I. Analysis of the general changes," *Acta Paediatrica Scandinavica*, vol. 64, no. 2, pp. 187–192, 1975.

[20] K. Albertsson-Wikland and J. Karlberg, "Natural growth in children born small for gestational age with and without catch-up growth," *Acta Paediatrica, Supplement*, vol. 83, no. 399, pp. 64–71, 1994.

[21] K. Karell, A. S. Louka, S. J. Moodie et al., "HLA types in celiac disease patients not carrying the DQA1*05-DQB1*02 (DQ2) heterodimer: results from the European genetics cluster on celiac disease," *Human Immunology*, vol. 64, no. 4, pp. 469–477, 2003.

[22] M. Bodd, S. Tollefsen, E. Bergseng, K. E. A. Lundin, and L. M. Sollid, "Evidence that HLA-DQ9 confers risk to celiac disease by presence of DQ9-restricted gluten-specific T cells," *Human Immunology*, vol. 73, no. 4, pp. 376–381, 2012.

[23] M. Hadjivassiliou, P. Aeschlimann, D. S. Sanders et al., "Transglutaminase 6 antibodies in the diagnosis of gluten ataxia," *Neurology*, vol. 80, no. 19, pp. 1740–1745, 2013.

[24] J. Stamnaes, S. Dorum, B. Fleckenstein, D. Aeschlimann, and L. M. Sollid, "Gluten T cell epitope targeting by TG3 and TG6; Implications for dermatitis herpetiformis and gluten ataxia," *Amino Acids*, vol. 39, no. 5, pp. 1183–1191, 2010.

[25] P. G. Lunn, C. A. Northrop-Clewes, and R. M. Downes, "Intestinal permeability, mucosal injury, and growth faltering in Gambian infants," *The Lancet*, vol. 338, no. 8772, pp. 907–910, 1991.

[26] P. G. Lunn, "The impact of infection and nutrition on gut function and growth in childhood," *Proceedings of the Nutrition Society*, vol. 59, no. 1, pp. 147–154, 2000.

[27] A. K. Dimitrova, R. C. Ungaro, B. Lebwohl et al., "Prevalence of migraine in patients with celiac disease and inflammatory bowel disease," *Headache*, vol. 53, no. 2, pp. 344–355, 2013.

[28] R. Francavilla, F. Cristofori, S. Castellaneta et al., "Clinical, serologic, and histologic features of gluten sensitivity in children," *Journal of Pediatrics*, vol. 164, no. 3, pp. 463–467, 2013.

[29] M. Hadjivassiliou, R. A. Grünewald, M. Lawden, G. A. B. Davies-Jones, T. Powell, and C. M. L. Smith, "Headache and CNS white matter abnormalities associated with gluten sensitivity," *Neurology*, vol. 56, no. 3, pp. 385–388, 2001.

[30] S. Currie, M. Hadjivassiliou, M. J. Clark et al., "Should we be "nervous" about coeliac disease? Brain abnormalities in patients with coeliac disease referred for neurological opinion," *Journal of Neurology, Neurosurgery and Psychiatry*, vol. 83, no. 12, pp. 1216–1221, 2012.

[31] J. F. Ludvigsson and M. Hadjivassiliou, "Can head trauma trigger celiac disease? Nation-wide case-control study," *BMC Neurology*, vol. 13, p. 105, 2013.

[32] S. Boscolo, A. Lorenzon, D. Sblattero et al., "Anti transglutaminase antibodies cause ataxia in mice," *PloS ONE*, vol. 5, no. 3, Article ID e9698, 2010.

[33] J. Wang, J. L. Wang, X. Yang et al., "TGM6 identified as a novel causative gene of spinocerebellar ataxias using exome sequencing," *Brain*, vol. 133, no. 12, pp. 3510–3518, 2010.

[34] M. Li, S. Y. Pang, Y. Song, M. H. Kung, S. L. Ho, and P. C. Sham, "Whole exome sequencing identifies a novel mutation in the transglutaminase 6 gene for spinocerebellar ataxia in a Chinese family," *Clinical Genetics*, vol. 83, no. 3, pp. 269–273, 2013.

15

Neuroantibody Biomarkers: Links and Challenges in Environmental Neurodegeneration and Autoimmunity

Hassan A. N. El-Fawal

Neurotoxicology Laboratory, Albany College of Pharmacy and Health Sciences, 106 New Scotland Avenue, Albany, NY 12208, USA

Correspondence should be addressed to Hassan A. N. El-Fawal; hassan.el-fawal@acphs.edu

Academic Editor: K. Michael Pollard

The majority of neurodegenerative (ND) and autoimmune diseases (AID) remain idiopathic. The contribution of environmental chemicals to the development of these disorders has become of great interest in recent years. A convergence of mechanism between of ND and AID development has also emerged. In the case of ND, including neurotoxicity, the focus of this review, work over the last two decade in the realm of biomarker development, indicates that the immune response provides a venue whereby humoral immunity, in the form of autoantibodies to nervous system specific proteins, or neuroantibodies (NAb), may provide, once validated, a sensitive high throughput surrogate biomarker of effect with the potential of predicting outcome in absence of overt neurotoxicity/neurodegeneration. In addition, NAb may prove to be a contributor to the progression of the nervous system pathology, as well as biomarker of stage and therapeutic efficacy. There is a compelling need for biomarkers of effect in light of the introduction of new chemicals, such as nanoengineered material, where potential neurotoxicity remains to be defined. Furthermore, the convergence of mechanisms associated with ND and AID draws attention to the neglected arena of angiogenesis in defining the link between environment, ND, and AID.

1. Introduction

Identification of etiological factors that precipitate autoimmune (AID) and neurodegenerative diseases (ND) continues to be a challenge. According to the World Health Organization (WHO), 1 in 6 individuals, worldwide, suffer from a neurological disorder, mostly idiopathic, while the prevalence of AID varies according to the organ/system affected. WHO has prioritized investigations of the link between the environmental factors (e.g., chemicals) and both these disease entities [1, 2]. This is paralleled by the recently formulated strategic plan of National Institute of Environmental Health Sciences (NIEHS) in the study of environmental links to both ND and AID [3, 4]. The debilitating impact, as well as social and economic burden, particularly in children and the elderly, is compelling reason to develop biomarkers that can translate to the clinical setting in order to diagnose, evaluate sequelae, and provide a means of measuring successful intervention and to the identification of etiological factors and defining the mechanisms involved in ND and AID. It has become evident in recent years that there is a convergence of mechanisms involved in the pathogenesis of many ND and AID. Central to both is the increased angiogenesis and autoinflammatory sequelae to tissue damage. Also relevant to both is the involvement of integrins and Th17 lymphocytes. Additionally, the involvement of oxidative stress and necrotic-apoptotic events with exposure of autoantigens and the ensuing inflammation strengthens the proposition that the immune system may be a major effector of neurodegeneration. What is acknowledged in ND and AID is the loss and/or alterations in structural proteins, organ/cell-specific or common antigens, and an autoimmune, often humoral, signature. Indeed, because many of these proteins are sequestered intracellular proteins, the presence of immune effectors at the site of injury results in a humoral immune response (i.e., immunoglobulins (Ig)) directed against these autoantigens has been demonstrated in response to environmental chemical exposures. Work in our laboratory over the course of two decades has demonstrated that autoantibodies to NS proteins (neuroantibodies) may provide biomarkers of injury and may possibly be pathogenic [5].

It should be noted that in the context of this review and neurotoxicity, the discussion focuses on the effects of known environmental and occupational chemicals known to directly cause nervous system damage and not the recently described autoimmune/inflammatory syndrome induced by adjuvants (ASIA). Yehuda Shoenfeld's [6] group coined the term ASIA, also known as Shoenfeld's syndrome, as an umbrella to describe the clinical conditions of siliconosis, Gulf War syndrome, macrophagic myofasciitis syndrome, sick building syndrome, and postvaccination phenomena which share similar signs or symptoms, some of which are neurological and may be associated with demyelination and the presence of autoantibodies to an adjuvant material. The premise in ASIA is that the adjuvant may set in motion biological and immunological events that, in susceptible individuals, ultimately lead to the development of autoimmune disease, whereas in neurotoxicity we are often dealing with chemicals that directly induce neuronal death, apoptotic and necrotic, glial dysfunction, and aberrant neurotransmission [5].

This review seeks to address a major challenge in the identification and diagnosis of neurotoxicity and, by extension, ND, which is the development and validation of biomarkers of nervous system insult. However, in so much that these suggested biomarkers rely on an immune response to autoantigen (i.e., an autoimmune response), a possible epiphenomenon secondary to insults, whether acute or chronic, it raises the question as to whether this response may prove to be pathogenic, contributing to progression of the neuropathology. It should be noted that the study of neurotoxicity provides a useful paradigm for the development and testing of potential biomarkers of nervous system insult, since the level of injury can be controlled by dose, in the case of preclinical models, and the etiological factor(s) with target selectivity (neuronal versus demyelination) can be defined based on the agents used.

2. The Generation of Neuroantibodies as Biomarkers

Since proteins, many of them intracellular, are invariably lost during the neurodegenerative process and/or neurotoxic insult, several studies have advocated for the detection of proteins in cerebrospinal fluid (CSF) and blood serum or plasma as biomarkers of neurodegeneration. This has been reviewed elsewhere [7, 8]. This approach assumes that the clinician is aware of the precipitating event (e.g., stroke, traumatic brain injury, toxic exposure). However, the reality is that functional deficits are often slow in development and indeed, in the case of Alzheimer's disease (AD), Parkinson's disease (PD), and amyotrophic lateral sclerosis (ALS), may take years before a diagnosis is made based on overt morphological and behavioral alterations, when intervention may be of limited benefit. Unfortunately, this approach has its limitations, most notably the short half-life of many of these proposed proteins in the periphery and/or their specificity for NS as shown in Table 1 [9-13]. In contrast, because many of these proteins are sequestered intracellular proteins, the presence of immune effectors *in situ* or following translocation to peripheral lymphoid tissue (i.e., cervical lymph nodes and spleen) results in a humoral immune response directed against these autoantigens. With the development of immunological memory (IgG) or chronic degeneration (IgM), these immunoglobulins are likely to persist. Thus, capitalizing on the immune response, work in the Neurotoxicology Laboratory has advocated and demonstrated that these autoantibodies (neuroantibodies or NAb) provide a stable signature of nervous system (NS) injury [5]. This hypothesis is summarized in Figure 1.

Table 1: Serum/plasma half-life of some proteins proposed as biomarkers of neurodegeneration.

Protein	Half-life	Reference
Neuron-specific enolase (NSE)	48 hr	[9]
S100β	20–120 minutes	[10, 11]
Glial fibrillary acidic protein (GFAP)	10–17 hr	[12]
Myelin basic protein (MBP)	4 hr (plasma) 12 minutes (serum)	[13]

However, once again, the question may be raised, if NAb are validated as biomarkers of effect, what advantage do they provide for the clinician and when would they be applied? In the context of exposure to known neurotoxicants, particularly occupational exposures, exposure monitoring, individual and environmental, is common as required by the Occupational Safety and Health Administration (OSHA) in the United States and the European Agency for Safety and Health at Work (EU-OSHA). This requires periodic monitoring of workers and their rotation within the industry based on exposure levels (e.g., blood Pb). It is conceivable that a validated high-throughput biomarker of effect may be a useful adjunct to routine exposure monitoring in occupational settings. This is particularly relevant with the increased evidence linking environment and ND, as well as gene-environmental interactions. In addition, many countries now require the determination of blood Pb levels in school aged children. Environmental and occupational chemicals, solvents, polychlorinated biphenyls (PCB), methyl mercury, lead, and pesticides are known to be neurotoxic in adults and developmental neurotoxicants in children, yet diagnosis of effects is often delayed until overt behavioral manifestations occur, despite knowledge of exposure histories. The availability of a validated biomarkers of insult would prove beneficial to detect early effects in vulnerable populations. Today, monitoring of blood cholesterol, hemoglobin A1C (HbA1c), and prostate-specific antigen (PSA), once validated, have become routine tests to evaluate risk of cardiovascular disease, diabetes, and prostate cancer, respectively. It is conceivable that a validated biomarker of nervous system insult, such as NAb, may come to enjoy such a status. Indeed, the need for routine, economical, relatively noninvasive blood-based biomarkers, with early testing, in absence of overt signs, has been advocated in the case of AD, as a result of a roundtable convened in 2012 by the Alzheimer's Association and the Alzheimer's Drug Discovery Foundation [14]. In this

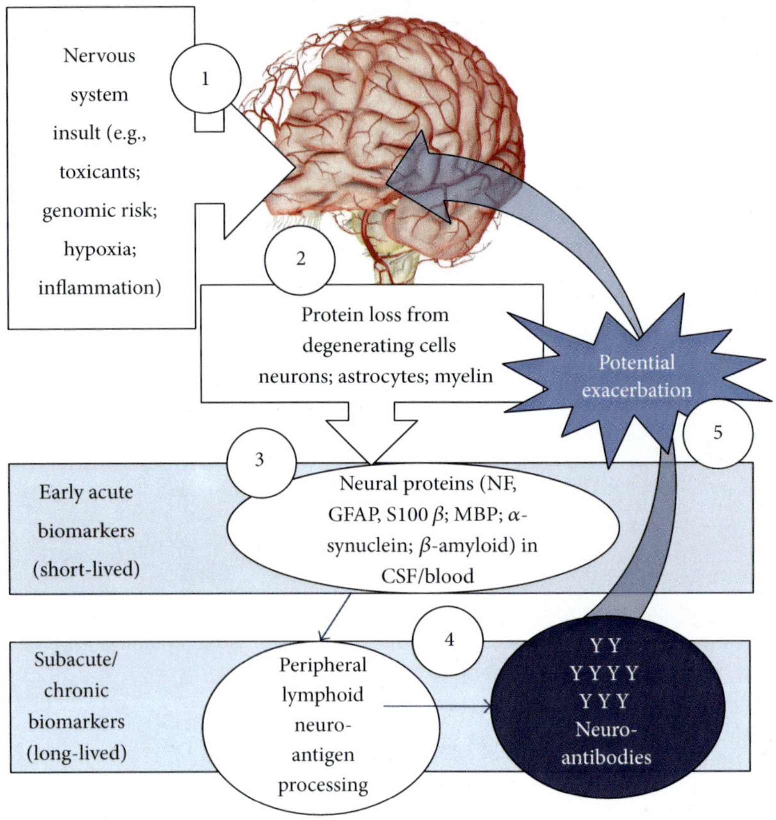

FIGURE 1: (1, 2) In the presence of toxicant-induced neurodegeneration, alterations in intracellular structural proteins and proteolysis, antigens (e.g., neuronal neurofilaments, α-synuclein, β-amyloid) are released into (3) the CSF and blood where (4) they are processed by antigen-presenting cells (APC) in the lymphoid tissue to induce humoral autoimmune responses. This autoimmune response, manifested in the form of autoantibodies, provides an accessible biomarker of neurotoxic effects [5]. These antibodies may propagate neurodegenerative changes through complement activation and direct targeting of the neural and vascular architecture, particularly in the presence of increased vascular permeability. Modified from [5].

context, it should be noted that the threshold (i.e., quantity of autoantigen) to produce an immune response is significantly less than the magnitude of neuronal loss to detect overt clinical manifestations (e.g., 60–80% nigrostriatal 3 dopaminergic neuronal loss in PD, [15]).

The parallels between neurodegeneration and neurotoxicities, including the generation of NAb, have recently been reviewed [5] and will not be detailed here. This has included preclinical and clinical studies of acute and chronic exposures to heavy metals (inorganic lead, methyl mercury, trimethyl tin) organic compounds (insecticides, solvents, and organophosphorus compounds) and in hemodialysis patients [16–24]. Rather, this review will use examples to highlight the utility of NAb and future challenges in the sphere of neurotoxicity, ND, and AID.

3. Approach

For the toxicologist, experimental and clinical, pursuing the development and use of biomarkers, it is of great benefit to bear in mind two guiding principles. The first of these is the association between the biomarker and the associated cellular substrate in terms of relevance. For the neurotoxicologist, even if evaluating an environmental exposure of unknown neurotoxic potential, proteins unique to the NS should be identified. While many investigations in the last two decades have measured blood cytokine levels with interest in a particular system insult, because of investigator specialty, the relevance of these cytokines can only be revealing if tied into that system of interest by a measure unique to that system. It also becomes incumbent on the investigator that she/he recognizes that, for environmental exposures, multiple organs may be targeted by toxic compounds. For examples, PCB or lead may target the liver, the kidney, reproductive system(s), and immune and nervous systems. The detection of biomarkers against the liver, the kidney, or reproductive system(s) does not minimize or preclude the relevance and toxicity of having detected biomarkers that indicate NS involvement, only because other organ systems are involved.

The second principle to bear in mind, particularly with the increased interest in gene-environment, environment-ND, and environment-AID associations, is that preclinical and prospective clinical toxicology studies provide a model paradigm to develop and validate emerging biomarkers for genetic/genomic risk, ND, and AID. While strides have been

TABLE 2: Protein antigens, their cellular source, and function.

Cell	Protein	Function
Neuron	Neurofilament (NF) Triplet*	Neuronal intermediate filaments (IF)
	NF-L (light; NF-68)	Mechanical stability of soma, dendrites, and axon
	NF-M (medium; NF-160)	Mechanical stability of soma, dendrites, and axon
	NF-H (heavy; NF-200)	Together with NF-L and NF-M, mechanical stability of the axon
Astrocyte	Glial fibrillary acidic protein (GFAP)	IF of mature astrocytes biomarker of reactive gliosis
	Vimentin	IF transiently expressed during development
Myelinating cells	Myelin basic protein (MBP)	Compaction protein of myelin in CNS and PNS
Oligodendroglia	Myelin oligodendrocyte protein (MOG)	CNS myelin
Schwann Cell	Peripheral myelin protein-22 (PMP-22)	PNS myelin

*Individual proteins differ in their immunogenicity.

made in developing biomarkers of ND, if one looks at the AD, PD, or ALS literature, these biomarkers are, more often than not, developed in patients with overt ND, robbing them of their predictive value as to disease outcome. However, with a "training set" of environmental chemicals, if a biomarker is developed that indicates the likelihood of neurodegenerative changes *prior* to emergence of frank deficits and pathology, such a biomarker would likely prove of benefit in defining idiopathic ND, as well.

A useful approach in the development and validation of NAb has been predicated on three tiers.

(1) Do NAb indicate neuropathology, regardless of a specific etiological factor (toxicity, physical trauma, ND)? This recognizes that there are common protein substrates (autoantigens) found in all neurons (e.g., neurofilaments (NF)), astrocytes (e.g., GFAP), and elaborated by myelinating cells (e.g., myelin basic protein (MBP)).

(2) Can NAb that identifies a unique cellular target (e.g., cholinergic versus catecholaminergic neurons)? This recognizes that there are neurotransmitter proteins, particularly enzymes (e.g., acetylcholinesterase (AChE), tyrosine hydroxylase), neuron-specific structural proteins (e.g., DARP-32 in dopaminergic neuron), or protein aggregates (α-synuclein, β-amyloid). It also recognizes that different neurotoxicants and neurodegenerative conditions target different populations of neural cells.

(3) Are NAb pathogenic? This recognizes that autoantibodies which may be epiphenomena, secondary to injury, have frequently been shown to have agonistic or antagonistic activity, bind (and penetrate) cells, as well as activate complement and other immune effectors.

Whenever possible, it is prudent to look for concordance between experimental and clinical studies. The study and figures below demonstrate the tiered approach using organophosphate-induced delayed polyneuropathy (OPIDP) as an example.

4. Application

In this proof of concept approach, the Neurotoxicology Laboratory has chosen the detection of NAb against proteins representing the cellular heterogeneity of the nervous system, while being common to all neurons, regardless of specialization based on neurotransmitters. Some of these protein antigens and the cellular substrates they represent are summarized in Table 2.

Organophosphorus compounds represent a large class of chemical agents that include insecticides and nerve agents, as well as chemicals that are used as lubricants, fuel, and industrial additives. The acute toxicity of the insecticides and nerve agents due to severe AChE and pseudoesterase inhibition has long been recognized. Chronic low level exposure may induce what is known as an intermediate syndrome, whereas acute single exposures of lubricant, fuel, and industrial additives may induce a central-peripheral neuropathy known as OPIDP. This is believed to be independent of anti-AChE activity, although some AChE inhibitors may also precipitate OPIDP. We have previously published result of NAb utility in OPIDP induced by phenyl saligenin phosphate (PSP) and amelioration with calcium channel blockade in the hen, the Environmental Protection Agency's (EPA) mandated model [23]. These results have been confirmed in humans by AbouDonia and colleagues [25].

In a study confirming our 2008 [23] findings, NAb, IgG (avian IgY), against NF, GFAP, and MBP were detected in hens as early as 7 days following a single dose of PSP (Figure 2). Titers of anti-NF, but not GFAP or MBP, NAb significantly correlated with changes in gait considered indicative of ataxia in OPIDP, decrease in stride length, and increase in width (Table 3). The lack of associations with GFAP and MBP is consistent with the primary targeting of neurons in OPIDP, although the earlier study did show associations with anti-MBP, secondary myelin involvement, and scored clinical ataxia [23, 26]. In addition, IgG against AChE was detected in sera of these hens (Figure 3). In a preliminary study, Ig fraction separated by dialysis, when incubated with the biventer cervicis nerve-muscle preparation [26] increased the magnitude of twitch responses of fast muscle fibers to electrical stimulation, as well as the response of slow muscle

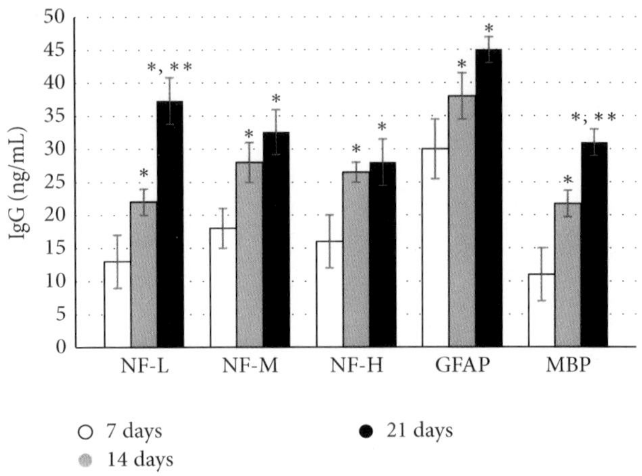

FIGURE 2: Serum titers of IgG against neurotypic (NF) and gliotypic (GFAP and MBP) proteins in hens ($n = 7$) administered a single dose of OPIDP-inducing phenyl saligenin phosphate (2.5 mg/kg, im). Serum was collected at 7, 14, and 21 days. Mean levels of IgG (±S.E.) were significantly ($^*P < 0.05$) higher at 14 and 21 days compared to 7 days. With the exception of anti-NF-L and anti-MBP titers, there were no statistical differences between 14 and 21 days, suggesting peaking of the anti-NF-M, anti-NF-H, and anti-GFAP titers against these antigens. There was no detectable titer of antibodies against these antigens in control hens or in sera of hens prior to PSP administration.

TABLE 3: Pearson's correlation coefficients for antineurofilament IgG titers and changes in gait length and width of hens monitored for 21 days*.

IgG	Stride length		Stride width	
	r	P	r	P
Anti-NF-L	−0.45	0.04	0.52	0.01
Anti-NF-M	−0.47	0.04	0.48	0.03
Anti-NF-H	−0.33	0.10	0.42	0.05
Anti-GFAP	−0.11	0.63	0.21	0.36
Anti-MBP	−0.23	0.31	0.34	0.13

*Total gait measurements; $n = 21$ measured gaits.

fibers to exogenous acetylcholine (Figure 4). This indicates that serum elements may have had inhibitory activity on catabolic enzyme or agonistic activity. This was further confirmed, in part, by measuring muscle homogenate AChE activity in the absence and presence of dialysis fractions of pooled sera with detectable anti-AChE antibodies (Figure 5).

It is important to insert a word of caution regarding the use of autoantibody detection in the context of toxicological studies, in general, and for neurotoxicology, in particular. Classical toxicology (and pharmacology) is quite often wed to dose, where an increase in dose beyond threshold is predicted to result in an increase in response and by extension deficits. While, in our experience, this is frequently the case, it quite often may not hold true when measuring an immune response. Several factors are likely to account for this. In brief, the following should be recognized.

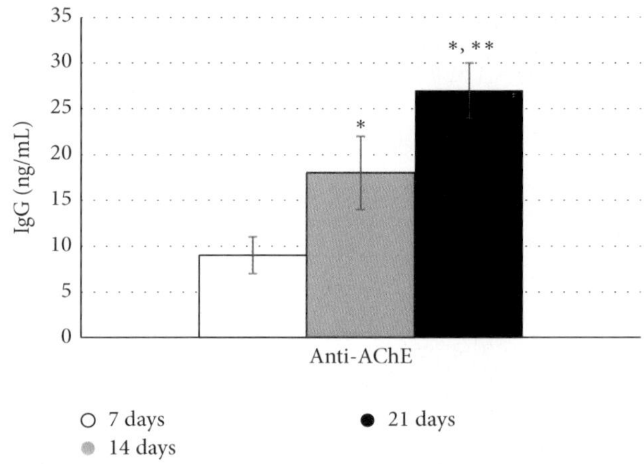

FIGURE 3: Serum titers of IgG against AChE, the enzyme responsible for acetylcholine hydrolysis, in hens ($n = 7$) administered a single dose of OPIDP-inducing phenyl saligenin phosphate (PSP, 2.5 mg/kg, im). Serum was collected at 7, 14, and 21 days. Mean levels of IgG (±S.E.) were significantly ($^*P < 0.05$) higher at 14 and 21 days compared to 7 days and at 21 days compared to 14 days ($^{**}P < 0.05$). Although OPIDP development is believed to be independent of AChE inhibition, some organophosphates may induce acute inhibition and phosphorylation of the enzyme.

(1) Traditional measurements of internal dose, exposure biomarkers, to an environmental agent often reflect cross-sectional measurements (single time point), ignoring the kinetics and accumulation of the agent and where it may be sequestered (e.g., blood lead). They do not necessarily reflect past exposures or biological response. Borrowing from the virology and vaccine literature [27], in developing and validating NAb as biomarkers of neurotoxicity, the question is that given a particular exposure are these autoantibodies present and do they exceed background or the "natural repertoire" of antibodies. In the latter case, determination of antibody class and subclass is also likely to be useful.

(2) The immune response, cellular and humoral, is a dynamic processes, but not infinite. Classical studies of immunoglobulin responses to vaccines recognize fluctuations and peaking of immunoglobulin production to a given antigen. It is likely that autoantibody levels peak even in the presence of continued exposure or accumulation of toxic chemicals.

(3) Antibodies changes in affinity and avidity with repeated exposure to antigen and the development of immunological memory. It is useful in preclinical studies to harvest lymphoid tissue for cell isolation and *in vitro* challenge. It should also be recognized that antigens have multiple epitopes which impacts on polyclonal titer levels, as well as the exposure of new epitopes that may not be exposed in the native protein(s).

(4) In the presence of high levels of circulating released antigens, including autoantigens, due to progressive

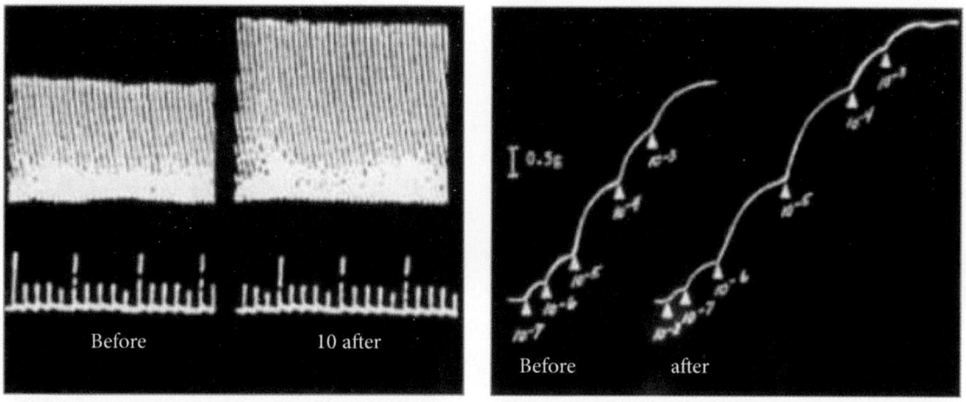

FIGURE 4: Representative original polygraph tracings of chicken biventer cervicis nerve-muscle preparation (in Krebs-Henseleit solution aerated with 95% O_2/5% CO_2) in response to electrical stimulation of fast twitch fibers and contraction to exogenous acetylcholine (slow muscle fibers) in the presence (after) and absence (before) of pooled immunoglobulin fraction (21 days after PSP administration). This suggests that these serum immunoglobulins may alter neuromuscular function.

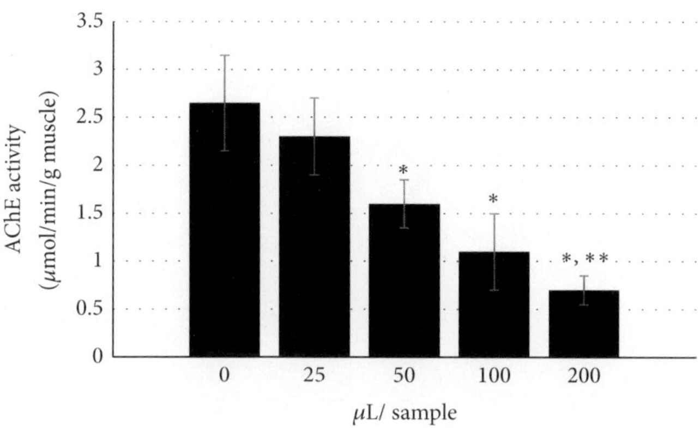

FIGURE 5: Activity of skeletal muscle homogenate AChE in the in the presence of different volumes of pooled serum Ig fraction from hens ($n = 7$) at 21 days following a single exposure to OPIDP-inducing phenyl saligenin phosphate (PSP, 2.5 mg/kg, im). This confirms that serum elements, possibly the detected anti-AChE, may interfere with neuromuscular function as observed in the isolated muscle preparations (see Figure 4).

and significant insult, antigen-antibody complexes are formed which gives misleading low titer levels in traditional assays (i.e., ELISA and microarray), since the Ig is already bound in the serum. It may also suggest that these autoantibodies are bound to cellular targets *in vivo*. In our own work, we have noted these decreases followed by rebound in chronic progressive neuropathologies.

It should be noted that in the context of environment-AID and environment-NAb interactions many of these issues remain to be addressed.

5. Challenges

5.1. Neurotoxicity of Nanoparticles. Linking environmental exposures to ND and AID is a challenge, particularly with the increase in both disorders. Ironically, the development of biomarkers of effects for the vast number of industrial and pharmaceutical chemicals remains a work in progress, yet with technological progress we continue to introduce new materials. The emergence of nanotechnology, which takes advantage of the unique physicochemical properties of submicron-sized nanomaterials, has profoundly impacted every aspect of daily life in the 21st century. In biomedical fields, the demand for nanotechnology and its applications is rapidly growing. Evidence for rapid growth of nanotechnology is reflected by the increase in the annual budget for the National Nanotechnology Initiative from \$650 million in 2005 to \$1.7 billion in 2014 [27] and by its annual growth rate of more than 17% [28, 29]. The National Science Foundation estimated that in the near future half of all pharmaceutical industry products will have some association with nanotechnology [30]. In spite of public concerns over their potential health impacts [31–35], comparatively little effort has been devoted to understanding the safety profiles of these nanomaterials. From a toxicology perspective, nanoparticles (NPs) possess important characteristic features, which differ from the features of their native parent materials and are greatly influenced by the formulation of NPs. Hence, there is a clear need to better understand the potential adverse health effects associated with emerging nanotechnologies, their biocompatibility, and potential toxicity.

Oberdörster and his collaborators [36–38] and Elder et al. [39] have demonstrated and reviewed studies that inhaled and possibly ingested or topically applied ultrafine particles can be translocated to the brain and nervous system. This translocation is likely to be via the olfactory bulbs and/or the systemic circulation. In the latter case this would involve movement across the blood-brain barrier (BBB), a key strategy for drug delivery using NP [40, 41]. Because of their size, which falls within the same range as viruses, it is possible that systemically distributed NP may also gain access to the nervous system at the neuromuscular junction (NMJ), similar to the poliovirus [42]. Transport whether from the olfactory nerves, the NMJ, or within the brain would

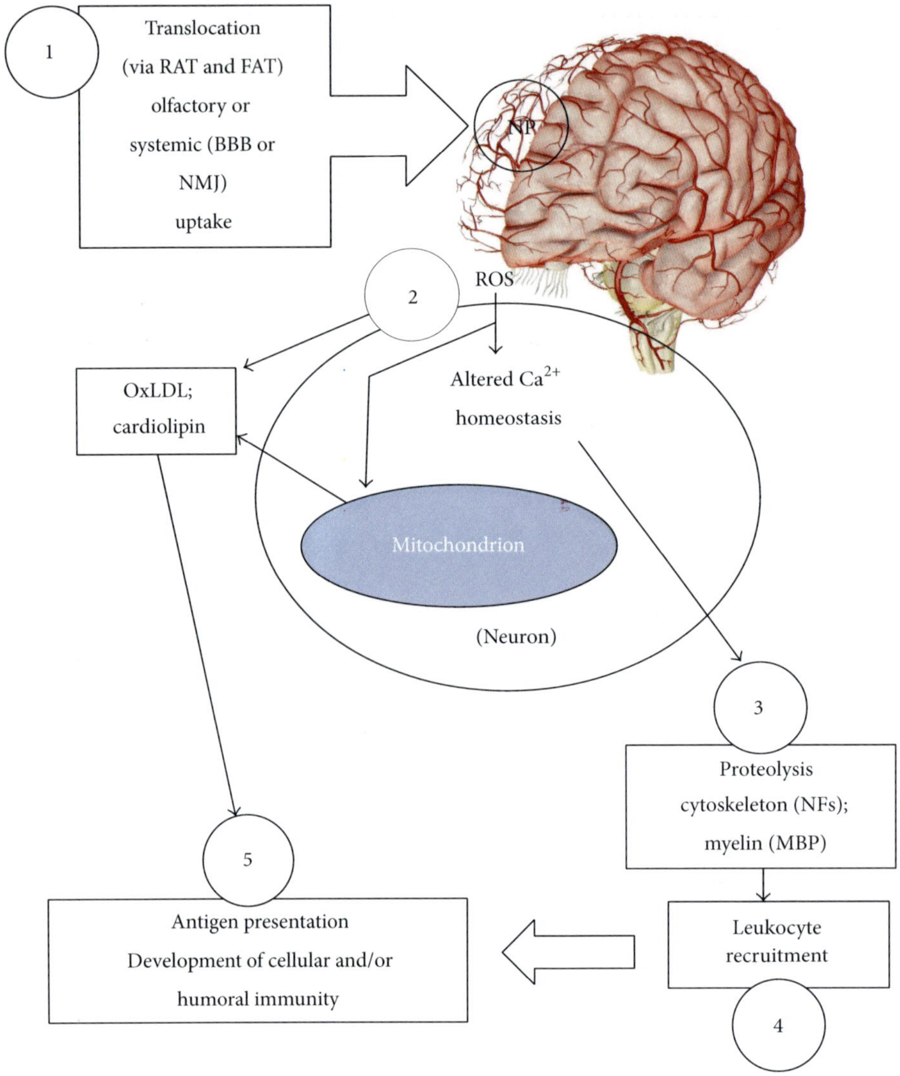

FIGURE 6: Mechanisms by which NP produce neurotoxicity and resulting autoantibody generation. (1) Translocation of NP introduced via the olfactory bulbs (or neuromuscular junction: NMJ) to the nervous system via retrograde (RAT) and fast anterograde (FAT) transport; (2) translocated NP may induce lipid peroxidation (e.g., LDL) and oxidative stress, as well as Ca^{2+} overload and displacement from ER/mitochondria; (3) cytoskeletal proteolysis, as a result of Ca^{2+} overload, which also results in mitochondrial derangement (e.g., cardiolipin dissociation). These events result in exposure of autoantigens; (4) recruitment of immune effectors, including microglia, *in situ*, and peripheral leukocytes; (5) antigen processing, presentation, and antibody production in lymphoid tissue.

likely rely on retrograde axonal transport (RAT) and fast anterograde axonal transport (FAT). Assessment of possible neurodegenerative changes or neurotoxic potential of NP is relatively new. Combustion-derived NPs are capable of being translocated to the brain. One example, manganese oxide, generated during arc welding, may be an occupational contributor to PD in susceptible individuals [43].

In several reviews and opinion papers [44, 45], it has been suggested that NP may precipitate autoimmune responses in exposed individuals by acting as haptens, exposing cytoskeletal elements, or promoting degeneration as a consequence of calcium overload. Based on published evidence, we have hypothesized that NPs and agents not normally considered neurotoxic may induce NS insult if generated as NPs (Figure 6).

In a preliminary study using arc-spark generated nickel NPs (≤40 nm; Ni-NP), a metal not typically associated with neurotoxicity, mice were assessed for the generation of NAb against NF, GFAP and MBP following chronic inhalation exposure of 6 weeks. The mice used included wild type C57BL/6 and their $APO^{-/-}$ (knockout counterpart). The choice of this model for neurotoxicity studies of NP is to provide a model of a human population susceptible to neurodegeneration. $ApoE^{-/-}$ mice have been shown to be susceptible to excitotoxicity in models of AD [44, 45], hyperphosphorylation of *tau* [46, 47], sensitivity to synaptic derangement [48, 49], and an increased susceptibility to oxidative damage [50]. These are believed to mimic changes associated with aging and increased susceptibility to nervous system damage following trauma and stroke. In addition,

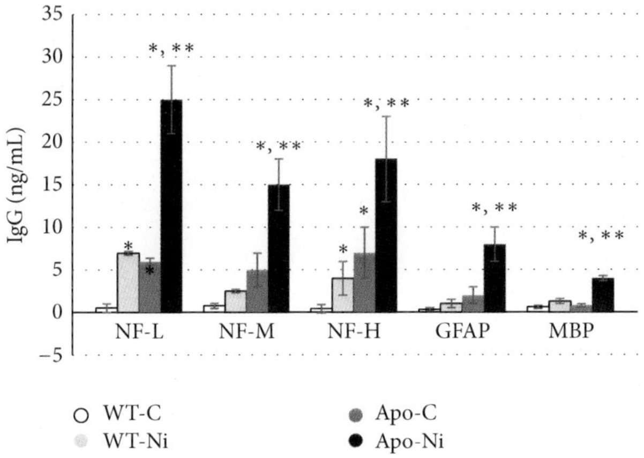

FIGURE 7: Inhalation exposure of wild-type C57BL/6 (WT) and ApoE knock out male mice to arc-spark generated Ni-NP (≤40 nm; 5 h/wk for 6 wks) resulted in detectable levels of IgG against neurotypic (NF) and gliotypic (GFAP and MBP) proteins. Levels of IgG were significantly ($P < 0.05$) higher in ApoE$^{-/-}$ mice exposed to Ni-NP compared to WT controls, WT exposed to Ni-NP (∗) or ApoE$^{-/-}$ control mice (∗∗) (inhalation exposures conducted by L. C. Chen and P. Gillespie at New York University Institute of Environmental Medicine).

although there are apparently no differences in lymphocyte populations, ApoE$^{-/-}$ mice tend to respond stronger to antigen challenge and may be predisposed to autoimmunity [51], including the development of autoantibodies to nervous system antigens [52].

Titer levels, both IgM and IgG, were detected in sera of mice. Levels of NAb and IgG are shown in Figure 7. While wild type mice exposed to Ni-NP had detectable levels of NAb against all antigens, the more susceptible ApoE null mice had significantly higher titers. In addition titers of anticardiolipin (ACA) and antioxidized LDL (oxLDL) were also detected (not shown).

OxLDL has been shown to accumulate in astrocytes following cerebral infarcts and stimulates IL6 release from astrocytes in culture [53], while ACA have been shown to reduce viability of neuronal cultures [54] and damage to cerebral white and gray matter and inhibit astrocyte function [55, 56].

With the increased development and use of NP in industry and as therapeutic delivery systems, the safety of nanoengineered particles and anthropogenic NP (i.e., ultrafine particle pollutants) should be a priority. Utilizing NAb detection, particularly with inhalation exposure, would provide a cost-effective option in determining neurotoxicity.

5.2. Angiogenesis, Neurodegeneration, and Autoimmunity. Angiogenesis, the elaboration of neovasculature, has emerged as playing a central role on both ND and AID. Despite this and the significant role played by vascularization in neurodevelopment, maintenance of the nervous system, and inflammatory autoimmunity, it remains a neglected area of research in the field of toxicology, outside the sphere of carcinogenesis.

Recently completed studies from the Neurotoxicology Laboratory and Pharmaceutical Research Institute have demonstrated that neurotoxic thyromimetic PCB induce angiogenesis through the $\alpha v\beta 3$ integrin receptor. Not only is this receptor responsible for mediating proangiogenic activity of thyroid hormone, but it is also targeted by vascular endothelial growth factor (VEGF) and basic fibroblast growth factor (bFGF). The $\alpha v\beta 3$ integrin receptor also activates Th17 lymphocytes. The role of these cells in neuroinflammation and neuroimmunity has recently been reviewed by Vojdani et al. and Marwaha et al. [57, 58]. Th17, designated as such because of the production of IL-17, may be major effector of autoimmunity [59, 60], including the production of antibodies, where they provide B help [61, 62]. In addition, recent evidence implicates Th17 and ND such as PD, AD, and MS [63, 64]. Relevant to the toxicity of PCB is evidence that Th17 differentiation and activity may be mediated via $\alpha v\beta 3$ integrin receptors in experimental autoimmune encephalopathy [65] or via the aryl-hydrocarbon receptor (AHR) [66], of which several PCB congeners are agonists. In addition, IL-17 has been shown to induce VEGF release, thereby contributing to encephalopathy in SLE [67]. Furthermore, the participation of VEGF and angiogenesis in AID, reviewed by Shoenfeld's group [68], plays a significant role in SLE, RA, and MS. In ND, angiogenesis and hypervascularization mediated by VEGF and $\alpha v\beta 3$ integrin receptor-dependent process with ensuing hyperpermeability has been reported [69–77]. In addition, activation of the $\alpha v\beta 3$ receptor plays a role in recruitment of leukocytes in response to CCL2 (aka MCP-1) produced from astrocytes [78] and in response to ICAM and VCAM [79]. This is consistent with the localization of $\alpha v\beta 3$ integrin to T and B lymphocytes for interaction with the vitronectin matrix during migration and endothelial interactions [80]. The participation of $\alpha v\beta 3$ integrin receptor in angiogenesis and immune cell migration and activation in AID underlies its promising potential as a therapeutic target in RA [81] and experimental glomerulonephritis [82].

In the context of the NS, aside from angiogenesis, $\alpha v\beta 3$ is implicated in upregulation of glutamate receptor production and excitotoxicity [83, 84], major effector of neurotoxicity and ND [5]. It is relevant that some PCB increase extracellular glutamate availability by inhibiting its uptake into astrocytes [85]. $\alpha v\beta 3$ integrin is also implicated in reactive astrogliosis, a hallmark of neurotoxicity, and inhibition of neurite growth and process retraction [86], while $\alpha v\beta 3$ integrin receptors play a role in microglia-induced neuroinflammation models of AD, PD, MS, and ALS [87–89].

Taken together, hypervascularization in the nervous system, as demonstrated in the pathogenesis of ND, and increased permeability may provide opportunities for toxicant entry and NAb penetration into the CNS, thereby exacerbating neuropathology.

6. Conclusion

Emerging recognition that environmental agents may play a role in ND and AID and that many ND have an autoimmune and/or autoinflammatory component provides not only potential targets of intervention but also biomarkers of effect. Defining these interactions and capitalizing on the humoral immune response, in the form of autoantibodies, provide accessible markers for predicting and diagnosing neurological outcome. As epiphenomena, secondary to initial insult, regardless of etiological factor(s), these NAbs may be indices of neurotoxicity and neurodegenerative processes, as well as a means of monitoring therapeutic efficacy. The potential contribution of NAb to the pathogenesis of ND and neurotoxicity, whether through complement activation, activation of phagocytes, or exacerbation of neuroinflammation, needs to be delineated. This may be a key to understanding disease progression and developing effective interventions in environmentally induced disease. Work over the last two decades in neurotoxicology has concentrated, for the most part, on the use of NAb in preclinical studies and remains to be validated in large cohorts of at-risk humans. In attempts at clinical translation, it should be recognized that immune responses in the presence of exposure may not adhere to the dogma of dose response. It is also important that one should not lose sight of the reality that environmental agents often demonstrate pleiotropic activity, impacting multiple systems. It should also be noted that cellular immune response remains unexplored in the context of neurotoxicology.

In tandem with the use NAb of as potential biomarkers, initial studies have begun to explore the pathogenicity of NAb generated in response to some environmental chemicals. It is also believed that development and validation of biomarkers that capitalize on the immune response may prove useful for determining the safety and/or potential toxicity of emerging technologies (i.e., nanoengineered materials).

Finally, for both the neurotoxicologist and immunotoxicologist, a long neglected area of research at the crossroads of ND and AID is angiogenesis and the effect of chemicals, directly and indirectly, in promoting increased vascular permeability and providing an avenue of disease exacerbation.

Conflict of Interests

The author declares that there is no conflict of interests regarding the publication of this paper.

References

[1] "Neurological disorders: public health challenges," World Health Organization, 2006.

[2] "Environmental Health Criteria 236. Principles and Methods for Assessing Autoimmunity Associated with Exposure to Chemicals," WHO Task Group on Environmental Health Criteria. WHO Report, 2006.

[3] C. Selmi, P. S. C. Leung, D. H. Sherr et al., "Mechanisms of environmental influence on human autoimmunity: a national institute of environmental health sciences expert panel workshop," *Journal of Autoimmunity*, vol. 39, no. 4, pp. 272–284, 2012.

[4] F. W. Miller, L. Alfredsson, K. H. Costenbader et al., "Epidemiology of environmental exposures and human autoimmune diseases: findings from a National Institute of Environmental Health Sciences Expert Panel Workshop," *Journal of Autoimmunity*, vol. 39, no. 4, pp. 259–271, 2012.

[5] H. A. N. El-Fawal, "Neurotoxicology," in *Encyclopedia of Environmental Health*, J. O. Nriagu, Ed., vol. 4, pp. 87–106, Elsevier, Burlington, Mass, USA, 2011.

[6] C. Perricone, S. Colafrancesco, R. D. Mazor, A. Soriano, N. Agmon-Levin, and Y. Shoenfeld, "Autoimmune/inflammatory syndrome induced by adjuvants (ASIA) 2013: unveiling the pathogenic, clinical and diagnostic aspects," *Journal of Autoimmunity*, vol. 47, pp. 1–16, 2013.

[7] H. Tumani, C. Teunissen, S. Süssmuth, M. Otto, A. C. Ludolph, and J. Brettschneider, "Cerebrospinal fluid biomarkers of neurodegeneration in chronic neurological diseases," *Expert Review of Molecular Diagnostics*, vol. 8, no. 4, pp. 479–494, 2008.

[8] L. M. Shaw, M. Korecka, C. M. Clark, V. M.-Y. Lee, and J. Q. Trojanowski, "Biomarkers of neurodegeneration for diagnosis and monitoring therapeutics," *Nature Reviews Drug Discovery*, vol. 6, no. 4, pp. 295–303, 2007.

[9] L. E. Pelinka, M. Jafarmadar, H. Redl, and S. Bahrami, "Neuron-specific-enolase is increased in plasma after hemorrhagic shock and after bilateral femur fracture without traumatic brain injury in the rat," *Shock*, vol. 22, no. 1, pp. 88–91, 2004.

[10] G. Ghanem, B. Loir, R. Morandini et al., "On the release and half-life of S100B protein in the peripheral blood of melanoma patients," *International Journal of Cancer*, vol. 94, no. 4, pp. 586–590, 2001.

[11] W. Townend, C. Dibble, K. Abid, A. Vail, R. Sherwood, and F. Lecky, "Rapid elimination of protein S-100B from serum after minor head trauma," *Journal of Neurotrauma*, vol. 23, no. 2, pp. 149–155, 2006.

[12] M. C. C. Lim, G. Maubach, and L. Zhuo, "Glial fibrillary acidic protein splice variants in hepatic stellate cells—expression and regulation," *Molecules and Cells*, vol. 25, no. 3, pp. 376–384, 2008.

[13] J. R. McDermott and A. B. Keith, "Relative effectiveness of spinal cord and purified myelin basic protein in producing resistance to experimental allergic encephalomyelitis," *European Neurology*, vol. 18, no. 2, pp. 136–139, 1979.

[14] H. M. Snyder, M. C. Carrillo, F. Grodstein et al., "Developing novel blood-based biomarkers for Alzheimer's disease," *Alzheimers and Dementia*, vol. 10, pp. 109–114, 2014.

[15] S. Fahn, "Description of Parkinson's disease as a clinical syndrome," *Annals of the New York Academy of Sciences*, vol. 991, pp. 1–14, 2003.

[16] S. J. Waterman, H. A. N. El-Fawal, and C. A. Snyder, "Lead alters the immunogenicity of two neural proteins: a potential mechanism for the progression of lead-induced neurotoxicity," *Environmental Health Perspectives*, vol. 102, no. 12, pp. 1052–1056, 1994.

[17] H. A. N. El-Fawal, Z. Gong, A. R. Little, and H. L. Evans, "Exposure to methylmercury results in serum autoantibodies to neurotypic and gliotypic proteins," *NeuroToxicology*, vol. 17, no. 2, pp. 531–540, 1996.

[18] R. McConnell, E. Delgado-Téllez, R. Cuadra et al., "Organophosphate neuropathy due to methamidophos: biochemical and neurophysiological markers," *Archives of Toxicology*, vol. 73, no. 6, pp. 296–300, 1999.

[19] I. A. Moneim, M. Y. Shamy, R. M. el-Gazzar, and H. A. el-Fawal, "Autoantibodies to neurofilaments (NF), glial fibrillary acidic protein (GFAP) and myelin basic protein (MBP) in workers exposed to lead," *The Journal of the Egyptian Public Health Association*, vol. 74, no. 1-2, pp. 121–138, 1999.

[20] H. A. N. El-Fawal, S. J. Waterman, A. De Feo, and M. Y. Shamy, "Neuroimmunotoxicology: humoral assessment of neurotoxicity and autoimmune mechanisms," *Environmental Health Perspectives*, vol. 107, no. 5, supplement, pp. 767–775, 1999.

[21] H. A. N. El-Fawal and J. P. O'Callaghan, "Autoantibodies to neurotypic and gliotypic proteins as biomarkers of neurotoxicity: assessment of trimethyltin (TMT)," *NeuroToxicology*, vol. 29, no. 1, pp. 109–115, 2008.

[22] G. Surendran and H. A. N. El-Fawal, "Neuroimmune responses to toxic agents: comparison of organometal electrophiles using detection of antibodies to neural cytoskeleton and myelin as biomarkers," *Journal of Pharmacology and Toxicology*, vol. 3, no. 3, pp. 173–189, 2008.

[23] H. A. N. El-Fawal and W. C. McCain, "Monitoring the development of organophosphorusinduced delayed neuropathy (OPIDN) and its amelioration," *Neurotoxicology and Teratology*, vol. 30, no. 3, pp. 161–166, 2008.

[24] D. L. Mason, M. M. Assimon, J. R. Bishop, and H. A. N. El-Fawal, "Nervous system autoantibodies and vitamin D receptor gene polymorphisms in hemodialysis patients," *Hemodialysis International*, vol. 17, no. 1, pp. 3–11, 2013.

[25] M. B. Abou-Donia, M. M. Abou-Donia, E. M. Elmasry, J. A. Monro, and M. F. A. Mulder, "Autoantibodies to nervous system-specific proteins are elevated in sera of flight crew members: biomarkers for nervous system injury," *Journal of Toxicology and Environmental Health A*, vol. 76, no. 6, pp. 363–380, 2013.

[26] H. A. N. El-Fawal, B. S. Jortner, P. Eyre, and M. Ehrich, "The biventer cervicis nerve-muscle preparation of adult hens: effects of phenyl saligenin phosphate administration," *NeuroToxicology*, vol. 9, no. 4, pp. 625–636, 1988.

[27] C. A. Siegrist, "Vaccine immunology," in *Vaccines*, S. A. Plotkin, W. A. Orenstein, and P. A. Offit, Eds., pp. 17–36, Elsevier, 6th edition, 2013.

[28] National Nanotechnology Initiative, 2013, http://www.nano.gov/about-nni/what/funding.

[29] T. F. Group, "Nanotechnology in Health Care, US Industry Study with Forecasts to 2011, 2016 & 2021," The Freedonia Group, Cleveland, Ohio, USA, 2007.

[30] Lux Research, *The Nanotech Report: Investment Overview and Market Research for Nanotechnology*, Lux Research, New York, NY, USA, 4th edition, 2007.

[31] D. J. Bharali and S. A. Mousa, "Emerging nanomedicines for early cancer detection and improved treatment: current perspective and future promise," *Pharmacology and Therapeutics*, vol. 128, no. 2, pp. 324–335, 2010.

[32] S. T. Stern and S. E. McNeil, "Nanotechnology safety concerns revisited," *Toxicological Sciences*, vol. 101, no. 1, pp. 4–21, 2008.

[33] P. Borm, F. C. Klaessig, T. D. Landry et al., "Research strategies for safety evaluation of nanomaterials—part V: role of dissolution in biological fate and effects of nanoscale particles," *Toxicological Sciences*, vol. 90, no. 1, pp. 23–32, 2006.

[34] R. Dagani, "Nanomaterials: safe or unsafe?" *Chemical and Engineering News*, vol. 81, no. 17, pp. 30–33, 2003.

[35] B. Fadeel and A. E. Garcia-Bennett, "Better safe than sorry: understanding the toxicological properties of inorganic nanoparticles manufactured for biomedical applications," *Advanced Drug Delivery Reviews*, vol. 62, no. 3, pp. 362–374, 2010.

[36] G. Oberdörster, Z. Sharp, V. Atudorei et al., "Extrapulmonary translocation of ultrafine carbon particles following whole-body inhalation exposure of rats," *Journal of Toxicology and Environmental Health A*, vol. 65, no. 20, pp. 1531–1543, 2002.

[37] G. Oberdörster, E. Oberdörster, and J. Oberdörster, "Nanotoxicology: an emerging discipline evolving from studies of ultrafine particles," *Environmental Health Perspectives*, vol. 113, no. 7, pp. 823–839, 2005.

[38] G. Oberdörster, Z. Sharp, V. Atudorei et al., "Translocation of inhaled ultrafine particles to the brain," *Inhalation Toxicology*, vol. 16, no. 6-7, pp. 437–445, 2004.

[39] A. Elder, R. Gelein, V. Silva et al., "Translocation of inhaled ultrafine manganese oxide particles to the central nervous system," *Environmental Health Perspectives*, vol. 114, no. 8, pp. 1172–1178, 2006.

[40] A. Peters, B. Veronesi, and L. Calderón-Garcidueñas, "Translocation and potential neurological effects of fine and ultrafine particles a critical update," *Particle and Fibre Toxicology*, vol. 3, pp. 13–26, 2006.

[41] K. Ringe, C. M. Walz, and B. A. Sabel, "Nanoparticle drug delivery to the brain," *Encyclopedia of Nanoscience and Nanotechnology*, vol. 7, pp. 91–104, 2005.

[42] J.-C. Olivier, "Drug transport to brain with targeted nanoparticles," *NeuroRx*, vol. 2, no. 1, pp. 108–119, 2005.

[43] S. Ohka, N. Matsuda, K. Tohyama et al., "Receptor (CD155)-dependent endocytosis of poliovirus and retrograde axonal transport of the endosome," *Journal of Virology*, vol. 78, no. 13, pp. 7186–7198, 2004.

[44] G. McMillan, "Is electric arc welding linked to manganism or Parkinson's disease?" *Toxicological Reviews*, vol. 24, no. 4, pp. 237–257, 2005.

[45] P. J. A. Borm and W. Kreyling, "Toxicological hazards of inhaled nanoparticles—potential implications for drug delivery," *Journal of Nanoscience and Nanotechnology*, vol. 4, no. 5, pp. 521–531, 2004.

[46] M. Buttini, M. Orth, S. Bellosta et al., "Expression of human apolipoprotein E3 or E4 in the brains of Apoe(-/-) mice: isoform-specific effects on neurodegeneration," *Journal of Neuroscience*, vol. 19, no. 12, pp. 4867–4880, 1999.

[47] I. Genis, I. Gordon, E. Sehayek, and D. M. Michaelson, "Phosphorylation of tau in apolipoprotein E-deficient mice," *Neuroscience Letters*, vol. 199, no. 1, pp. 5–8, 1995.

[48] W. J. Brecht, F. M. Harris, S. Chang et al., "Neuron-specific apoplipoprotein E4 proteolysis is associated with increased tau phosphorylation in brains of transgenic mice," *Journal of Neuroscience*, vol. 24, no. 10, pp. 2527–2534, 2004.

[49] E. Masliah, M. Mallory, N. Ge, M. Alford, I. Veinbergs, and A. D. Roses, "Neurodegeneration in the central nervous system of apoE-deficient mice," *Experimental Neurology*, vol. 136, no. 2, pp. 107–122, 1995.

[50] S. Chapman and D. M. Michaelson, "Specific neurochemical derangements of brain projecting neurons in apolipoprotein E-deficient mice," *Journal of Neurochemistry*, vol. 70, no. 2, pp. 708–714, 1998.

[51] T. B. Shea, E. Rogers, D. Ashline, D. Ortiz, and M.-S. Sheu, "Apolipoprotein E deficiency promotes increased oxidative stress and compensatory increases in antioxidants in brain tissue," *Free Radical Biology and Medicine*, vol. 33, no. 8, pp. 1115–1120, 2002.

[52] Y. Zhou, A. Cheshire, L. A. Howell, D. H. Ryan, and R. B. S. Harris, "Neuroautoantibody immunoreactivity in relation to aging and stress in apolipoprotein E-deficient mice," *Brain Research Bulletin*, vol. 49, no. 3, pp. 173–179, 1999.

[53] S. Yu, R.-S. Duan, Z. Chen et al., "Increased susceptibility to experimental autoimmune neuritis after upregulation of the

autoreactive T cell response to peripheral myelin antigen in apolipoprotein E-deficient mice," *Journal of Neuropathology and Experimental Neurology*, vol. 63, no. 2, pp. 120–128, 2004.

[54] F.-S. Shie, M. D. Neely, I. Maezawa et al., "Oxidized low-density lipoprotein is present in astrocytes surrounding cerebral infarcts and stimulates astrocyte interleukin-6 secretion," *American Journal of Pathology*, vol. 164, no. 4, pp. 1173–1181, 2004.

[55] C. Andreassi, A. Zoli, A. Riccio et al., "Anticardiolipin antibodies in patients with primary antiphospholipid syndrome: a correlation between IgG titre and antibody-induced cell dysfunctions in neuronal cell cultures," *Clinical Rheumatology*, vol. 20, no. 5, pp. 314–318, 2001.

[56] K.-H. Sun, W.-T. Liu, C.-Y. Tsai, T.-S. Liao, W.-M. Lin, and C.-L. Yu, "Inhibition of astrocyte proliferation and binding to brain tissue of anticardiolipin antibodies purified from lupus serum," *Annals of the Rheumatic Diseases*, vol. 51, no. 6, pp. 707–712, 1992.

[57] A. Vojdani, J. Lambert, and G. Kellermann, "The role of th17 in neuroimmune disorders: a target for cam therapy—part III," *Evidence-Based Complementary and Alternative Medicine*, vol. 2011, Article ID 548086, 11 pages, 2011.

[58] A. K. Marwaha, N. J. Leung, A. N. McMurchy, and M. K. Levings, "TH17 cells in autoimmunity and immunodeficiency: protective orpathogenic?" *Frontiers in Immunology*, vol. 3, Article ID Article 129, 2012.

[59] M. Mitsdoerffer, Y. Lee, A. Jäger et al., "Proinflammatory T helper type 17 cells are effective B-cell helpers," *Proceedings of the National Academy of Sciences of the United States of America*, vol. 107, no. 32, pp. 14292–14297, 2010.

[60] C. L. Hickman-Brecks, J. L. Racz, D. M. Meyer, T. P. LaBranche, and P. M. Allen, "Th17 cells can provide B cell help in autoantibody induced arthritis," *Journal of Autoimmunity*, vol. 36, no. 1, pp. 65–75, 2011.

[61] A. D. Reynolds, D. K. Stone, J. A. L. Hutter, E. J. Benner, R. L. Mosley, and H. E. Gendelman, "Regulatory T cells attenuate Th17 cell-mediated nigrostriatal dopaminergic neurodegeneration in a model of Parkinson's disease," *Journal of Immunology*, vol. 184, no. 5, pp. 2261–2271, 2010.

[62] J. Zhang J, K. F. Ke, Z. Liu, Y. H. Qiu, and Y. P. Peng, "Th17 cell-mediated neuroinflammation is involved in neurodegeneration of aβ1-42-induced Alzheimer's disease model rats," *PLoS ONE*, vol. 4, Article ID e75786, 2013.

[63] M. Acharya, S. Mukhopadhyay, H. Païdassi et al., "αv Integrin expression by DCs is required for Th17 cell differentiation and development of experimental autoimmune encephalomyelitis in mice," *Journal of Clinical Investigation*, vol. 120, no. 12, pp. 4445–4452, 2010.

[64] M. Veldhoen, K. Hirota, A. M. Westendorf et al., "The aryl hydrocarbon receptor links TH17-cell-mediated autoimmunity to environmental toxins," *Nature*, vol. 453, no. 7191, pp. 106–109, 2008.

[65] S. J. Park, K. S. Pai, J. H. Kim, and J. I. Shin, "Could increased vascular endothelial growth factor induced by interleukin 17 be the cause of posterior reversible encephalopathy syndrome in systemic lupus erythematosus?" *Journal of Rheumatology*, vol. 39, no. 4, p. 870, 2012.

[66] J. F. Carvalho, M. Blank, and Y. Shoenfeld, "Vascular endothelial growth factor (VEGF) in autoimmune diseases," *Journal of Clinical Immunology*, vol. 27, no. 3, pp. 246–256, 2007.

[67] O. O. Ogunshola and X. Antoniou, "Contribution of hypoxia to Alzheimer's disease: is HIF-1α a mediator of neurodegeneration?" *Cellular and Molecular Life Sciences*, vol. 66, no. 22, pp. 3555–3563, 2009.

[68] P. Grammas, D. Tripathy, A. Sanchez, X. Yin, and J. Luo, "Brain microvasculature and hypoxia-related proteins in Alzheimer's disease," *International Journal of Clinical and Experimental Pathology*, vol. 4, no. 6, pp. 616–627, 2011.

[69] Z. Zhang, J. Yan, Y. Chang, S. ShiDu Yan, and H. Shi, "Hypoxia inducible factor-1 as a target for neurodegenerative diseases," *Current Medicinal Chemistry*, vol. 18, no. 28, pp. 4335–4343, 2011.

[70] I. Unal-Cevik, Y. Gursoy-Ozdemir, M. Yemisci et al., "Alpha-synuclein aggregation induced by brief ischemia negatively impacts neuronal survival in vivo: a study in A30Palpha-synuclein transgenic mouse," *Journal of Cerebral Blood Flow and Metabolism*, vol. 31, no. 3, pp. 913–923, 2011.

[71] X. Hu, H. C. Rea, J. E. Wiktorowicz, and J. R. Perez-Polo, "Proteomic analysis of hypoxia/ischemia-induced alteration of cortical development and dopamine neurotransmission in neonatal rat," *Journal of Proteome Research*, vol. 5, no. 9, pp. 2396–2404, 2006.

[72] K. E. Biron, D. L. Dickstein, R. Gopaul, and W. A. Jefferies, "Amyloid triggers extensive cerebral angiogenesis causing blood brain barrier permeability and hypervascularity in alzheimer's disease," *PLoS ONE*, vol. 6, no. 8, Article ID e23789, 2011.

[73] K. Wada, H. Arai, M. Takanashi et al., "Expression levels of vascular endothelial growth factor and its receptors in Parkinson's disease," *NeuroReport*, vol. 17, no. 7, pp. 705–709, 2006.

[74] K. E. Ohlin, V. Francardo, H. S. Lindgren et al., "Vascular endothelial growth factor is upregulated by l-dopa in the parkinsonian brain: implications for the development of dyskinesia," *Brain*, vol. 134, no. 8, pp. 2339–2357, 2011.

[75] A. Brockington, S. B. Wharton, M. Fernando et al., "Expression of vascular endothelial growth factor and its receptors in the central nervous system in amyotrophic lateral sclerosis," *Journal of Neuropathology and Experimental Neurology*, vol. 65, no. 1, pp. 26–36, 2006.

[76] M. A. Carrillo-de Sauvage, A. Gómez, C. M. Ros et al., "CCL2-Expressing astrocytes mediate the extravasation of T lymphocytes in the brain. Evidence from patients with glioma and experimental models in vivo," *PLoS ONE*, vol. 7, no. 2, Article ID e30762, 2012.

[77] B. A. Imhof, D. Weerasinghe, E. J. Brown et al., "Cross talk between $\alpha v\beta 3$ and $\alpha 4\beta 1$ integrins regulates lymphocyte migration on vascular cell adhesion molecule 1," *European Journal of Immunology*, vol. 27, no. 12, pp. 3242–3252, 1997.

[78] J. S. Bennett, C. Chan, G. Vilaire, S. A. Mousa, and W. F. Degrado, "Agonist-activated $\alpha v\beta 3$ on platelets and lymphocytes binds to the matrix protein osteopontin," *Journal of Biological Chemistry*, vol. 272, no. 13, pp. 8137–8140, 1997.

[79] R. L. Wilder, "Integrin alpha V beta 3 as a target for treatment of rheumatoid arthritis and related rheumatic diseases," *Annals of the Rheumatic Diseases*, vol. 61, no. 2, pp. ii96–ii99, 2002.

[80] K. Amann, C. S. Haas, J. Schüssler, C. Daniel, A. Hartner, and H. O. Schöcklmann, "Beneficial effects of integrin $\alpha v\beta 3$-blocking RGD peptides in early but not late phase of experimental glomerulonephritis," *Nephrology, Dialysis, Transplantation*, vol. 27, no. 5, pp. 1755–1768, 2012.

[81] P. M. D. Watson, M. J. Humphries, J. Relton, N. J. Rothwell, A. Verkhratsky, and R. M. Gibson, "Integrin-binding RGD

peptides induce rapid intracellular calcium increases and MAPK signaling in cortical neurons," *Molecular and Cellular Neuroscience*, vol. 34, no. 2, pp. 147–154, 2007.

[82] L. A. Cingolani, A. Thalhammer, L. M. Y. Yu et al., "Activity-dependent regulation of synaptic AMPA receptor composition and abundance by beta3 integrins," *Neuron*, vol. 58, no. 5, pp. 749–762, 2008.

[83] L. Struzyńska, G. Sulkowski, and B. Dabrowska-Bouta, "Aroclor 1254 selectively inhibits expression of glial GLT-1 glutamate transporter in the forebrain of chronically exposed adult rat," *Toxicology*, vol. 300, no. 1-2, pp. 12–18, 2012.

[84] R. Herrera-Molina, R. Frischknecht, H. Maldonado et al., "Astrocytic α vβ 3 integrin inhibits neurite outgrowth and promotes retraction of neuronal processes by clustering thy-1," *PLoS ONE*, vol. 7, no. 3, Article ID e34295, 2012.

[85] H.-Y. Han, J.-P. Zhang, S.-Q. Ji et al., "αv and $\beta 1$ integrins mediate Aβ-induced neurotoxicity in hippocampal neurons via the FAK signaling pathway," *PLoS ONE*, vol. 8, no. 6, Article ID e64839, 2013.

[86] S. V. More, H. Kumar, I. S. Kim, S.-Y. Song, and D.-K. Choi, "Cellular and molecular mediators of neuroinflammation in the pathogenesis of Parkinson's disease," *Mediators of Inflammation*, vol. 2013, Article ID 952375, 12 pages, 2013.

[87] J. V. Welser-Alves, A. Boroujerdi, U. Tigges, and R. Milner, "Microglia use multiple mechanisms to mediate interactions with vitronectin; non-essential roles for the highly-expressed $\alpha v\beta 3$ and $\alpha v\beta 5$ integrins," *Journal of Neuroinflammation*, vol. 8, article 157, 2011.

[88] T. M. Zielonka, U. Demkow, K. Zycinska et al., "Angiogenic activity of sera from patients with systemic autoimmune diseases in relation to clinical, radiological, and functional pulmonary status," *Journal of Physiology and Pharmacology*, vol. 59, no. 6, pp. 791–800, 2008.

[89] P. Karczewski, A. Pohlmann, B. Wagenhaus et al., "Antibodies to the $\alpha 1$-Adrenergic receptor cause vascular impairments in rat brain as demonstrated by magnetic resonance Angiography," *PLoS ONE*, vol. 7, no. 7, Article ID e41602, 2012.

16

Idiopathic Uveitis and Familial Mediterranean Fever: Is There Any Relationship?

Farhad Salehzadeh,[1] Ozra Yasrebi,[2] Mahsa Hosseini Khotbesara,[2] and Maryam Hosseini Khotbesara[2]

[1] *Pediatric Department, Ardabil University of Medical Sciences (ARUMS), Ardabil 56157, Iran*
[2] *Department of Pediatrics, Ardabil University of Medical Sciences (ARUMS), Bouali Hospital, Iran*

Correspondence should be addressed to Farhad Salehzadeh; salehzadeh_f@yahoo.com

Academic Editor: Nalini S. Bora

Introduction. Familial Mediterranean fever (FMF) is an auto-inflammatory disease characterized by attacks of fever and polyserositis. FMF is often associated with other autoimmune diseases such as rheumatoid arthritis, polyarteritis nodosa (PAN), and Behcet. Uveitis is an inflammatory process caused by underlying infectious and inflammatory disorders. This study investigates the probable relationship between idiopathic uveitis and FMF. *Methods*. Patients with idiopathic uveitis were analyzed for the 12 most common MEFV mutations (P369S, F479L, M680I(G/C), M680I(G/A), I692del, M694V, M694I, K695R, V726A, A744S, R761H, E148Q) by a reverse hybridization assay (FMF StripAssay,Vienna lab,Vienna, Austria). *Results*. 12 patients with idiopathic uveitis were enrolled in this study. 10 of them were female. The youngest patient was a 7-year-old child and the oldest was 57. The most common complaints of patients were blurred vision and then eye redness. One patient was heterozygous for R761H. Genetic analysis of the 12 most common MEFV mutations in the patients with idiopathic uveitis didnot have any positive results. *Conclusion*. According to the analysis of the 12 most common MEFV gene mutations, FMF is not an underlying cause of idiopathic uveitis. On the other hand, uveitis merely could not be the first presentation of FMF.

1. Introduction

FMF is a Mendelian autosomal recessive disease that is highly prevalent in the Mediterranean population [1, 2] characterized by attacks of fever and painful manifestations [3]. The disease is characterized mainly by fever, abdominal pain, arthritis, and erysipelas [4]. The MEFV gene with more than 240 mutations is responsible for FMF [5].

Uveitis is defined as an inflammation of the uveal tract (the iris, ciliary body, choroid) [6, 7] and may involve the optic nerve, sclera, retina, and vitreous humor [8]. Idiopathic uveitis is a condition in which no cause is identified. The uveitis was classified in different ways, based on the anatomical location of the inflammation: anterior, intermediate, posterior, and panuveitis and based on the course of uveitis: acute, chronic, and recurrent, and on etiology it was classified as infectious, autoimmune, and idiopathic, [6, 8]. Uveitis is a very serious and potentially blinding disease [9]. In the uveitis, different patterns of etiology, disease presentation, and progression are associated with difference of race and ethnicity [10].

In Ozdal study, ocular toxoplasmosis was the main cause of infectious uveitis. Other causes of infectious uveitis were herpes, toxocara, and brucella [11]. One common disease that associated with idiopathic uveitis, is Behcet's disease. This disease has a low proportion as an etiologic agent in nonendemic areas but it is one of the common causes of uveitis in endemic areas. Behcet has been observed in 0.5–2.2% of the patients with childhood-onset uveitis in nonendemic areas [12–14]. But in a study in Turkey, Behcet's disease was reported to be the cause of 16.5% of cases with uveitis [15].

FMF is often associated with other autoimmune diseases such as ankylosing spondylitis, rheumatoid arthritis, PAN,

Table 1: Patients' findings.

No.	Sex	Age (yr)	Main symptom	Other symptoms	Age of onset (yr)	Duration of symptoms (yr)	MEFV gene
1	F	25	Redness	Blurred vision	22	3	Wt/wt
2	F	39	Redness	Blurred vision	34	5	Wt/wt
3	F	28	Blurred vision	Headache	24	4	Wt/wt
4	F	20	Blurred vision	—	17	3	Wt/wt
5	M	12	Blurred vision	—	6	6	Wt/wt
6	F	57	Blurred vision	Pain	54	3	R761H/wt
7	F	23	Blurred vision	—	21	1.5	Wt/wt
8	F	19	Blurred vision	—	15	4	Wt/wt
9	F	22	Blurred vision	—	19	3	Wt/wt
10	F	7	Accidental	—	5	2	Wt/wt
11	F	31	Redness	Pain	21	10	Wt/wt
12	M	14	Redness	Blurred vision	2	1.5	Wt/wt

Behcet and MS; all are chronic progressive with unknown etiology [16].

Ophthalmological manifestations of FMF are few and include retinal colloid-like bodies, panuveitis, anterior uveitis, scleritis, episcleritis, and papillitis. Michaelson's team published the first report of eye manifestations in FMF in 1959 [17].

According to the influence of geographical factors in the etiology of idiopathic uveitis and since FMF is highly prevalent in this area [2], the present study was designed to answer these questions, does FMF play a role in the etiology of idiopathic uveitis? And whether uveitis would be the only manifestation of FMF?

2. Material and Methods

12 patients with idiopathic uveitis were enrolled in this study. All patients had no underlying cause for the uveitis on the basis of clinical and paraclinical evaluation (complete blood count CBC diff, Erythrocyte sedimentation rate (ESR), C reactive protein (CRP), Tuberculin test (PPD), Renal Tests, Liver Functions, ANA (profile), RF, HLA-B27, HLA-B5-B51, Angiotensin converting enzyme (ACE), Chest X-Ray, ANCA, Lyme (Ig), Toxoplasma (antibody), Borrelia (antibody), Wright, 2Mercapto ethanol) when they enrolled in this study.

All the patients were screened for 12 common MEFV mutations by a reverse hybridization assay (FMF StripAssay, Vienna lab, Vienna, Austria) according to the instructions provided by the manufacturer. About 10 mL of peripheral blood was used for extracting DNA by boiling-based method. In a first step, exons 2, 3, 5, and 10 were amplified for each patient in a single, multiplex PCR, with primers supplied by the noted RDB kit. The thermocycling program of amplification was 35 cycles including (94 c for 15 sec, 58 c for 45 sec, and 72 c for 45 sec) and a final extension at 72 c for 7 min. Agarose electrophoresis revealed the accuracy of amplification by detecting four amplified DNA fragments including 206, 236, 295, and 318 bp. Biotinylated PCR products were selectively hybridized to a test strip presenting a parallel array of allele-specific oligonucleotide Probes. Thereby, the twelve common mutations E148Q in exon 2, P369S in exon 3, F479L in exon 5 and M680I (G/C), M680I (G/A), I692del, M694V, M694I, K695R, V726A, A744S, and R761H in exon 10 were determined.

Statistical analysis was performed using SPSS V 15.0. A P value of 0.05 was accepted as statistically significant.

3. Results

Among 12 patients, 10 of them were female and the remaining 2 were male. The youngest patient was a 7-year-old child and and the oldest was 57. The most common complaints of patients were blurred vision in 7 cases. Among these 7 patients, three had bilateral blurred vision, two had blurred vision in left eye, and two had blurred vision in right eye. The most commonly associated symptoms were gastrointestinal and musculoskeletal symptoms. The MEFV genetic analyses were performed in these 12 patients. No mutations were found in 11 patients (91.66%). One patient was found to be heterozygous for Wt/R761H (Table 1).

4. Discussion

FMF is often associated with other autoimmune diseases such as hepatitis, PAN, Behcet, and Multiple Sclerosis (MS). The association of familial Mediterranean fever with juvenile idiopathic arthritis (JIA) or ankylosing spondylitis and Systemic Lupus (SLE) has been described in several previous reports [9]. Michaelson reported eye manifestations of FMF as colloid-like bodes, in 56% of their Jewish patients (compared to 11% of the nonJewish ones). Subsequent studies from the same center of a larger group of patients yielded a lower prevalence (20%), and a later review of 50 Armenian and Arab patients with FMF revealed colloid-like bodies in only 4. Consequently, ophthalmic manifestations were dropped from the clinical criteria of FMF and are only used as findings to rule out this diagnosis [18].

In 1982, Yazici and Pazarli reported a case of anterior uveitis in a woman with FMF who later developed episcleritis. Several years later, four additional cases were described, making a total of five reports of seven cases of uveitis and episcleritis in FMF patients. Overall, four cases of episcleritis, two cases of panuveitis, and two cases of anterior uveitis associated FMF have been reported [18]. On the basis of these studies, looking for the relationship between varieties of eye involvement such as uveitis and FMF will not be unreasonable. Although these studies discussed different eye involvements in FMF patients, we investigated FMF as a background of idiopathic uveitis.

Recently, genetic criteria have been used for the diagnosis of FMF. According to genetic study and analysis of 12 common MEFV gene mutations in the present study, it seems that when we encounter idiopathic uveitis in an especial area with high prevalence of FMF, it could not be considered as an underlying cause of idiopathic uveitis, although we need all mutations (nearly 250 mutations) of MEFV genes analysis to confirm this result. On the other hand, these results showed that uveitis merely could not be probably the only and first presentation of FMF.

Conflict of Interests

There is no conflict of interests in this paper.

References

[1] N. Imirzalioglu, A. Dursun, B. Tastan, Y. Soysal, and M. C. Yakicier, "MEFV gene is a probable susceptibility gene for Behçet's disease," *Scandinavian Journal of Rheumatology*, vol. 34, no. 1, pp. 56–58, 2005.

[2] I. Touitou, X. Magne, N. Molinari et al., "MEFV mutations in Behçet's disease," *Human Mutation*, vol. 16, no. 3, pp. 271–272, 2000.

[3] T. Schwartz, P. Langevitz, D. Zemer, E. Gazit, M. Pras, and A. Livneh, "Behcet's disease in Familial Mediterranean fever: characterization of the association between the two diseases," *Seminars in Arthritis and Rheumatism*, vol. 29, no. 5, pp. 286–295, 2000.

[4] E. Ozalkaya, S. Mir, B. Sozeri, A. Berdeli, F. Mutlubas, and A. Cura, "Familial Mediterranean fever *gene* mutation frequencies and genotype-phenotype correlations in the Aegean region of Turkey," *Rheumatology International*, vol. 31, no. 6, pp. 779–784, 2011.

[5] M. Bonyadi, M. Esmaeili, A. Karimi, and S. Dastgiri, "Common mediterranean fever *gene* mutations in the Azeri Turkish population of Iran," *Genetic Testing and Molecular Biomarkers*, vol. 14, no. 1, pp. 149–151, 2010.

[6] H. Patel and D. Goldstein, "Pediatric uveitis," *Pediatric Clinics of North America*, vol. 50, no. 1, pp. 125–136, 2003.

[7] R. Bansal, V. Gupta, and A. Gupta, "Current approach in the diagnosis and management of panuveitis," *Indian Journal of Ophthalmology*, vol. 58, no. 1, pp. 45–54, 2010.

[8] R. V. Agrawal, S. Murthy, V. Sangwan, and J. Biswas, "Current approach in diagnosis and management of anterior uveitis," *Indian Journal of Ophthalmology*, vol. 58, no. 1, pp. 11–19, 2010.

[9] G. Yildiz, M. Kayataş, Y. Uygun, M. Timuçin, and F. Candan, "Coexistence of systemic lupus erythematosus and familial mediterranean fever," *Internal Medicine*, vol. 49, no. 8, pp. 767–769, 2010.

[10] J. A. Smith, F. Mackensen, H. N. Sen et al., "Epidemiology and course of disease in childhood uveitis," *Ophthalmology*, vol. 116, no. 8, pp. 1544.e1–1551.e1, 2009.

[11] P. Ozdal, E. Sen, A. Yazici, and F. Ozturk, "Patterns of childhood-onset uveitis in a referral center in Turkey," *Journal of Ophthalmic Inflammation and Infection*, vol. 2, no. 1, pp. 13–19, 2012.

[12] J. J. Kanski and G. A. Shun-Shin, "Systemic uveitis syndromes in childhood: an analysis of 340 cases," *Ophthalmology*, vol. 91, no. 10, pp. 1247–1251, 1984.

[13] I. Tugal-Tutkun, K. Havrlikova, W. J. Power, and C. S. Foster, "Changing patterns in uveitis of childhood," *Ophthalmology*, vol. 103, no. 3, pp. 375–383, 1996.

[14] P. Pivetti-Pezzi, "Uveitis in children," *European Journal of Ophthalmology*, vol. 6, no. 3, pp. 293–298, 1996.

[15] M. Soylu, G. Özdemir, and A. Anli, "Pediatric uveitis in Southern turkey," *Ocular Immunology and Inflammation*, vol. 5, no. 3, pp. 197–202, 1997.

[16] K. Aksu and G. Keser, "Coexistence of *vasculitis* with familial Mediterranean fever," *Rheumatology International*, vol. 31, no. 10, pp. 1263–1274, 2011.

[17] S. Berestizschevsky, D. Weinberger, I. Avisar, and R. Avisar, "Episcleritis associated with Familial Mediterranean fever," *Israel Medical Association Journal*, vol. 10, no. 4, pp. 318–319, 2008.

[18] H. Yazici and H. Pazarli, "Eye involvement in a patient with familial Mediterranean fever," *Journal of Rheumatology*, vol. 9, no. 4, pp. 644–645, 1982.

17

A Comparison of Anti-Nuclear Antibody Quantification Using Automated Enzyme Immunoassays and Immunofluorescence Assays

Renata Baronaite,[1,2] Merete Engelhart,[2] Troels Mørk Hansen,[2] Gorm Thamsborg,[3] Hanne Slott Jensen,[2] Steen Stender,[1] and Pal Bela Szecsi[1]

[1] *Department of Clinical Biochemistry, Gentofte Hospital, University of Copenhagen, 2900 Hellerup, Denmark*
[2] *Department of Rheumatology, Gentofte Hospital, University of Copenhagen, 2900 Hellerup, Denmark*
[3] *Department of Rheumatology, Glostrup Hospital, University of Copenhagen, 2600 Glostrup, Denmark*

Correspondence should be addressed to Pal Bela Szecsi; pal.szecsi@regionh.dk

Academic Editor: I. R. Mackay

Anti-nuclear antibodies (ANA) have traditionally been evaluated using indirect fluorescence assays (IFA) with HEp-2 cells. Quantitative immunoassays (EIA) have replaced the use of HEp-2 cells in some laboratories. Here, we evaluated ANA in 400 consecutive and unselected routinely referred patients using IFA and automated EIA techniques. The IFA results generated by two independent laboratories were compared with the EIA results from antibodies against double-stranded DNA (dsDNA), from ANA screening, and from tests of the seven included subantigens. The final IFA and EIA results for 386 unique patients were compared. The majority of the results were the same between the two methods (n = 325, 84%); however, 8% (n = 30) yielded equivocal results (equivocal-negative and equivocal-positive) and 8% (n = 31) yielded divergent results (positive-negative). The results showed fairly good agreement, with Cohen's kappa value of 0.30 (95% confidence interval (CI) = 0.14–0.46), which decreased to 0.23 (95% CI = 0.06–0.40) when the results for dsDNA were omitted. The EIA method was less reliable for assessing nuclear and speckled reactivity patterns, whereas the IFA method presented difficulties detecting dsDNA and Ro activity. The automated EIA method was performed in a similar way to the conventional IFA method using HEp-2 cells; thus, automated EIA may be used as a screening test.

1. Introduction

Visual inspection via indirect immunofluorescence microscopy has been the gold standard for detecting anti-nuclear antibodies (ANA) since their discovery more than 50 years ago [1, 2], and this method continues to be performed virtually with no modifications. Rodent tissue (stomach, liver, and/or kidney) was used as a substrate in early ANA testing but was subsequently replaced by the human epithelial-like cell line HEp-2 (HEp-2). Some laboratories have replaced HEp-2 cells with commercial cells (HEp-2000 cells) that overexpress Sjögren's Syndrome A antigen/small ribonucleoprotein particle (SSA/Ro) because HEp-2 cells lack sensitivity for the detection of the SSA/Ro antigens [3]. The intensity and staining patterns of antibodies that bind to cellular components allow a skilled observer to distinguish between numerous nuclear staining patterns: homogeneous, speckled, nuclear membranous, centromeric, nuclear dot, pleomorphic, SSA/Ro-positive, and other mixed or atypical patterns [4]. The IFA method is influenced by cell type, fixation procedure, dilution of patient serum, inspection time, day-to-day performance, experience level of the microscopist, and the microscope itself [5, 6]. Although the presence of ANA is associated with various rheumatic and nonrheumatic diseases, its highest sensitivity lies in identifying cases of systemic lupus erythematosus (SLE) (93–95%), systemic sclerosis (85%), juvenile idiopathic arthritis (61–80%), Sjögren's syndrome (48%), and mixed connective tissue disease (MCTD). ANA is also apparent in other autoimmune diseases and various nonrheumatologic conditions [4, 7–10]. Furthermore, a low ANA titer (1 : 40) is present in up to 32% of healthy individuals, whereas 3–5% exhibit a higher titer (1 : 160–1 : 320) [7]. The commercial availability of standardized kits has made IFA tests superior compared with homemade preparations. However, such kits remain at best only semiquantitative and cumbersome to perform despite attempts to automate IFA techniques [6, 8]. Several ANA antigens have been identified, and quantitative enzyme immunoassays (EIA) have been developed using either purified extracts or recombinant antigens. Most of the early manual EIA techniques have been widely replaced by automated versions. These newer methods are amenable to modern laboratories with high-throughput platforms, and they provide quantitative, reproducible results with minimal hands-on time and require less operator skill. In contrast to classical IFA methods using HEp-2 cells, which contain several hundred different antigens, the reactivity of EIA methods is limited to the relatively few individual antigens included in the assays. Although this factor may reduce EIA reactivity to some relevant antigens, it could also diminish reactivity toward irrelevant antigens.

Much of our experience with the clinical utility of ANA is based on standard IFA methodology. Thus, some reservations exist among clinicians as to whether EIA methods can replace conventional HEp-2 IFA techniques [1, 11, 12]. In this study, we compared conventional IFA with automated EIA for evaluating blood samples from 400 consecutive patients who were referred for routine ANA testing.

2. Materials and Methods

2.1. Patients. Between August and November 2007, serum samples were collected from 400 consecutive patients who were referred for routine ANA testing from hospital wards and outpatient clinics at three hospitals in the Copenhagen suburbs (Gentofte, Herlev, and Glostrup Hospitals). Information on the patients' age, sex, diagnosis, disease status, and any medications was collected one year after the ANA testing (registered anonymously). The study was conducted in accordance with the principles of the Declaration of Helsinki, but it was not considered a bioethics project according to the definition of the Danish Act on the Bioethics Committee System and the Processing of Bioethics Projects. Thus, no application for a review was submitted, and written informed consent was not obtained. The Danish Bioethics Committees for the Capital Region have approved the classification of this study.

2.2. Assays. An analytical flowchart for this study is shown in Figure 1. IFA was performed by incubating a 1 : 160 dilution of serum with HEp-2000 cells, which overexpress the 60-kDa SSA/Ro antigen [3], according to the manufacturer's protocol (Immuno Concepts, Sacramento, CA, USA). In cases of positive or ambiguous results from the primary laboratory, the samples were reanalyzed and titrated blindly at a secondary laboratory (Statens Serum Institut, Copenhagen, Denmark) using the same IFA assay. Automated EIA for ANA (Symphony, a mixture of the following seven subantigens: purified recombinant SmD; SSA/Ro (52- and 60-kDa); SSB/La; Scl-70; CENP-B; U1RNP (RNP70, A, C); and Jo-1 proteins) and anti-dsDNA measurements were performed using EliA reagents and a UniCAP 100 instrument (Phadia, Freiburg, Germany). All antibody levels were classified according to the manufacturer's recommendations: anti-dsDNA < 10 IU/mL was considered negative, >15 IU/mL was positive, and 10–15 IU/mL was equivocal; and an ANA Symphony test sample to calibrator ratio < 0.7 was negative, >1.0 was positive, and =0.7–1.0 was equivocal. Samples with a positive or equivocal Symphony result were reflex-tested by analyzing their individual reactivity to each of the seven subantigens included in the screening test. CENP-B, Jo-1, SSA/Ro, SSB/La, and Scl-70 levels < 7.0 U/mL and U1RNP and SmD levels < 5.0 U/mL were considered to be negative. CENP-B, Jo-1, SSA/Ro, SSB/La, and Scl-70 levels between 7.0 and 10.0 U/mL and U1RNP and SmD levels between 5.0 and 10.0 U/mL were considered equivocal. The final, combined EIA results (negative, equivocal, and positive) were derived from the data from the anti-dsDNA, ANA Symphony, and seven individual subantigen tests. The IFA results (negative, equivocal, and positive) were based on the data obtained from both the primary and the secondary laboratories. For the 14 patient serum samples that were tested in duplicate, only the results obtained from the first replicate were used.

2.3. Statistics. The VassarStats calculator (Vassar College, Poughkeepsie, NY, USA) was used to calculate the agreement between tests using Cohen's unweighted kappa with confidence intervals. A Kappa statistic < 0.2 was considered to indicate a "poor" strength of agreement; 0.21–0.40 was "fair," 0.41–0.60 was "moderate," 0.61–0.80 was "good," and >0.8 was "very good" [13]. All the other data analyses were performed using SPSS, release 20.0 (IBM, Armonk, NY, USA).

3. Results

The study population consisted of 241 females with a mean age of 52.4 years (range: 3–92) and 145 males with a mean age of 52.2 years (range: 1–89). The diagnoses are listed in Table 1.

The median anti-dsDNA level was 1.7 IU/mL, with a 90% interpercentile range of 0.6–11.1. A total of 365 samples (94.6%) were found to be anti-dsDNA-negative, six (1.6%) were equivocal, and 15 (3.9%) were positive. The female patients exhibited a statistically nonsignificant trend toward higher anti-dsDNA values (mean: 5.3 versus 2.4 IU/mL). Four of the 28 Symphony-positive serum samples were also positive for anti-dsDNA.

The primary laboratory generally reported weak, homogenous results that were found to be negative in the secondary laboratory (Table 2). Nonetheless, the 76 samples analyzed via IFA at both the primary and secondary laboratories exhibited moderately good agreement, with Cohen's unweighted kappa value of 0.45 (95% CI = 0.28–0.62).

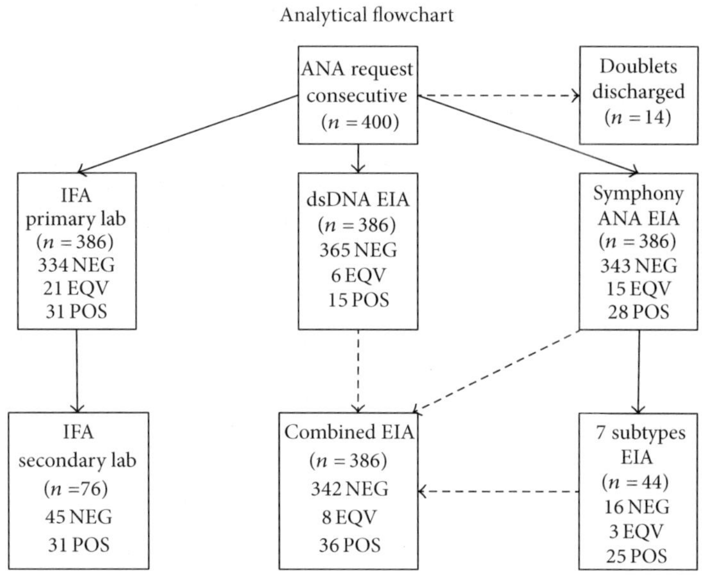

Figure 1: Analytical flowchart. EIA with a combination of dsDNA, ANA Symphony, and the 7 subantigens (SmD, U1RNP, SSA/Ro, SSB/La, Scl-70, CENP-B, and Jo-1) is referred to as "Combined EIA." IFA tests were performed at a primary laboratory (Gentofte Hospital) and a secondary laboratory (Statens Serum Institut). NEG: negative, EQV: equivocal, POS: positive, and ND: not determined.

The final assessments of the 386 samples obtained via EIA (the combined anti-dsDNA, Symphony, and seven subantigen results) and via IFA (the combined results from the primary and secondary laboratories) were compared (Table 3). The majority of the results were in agreement (n = 325, 84%), whereas 8% (n = 30) yielded equivocal results (equivocal-negative and equivocal-positive) and 8% (n = 31) yielded divergent results (positive-negative) (Table 4). The results exhibited fairly good agreement, with a Cohen's kappa value of 0.30 (95% CI = 0.14–0.46). The kappa value decreased to 0.23 (95% CI = 0.06–0.40) when the results of the anti-dsDNA analyses were omitted from the calculation despite the few solitary reactions for dsDNA.

Of the 333 samples that were negative using IFA, 24 were found to be reactive with EIA (anti-dsDNA and/or Symphony) without a clear pattern. However, the IFA testing missed several positive samples with significant anti-dsDNA reactivity via EIA screening. Furthermore, the IFA exhibited decreased reliability for detecting Ro reactivity, either alone or in combination with the other antigens. In contrast, the IFA method detected 14 positive and 19 equivocal samples that were negative when screened using the EIA method. Although most of these IFA reactions were weak, six of the samples had clear nuclear reactivity and four had clear speckled reactivity.

The IFA and EIA results for patients with SLE or MCTD exhibited fair agreement, and the results for patients with scleroderma demonstrated good agreement. The IFA produced equivocal results for rheumatoid arthritis (RA) patients, primarily due to weak, homogeneous IFA reactions at the primary laboratory and negative reactions in both EIA and IFA methods at the secondary laboratory. The sera from an unexpectedly large proportion (3/12) of patients with osteoporosis reacted positively in EIA and/or IFA, and two of these cases were Ro-positive.

Of the 388 samples evaluated, 36 were positive for ANA using EIA, and 11 of these were solely reactive to anti-dsDNA. A total of 30 samples reacted positively using IFA, and 15 of these also reacted positively in the EIA tests. Only one of the samples that reacted positively using both IFA and EIA exhibited anti-dsDNA reactivity, and the degree of reactivity was borderline. Among the patients diagnosed with ANA-associated disease, 23% (16/70) had positive EIA results (two samples had equivocal results) and 24% (17/70) had positive IFA results (two samples had equivocal results). Seven patients with nonANA-associated rheumatic disease reacted positively in both EIA and IFA, and 12 samples showed equivocal results via IFA compared with only two via EIA. Both the EIA and IFA methods yielded positive results in four of the eight patients with SLE (in three cases, both tests were positive). The EIA-negative and IFA-positive samples exhibited a nuclear staining pattern via IFA at a titer of 1 : 160, and the IFA-negative and EIA-positive samples had relatively high reactivity to both dsDNA (38 IU/mL) and Ro (38.2 U/mL). Both assays yielded negative results in three cases, one of which represented an overlapping syndrome with MCTD. Of the three patients with undifferentiated connective tissue disease (UCTD), all reacted positively via IFA (high-titer speckled patterns in two cases and a high-titer homogeneous pattern in one case), whereas only one case reacted positively in the EIA tests (U1RNP and SmD). Of the remaining two cases, only one exhibited weak anti-dsDNA reactivity. Out of eight patients with juvenile RA, only one had a positive IFA result (a speckled pattern at a titer > 1,280), whereas that patient's EIA result was negative. Of the 48 adult cases of RA, four and three reacted positively via EIA and

TABLE 1: Clinical diagnoses and results of EIA and IFA. The combined results of anti-dsDNA, ANA screening, and the seven individual antigens are referred to as "EIA-combined." The IFA classification was based on the results from the primary laboratory and (if performed) from the secondary laboratory.

Diagnosis	dsDNA EIA			ANA screen EIA			EIA-combined			IFA		
	NEG	EQV	POS	NEG	EQV	POS	NEG	EQV	POS	NEG	EQV	POS
ANA-associated disease (n = 44, 18%)	38	2	4	26	2	16	28	1	15	28	2	14
SLE (n = 8)	5		3	4	1	3	4		4	4		4
Juvenile RA (n = 8)	8			7	1		8			6	1	1
Raynaud (n = 5)	5			2		3	3		2	4		
Vasculitis (n = 5)	5			4		1	5			5		
Autoimmune hepatitis (n = 4)	3	1		2		2	2		2	3	1	
Dermatomyositis/polymyositis (n = 3)	3			3			3			3		
Scleroderma (n = 3)	3			1		2	1		2	1		2
UCTD (n = 3)	2	1		2		1	1	1	1			3
MCTD (n = 3)	2		1			3			3			3
Discoid lupus (n = 2)	2			1		1	1		1	2		
Non-ANA-associated disease (n = 157, 46%)	150	2	5	149	5	3	149	2	7	137	12	8
Rheumatoid arthritis (n = 48)	46		2	44	2	2	44		4	36	9	3
Back pain (n = 36)	34		2	34	2		34		2	35	1	
Arthritis (n = 34)	32	1	1	32	1	1	32	1	1	29	1	4
Osteoarthrosis (n = 13)	13			13			13			13		
Polymyalgia rheumatica (n = 11)	10	1		11			10	1		10	1	
Arthralgia/myalgia (n = 7)	7			7			7			7		
Ankylosing spondylitis (n = 5)	5			5			5			4		1
Giant cell arthritis (n = 3)	3			3			3			3		
Other diseases (n = 185, 36%)	177	2	6	168	8	9	166	5	14	169	8	8
Neurological disorder (n = 58)	53			56	2		52	1	5	56	2	
Miscellaneous (n = 50)	50			44	3	3	46	1	3	43	4	3
Malignancy (n = 13)	13			12	1		12			13		
Renal disorder (n = 12)	11	1		12			11	1		12		
Osteoporosis (n = 12)	11		1	9	1	2	9	1	2	9	1	2
Inflammatory bowel disease (n = 10)	10			10			10			9		1
Infection (n = 10)	10			10			10			9		
Liver disease (n = 9)	8	1		8	1		8	1		9		
Vitamin D deficiency (n = 5)	5			1		4	2		3	3	1	1
Lung disease (n = 4)	4			4			4			4		
Endocrine disorder (n = 2)	2			2			2			2		
All (n = 386)	365	6	15	343	15	28	342	8	36	334	22	30

NEG: negative; EQV: equivocal; and POS: positive; MCTD: mixed connective tissue disease; RA: rheumatoid arthritis; SLE: systemic lupus erythematosus; and UCTD: undifferentiated connective tissue disease.

IFA, respectively. Both EIA and IFA yielded positive results in all three MCTD patients. All of these patients had high anti-U1RNP titers; one reacted positively to Ro, and one exhibited positive anti-SmD and anti-dsDNA reactivity. In these cases, the IFA pattern was observed at a high titer (>1 : 1,280) and was speckled or homogenous. Both the IFA and EIA results were negative for the single dermatomyositis patient and the two polymyositis patients.

Among the 316 patients without ANA-associated disease, 33 exhibited positive ANA reactivity (IFA, EIA, or both) with no obvious pattern. Among the 56 RA patients, four tested positive via EIA and four via IFA, with a single overlap. However, nine RA patients received weak, equivocal results via IFA.

There were unexpectedly large proportions of ANA-positive results among the patients with osteoporosis (3/12), vitamin D deficiency (3/5), and optic neuritis (3/13). Optic neuritis patients tested positive for anti-dsDNA only via EIA, whereas vitamin D-deficient patients showed reactivity to Ro and CENP-B via EIA and strongly speckled reactivity via IFA. The osteoporotic patients showed anti-dsDNA and anti-Ro reactivity via EIA; however, their IFA results included predominantly speckled and homogenous patterns.

Table 2: Comparison of the immunofluorescence patterns and titers of HEp-2000 ANA testing at two independent laboratories.

Secondary laboratory	NEG	POS?	CEN?	CEN	HOM+	HOM	NUC?	NUC and HOM	NUC	SPE?	SPE+	SPE	MIT
NEG	**22**	*3*	*1*		*11*	3			2		2		*1*
CEN > 1280				**1**									
CEN > 1280 and MEM				**1**									
CEN > 1280 and SPE > 1280				**1**									
HOM+						**1**							
HOM > 1280						**2**							
HOM > 1280 and SPE > 1280						**1**							
HOM 1280						**1**							
HOM 160					**1**								
NUC++									**1**				
NUC 160	1					1			**2**				
NUC 320									**1**				
NUC 320 and SPE 160							*1*						
NUC 640						1		**1**	**1**				
SPE 320										*1*			
SPE												**1**	
SPE > 1280												**8**	
SPE+++												**1**	
MIT > 1280		*1*											

Primary laboratory: Gentofte Hospital, and secondary laboratory: Statens Serum Institut; NEG: negative; POS: positive; CEN: centromere; HOM: homogeneous; NUC: nuclear; SPE: speckled; MIT: mitochondria; ?: uncertain reaction; +: weak reaction; ++: intermediate reaction, and +++: strong reaction. Underlining and bold font indicate agreement, italics indicate acceptable agreement, and double underlining indicates disagreement.

Table 3: Comparison of immunofluorescence patterns and titers between HEp-2000 immunofluorescence (Immuno Concept) and combined ANA immunoassays (Phadia). The combined EIA results from dsDNA, ANA Symphony, and the 7 subantigens (SmD, U1RNP, SSA/Ro, SSB/La, Scl-70, CENP-B, and Jo-1) are shown.

EIA-combined	NEG	POS?	CEN?	CEN	HOM+	HOM	NUC?	NUC and HOM	NUC	SPE?	SPE+	SPE	MIT
NEG	308	1			12	5	1	1	6	1	2	3	1
CENP-B				2									
dsDNA	7	1	1			2							
dsDNA	4					1							
dsDNA, SSA/Ro	1												
dsDNA, SSA/Ro	1	1											
dsDNA, La, SSA/Ro												1	
dsDNA, RnpU1, SmD, SSA/Ro						1							
SSB/La	1												
SSB/La, SSA/Ro	1											1	
SSB/La, SSA/Ro, CENP-B				1									
RnpU1	2								1			2	
RnpU1	2												
RnpU1, SSA/Ro												1	
RnpU1, SmD												1	
SSA/Ro	4	1											
SSA/Ro, CENP-B	1												
Scl-70						1							
SmD	1												

Primary laboratory: Gentofte Hospital; NEG: negative; POS: positive; CEN: centromere; HOM: homogeneous; NUC: nuclear; SPE: speckled; MIT: mitochondria; ?: uncertain reaction; +: weak reaction; ++: intermediate reaction, and +++: strong reaction. Underlining and bold font indicate agreement, italics indicate acceptable agreement, and double underlining indicates disagreement.

Table 4: Comparison between combined ANA immunoassay (Phadia) and HEp-2000 cell immunofluorescence (Immuno Concept). The combined results of dsDNA, ANA Symphony, and the 7 subantigens constituted the EIA-combined assay, and the combined results of IFA using HEp-2000 cells from two laboratories constituted the HEp-2000-combined assay. The results of the immunoassays were considered equivocal if the anti-dsDNA levels were between 10–15 IU/mL or if the Symphony results were between 0.7–1.0; however, the 7 subantigen results overruled those of the Symphony. The HEp-2000 results were considered equivocal if the two laboratories' results were discordant. The degree of agreement was fair (Kappa statistic = 0.29).

EIA-combined	IFA-combined			
	NEG	EQV	POS	Total
NEG	**310**	*18*	14	342
EQV	7	**0**	*1*	8
POS	17	*4*	**15**	36
Total	334	22	30	388

4. Discussion

Our results demonstrate that at best using HEp-2000 cells as a substrate for IFA ANA testing only improves upon the insufficient sensitivity of SSA/Ro antibodies; this method still fails to detect even the extremely high antibody levels that are detected using the specific Ro EIA (Table 3). Both the screening and the solitary SSA/Ro EIA methods employ a mixture of the 52- and 60-kDa Ro protein isoforms; thus, they cannot identify reactivity toward a single Ro isoform, which might be clinically useful. Our data also illustrate the difficulties in reproducing IFA results, which have been previously observed by others [14]. The analyses of 76 samples at both the primary and secondary laboratories produced only a moderately good agreement (Table 2). Notably, both laboratories used identical commercial assay systems; all the factors except the microscopist were eliminated. An even lower degree of agreement could be expected among laboratories that use different methods [15].

However, there were weaknesses in this study that should be addressed. First, IFA was not performed at the secondary laboratory in all cases. Most of the samples with negative results at the primary laboratory were not validated further, which may have resulted in an under- or overestimation of the degree of agreement. However, because only one of the 23 negative samples analyzed at the primary laboratory was found to be positive at the second laboratory, the overall conclusion is likely to stand. Second, relatively few patients with ANA-associated disease ($n = 44$) were evaluated; thus, predictive values cannot be calculated for individuals with this disease.

Taken together, our results are consistent with previous reports of similar findings using EIA [16–18]. Fenger et al. compared the results for three selected populations evaluated using IFA and seven different EIA methods [18], but they evaluated anti-dsDNA and Symphony reactivity separately. Notably, the authors did not test for the individual antigens when the screening test revealed positive or equivocal results. However, they found a degree of agreement between EIA and IFA tests that was comparable to our results, although the Phadia tests exhibited similar specificity but lower sensitivity compared with the other assays.

Other groups have produced results similar to ours when comparing a combination of Phadia Symphony EIA screening and anti-dsDNA testing with IFA; however, their performance when testing sera from SLE patients was relatively lower [17]. We did not observe significant differences among the relatively few SLE cases in our study, although neither EIA nor IFA identified all the relevant patients. However, other groups have found that IFA and EIA exhibited satisfactory specificity and sensitivity for assessing SLE patients, albeit with somewhat variable levels of agreement [19–22].

Bizzaro et al. compared the findings of 16 manufacturers and two university laboratories, which used different methods to analyze sera from 11 autoimmune patients [21]. The overall agreement, independent of method, was relatively good for ANA (95.5%) and was somewhat lower for anti-dsDNA (85.2%). However, considerable variation between the different methods was observed for both IFA and EIA. The IFA results revealed variability in both titer and pattern, and the EIA results showed variability in specificity for individual antigens. In all cases, the EIA results were at a low, borderline cut-off level. In agreement with these observations, a multicenter evaluation of nine EIA kits could not clearly demonstrate that one assay was superior to the others [23], particularly for anti-dsDNA and SmD antigen detection, although the newer versions yielded improved performance.

HEp-2 cells contain several hundred antigens; therefore, IFA should be the ultimate multiplexing screening assay and should be principally similar to the Phadia Symphony and other EIA kits. However, some of the antigens in HEp-2 cells are not relevant to autoimmune diseases, whereas other more relevant antigens are present in only minor amounts.

Although IFA can compensate for some of these limitations via pattern recognition and titer determination, EIA can only reveal reactivity toward the limited number of antigens included in the test by using a more standardized quantitative method.

Phadia has introduced a new screening assay that evaluates 17 antigens (the EliA CTD Screen), but some authors still consider the sensitivity of this assay to be insufficient, especially for assessing anti-fibrillin and anti-RNA polymerase III reactivity [20]. Op de Beeck et al. recently compared the CTD assay against an IFA method with a HEp-2000 substrate, using samples from autoimmune and chronic fatigue patients, blood donors, and disease control patients [24]. They found that the CTD assay yielded high specificity but with limited sensitivity. Furthermore, an excessive number of samples required additional testing with all the individual antigens. These shortcomings could be attributed to the inclusion of a dsDNA antigen in the CTD screening assay and to an overabundance of conjugated antigens on a single surface, resulting in dilution of specific, individual signals. As the clinical usefulness of rarer IFA patterns is established, these antigens may be included in future EIA methods [2]. One of these antigens might be the dense fine speckles

70 antigen (DFS70), which is associated with a dense fine speckled pattern in IFA that has promising discriminatory properties in systemic autoimmune diseases [25]. However, we did not observe any patients with this pattern in the present study, and this antigen was not included in our EIA method. A positive dense fine speckled pattern did not receive a separate classification, and positive sera may have been classified as simple speckled.

Weak positive reactions are less likely to yield concordant results between IFA and EIA techniques, as illustrated in Table 4. A two-step serial titration of positive IFA results allows for some degree of quantization. However, EIA directly provides quantitative results, simplifying the interpretation of clinically doubtful borderline reactions.

Newer methods, such as suspension arrays, simultaneously allow for multiplexing and the direct individual quantification of numerous antigens. Several companies have developed these assays, and their overall results correlate well with each other [19, 26–29]. A comparison between a multiplex assay with nine antigens and ELISA revealed 99% and 94.7% agreement in a cohort of 37 Sjögren's syndrome patients and 96 healthy controls, respectively [19]. However, a study comparing IFA against a fully automated multiplex assay with 13 antigens [29] revealed a discrepancy that was likely due to the choice of antigens and absence of standardization. The authors reported a kappa coefficient agreement of 0.31 when using IFA to assess an unselected hospital cohort of 1,004 patients; in comparison, an anti-dsDNA EIA yielded a kappa coefficient of agreement of 0.66.

5. Conclusions

In conclusion, quantitative EIA-based ANA techniques perform as well as (or as poorly as) IFA-based ANA techniques. The EIA methods appear to have limitations identifying nuclear and some speckled ANA reactivity, whereas the IFA techniques exhibit a limited detection of antibodies against dsDNA and SSA/Ro. The two methods are not equivalent, and both will likely produce false-negative or false-positive reactions in some cases. However, it is not clear whether these differences are clinically relevant. Quantitative automated systems for ANA screening could be used for primary screening. When more relevant antigens are identified, evaluated, and subsequently included into new EIA techniques, the use of classical IFA may diminish further.

Abbreviations

ANA:	Anti-nuclear antibodies
CENP-B:	Centromere protein B
CI:	Confidence interval
DFS70:	Dense fine speckles 70 antigen
dsDNA:	Double-stranded DNA
EIA:	Enzyme immunoassay
ELISA:	Enzyme-linked immunosorbent assay
HEp-2:	Human epidermoid cancer cells
IFA:	Indirect immunofluorescence assay
Jo-1:	Histidyl-t-RNA synthetase
MCTD:	Mixed connective tissue disease
RNP70 A, C:	Small nuclear ribonucleoprotein complexes, 70 kDa, A, C polypeptides
Scl-70:	DNA topoisomerase I
SLE:	Systemic lupus erythematosus
SmD:	Smith's antigen (a family of RNA-binding proteins)
SSA/Ro:	Sjögren's Syndrome A antigen/small ribonucleoprotein particle (Ro 52 and 60 kDa)
SSB/La:	Sjögren's Syndrome B antigen/Lupus antigen, La ribonucleoprotein domain family, member 3
U1RNP:	U1 nuclear ribonucleoprotein (mixture of recombinant RNP70, A, C)
UCTD:	Undifferentiated connective tissue disease
RA:	Rheumatoid arthritis.

Conflict of Interests

The authors declare that there is no conflict of interests regarding the publication of this paper.

Acknowledgments

Mrs. Lotte Heckmann and Mrs. Lis Nielsen are acknowledged for their technical assistance.

References

[1] P. L. Meroni and P. H. Schur, "ANA screening: an old test with new recommendations," *Annals of the Rheumatic Diseases*, vol. 69, no. 8, pp. 1420–1422, 2010.

[2] P. Vermeersch and X. Bossuyt, "Prevalence and clinical significance of rare antinuclear antibody patterns," *Autoimmunity Reviews*, vol. 12, no. 10, pp. 998–1003, 2013.

[3] M. J. Fritzler, C. Hanson, J. Miller, and T. Eystathioy, "Specificity of autoantibodies to SS-A/Ro on a transfected and overexpressed human 60 kDa Ro autoantigen substrate," *Journal of Clinical Laboratory Analysis*, vol. 16, no. 2, pp. 103–108, 2002.

[4] G. Servais, R. Karmali, M. P. Guillaume, V. Badot, J. Duchateau, and F. Corazza, "Anti DNA antibodies are not restricted to a specific pattern of fluorescence on HEp2 cells," *Clinical Chemistry and Laboratory Medicine*, vol. 47, no. 5, pp. 543–549, 2009.

[5] B.-N. Pham, S. Albarede, A. Guyard, E. Burg, and P. Maisonneuve, "Impact of external quality assessment on antinuclear antibody detection performance," *Lupus*, vol. 14, no. 2, pp. 113–119, 2005.

[6] A. Rigon, F. Buzzulini, P. Soda et al., "Novel opportunities in automated classification of antinuclear antibodies on HEp-2 cells," *Autoimmunity Reviews*, vol. 10, no. 10, pp. 647–652, 2011.

[7] E. M. Tan, T. E. W. Feltkamp, J. S. Smolen et al., "Range of antinuclear antibodies in "healthy" individuals," *Arthritis and Rheumatism*, vol. 40, no. 9, pp. 1601–1611, 1997.

[8] S. Kivity, B. Gilburd, N. Agmon-Levin et al., "A novel automated indirect immunofluorescence autoantibody evaluation," *Clinical Rheumatology*, vol. 31, no. 3, pp. 503–509, 2012.

[9] D. H. Solomon, A. J. Kavanaugh, P. H. Schur et al., "Evidence-based guidelines for the use of immunologic tests: antinuclear

antibody testing," *Arthritis Care and Research*, vol. 47, no. 4, pp. 434–444, 2002.

[10] I. Peene, L. Meheus, E. M. Veys, and F. de Keyser, "Detection and identification of antinuclear antibodies (ANA) in a large and consecutive cohort of serum samples referred for ANA testing," *Annals of the Rheumatic Diseases*, vol. 60, no. 12, pp. 1131–1136, 2001.

[11] H. Nossent and O. P. Rekvig, "Antinuclear antibody screening in this new millennium: farewell to the microscope?" *Scandinavian Journal of Rheumatology*, vol. 30, no. 3, pp. 123–126, 2001.

[12] W. Emlen and L. O'Neill, "Clinical significance of antinuclear antibodies: comparison of detection with immunofluorescence and enzyme-linked immunosorbent assays," *Arthritis and Rheumatism*, vol. 40, no. 9, pp. 1612–1618, 1997.

[13] J. R. Landis and G. G. Koch, "The measurement of observer agreement for categorical data," *Biometrics*, vol. 33, no. 1, pp. 159–174, 1977.

[14] C. González, P. Guevara, I. Alarcón, M. Hernando, J. A. Navajo, and J. M. González-Buitrago, "Antinuclear antibodies (ANA) screening by enzyme immunoassay with nuclear HEp-2 cell extract and recombinant antigens: analytical and clinical evaluation," *Clinical Biochemistry*, vol. 35, no. 6, pp. 463–469, 2002.

[15] P. Kern, M. Kron, and K. Hiesche, "Measurement of antinuclear antibodies: assessment of different test systems," *Clinical and Diagnostic Laboratory Immunology*, vol. 7, no. 1, pp. 72–78, 2000.

[16] P. A. J. M. Vos, E. J. E. G. Bast, and R. H. W. M. Derksen, "Cost-effective detection of non-antidouble-stra]nded DNA antinuclear antibody specificities in daily clinical practice," *Rheumatology*, vol. 45, no. 5, pp. 629–635, 2006.

[17] C. González, B. García-Berrocal, M. Pérez, J. A. Navajo, O. Herraez, and J. M. González-Buitrago, "Laboratory screening of connective tissue diseases by a new automated ENA screening assay (EliA Symphony) in clinically defined patients," *Clinica Chimica Acta*, vol. 359, no. 1-2, pp. 109–114, 2005.

[18] M. Fenger, A. Wiik, M. Høier-Madsen et al., "Detection of antinuclear antibodies by solid-phase immunoassays and immunofluorescence analysis," *Clinical Chemistry*, vol. 50, no. 11, pp. 2141–2147, 2004.

[19] B. Gilburd, M. Abu-Shakra, Y. Shoenfeld et al., "Autoantibodies profile in the sera of patients with sjogren's syndrome: the ANA evaluation—a homogeneous, multiplexed system," *Clinical and Developmental Immunology*, vol. 11, no. 1, pp. 53–56, 2004.

[20] J. C. Parker and C. C. Bunn, "Sensitivity of the Phadia EliA connective tissue disease screen for less common disease-specific autoantibodies," *Journal of Clinical Pathology*, vol. 64, no. 7, pp. 631–633, 2011.

[21] N. Bizzaro, R. Tozzoli, E. Tonutti et al., "Variability between methods to determine ANA, anti-dsDNA and anti-ENA autoantibodies: a collaborative study with the biomedical industry," *Journal of Immunological Methods*, vol. 219, no. 1-2, pp. 99–107, 1998.

[22] M. Hernando, C. González, A. Sánchez et al., "Clinical evaluation of a new automated anti-dsDNA fluorescent immunoassay," *Clinical Chemistry and Laboratory Medicine*, vol. 40, no. 10, pp. 1056–1060, 2002.

[23] E. M. Tan, J. S. Smolen, J. S. McDougal et al., "A critical evaluation of enzyme immunoassays for detection of antinuclear autoantibodies of defined specificities—I. Precision, sensitivity, and specificity," *Arthritis Care & Research*, vol. 42, no. 3, pp. 455–464, 1999.

[24] K. Op de Beeck, P. Vermeersch, P. Verschueren et al., "Detection of antinuclear antibodies by indirect immunofluorescence and by solid phase assay," *Autoimmunity Reviews*, vol. 10, no. 12, pp. 801–808, 2011.

[25] M. Miyara, R. Albesa, J. L. Charuel et al., "Clinical phenotypes of patients with anti-DFS70/LEDGF antibodies in a routine ANA referral cohort," *Clinical and Developmental Immunology*, vol. 2013, Article ID 703759, 8 pages, 2013.

[26] S. S. Copple, T. B. Martins, C. Masterson, E. Joly, and H. R. Hill, "Comparison of three multiplex immunoassays for detection of antibodies to extractable nuclear antibodies using clinically defined sera," *Annals of the New York Academy of Sciences*, vol. 1109, pp. 464–472, 2007.

[27] O. Shovman, B. Gilburd, G. Zandman-Goddard, A. Yehiely, P. Langevitz, and Y. Shoenfeld, "Multiplexed A the NA multilyte immunoassay for ANA screening in autoimmune diseases," *Autoimmunity*, vol. 38, no. 1, pp. 105–109, 2005.

[28] Y. Kim, Y. Park, E. Y. Lee, and H.-S. Kim, "Comparison of automated multiplexed bead-based ANA screening assay with ELISA for detecting five common anti-extractable nuclear antigens and anti-dsDNA in systemic rheumatic diseases," *Clinica Chimica Acta*, vol. 413, no. 1-2, pp. 308–311, 2012.

[29] S. Desplat-Jego, N. Bardin, B. Larida, and M. Sanmarco, "Evaluation of the BioPlex 2200 ANA screen for the detection of antinuclear antibodies and comparison with conventional methods," *Annals of the New York Academy of Sciences*, vol. 1109, pp. 245–255, 2007.

18

Role of Mast Cells in Oral Lichen Planus and Oral Lichenoid Reactions

Suganya Ramalingam,[1] Narasimhan Malathi,[1] Harikrishnan Thamizhchelvan,[1] Narasimhan Sangeetha,[2] and Sharada T Rajan[1]

[1]*Department of Oral Pathology, Faculty of Dental Sciences, Sri Ramachandra Medical College and Research Institute (Deemed to Be University), Chennai, India*
[2]*Oral and Craniofacial Health Sciences, College of Dental Medicine, University of Sharjah, Sharjah, UAE*

Correspondence should be addressed to Suganya Ramalingam; drsuganyapavendhan@yahoo.com

Academic Editor: Corrado Betterle

Introduction. Oral lichen planus (OLP) is a chronic T cell mediated disease of oral mucosa, skin, and its appendages with a prevalence of 0.5 to 2.6% worldwide. Oral lichenoid reactions (OLR) are a group of lesions with diverse aetiologies but have clinical and histological features similar to OLP, thereby posing a great challenge in differentiating both lesions. Mast cells are multifunctional immune cells that play a major role in the pathogenesis of lichen planus by release of certain chemical mediators. Increased mast cell densities with significant percentage of degranulation have been observed as a consistent finding in pathogenesis of oral lichen planus. *Aim*. The current study was aimed at quantifying the mast cells in histopathological sections of OLP and OLR thereby aiding a means of distinguishing these lesions. *Materials and Methods*. The study group involved 21 cases of oral lichen planus, 21 cases of oral lichenoid reactions, and 10 control specimens of normal buccal mucosa. All the cases were stained with Toluidine Blue and routine haematoxylin and eosin and the mast cells were quantified. *Statistical Analysis Used*. The results were analyzed using the Kruskal–Wallis test and an intergroup analysis was performed using Mann–Whitney *U* test. *Conclusion*. The number of mast cells showed an increased value in oral lichen planus when compared to oral lichenoid reaction and thus an estimation of mast cells count could aid in distinguishing OLP from OLR histopathologically.

1. Introduction

Lichen planus is a chronic mucocutaneous T cell mediated disease that usually involves the oral mucosa [1]. An antigen specific cell mediated immune response initiated by various chemokines and extracellular matrix proteins act through different pathways to cause degeneration of basal keratinocytes in the oral epithelium [2]. Clinically, OLP almost always occurs bilaterally. Though these lesions exhibit various clinical forms, namely, ulcerated, papular, atrophic, bullous, plaque-like, and reticular lesions, the highly characteristic feature of OLP showing fine white lines forming a lace-like network called Wickham's striae should always be present to define it as LP [3]. However, the presence of Wickham's striae alone does not usually designate the lesion as oral lichen planus, because the diagnosis of OLP is always clinicopathological [4].

The WHO criteria (1978) for histopathological diagnosis of OLP include thickened ortho- or parakeratinised epithelium, liquefaction degeneration of basal layer, well-defined juxtaepithelial lymphocytic infiltration, and Civatte bodies in basal epithelium and lamina propria [3].

Oral lichenoid reactions are clinical and histological analogues to oral lichen planus. They appear as white hyperkeratotic thickened lesions often related to drugs, dental restorative materials, graft versus host disease, and medications. These lesions occur in atypical sites that usually has straight topographic relation to the causative agent. Similar to oral lichen planus, the lichenoid reactions also occur in various forms like erythematous, reticular, plaque-like, and atrophic [5].

Histopathologically oral lichenoid reactions show more diffuse subepithelial inflammatory infiltrate which extends much below into the connective tissue and is more lymphohistiocytic compared to mixed inflammatory infiltration [5].

Mast cells are granular, bone-marrow derived, mobile leucocytes with wide range of functions including inflammation, immune modulation, tissue repair, and remodelling. On response to immunologic and nonimmunologic stimuli, they release preformed mediators, vasoactive amines, cytokines, and enzymes via granules [6]. The interaction between T cells and secretions from mast cells plays an important role in the regulation of immune responses emphasizing the immunopathogenesis of OLP.

Antigenically altered basal epithelial cells stimulate the mucosal mast cells through RANTES. Stimulation of mast cells presents the antigen to the T cells which in sequence causes activation and degranulation of mast cell and release of various factors like TNF-α, a series of interleukins (IL-3, IL-4, IL-5, IL-6, IL-8, IL-10, IL-11, IL-13, and IL-16), chymase, and tryptase. Both chymase and tryptase which are derivative of mast cell along with matrix metalloproteinase which is derivative of T cell lead to the breakup of basement membrane of the epithelium thereby exposing the basal keratinocytes to the cytotoxic CD8+ T cells leading to their apoptosis [7].

One of the important causes for oral lichenoid reactions could be allergic hypersensitivity reaction in which main causative phenomena occur by degranulation of mast cells [8].

The present study was designed for quantifying mast cells in oral lichenoid reactions and oral lichen planus to understand the potential function of mast cells in the pathogenesis of these diseases.

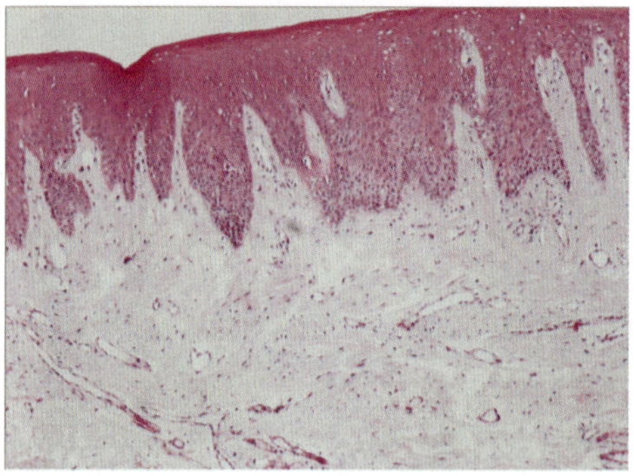

FIGURE 1: Photomicrograph of the section shows normal buccal mucosa (H&E 10x).

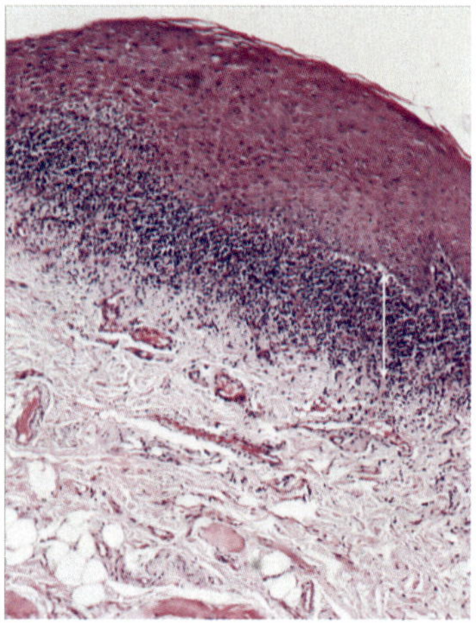

FIGURE 2: Photomicrograph of the section shows parakeratotic stratified squamous epithelium with juxtaepithelial band of inflammatory infiltration in oral lichen planus (H&E 10x). The arrows refer to juxtaepithelial band of inflammatory infiltration in oral lichen planus.

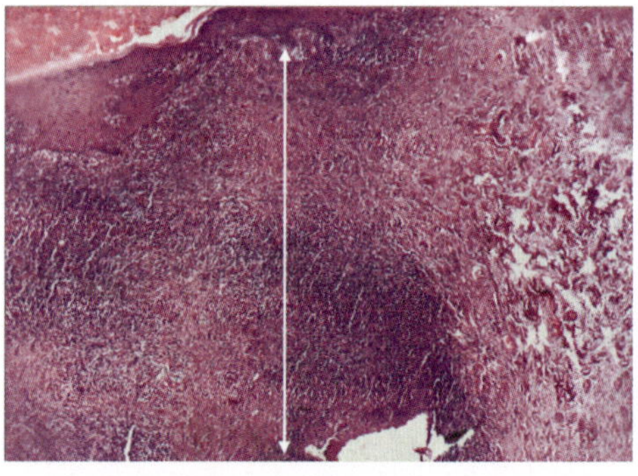

FIGURE 3: Photomicrograph of the section shows parakeratotic stratified squamous epithelium with basal cell degeneration. The arrows refer to inflammatory infiltration extending deep into reticular zone of lamina propria in oral lichenoid reaction (H&E 20x).

2. Materials and Methods

The current study involved formalin-fixed paraffin-embedded tissue sections of histopathologically diagnosed cases of oral lichen planus ($n = 21$) and oral lichenoid reactions ($n = 21$) from the archives of Department of Oral Pathology. Demographic data and history of the cases were also retrieved from Department of Medical Records. Normal buccal mucosa tissues ($n = 10$) from volunteers with no oral lesions and no associated oral habits were also obtained after taking informed consent and processed in the same way as routine pathological specimens. All study samples were stained with routine histopathological haematoxylin and eosin stain (Figures 1–3) and a special Toluidine Blue stain (Figures 4–6).

2.1. Special Stain: Toluidine Blue. 1 gm of Toluidine Blue O (sigma) and 100 mL of 70% alcohol were used to prepare Toluidine Blue stock solution. One percent sodium chloride was freshly prepared and pH was adjusted to 2.0–2.5 using glacial acetic acid. Working solution with pH of 2.3 was prepared with 5 mL of Toluidine Blue stock solution and 45 mL of 1% sodium chloride. The working solution was prepared fresh and was discarded after use each time.

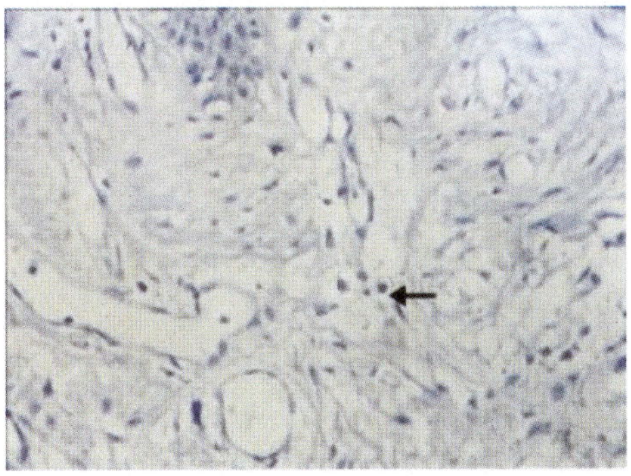

FIGURE 4: Photomicrograph of the section shows normal buccal mucosa (Toluidine Blue 10x). The arrows refer to mast cells.

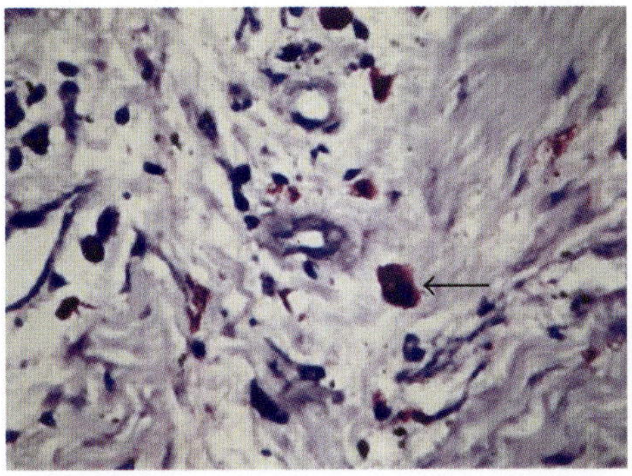

FIGURE 5: Photomicrograph of the section shows intact mast cells in oral lichen planus (Toluidine Blue 40x). The arrows refer to intact mast cells in oral lichen planus.

By using rotary microtome, 4 μm tissue sections were cut and transferred to egg albumin coated microscopic slides. The slides were kept on the slide warmer at 58°C for 15 minutes and were deparaffinised by immersing in 3 changes of fresh xylene each for 10 minutes. Further they were dehydrated in 3 changes of absolute alcohol for 5 minutes each and washed in running tap water for 10 minutes. The sections were treated with working solution of Toluidine Blue for 2-3 minutes followed by three changes of distilled water wash. The slides were then dehydrated quickly in 95% alcohol and 2 changes of absolute alcohol and were cleared in 2 changes of xylene and mounted with DPX. The mast cells stained deep purple against a blue background. Ten higher magnifications fields (40x) were selected at random and mast cells were counted using a compound light microscope.

3. Observation and Results

The age group of study samples range from 18 to 70 years. The mean age of the patients in Group I, Group II, and Group II was 29.2 years, 43.2 years, and 43.8 years, respectively. The male: female ratio among Group I, Group II, and Group III was 1 : 1, 1.6 : 1, and 1 : 1.6, respectively. The study sample included 4 different sites, buccal mucosa, tongue, lip, and

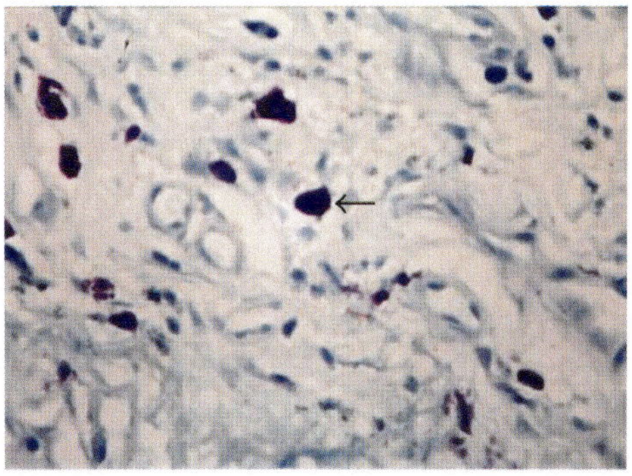

FIGURE 6: Photomicrograph of the section shows intact mast cells in oral lichenoid reaction (H&E 40x). The arrow refers to intact mast cells.

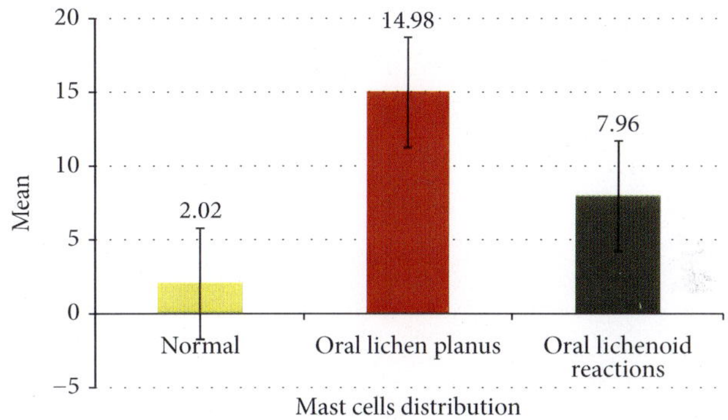

FIGURE 7: Mast cells distribution between study group.

TABLE 1: Chi-square test.

Variable	Chi-square value	p value
Wickham's striae	8.4	0.004 (significant)

gingiva. All the normal tissues were from the buccal mucosa. Wickham's striae were present in 95.2% of oral lichen planus and 57.1% of oral lichenoid reactions which were statistically significant (p value: 0.004) (Table 1).

The numbers of mast cells were significantly high in oral lichen planus (mean: 14.98) compared to oral lichenoid reactions (mean: 7.96) and normal oral mucosal tissues (mean: 2.02) (Figure 7). Comparisons of mean number of mast cells among three groups were done using Kruskal–Wallis test and it was statistically significant (p value: 0.001) (Table 2). Intergroup analysis was done using Mann–Whitney U test which was also statistically significant (p value: 0.0002, 0.0004, and 0.000001) (Table 3).

4. Discussion

Oral lichen planus is a T cell mediated autoimmune disease in which autocytotoxic CD8+ T cells activate the apoptosis of oral epithelial cells [9]. Clinically, oral lichenoid reactions

TABLE 2: Comparison of mast cell distribution among study groups using Kruskal–Wallis test.

Group	N	Mean mast cell count	Range	Standard deviation	p value
Group I	10	2.02	0.9–3.1	1.18	
Group II	21	14.98	7.9–33.4	5.16	*0.001 (significant)*
Group III	21	7.96	1.2–17.4	5.04	

Note. p value is significant below the value of 0.05.

TABLE 3: Intergroup comparison of mast cell distribution using Mann–Whitney U test.

S. number	Comparison of groups	Median	Mann–Whitney U test	p value
(1)	*Group II versus Group III*			
	Group II	14.4	368.5	*0.0002 (significant)*
	Group III	6.6	72.5	
(2)	*Group III versus Group I*			
	Group III	6.6	188.5	*0.0004 (significant)*
	Group I	1.5	21.5	
(3)	*Group II versus Group I*			
	Group II	14.4	210	*0.000001 (significant)*
	Group I	1.5	0	

p value of <0.017 was considered as statistically significant.

may mimic OLP; nevertheless they are unilateral in distribution unlike bilateral occurrence in OLP. These lesions might be associated with a known aetiology; however they are analogous to oral lichen planus both clinically and histologically [10]. Mast cells have also been demonstrated in the lamina propria of oral lichenoid reaction but however the role of these cells in pathogenesis of OLR is not well understood like OLP. Various studies have provided substantial data to support the responsibility of mast cells in the pathogenesis of oral lichen planus and oral lichenoid reaction. Our study was aimed at quantifying mast cells as a distinguishing factor between OLP and OLR histopathologically. Toluidine Blue which has high affinity for the metachromatic granules in the mast cells was chosen to specifically recognize these cells in the study samples.

Oral lichen planus occurs mainly in adults above 40 years with female predilection [11]. However our sample showed slight increase in male predilection. This could be attributed to smaller sample size. A high female predilection is also noted in OLR irrespective of its etiology which matches in our study [12]. A wide variety of studies have concluded that the buccal mucosa is the most common site of occurrence of OLP and OLR in the oral cavity [13–15]. Among the 42 cases studied, about 73% of lesions were present on the buccal mucosa which is consistent with the above studies. A steady increase in the quantity of mast cells from normal oral tissues to OLR to OLP was noted among the samples. The mast cell count was highest in OLP cases compared to OLR suggesting a vital role demonstrated by mast cells in the pathogenesis of these lesions. Similar findings consistent with our study were noted in several other studies conducted by various authors [8, 16, 17]. In OLP, degranulation of mast cells releases proinflammatory mediators such as chymase, TNF-α, and tryptase. Release of TNF-α from degranulation of mast cells can upregulate RANTES from T cells leading to the activation and secretion of matrix metalloproteinases by T cells from lesions which are responsible for the degradation of basement membrane. At the areas of basement membrane disruption in OLP, presence of both mast cells and intraepithelial $CD8^+$ T cells suggests its role in pathogenesis of OLP. This concept emphasizes how mast cells and T cells work together for the growth of lesion chronicity in OLP; thus it recognizes that breakdown of matrix may help migration of T cell from the vasculature to epithelium and lamina propria [11, 16]. In OLR, the exposure to exogenic antigens triggers a hyperimmune type of response which mobilizes mast cells to the affected site, which in turn causes keratinocytes apoptosis. Therefore, from our study, the difficulties in separation of the two conditions in the perspective of overlapping in the range of the values have been clearly explained. However, unlike OLP, the withdrawal of the causative agent leads to a reduction in the mast cells in OLR justifying a decreased number of mast cells in OLR compared to OLP [18].

5. Conclusion

Our study revealed that mast cell count is increased in OLP compared to OLR thereby guiding us to propose that mast cell count can be used as one of the essential histopathological elements in the differentiation of OLP and OLR.

Conflicts of Interest

The authors declare that there are no conflicts of interest regarding the publication of this paper.

Acknowledgments

The authors are thankful to Dr. C. Ravindran, Professor at and Head of Department of Oral and Maxillofacial Surgery, for providing normal tissue samples towards the completion of this study.

References

[1] N. Lavanya, P. Jayanthi, U. Rao, and K. Ranganathan, "Oral lichen planus: An update on pathogenesis and treatment," *Journal of Oral and Maxillofacial Pathology*, vol. 15, no. 2, pp. 127–132, 2011.

[2] B. Dudhia, S. Dudhia, P. Patel, and Y. Jani, "Oral lichen planus to oral lichenoid lesions: Evolution or revolution," *Journal of Oral and Maxillofacial Pathology*, vol. 19, no. 3, pp. 364–370, 2015.

[3] K. Shirasuna, "Oral lichen planus: Malignant potential and diagnosis," *Oral Science International*, vol. 11, no. 1, pp. 1–7, 2014.

[4] E. H. van der Meij and I. van der Waal, "Lack of clinicopathologic correlation in the diagnosis of oral lichen planus based on the presently available diagnostic criteria and suggestions for modifications," *Journal of Oral Pathology & Medicine*, vol. 32, no. 9, pp. 507–512, 2003.

[5] V. V. Kamath, K. Setlur, and K. Yerlagudda, "Oral lichenoid lesions - A review and update," *Indian Journal of Dermatology*, vol. 60, no. 1, p. 102, 2015.

[6] L. J. Walsh, "Mast cells and oral inflammation," *Critical Reviews in Oral Biology & Medicine*, vol. 14, pp. 188–198, 2003.

[7] Z. Z. Zhao, N. W. Savage, P. B. Sugerman, and L. J. Walsh, "Mast cell/T cell interactions in oral lichen planus," *Journal of Oral Pathology & Medicine*, vol. 31, no. 4, pp. 189–195, 2002.

[8] D. Santhosh Reddy, B. Sivapathasundharam, T. R. Saraswathi, and G. Sriram, "Evaluation of mast cells, eosinophils, blood capillaries in oral lichen planus and oral lichenoid mucositis," *Indian Journal of Dental Research*, vol. 23, no. 5, pp. 695-696, 2012.

[9] S. B. Ismail, S. K. S. Kumar, and R. B. Zain, "Oral lichen planus and lichenoid reactions: etiopathogenesis, diagnosis, management and malignant transformation," *Journal of oral science*, vol. 49, no. 2, pp. 89–106, 2007.

[10] I. Al-Hashimi, M. Schifter, P. B. Lockhart et al., "Oral lichen planus and oral lichenoid lesions: diagnostic and therapeutic considerations," *Oral Surgery, Oral Medicine, Oral Pathology, Oral Radiology, and Endodontology*, vol. 103, supplement 1, pp. S25–S31, 2007.

[11] P. B. Sugerman, N. W. Savage, L. J. Walsh et al., "The pathogenesis of oral lichen planus," *Critical Reviews in Oral Biology & Medicine*, vol. 13, no. 4, pp. 350–365, 2002.

[12] D.-A. Cortés-Ramírez, M.-L. Gainza-Cirauqui, M.-A. Echebarria-Goikouria, and J. M. Aguirre-Urizar, "Oral lichenoid disease as a premalignant condition: The controversies and the unknown," *Medicina Oral Patología Oral y Cirugía Bucal*, vol. 14, no. 3, pp. E118–E122, 2009.

[13] D. Eisen, M. Carrozzo, J.-V. B. Sebastian, and K. Thongprasom, "Number V. Oral lichen planus: clinical features and management," *Oral Diseases*, vol. 11, no. 6, pp. 338–349, 2005.

[14] S. L. Myers, N. L. Rhodus, H. M. Parsons, J. S. Hodges, and S. Kaimal, "A retrospective survey of oral lichenoid lesions: Revisiting the diagnostic process for oral lichen planus," *Oral Surgery, Oral Medicine, Oral Pathology, Oral Radiology, and Endodontology*, vol. 93, no. 6, pp. 676–681, 2002.

[15] J. J. Jacobson, P.-J. Lamey, B. E. McCartan, D. G. MacDonald, and R. M. MacKie, "Basal cell cytoplasmic autoantibodies in oral lichenoid reactions," *Oral Surgery, Oral Medicine, Oral Pathology, Oral Radiology, and Endodontology*, vol. 79, no. 1, pp. 44–49, 1995.

[16] L. J. Walsh, M. F. Davis, L. J. Xu, and N. W. Savage, "Relationship between mast cell degranulation and inflammation in the oral cavity," *Journal of Oral Pathology & Medicine*, vol. 24, no. 6, pp. 266–272, 1995.

[17] R. Sharma, K. Sircar, S. Singh, and V. Rastogi, "Role of mast cells in pathogenesis of oral lichen planus," *Journal of Oral and Maxillofacial Pathology*, vol. 15, no. 3, pp. 267–271, 2011.

[18] G. Jahanshahi and A. Aminzadeh, "A histochemical and immunohistochemical study of mast cells in differentiating oral lichen planus from oral lichenoid reactions," *Quintessence International*, vol. 41, no. 3, pp. 221–227, 2010.

19

Immunotherapy of Neuromyelitis Optica

Benjamin Bienia and Roumen Balabanov

Department of Neurological Sciences, Multiple Sclerosis Center, Rush University Medical Center, 1725 W. Harrison Street, Suite 309, Chicago, IL 60612, USA

Correspondence should be addressed to Roumen Balabanov; roumen_balabanov@rush.edu

Academic Editor: Daniel Menkes

Neuromyelitis optica (NMO) is a chronic inflammatory disease of the central nervous system that affects the optic nerves and spinal cord resulting in visual impairment and myelopathy. There is a growing body of evidence that immunotherapeutic agents targeting T and B cell functions, as well as active elimination of proinflammatory molecules from the peripheral blood circulation, can attenuate disease progression. In this review, we discuss the immunotherapeutic options and the treatment strategies in NMO. We also analyze the pathogenic mechanisms of the disease in order to provide recommendations regarding treatments.

1. Introduction

Neuromyelitis optica (NMO), also known as Devic's disease, is a chronic inflammatory disease of the central nervous system (CNS) that preferentially targets the optic nerves and spinal cord [1]. The overall disease incidence has been estimated at 1 : 100,000 and that it has a predilection for middle-aged, non-Caucasian females [2]. NMO spectrum disorders (NMOSD) encompass a variation of this classical picture in that patients may have brain involvement or a more limited presentation such as isolated transverse myelitis or an optic neuritis [3]. Historically, many thought of NMO as a rare variant of multiple sclerosis (MS). Given the identification of unique clinical and radiological differences and the discovery of the NMO-IgG, an autoantibody against aquaporin-4 (aqp4), it is now understood to be its own entity with distinct pathogenesis, diagnostic criteria, prognosis, and treatment [1–5].

Until recently, NMO was considered a disease of limited therapeutic options and poor prognosis. Research over the last decade brought new understanding of the disease pathogenesis that translated into immunotherapy directed against this disease. Moreover, there is a growing body of evidence that NMO can be controlled by immunotherapeutics targeting its cellular and humoral immune mechanisms. We review the immunotherapy of NMO, the various treatment options, and the clinical strategies that are typically encountered in practice.

2. Neuromyelitis Optica: An Overview

NMO is a neurological disorder that classically presents as a case of severe bilateral optic neuritis associated with a transverse myelitis [1–5]. The typical disease onset is either acute or subacute, and the symptoms are likely to persist without treatment. Optic neuritis results in decreased or a complete loss of vision. Transverse myelitis is usually extensive and spans more than 3 consecutive vertebral segments. Deficits related to myelitis include paralysis and sensory loss below the lesion level along with gait impairment. Additional complications may include phrenic nerve paralysis, loss of sphincter control, dysautonomia, and painful tonic spasms. Brainstem (medulla oblongata and area postrema) can be involved at times with resultant persistent nausea and hiccups [6].

Magnetic resonance imaging (MRI) is used for diagnosis and monitoring of the disease [1, 4]. Optic nerve and spinal cord lesions appear as hyperintense on T2- and hypointense on T1-weighted images and enhance with gadolinium when they are inflamed. In the acute phase, the inflamed lesions also enlarge in size secondary to tissue edema. Inflammation may persist for months and result in tissue atrophy [7]. MRI lesions involving the brainstem, hypothalamus, and periventricular white matter may be seen in typical NMOSD and sometimes late in the disease course of NMO [1–3]. Independent of imaging, visual evoked potentials and CSF studies can be helpful in establishing the diagnosis [4, 8]. Optic coherence tomography (OCT) may also be used to monitor the extent and the degree of progression of optic neuropathy [9].

NMO follows a relapsing-remitting clinical course in 70–90% of all patients [2]. Such a clinical course is correlated with female gender, older age of disease onset, longer (>3 months) optic neuritis-myelitis interval, and presence of systemic autoimmunity [2, 3]. Seropositivity for anti-aqp4 antibody is also a strong predictor for future disease relapses [10]. A monophasic clinical course tends to occur in young males. Neurological disability in relapsing-remitting disease appears to be a cumulative result of disease relapses [2]. After five years, approximately 50% of affected individuals have significant visual or motor impairment and require assistive devices for ambulation [2]. This time frame of five years is also notable for a mortality rate of 32% with the relapsing-remitting disease and 10% with the monophasic disease. Most patients expire from disease complications such as respiratory failure, urosepsis, and pulmonary embolism [2–4].

The etiology of NMO is unknown but it is believed to be an autoimmune disorder triggered by an environmental factor, possibly an infection, in genetically susceptible individuals [11–13]. The principal effector in NMO is the self-reactive, complement-activating anti-aqp4 antibody [14]. Aqp4 is a transmembrane protein that regulates the flow of water in cells. It is expressed by CNS astrocytes and astrocytic processes surrounding small blood vessels at the glia limitans [15]. The autoantibody has the capacity to bind to aqp4 on the astrocytic foot processes and then recruit and activate complement. This leads to the mobilization of polymorphonuclear cells (neutrophils and eosinophils), inflammation, and tissue swelling [16, 17].

Recent studies indicate that Th17 cells (a T cell subset producing interleukin 17) specific to aqp4 may also be involved in the disease pathogenesis [18]. They are implicated in the breakdown of the blood-brain barrier allowing extravasation of anti-aqp4 antibody and complement, along with recruitment of polymorphonuclear cells to the lesion sites. Pathologically, NMO lesions involve both the white and gray matter. They contain perivascular deposits of immune complexes, activated complement, and inflammatory cellular infiltrates [19]. The cellular infiltrates are composed of mononuclear and polymorphonuclear cells. Astrocytes targeted by the autoimmune response display cytopathic changes and downregulate the expression of aqp4 in a vasculocentric pattern [20]. Vascular hyalinization, tissue necrosis, demyelination, and gliosis commonly accompany the inflammatory process [18–22].

3. Immunotherapy of NMO

Immunotherapy of NMO is based on the current understanding of its pathogenesis. As summarized above, lesion formation involves interplay between cellular and humoral immune responses. It appears that the autoimmune reaction arises in the periphery with the appearance of anti-aqp4 antibodies and Th17 cells; then it progresses in cascade-like fashion. There are several points of augmentation and diversification of the autoimmune reaction, including complement activation and release of interleukin 17, which have proinflammatory and chemotactic effects. This contributes to the recruitment of mononuclear and polymorphonuclear cells to the sites of initial inflammation. As the inflammatory reaction unfolds, a number of nonspecific injurious mechanisms become involved including vascular damage, tissue swelling, oxidative stress, astrocyte injury, and secondary demyelination. These processes can be suppressed by using immunotherapeutic agents targeting T and B cells (immunosuppressant, cytotoxic, and biologic agents) or by actively removing the pro-inflammatory factors from the peripheral blood circulation (therapeutic plasma exchange) (Figure 1). These therapeutic approaches are nonspecific to the self-reactive cells or antibodies but affect the immune system globally. Inflammation in NMO is necrotizing in nature and cannot be reversed; it can only be prevented or minimized with effective treatment.

Immunotherapy of NMO is divided into two parts: rescue therapy of an acute disease relapse and disease-modifying therapy. The goal of rescue therapy is to suppress the acute inflammatory process in order to achieve functional recovery in patients. Early and effective rescue therapy is essential in minimizing the degree of permanent tissue damage and neurological disability. Corticosteroids and plasma exchange (PLEX) are the most commonly used therapeutic modalities in acute settings. Corticosteroids exert global immunosuppressive and anti-inflammatory effects, whereas PLEX removes antibodies, complement, and cytokines from the blood. The effects of both treatment modalities are rapid and can be appreciated within days of their initiation. Corticosteroids are administered intravenously. The usual treatment regimen is that of methylprednisolone 1000 mg daily for 5 days, followed by an extended oral prednisone taper starting at 60–100 mg per day [23]. If the disease is refractory to corticosteroids, PLEX therapy should be considered. PLEX can be beneficial to patients with acute NMO and is frequently recommended as a second line therapy in refractory cases [24, 25]. In practice, methylprednisolone is administered first and if there is no treatment response within three to four days, PLEX may be initiated. PLEX is administered every other day (1.5x plasma volume per each exchange) over the course of two weeks. In our clinical experience, most patients exhibited functional improvement after four to six PLEX treatments. The patient's response to initial rescue therapy may not be immediate and should be reevaluated within a few weeks after its completion. In cases of a poor response or an early disease relapse, one may consider repeating the corticosteroid/PLEX treatment or using cytotoxic agents such as cyclophosphamide. The latter is administered as several monthly infusions at $0.5–1\,g/m^2$ and can be beneficial in refractory cases, particularly in patients with concomitant systemic autoimmune diseases [26].

The goal of disease-modifying treatment is to maintain disease remission and prevent future relapses. It is important to keep in mind that the majority of NMO patients are likely to have a relapsing-remitting disease. As such, their neurological disability will be cumulative and related to the frequency and severity of their disease relapses [27]. As many as 60% of all patients are likely to develop a disease relapse

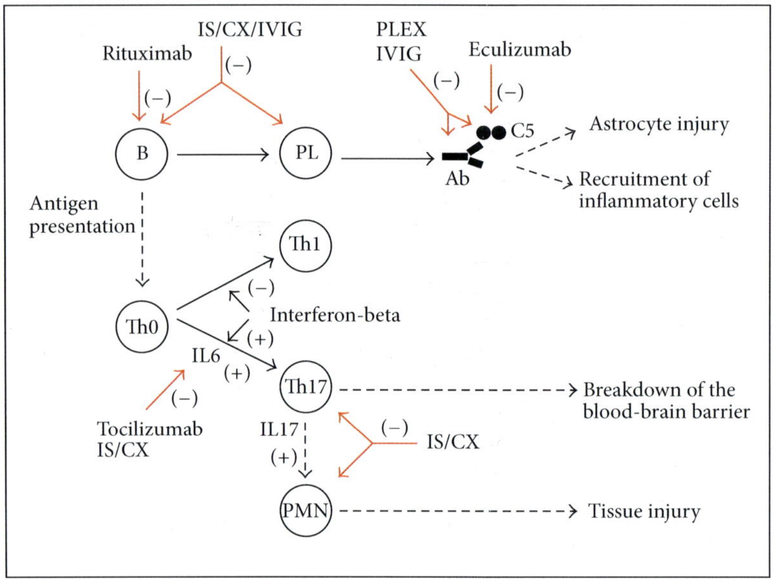

FIGURE 1: Summary of the mechanisms of action of immunotherapies in NMO. Abbreviations: B = B cell, C5 = protein 5 of complement, CX = cytotoxic agent, IL = interleukin, IS = immunosuppressant, IVIG = intravenous immunoglobulin, PL = plasma cell, PMN = polymorphonuclear cell, Th = T helper cell.

in the first year and 95% within three years of diagnosis [2]. In this respect early recognition of the predictors of relapsing-remitting disease is important. There are no randomized double blind placebo-controlled studies that have demonstrated the efficacy of any of the aforementioned treatment options. Most of the current knowledge is derived from anecdotal or small retrospective studies. Therefore, recommended treatments are based on the current understanding of disease pathogenesis, observed responses to treatment, tolerability, and the availability of resources.

Immunosuppressant agents interfering with the function of T and B cells have been shown to prevent disease relapses and reduce neurological disability in NMO. They can be viewed as steroid-sparing agents extending the beneficial effect of the rescue corticosteroid therapy. Azathioprine, perhaps the most commonly used oral immunosuppressant agent in NMO, primarily suppresses T cell function [23, 28]. The largest retrospective study involving 99 patients reported that azathioprine decreased the annualized relapse rate by 76% and either improved or stabilized disability in 40% of patients in a twelve-month period [28]. Azathioprine may be initiated at a dose of 50 mg daily or less and subsequently increased as tolerated to a target dose of 2-3 mg/kg/day (approximately 200–300 mg daily) either during or immediately after the intravenous methylprednisolone treatment. Doses lower than 2 mg/kg/day may have a limited effect on disease activity [28]. Prednisone in a prolonged tapering regimen from a dose of 100 mg down to 10 mg over a year may be added in order to compensate for the slow mechanism of action of azathioprine and to broaden the spectrum of immunosuppression. Once disease remission is achieved, then the medication can be continued as monotherapy for years at the lowest effective dose [23, 28].

Mycophenolate mofetil is another oral immunosuppressant that has the advantage of suppressing the proliferation of both T and B cells, as well as the production of antibodies by plasma cells [29]. It is effective in patients with NMO at an average dose of 2000 mg daily and is generally well tolerated [29]. In a retrospective study involving 25 patients, treatment with mycophenolate mofetil was reported to decrease the annualized relapse rate in 71% of patients and improves disability in 91% of patients over a median follow-up of twenty-eight months [29]. Similar to azathioprine, adding corticosteroids (intravenous or oral) to mycophenolate mofetil treatment can potentiate its efficacy, particularly in the first several months of treatment. In addition, prednisone can prevent disease relapses in some cases as a sole disease-modifying agent. In these instances, doses at 25 mg or above every other day are necessary to maintain disease remission [30].

A few small case studies reported the disease-modifying effect of intermittent PLEX on NMO relapses [31, 32]. This approach may be used as a long-term extension of the rescue PLEX, especially in patients who have had a dramatic initial treatment response. It can be also considered as an alternative to immunosuppressants in the setting of treatment failure or significant side effects. While the frequency of intermittent PLEX sessions should be established empirically based on the duration of treatment-induced disease remissions, it is usually administered once every two to three months [31]. More frequent regimens on a weekly basis can be considered as well [32]. As previously noted, a small dose of daily prednisone of 5–20 mg daily can provide an add-on therapeutic benefit [31].

Rituximab is a monoclonal antibody against B cells (anti-CD 20), which can directly deplete this cell population from the peripheral blood circulation in a matter of a few weeks. This effect is global as B cells serve as precursors of antibody-producing plasma cells and are involved in the processes of antigen presentation and T cell activation. Rituximab has been reported to be effective, particularly in patients who have failed oral immunosuppressant therapy [33–35]. The two largest retrospective studies, which included more than 20 patients, each reported significant reduction in the annualized relapse rate and improvement in neurological disability in more than 80%–90% of cases in nearly a two-year period [34, 35]. The drug can be administered intravenously at 375 mg/m once weekly for four weeks or at a flat dose of 1 g two weeks apart. Periodic retreatments are often necessary depending on the clinical response [36, 37]. Notably, the rituximab dose and frequency of administration can be tailored to the level of peripheral B cells, which should be maintained at zero.

Eculizumab is another monoclonal antibody that neutralizes complement protein 5 (anti-C5), thereby inhibiting the propagation of the complement cascade, the recruitment of inflammatory cells, and the formation of the membrane-attack complex. Recently, a small open-label study involving 14 NMO-IgG seropositive patients reported that biweekly intravenous administration of 900 mg of eculizumab (after a titration period) had a significant impact on the disease [38]. Twelve of 14 patients became relapse free after twelve months of treatment. Significant improvements in visual acuity and median disability scores were reported as well. None of the patients developed disease worsening. However, a return of disease activity was observed in 5 patients following discontinuation of the medication. Eculizumab administration was associated with significant suppression of serum complement activity and reduction of C5 levels in CSF, whereas medication discontinuation was associated with their normalization. NMO-IgG titers measured throughout the study remained unchanged.

Other authors reported benefit with other agents including cyclosporine, mitoxantrone, methotrexate, intravenous immunoglobulin (IVIG), and tocilizumab (anti-interleukin 6) [39–43]. For instance, intermittent administration of IVIG may be useful as an acute and chronic treatment in patients who have failed standard immunosuppressive therapy [42]. Tocilizumab blockade of interleukin 6, a cytokine that potentiates B cell survival and Th17 immune responses, may be effective in patients with highly active disease that are unresponsive to multiple immunosuppressive and cell depleting therapies [43]. Overall, these studies are retrospective, anecdotal, or small in size [39–43]. Nonetheless, NMO is a rare autoimmune disease that can be refractory to multiple treatments and every positive experience can be of potential value in clinical practice.

4. Additional Considerations

Currently, there is no biomarker for therapeutic response in NMO. There are observations correlating effective immunotherapy to a decrease in anti-aqp4 antibody levels of patients [44]. However, there are no definitive studies establishing the significance of this autoantibody as a biomarker of treatment response. Moreover, it appears that seropositive and seronegative NMO patients do not differ in their responses to immunotherapy [45, 46]. Most of the treatment assessments are based on general neurologic or empirical principles. These include change in relapse rate or neurological disability and appearance of new or gadolinium-enhancing lesions on MRI. In a few studies neurological improvement in patients treated with PLEX was reported to be associated with early treatment, rapid initial response, male gender, preserved leg reflexes, and absence of atrophy on MRI [46, 47]. In addition, there is evidence that preservation of retinal nerve fiber layer on OCT can be associated with a good treatment response to corticosteroids and PLEX [9, 32].

Certain laboratory tests reflecting the mechanism of action of medications may be useful in monitoring and predicting treatment responses in patients. For instance, a slight elevation of the erythrocyte mean corpuscular volume (MCV) more than 5 points above baseline following treatment with azathioprine may correlate with effective immune suppression and associated decline in patients' annualized relapse rate [28]. This increase in size of red blood cells is a metabolic effect of the medication and in fact some of its metabolites can be directly measured in these cells [48]. Elevation of MCV is well tolerated and is reversible with discontinuation of azathioprine [48]. Levels of mycophenolate mofetil metabolites such as mycophenolic acid and mycophenolic acid glucuronide can be directly measured in patient's blood [49]. Even though there are studies indicating the significance of therapeutic monitoring of mycophenolic acid in organ transplantation, its value in NMO remains to be established.

Rituximab is a cell depleting monoclonal antibody whose clinical benefit negatively correlates with levels of peripheral B cells [36, 50]. In some reported cases, rituximab failure was associated with rapid recovery of B cells after treatment. However, disease worsening on rituximab may have a more complex nature. Initial response to corticosteroids was identified as a negative predictor in some patients. This was hypothesized as being due to predominant T cell involvement with relatively less B cell involvement in the disease's pathogenesis [50]. Early disease worsening can be also due to extensive B cell death and secondary nonspecific activation of the immune system or by transient elevation of the anti-aqp4 antibody [50–52]. It is also important to mention that rituximab exerts little effect on certain CD20 negative B cells and on mature antibody-producing plasma cells, which may maintain the disease activity despite its presence.

Even though most of the immunotherapies are new to the NMO field, they are widely used in other autoimmune diseases and their side effects are well described in the medical literature. In general, NMO patients tolerate these therapies similarly to other patient populations. However, treatment of NMO patients with long-term immunosuppressants is complicated by their neurological disability and coexistent medical conditions. Therefore, systemic and organ-specific adverse effects should be expected and frequent monitoring is recommended. The most important adverse effects are myelosuppression and secondary leucopenias and lymphopenias. Significant myelosupperssion associated with azathioprine use can occur in patients in whom the critical metabolizing enzyme thiopurine S-methyltransferase (TPMT) is either partially or completely inactivated [28, 53]. The latter can be seen in patients with homozygous or heterozygous mutations in the TPMT gene. These mutations may be found in 10% of the population or associated with intake of enzyme inhibitors such as aspirin, allopurinol, and furosemide. Independently, myelosuppression can also be potentiated by carbamazepine, an anticonvulsant that is commonly used for neuropathic pain [54]. Finally, NMO patients are likely to be treated with multiple immunosuppressive and cytotoxic agents raising concerns about secondary malignancies as well as systemic or opportunistic infections [28, 29, 34, 38].

One should be aware that certain therapeutic agents that are commonly used in MS could actually worsen NMO. In particular, treatment with interferon-beta has been shown to increase disease activity in NMO, as well as to increase anti-aqp-4 antibody titers [55]. It is now recognized that disease mechanisms of MS and NMO involve different T cell subsets. Autoimmunity in MS is driven predominantly by Th1 cells (a T cell subset producing interferon-gamma), whose function is suppressed by interferon-beta. In contrast, NMO is a predominantly Th17-driven disease and administration of interferon-beta potentiates its pro-inflammatory effect on neutrophils and antibody production [56]. In addition, fingolimod and natalizumab may be associated with persisting or worsening NMO activity [57, 58]. Therefore, these medications should be avoided in patients suspected of having NMO. In clinical practice, NMO and NMOSD should be on the differential diagnosis in patients with suspected MS who worsen on interferon-beta, natalizumab, or fingolimod treatment. As a corollary, NMO patients with coexisting systemic autoimmune diseases should be carefully monitored for unintended treatment-induced disease worsening, as more than 30% of all NMO patients may have another autoimmune disease [59].

There is circumstantial evidence of an association between infections and NMO. Disease onset may be preceded by an infectious prodrome in up to 30% of all patients [2]. Chronic infections such as Mycobacterium tuberculosis, human immunodeficiency virus, Helicobacter pylori, and others may be present in patients with NMO [12, 60, 61]. One should consider investigating patients for chronic infections, particularly if environmental or personal risk factors for such infections can be identified. One may also consider the possibility of disease relapses being triggered by more ubiquitous microbial species. These can express immune epitopes with the capacity to cross-react and activate anti-aqp4 specific T and B cells [62–65]. The latter may be relevant to patients with chronic respiratory or bladder problems and decubitus ulcers, who are more prone for infectious complications. Clinical vigilance and at times prophylactic use of antibiotics and changes in immunotherapy may be warranted. In some NMO cases, specific antibiotic (antituberculosis) treatment has been reported to induce disease remission [66]. At this point, there is no available information regarding whether or not vaccination planning should be applied differently to NMO patients. Nonetheless, a clinician should consider a patients' general health status and their current immunosuppressive therapy.

Despite the fact that immunotherapy of NMO takes into account the relative predominance of certain humoral and cellular processes in the disease pathogenesis, it remains nonspecific in nature and produces global immunosuppression. Recently, new experimental approaches directed against more disease-specific immune mechanisms were proposed [67]. Among these is the use of inhibitors of anti-aqp4 antibody binding. An example of this approach is aquaporumab, a nonpathogenic monoclonal antibody against aqp4, which can function as a competitive inhibitor of the disease-associated NMO IgG. This strategy has generated promising results in some of the *in vitro* and *in vivo* models of NMO [68]. Another example is the treatment of patient sera with bacteria-derived endoglycosidase S. Such treatment causes IgG deglycosylation and converts the pathogenic anti-aqp4 antibodies into nonpathogenic target-blocking antibodies [69]. Development and implementation of disease-specific therapeutics may be an important step towards improving the treatment outcomes of the disease and solving some of the clinical dilemmas associated with chronic immunosuppression.

5. Conclusion

Clinical and basic science knowledge of NMO has dramatically increased over the last decade. Immunotherapy of NMO is still in its naissance but appears promising and certainly has changed the perception of NMO as an inevitably disabling or fatal disease. Perhaps, the most encouraging aspect is that a large number of treatment options may be used depending on the specific clinical settings. Issues that remain to be addressed include better and earlier recognition of patients with relapsing-remitting disease, identification of prognostic factors of treatment response, development of a biomarker of disease activity, and research on the infectious triggers of the disease. This is complicated by the fact that NMO is a rare disease such that the clinical experience with immunotherapies is still anecdotal. Multicenter, prospective, and controlled studies are required in order to identify the optimal immunotherapies for this disease.

Conflict of Interests

The authors declare that there is no conflict of interests regarding the publication of this paper.

References

[1] D. M. Wingerchuk, V. A. Lennon, S. J. Pittock, C. F. Lucchinetti, and B. G. Weinshenker, "Revised diagnostic criteria for neuromyelitis optica," *Neurology*, vol. 66, no. 10, pp. 1485–1489, 2006.

[2] D. M. Wingerchuk, W. F. Hogancamp, P. C. O'Brien, and B. G. Weinshenker, "The clinical course of neuromyelitis optica (Devic's syndrome)," *Neurology*, vol. 53, no. 5, pp. 1107–1114, 1999.

[3] D. M. Wingerchuk, V. A. Lennon, C. F. Lucchinetti, S. J. Pittock, and B. G. Weinshenker, "The spectrum of neuromyelitis optica," *The Lancet Neurology*, vol. 6, no. 9, pp. 805–815, 2007.

[4] J. I. O'Riordan, H. L. Gallagher, A. J. Thompson et al., "Clinical, CSF, and MRI findings in Devic's neuromyelitis optica," *Journal of Neurology Neurosurgery and Psychiatry*, vol. 60, no. 4, pp. 382–387, 1996.

[5] P. V. A. Lennon, D. M. Wingerchuk, T. J. Kryzer et al., "A serum autoantibody marker of neuromyelitis optica: distinction from multiple sclerosis," *The Lancet*, vol. 364, no. 9451, pp. 2106–2112, 2004.

[6] T. Misu, K. Fujihara, I. Nakashima, S. Sato, and Y. Itoyama, "Intractable hiccup and nausea with periaqueductal lesions in neuromyelitis optica," *Neurology*, vol. 65, no. 9, pp. 1479–1482, 2005.

[7] K. Tashiro, K. Ito, and Y. Maruo, "MR imaging of spinal cord in Devic disease," *Journal of Computer Assisted Tomography*, vol. 11, no. 3, pp. 516–517, 1987.

[8] F. Masuhr, M. Busch, K. Wetzel, L. Harms, and E. Schielke, "Relapsing myelitis with pathological visual evoked potentials: a case of neuromyelitis optica?" *European Journal of Neurology*, vol. 9, no. 4, pp. 430–432, 2002.

[9] D. B. Fernandes, A. S. Raza, R. G. Nogueira et al., "Evaluation of inner retinal layers in patients with multiple sclerosis or neuromyelitis optica using optical coherence tomography," *Ophthalmology*, vol. 57, no. 3, pp. 387–394, 2012.

[10] B. G. Weinshenker, D. M. Wingerchuk, S. Vukusic et al., "Neuromyelitis optica IgG predicts relapse after longitudinally extensive transverse myelitis," *Annals of Neurology*, vol. 59, no. 3, pp. 566–569, 2006.

[11] J. E. Cosnett, "Multiple sclerosis and neuromyelitis optica in tropical and subtropical countries," *Medical Hypotheses*, vol. 7, no. 1, pp. 61–63, 1981.

[12] S. Yoshimura, N. Isobe, T. Matsushita et al., "Distinct genetic and infectious profiles in Japanese neuromyelitis optica patients according to anti-aquaporin 4 antibody status," *Journal of Neurology, Neurosurgery and Psychiatry*, vol. 84, no. 1, pp. 29–34, 2013.

[13] H. Zéphir, I. Fajardy, O. Outteryck et al., "Is neuromyelitis optica associated with human leukocyte antigen?" *Multiple Sclerosis*, vol. 15, no. 5, pp. 571–579, 2009.

[14] V. A. Lennon, T. J. Kryzer, S. J. Pittock, A. S. Verkman, and S. R. Hinson, "IgG marker of optic-spinal multiple sclerosis binds to the aquaporin-4 water channel," *Journal of Experimental Medicine*, vol. 202, no. 4, pp. 473–477, 2005.

[15] P. Agre and D. Kozono, "Aquaporin water channels: molecular mechanisms for human diseases," *FEBS Letters*, vol. 555, no. 1, pp. 72–78, 2003.

[16] L. Sabater, A. Giralt, A. Boronat et al., "Cytotoxic effect of neuromyelitis optica antibody (NMO-IgG) to astrocytes: an in vitro study," *Journal of Neuroimmunology*, vol. 215, no. 1-2, pp. 31–35, 2009.

[17] T. Vincent, P. Saikali, R. Cayrol et al., "Functional consequences of neuromyelitis optica-IgG astrocyte interactions on blood-brain barrier permeability and granulocyte recruitment," *Journal of Immunology*, vol. 181, no. 8, pp. 5730–5737, 2008.

[18] Y. Li, H. Wang, Y. Long, Z. Lu, and X. Hu, "Increased memory Th17 cells in patients with neuromyelitis optica and multiple sclerosis," *Journal of Neuroimmunology*, vol. 234, no. 1-2, pp. 155–160, 2011.

[19] C. F. Lucchinetti, R. N. Mandler, D. McGavern et al., "A role for humoral mechanisms in the pathogenesis of Devic's neuromyelitis optica," *Brain*, vol. 125, no. 7, pp. 1450–1461, 2002.

[20] S. F. Roemer, J. E. Parisi, V. A. Lennon et al., "Pattern-specific loss of aquaporin-4 immunoreactivity distinguishes neuromyelitis optica from multiple sclerosis," *Brain*, vol. 130, no. 5, pp. 1194–1205, 2007.

[21] D. Lefkowitz and J. N. Angelo, "Neuromyelitis optica with unusual vascular changes," *Archives of Neurology*, vol. 41, no. 10, pp. 1103–1105, 1984.

[22] R. N. Mandler, L. E. Davis, D. R. Jeffery, and M. Kornfeld, "Devic's neuromyelitis optica: a clinicopathological study of 8 patients," *Annals of Neurology*, vol. 34, no. 2, pp. 162–168, 1993.

[23] R. N. Mandler, W. Ahmed, and J. E. Dencoff, "Devic's neuromyelitis optica: a prospective study of seven patients treated with prednisone and azathioprine," *Neurology*, vol. 51, no. 4, pp. 1219–1220, 1998.

[24] B. G. Weinshenker, P. C. O'Brien, T. M. Petterson et al., "A randomized trial of plasma exchange in acute central nervous system inflammatory demyelinating disease," *Annals of Neurology*, vol. 46, no. 6, pp. 878–886, 1999.

[25] M. Bonnan and P. Cabre, "Plasma exchange in severe attacks of neuromyelitis optica," *Multiple Sclerosis International*, vol. 2012, Article ID 787603, 9 pages, 2012.

[26] A. Polgár, C. Rózsa, V. Müller, J. Matolcsi, G. Poór, and E. V. Kiss, "Devic's syndrome and SLE. Challenges in diagnosis and therapeutic possibilities based on two overlapping cases," *Autoimmunity Reviews*, vol. 10, no. 3, pp. 171–174, 2011.

[27] D. M. Wingerchuk, S. J. Pittock, C. F. Lucchinetti, V. A. Lennon, and B. G. Weinshenker, "A secondary progressive clinical course is uncommon in neuromyelitis optica," *Neurology*, vol. 68, no. 8, pp. 603–605, 2007.

[28] C. Costanzi, M. Matiello, C. F. Lucchinetti et al., "Azathioprine: tolerability, efficacy, and predictors of benefit in neuromyelitis optica," *Neurology*, vol. 77, no. 7, pp. 659–666, 2011.

[29] A. Jacob, M. Matiello, B. G. Weinshenker et al., "Treatment of neuromyelitis optica with mycophenolate mofetil: retrospective analysis of 24 patients," *Archives of Neurology*, vol. 66, no. 9, pp. 1128–1133, 2009.

[30] S. Watanabe, T. Misu, I. Miyazawa et al., "Low-dose corticosteroids reduce relapses in neuromyelitis optica: a retrospective analysis," *Multiple Sclerosis*, vol. 13, no. 8, pp. 968–974, 2007.

[31] K. Miyamoto and S. Kusunoki, "Intermittent plasmapheresis prevents recurrence in neuromyelitis optica," *Therapeutic Apheresis and Dialysis*, vol. 13, no. 6, pp. 505–508, 2009.

[32] B. O. Khatri, J. Kramer, M. Dukic, M. Palencia, and W. Verre, "Maintenance plasma exchange therapy for steroid-refractory neuromyelitis optica," *Journal of Clinical Apheresis*, vol. 27, no. 4, pp. 183–192, 2012.

[33] B. A. C. Cree, S. Lamb, K. Morgan, A. Chen, E. Waubant, and C. Genain, "An open label study of the effects of rituximab in neuromyelitis optica," *Neurology*, vol. 64, no. 7, pp. 1270–1272, 2005.

[34] A. Jacob, B. G. Weinshenker, I. Violich et al., "Treatment of neuromyelitis optica with rituximab: retrospective analysis of 25 patients," *Archives of Neurology*, vol. 65, no. 11, pp. 1443–1448, 2008.

[35] G. S. Bedi, A. D. Brown, S. R. Delgado, N. Usmani, B. L. Lam, and W. A. Sheremata, "Impact of rituximab on relapse rate and disability in neuromyelitis optica," *Multiple Sclerosis*, vol. 17, no. 10, pp. 1225–1230, 2011.

[36] S.-H. Kim, W. Kim, X. F. Li, I.-J. Jung, and H. J. Kim, "Repeated treatment with rituximab based on the assessment of peripheral circulating memory B cells in patients with relapsing neuromyelitis optica over 2 years," *Archives of Neurology*, vol. 68, no. 11, pp. 1412–1420, 2011.

[37] H. L. Pellkofer, M. Krumbholz, A. Berthele et al., "Long-term follow-up of patients with neuromyelitis optica after repeated

therapy with rituximab," *Neurology*, vol. 76, no. 15, pp. 1310–1315, 2011.

[38] S. J. Pittock, V. A. Lennon, A. McKeon et al., "Eculizumab in AQP4-IgG-positive relapsing neurolmyelitis optica spectrum disorders: an open-label study," *The Lancet Neurology*, vol. 12, no. 6, pp. 554–562, 2013.

[39] T. Kageyama, M. Komori, K. Miyamoto et al., "Combination of cyclosporine A with corticosteroids is effective for the treatment of neuromyelitis optica," *Journal of Neurology*, vol. 260, no. 2, pp. 627–634, 2012.

[40] B. Weinstock-Guttman, M. Ramanathan, N. Lincoff et al., "Study of mitoxantrone for the treatment of recurrent neuromyelitis optica (Devic disease)," *Archives of Neurology*, vol. 63, no. 7, pp. 957–963, 2006.

[41] A. Minagar and W. Sheramata, "Treatment of Devic's with methotrexate and prednisone," *International Journal of Multiple Sclerosis Care*, vol. 2, pp. 39–43, 2000.

[42] J. Bakker and L. Metz, "Devic's neuromyelitis optica treated with intravenous gamma globulin (IVIG)," *Canadian Journal of Neurological Sciences*, vol. 31, no. 2, pp. 265–267, 2004.

[43] B. C. Kieseier, O. Stüve, T. Dehmel et al., "Disease amelioration with tocilizumab in a treatment-resistant patient with neuromyelitis optica: implication for cellular immune responses," *Archives of Neurology*, vol. 7, no. 3, pp. 390–393, 2012.

[44] T. Takahashi, K. Fujihara, I. Nakashima et al., "Anti-aquaporin-4 antibody is involved in the pathogenesis of NMO: a study on antibody titre," *Brain*, vol. 130, no. 5, pp. 1235–1243, 2007.

[45] M. Bonnan, R. Valentino, M. Bonnan, H. Mehdaoui, D. Smadja, and P. Cabre, "Plasma exchange in severe spinal attacks associated with neuromyelitis optica spectrum disorder," *Multiple Sclerosis*, vol. 15, no. 4, pp. 487–492, 2009.

[46] Y. M. Lim, S. Y. Pyun, B. H. Kang, J. Kim, and K. K. Kim, "Factors associated with the effectiveness of plasma exchange for the recruitment of NMO-IgG positive neuromyelitis optica spectrum disorders," *Multiple Sclerosis Journal*, vol. 19, no. 9, pp. 1216–1218, 2012.

[47] M. Keegan, A. A. Pineda, R. L. McClelland, C. H. Darby, M. Rodriguez, and B. G. Weinshenker, "Plasma exchange for severe attacks of CNS demyelination: predictors of response," *Neurology*, vol. 58, no. 1, pp. 143–148, 2002.

[48] C. Cuffari, "A physician's guide to azathioprine metabolite testing," *Gastroenterology and Hepatology*, vol. 2, no. 1, pp. 58–63, 2006.

[49] H. Jeong and B. Kaplan, "Therapeutic monitoring of mycophenolate mofetil," *Clinical Journal of the American Society of Nephrology*, vol. 2, no. 1, pp. 184–191, 2007.

[50] B. M. Greenberg, D. Graves, G. Remington et al., "Rituximab dosing and monitoring strategies in neuromyelitis optica patients: creating strategies for therapeutic success," *Multiple Sclerosis Journal*, vol. 18, no. 7, pp. 1022–1026, 2012.

[51] J. W. Lindsey, K. M. Meulmester, S. A. Brod, F. Nelson, and J. S. Wolinsky, "Variable results after rituximab in neuromyelitis optica," *Journal of the Neurological Sciences*, vol. 317, no. 1-2, pp. 103–105, 2012.

[52] I. Nakashima, T. Takahashi, B. A. C. Cree et al., "Transient increases in anti-aquaporin-4 antibody titers following rituximab treatment in neuromyelitis optica, in association with elevated serum BAFF levels," *Journal of Clinical Neuroscience*, vol. 18, no. 7, pp. 997–998, 2011.

[53] H. L. McLeod and C. Siva, "The thiopurine S-methyltansferase gene locus—implications for clinical pharmacogenomics," *Pharmacogenomics*, vol. 3, no. 1, pp. 89–98, 2002.

[54] R. J. Flanagan and L. Dunk, "Haematological toxicity of drugs used in psychiatry," *Human Psychopharmacology*, vol. 23, no. 1, pp. 27–41, 2008.

[55] J. Palace, M. I. Leite, A. Nairne, and A. Vincent, "Interferon beta treatment in neuromyelitis optica: increase in relapses and aquaporin 4 antibody titers," *Archives of Neurology*, vol. 67, no. 8, pp. 1016–1017, 2010.

[56] R. C. Axtell, C. Raman, and L. Steinman, "Interferon-β exacerbates Th17-mediated inflammatory disease," *Trends in Immunology*, vol. 32, no. 6, pp. 272–277, 2011.

[57] J.-H. Min, B. J. Kim, and K. H. Lee, "Development of extensive brain lesions following fingolimod (FTY720) treatment in a patient with neuromyelitis optica spectrum disorder," *Multiple Sclerosis*, vol. 18, no. 1, pp. 113–115, 2012.

[58] A. Jacob, M. Hutchinson, L. Elsone et al., "Does natalizumab therapy worsen neuromyelitis optica?" *Neurology*, vol. 79, no. 10, pp. 1065–1066, 2012.

[59] S. J. Pittock, V. A. Lennon, J. De Seze et al., "Neuromyelitis optica and non-organ-specific autoimmunity," *Archives of Neurology*, vol. 65, no. 1, pp. 78–83, 2008.

[60] J. Sellner, B. Hemmer, and M. Mühlau, "The clinical spectrum and immunobiology of parainfectious neuromyelitis optica (Devic) syndromes," *Journal of Autoimmunity*, vol. 34, no. 4, pp. 371–379, 2010.

[61] W. Li, M. Minohara, H. Piao et al., "Association of anti-Helicobacter pylori neutrophil-activating protein antibody response with anti-aquaporin-4 autoimmunity in Japanese patients with multiple sclerosis and neuromyelitis optica," *Multiple Sclerosis*, vol. 15, no. 12, pp. 1411–1421, 2009.

[62] M. Koga, T. Takahashi, M. Kawai, K. Fujihara, and T. Kanda, "A serological analysis of viral and bacterial infections associated with neuromyelitis optica," *Journal of the Neurological Sciences*, vol. 300, no. 1-2, pp. 19–22, 2011.

[63] Z. Ren, Y. Wang, T. Duan et al., "Cross-immunoreactivity between bacterial aquaporin-Z and human aquaporin-4: potential relevance to neuromyelitis optica," *Journal of Immunology*, vol. 189, no. 9, pp. 4602–4611, 2012.

[64] P. O. Barros, U. C. Linhares, B. Teixeira et al., "High in vitro immune reactivity to *Escherichia coli* in neuromyelitis optica patients is correlated with both neurological disabilities and elevated plasma lipopolysaccharide levels," *Human Immunology*, vol. 74, no. 9, pp. 1080–1087, 2013.

[65] M. Varrin-Doyer, C. M. Spencer, U. Schulze-Topphoff et al., "Aquaporin 4-specific T cells in neuromyelitis optica exhibit a Th17 bias and recognize Clostridium ABC transporter," *Annals of Neurology*, vol. 72, no. 1, pp. 53–64, 2012.

[66] Y.-Q. Feng, N. Guo, F. Huang, X. Chen, Q.-S. Sun, and J.-X. Liu, "Anti-tuberculosis treatment for Devic's neuromyelitis optica," *Journal of Clinical Neuroscience*, vol. 17, no. 11, pp. 1372–1377, 2010.

[67] M. C. Papadopoulos and A. S. Verkman, "Aquaporin 4 and neuromyelitis optica," *The Lancet Neurology*, vol. 11, no. 6, pp. 535–544, 2012.

[68] L. Tradtrantip, H. Zhang, S. Saadoun et al., "Anti-aquaporin-4 monoclonal antibody blocker therapy for neuromyelitis optica," *Annals of Neurology*, vol. 71, no. 3, pp. 314–322, 2012.

[69] L. Tradtrantip, J. Ratelade, H. Zhang, and A. S. Verkman, "Enzymatic deglycosylation converts pathogenic neuromyelitis optica anti-aquaporin-4 immunoglobulin G into therapeutic antibody," *Annals of Neurology*, vol. 73, no. 1, pp. 77–85, 2013.

20

Therapeutic Effect of Saponin Rich Fraction of *Achyranthes aspera* Linn. on Adjuvant-Induced Arthritis in Sprague-Dawley Rats

Pankaj S. Kothavade, Vipin D. Bulani, Dnyaneshwar M. Nagmoti, Padmini S. Deshpande, Nitin B. Gawali, and Archana R. Juvekar

Department of Pharmaceutical Science and Technology, Institute of Chemical Technology, N. P. Marg, Matunga, Mumbai, Maharashtra 400 019, India

Correspondence should be addressed to Archana R. Juvekar; juvekar.archana@gmail.com

Academic Editor: Maria Bokarewa

Objective. Achyranthes aspera Linn. (AA) is used in folklore for the treatment of various inflammatory ailments and arthritis like conditions. Anti-inflammatory activity of saponin rich (SR) fraction of AA has been previously reported. The objective of this study was to assess the antiarthritic effect of SR fraction of *Achyranthes aspera* in adjuvant-induced arthritic rats. *Methods.* Arthritis was assessed by arthritis score, paw volume, changes in tibiotarsal joint thickness, hyperalgesic parameters, and spleen and thymus index. Haematological, serum, biochemical, and inflammatory cytokine and *in vivo* antioxidant parameters were measured on the last day of the study. *Results.* SR fraction significantly suppressed paw swelling and arthritic score and improved the pain threshold in motility and stair climbing tests. There was a reversal in the levels of altered parameters, alanine aminotransferase, aspartate aminotransferase, alkaline phosphatase, and antioxidant parameters like superoxide dismutase, catalase, glutathione, malondialdehyde, and nitric oxide. SR fraction significantly decreased plasma levels of tumor necrosis factor-alpha and interleukin-6. Moreover, histopathology revealed a significant reduction in synovial hyperplasia, inflammatory cell infiltration, and bone destruction in the joints. *Conclusion.* These observations explain the therapeutic benefit of SR fraction of AA in suppressing the progression of adjuvant-induced arthritis in rats.

1. Introduction

Rheumatoid arthritis (RA) is a chronic autoimmune disease that comprises a syndrome of pain, stiffness, and symmetrical synovitis of diarthrodial joints lead to slowly progressive disease characterized by a continual breakdown of articular cartilage and changes in the subchondral bone. RA affects about 1% of the world population and more common in women than in men 3 : 1 ratio [1, 2]. Currently, RA is clinically treated mainly by disease-modifying antirheumatic drugs (DMARDs), such as methotrexate and sulfasalazine, and nonsteroidal anti-inflammatory drugs (NSAIDs) including ibuprofen, aceclofenac, and naproxen combined with steroid hormones like cortisone and prednisone [3]. However, these drugs only transiently suppress inflammation and ameliorate symptoms as curable treatment is not available in the market for the consequences associated with arthritis. Hence, exploration of new antirheumatic drugs with high efficacy and less toxicity is needed.

Achyranthes aspera (AA) Linn. (Amaranthaceae) is widely distributed throughout Asia, South America, and Africa [4]. It is an annual, perennial, stiff, and erect herb growing up to one meter in height [5]. *A. aspera* is traditionally used for treatment of piles, renal dropsy, cough, pneumonia, kidney stone, skin eruptions, snake bite, gonorrhea, dysentery, asthma, hypertension, and diabetes [4, 6]. AA has been reported for its preliminary anti-inflammatory and antiarthritic activity, antinociceptive, antifungal, immunomodulatory antifertility and abortifacient, antiurolithiatic, and anxiolytic activities [6–12].

Our previous research exhibits saponin rich (SR) fraction of AA possessed anti-inflammatory effect through activity-guided fractionation [13]. Triterpenoid saponins from herbs attracted attention due to their structural diversity and biological activities like antitumor, antifungal, antiviral, and anticoronary heart dieseaes [3]. Therefore, our current study was designed to confirm antiarthritic effect of saponin rich fraction of *A. aspera* and to explore its potential mechanism by ajuvant-induced arthritis in rats.

2. Material and Methods

2.1. Plant Materials. Whole plant of *Achyranthes aspera* was collected during the month of October 2013 from Thane District, Maharashtra, India. The plant material was authenticated by Professor Ganesh Iyer, Ramnarain Ruia College, Matunga (East), Mumbai. A voucher specimen (2012/02) of the plant was deposited at the Herbarium of the Department of Pharmaceutical Science and Technology, Institute of Chemical Technology, Mumbai, India.

2.2. Reagents. Fraud's complete adjuvant (FCA) and indomethacin were purchased from Sigma-Aldrich (St Louis, MO, USA). ELISA test kits were purchased from KRISHGEN BioSystems, India. All other chemicals and reagents used for study were of analytical grade procured from Sigma-Aldrich (St Louis, MO, USA).

2.3. Fraction Preparation. The dried whole plant (3.5 kg) was extracted with methanol and filtered. The extract (418 g) was dissolved in water and portioned with petroleum ether, chloroform, ethyl acetate, and *n*-butanol, successively. The bioactive petroleum ether fraction was partitioned with methanol. Methanolic fraction was further taken up in water and reextracted with diethyl ether until all chlorophyll pigments were removed. Then aqueous phase was partitioned with *n*-butanol. The *n*-butanol fraction concentrated to dryness and saponin mixture (5.60 g) was obtained.

2.4. Animals. Sprague-Dawley adult female rats (180–200 g) were obtained from the Animals house, Haffkine Bio-Pharmaceutical Corporation Ltd., Mumbai. The animals were maintained, under a 12 hr light/dark cycle, at controlled room temperature (25 ± 1°C) and relative humidity (55 ± 5%). The animals were fed with a rodent standard diet with free access water *ad libitum*. All the animals were acclimatized to the laboratory environment for a week before the experiment. The Animal Ethics Committees of the Department of Pharmaceutical Science and Technology, Institute of Chemical Technology, Mumbai, approved all experimental protocols in accordance with Committee for the Purpose of Control and Supervision of Experiments on Animals (CPCSEA) guidelines.

2.5. Adjuvant-Induced Arthritis in Rats. SD rats were randomly divided into five groups, namely, control group, FCA control group, positive control group of indomethacin (1 mg/kg), and SR fraction (50 and 100 mg/kg) groups with six rats in each group. Except the control group, the arthritis was induced by a single injection of 0.1 mL of FCA into the left hind paw on day 0. After this primary immunization, treated groups were orally administered with SR fraction (50 and 100 mg/kg), indomethacin (1 mg/kg), while normal control group and FCA control group were given equal volume of normal saline. All groups were orally administered those doses daily after arthritis induction until the end of experiment (day 28).

2.6. Measurement of Arthritic Progression

2.6.1. Measurement of Paw Volume and Tibiotarsal Joint Thickness and Arthritis Score. Paw volume and tibiotarsal joint thickness of the injected paw was measured using plethysmometer (Model no. 7140, UGO Basile, Italy) and digital calliper (Mitutoya, Japan) on days 0, 7, 14, 21, and 28 days after vehicle/drug administration, respectively [14]. The severity of arthritis was assessed on a scale of 0–4 with the following criteria: 0 menas no edema or swelling, 1 means slight edema and limited erythema, 2 means slight edema and erythema from the ankle to the tarsal bone, 3 means moderate edema and erythema from the ankle to the tarsal bone, and 4 means edema and erythema from the ankle to the entire leg. The sum of the scores for all 4 limbs was calculated as the arthritic index, with a maximum possible score of 16 per rat [15].

2.6.2. Dorsal Flexion Pain, Motility Test, and Stair Climbing Ability [16]. In dorsal flexion pain (DFP), FCA injected paw was scored based on squeaking and leg withdrawal after the ankle joint of the rat was flexed five times until the toes touched the front of the leg. The DFP was scored from 0 to 2: score 0, if there were no squeaking and leg withdrawal; score 1, if there is either squeaking or leg withdrawal; score 2, if both squeaking and leg withdrawal were present. Motility was observed for the period of 5 min and scored from 0 to 2 points. Score 0: rats avoided touching the feet to ground; score 1: rats walked with difficulty with toes touching the ground; score 2: rats walked easily. In stair climbing ability test, trained rats were allowed to climb on a staircase with steps at 5, 10, and 15 cm having water at second and food on third step. This stair climbing ability was scored from 0 to 3, score 0 if the rats did not climb any step, score 1 if they climbed onto step 1, score 2 if they climbed onto step 2, and score 3 if they climbed onto step 3.

2.6.3. Thymus and Spleen Index. At the day 28 after immunization, the animals were sacrificed and thymus and spleen were promptly removed and weighed. The index of thymus and spleen was expressed as the ratio of thymus and spleen wet weight versus body weight (mg/g), respectively [14].

2.6.4. Haematological Analyses. On day 28 after FCA injection, blood sample of rat was collected in EDTA containing tubes from retroorbital vein puncture. The total and differential leukocyte counts were determined from blood sample.

2.6.5. Biochemical Analysis in Liver. Animals were sacrificed on day 28 after immunization; the liver was promptly

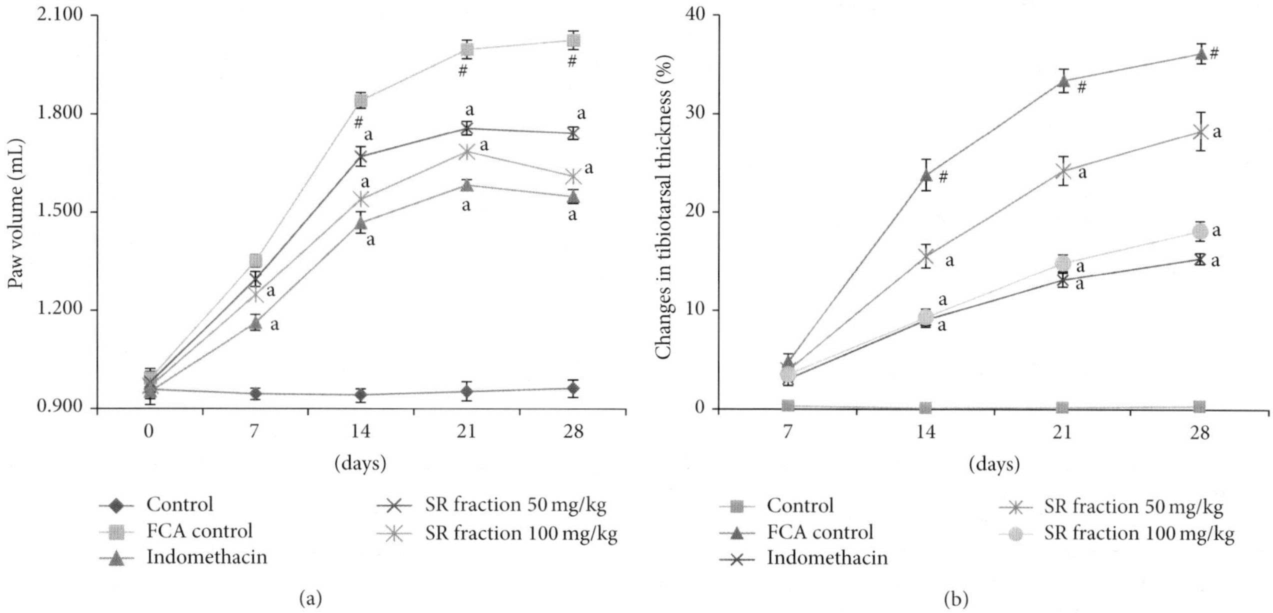

FIGURE 1: Effect of saponin rich (SR) fraction on (a) paw swelling and (b) % changes in tibiotarsal thickness. All data were expressed as mean ± SEM ($n = 6$). $^{a}P < 0.05$ compared to the FCA control group. $^{\#}P < 0.05$ compared with vehicle control.

removed and stored at −70°C. Portion of livers was homogenized. The homogenate was centrifuged at 6000 x g at 4°C for 20 min and the supernatant was collected. The supernatant was used to measure superoxide dismutase (SOD), catalase (CAT), reduced glutathione (GSH), malondialdehyde (MDA), and nitric oxide (NO) activity [14].

2.6.6. Biochemical Analysis in Serum and Cytokines Levels in Plasma. The levels of alkaline phosphatase (ALP), aspartate transaminase (AST), and alanine transaminase (ALT) in serum were determined by using quantitative colorimetric assay kits (manufacture name), according to the manufacturer instructions. Interleukin-1 (IL-1) and tumor necrosis factor alpha (TNF-α) in plasma were determined by using commercially available rat cytokine ELISA kits, according to the manufacturer instructions [14].

2.6.7. Histopathological Evaluation of Knee Joints. On day 28 after FCA injection, all rats were sacrificed after blood collection. Knee joint of injected paw was removed for histopathological examination. The joints were fixed in 10% phosphate buffer formalin, decalcified in 10% EDTA for 30 days at 4°C, and then embedded in paraffin. Sections of 5 μm were stained with hematoxylin and eosin (H&E) and examined under the light microscope.

2.7. Statistical Analysis. Data are expressed as mean ± SEM, and statistical comparisons were carried out using one-way analysis of variance (ANOVA) followed by post hoc Dunnett's test for comparison between control and test groups. The Dorsal flexion pain, stair climbing ability test, and motility are expressed as median scores and the Kruskal-Wallis test was used to compare the groups. The minimal level of significance was identified at $P < 0.05$.

3. Result

3.1. Effect of SR Fraction on Rat Hind Paw Volume, Tibiotarsal Joints Thickness, and Arthritis Score. Rat paw swelling trend is shown in Figure 1(a), in which the swelling of the right hind paw increased over time up to day 28. SR fraction (50 and 100 mg/kg) and indomethacin (1 mg/kg) treated group with significantly reduced paw edema compared with FCA control ($P < 0.05$). After day 14, clearly recognizable changes in tibiotarsal joint thickness were observed in the treated groups as compared to FCA untreated group. At day 7, no significant difference was found in tibiotarsal joints thickness of all groups (Figure 1(b)). Arthritis was scored on days 7, 14, 21, and 28 by physical observation. Treatment with SR fraction (100 mg/kg) significantly ($P < 0.05$) suppressed the arthritic score of FCA injected rat hind paw from day 14 to day 28. However, SR fraction 50 mg/kg significantly reduced the arthritic score on day 28 (Table 1).

3.2. Effect of SR Fraction on Dorsal Flexion Pain, Motility Test, and Stair Climbing Ability. As shown in Figure 2, FCA-induced arthritic rats exhibited low threshold of pain in hyperalgesic parameters such as dorsal flexion pain, motility, and stair climbing ability. In dorsal flexion pain treatment with SR fraction at dose of 100 mg/kg showed significance reduction in median score on day 28 compared to untreated arthritic rats ($P < 0.05$). Treatment indomethacin and SR fraction showed improvement in impaired motility pattern compared to untreated arthritic group. Moreover, SR fraction at dose of 100 mg/kg exhibited a significant ($P < 0.05$)

TABLE 1: Effect of saponin rich (SR) fraction of *Achyranthes aspera* on arthritis score in arthritic rats.

Treatment	Dose (mg/kg)	Arthritic score ± SEM Day 7	Day 14	Day 21	Day 28
Control	—	0.00	0.00	0.00	0.00
FCA control	—	6.17 ± 0.477	11.50 ± 0.563	13.33 ± 0.494	13.50 ± 0.619
Indomethacin	1	5.67 ± 0.333	8.67 ± 0.333***	9.17 ± 0.477***	7.83 ± 0.307***
SR fraction	50	6.17 ± 0.307	10.83 ± 0.654	11.83 ± 0.477	10.83 ± 0.477**
	100	5.83 ± 0.307	9.33 ± 0.333*	8.50 ± 0.428***	8.00 ± 0.365***

Values are expressed as means ± SEM, $n = 6$.
$^{*}P < 0.05$, $^{**}P < 0.01$, and $^{***}P < 0.001$ compared to the FCA control group.

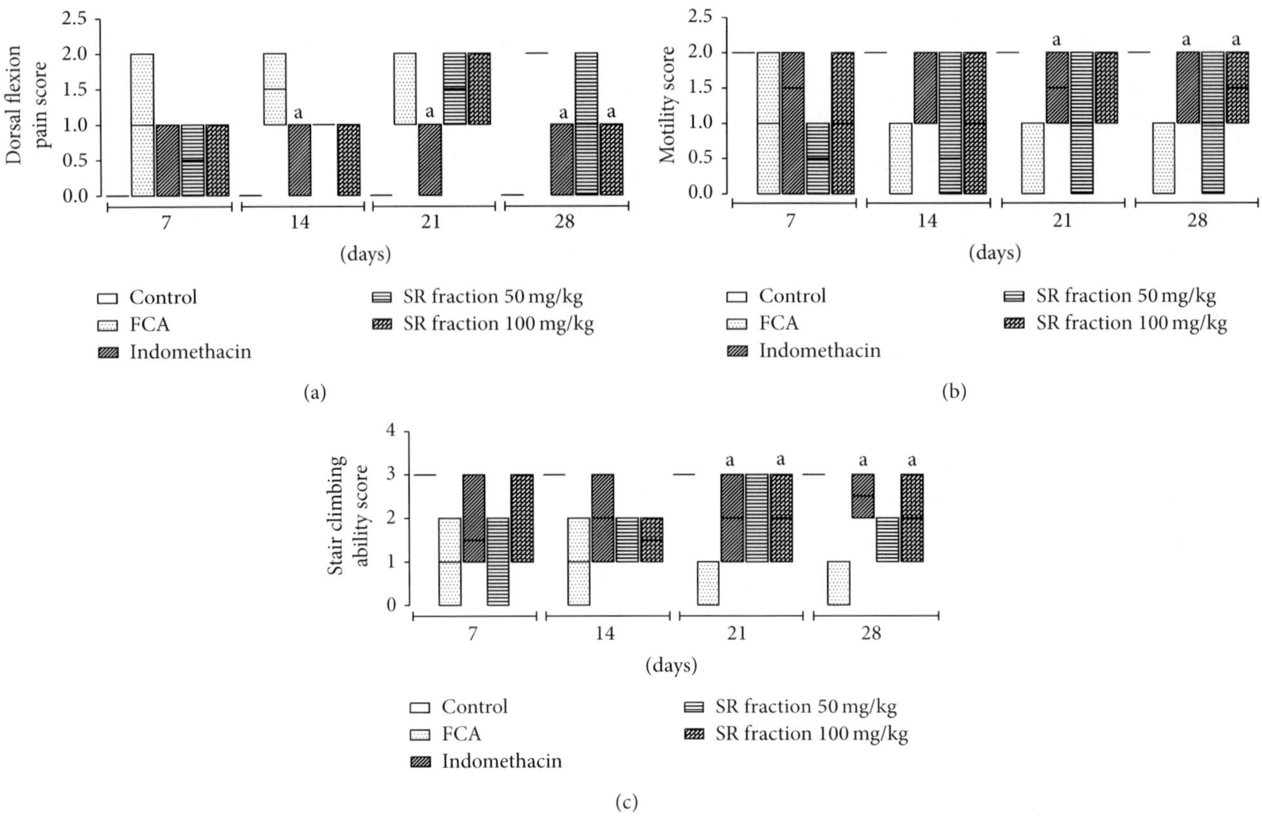

FIGURE 2: Effect of saponin rich (SR) fraction on inflammatory hyperalgesia in arthritic rats. The scores of (a) dorsal flexion pain, (b) motility, and (c) stair climbing ability is illustrated as box plots where bold line represents median values ($n = 6$) and boxes represent interquartile ranges (25th and 75th percentiles), $^{a}P < 0.05$ compared with FCA control.

increase in stair climbing score on day 21 and day 28 compared to arthritic control group.

3.3. Thymus and Spleen Index. The index of thymus and spleen was assayed on day 28. Results report an increase in thymus and spleen index of FCA control group compared to normal control group. There was significantly ($P < 0.05$) reduction of index of thymus and spleen in SR fraction treatment group (Table 2).

3.4. Haematological Examinations. Changes in peripheral blood profile were observed on day 28 after injection of FCA into the hind paw of rats. Indomethacin (1 mg/kg) showed significant decreases in total WBCs count. However, there were no significance differences in the haematological profile of SR fraction treated rats (Table 3).

3.5. Biochemical Examination in Liver Homogenate. The effects of SOD, CAT, GSH, MDA, and NO are summarized in Table 4. SOD, CAT, and GSH activities were significantly decreased, whereas MDA and NO level increased significantly in FCA control group compared to normal control ($P < 0.05$). Treatment with SR fraction (50 and 100 mg/kg) and indomethacin (1 mg/kg) showed significant modulation in all above antioxidant indexes. Thus SR fraction has potentially antioxidant effect.

TABLE 2: Effect of saponin rich (SR) fraction of *Achyranthes aspera* on immune organs in arthritic rats.

Treatment	Dose (mg/kg)	Thymus index	Spleen index
Control	—	0.44 ± 0.008	2.88 ± 0.046
FCA control	—	$0.62 \pm 0.017^{\#}$	$3.80 \pm 0.055^{\#}$
Indomethacin	1	$0.48 \pm 0.011^{***}$	$3.10 \pm 0.089^{***}$
SR fraction	50	$0.56 \pm 0.014^{*}$	$3.30 \pm 0.083^{***}$
	100	$0.52 \pm 0.009^{***}$	$3.14 \pm 0.056^{***}$

Values are presented as mean ± SEM, $n = 6$.
$^{*}P < 0.05$ and $^{***}P < 0.001$ compared with the FCA control group.
$^{\#}P < 0.05$ compared with vehicle control.

TABLE 3: Effect of saponin rich (SR) fraction of *Achyranthes aspera* on total and differential leucocyte count of arthritic rats.

Treatment	Dose (mg/kg)	Haematological parameters ± SEM					
		Total count ($\times10^3$/cmm)	Neutrophils (%)	Eosinophils (%)	Lymphocytes (%)	Monocytes (%)	Platelets ($\times10^5/\mu$L)
Control	—	9.03 ± 0.625	22.17 ± 2.136	2.33 ± 0.333	75.00 ± 1.983	0.50 ± 0.224	8.98 ± 0.499
FCA control	—	10.65 ± 0.650	26.83 ± 2.522	3.17 ± 0.601	69.67 ± 2.578	0.33 ± 0.211	7.92 ± 0.317
Indomethacin	1	$7.92 \pm 0.529^{**}$	21.00 ± 1.155	2.67 ± 0.333	75.67 ± 1.116	0.67 ± 0.211	8.27 ± 0.438
SR fraction	50	9.38 ± 0.476	23.83 ± 1.641	3.00 ± 0.365	72.83 ± 1.621	0.33 ± 0.211	9.10 ± 0.593
	100	8.92 ± 0.456	21.83 ± 2.023	2.83 ± 0.601	74.83 ± 2.442	0.50 ± 0.342	8.98 ± 0.464

Values are presented as mean ± SEM, $n = 6$.
$^{**}P < 0.01$ compared with the FCA control group.

TABLE 4: Effect of saponin rich (SR) fraction of *Achyranthes aspera* on indexes of oxidative stress in liver of arthritic rats.

Treatment	Dose (mg/kg)	SOD (U/mL/mg of protein)	CAT (U/mL/mg of protein)	GSH (μg/mL/mg of protein)	MDA (nMol/mL/mg of protein)	Nitric oxide (μMol/mL/mg of protein)
Control	—	20.44 ± 0.64	179.62 ± 5.42	21.96 ± 1.32	7.06 ± 0.514	11.78 ± 0.91
FCA Control	—	$4.72 \pm 0.60^{\#}$	$88.83 \pm 1.83^{\#}$	$6.99 \pm 0.76^{\#}$	$16.61 \pm 0.742^{\#}$	$90.72 \pm 2.86^{\#}$
Indo	1	$10.34 \pm 0.50^{***}$	$122.98 \pm 3.51^{*}$	$12.83 \pm 0.82^{**}$	$10.64 \pm 0.102^{***}$	$32.22 \pm 1.66^{***}$
SR fraction	50	$13.37 \pm 0.91^{***}$	$127.85 \pm 2.80^{***}$	$15.65 \pm 0.95^{***}$	13.71 ± 0.858	$40.19 \pm 1.79^{***}$
	100	$16.75 \pm 1.41^{***}$	$139.08 \pm 2.54^{***}$	$15.92 \pm 1.21^{***}$	$9.22 \pm 0.735^{***}$	$33.81 \pm 2.21^{***}$

Values are presented as mean ± SEM, $n = 6$.
$^{*}P < 0.05$, $^{**}P < 0.01$, and $^{***}P < 0.001$ compared with the FCA control group.
$^{\#}P < 0.05$ compared with vehicle control.

3.6. Biochemical Analysis in Serum. Table 5 depicts the effect of SR fraction on levels of tissue marker enzyme in arthritic rat serum. A significant increase in the levels of AST, ALT, and ALP was observed in arthritic rats. The administration of SR fraction (50 and 100 mg/kg) and indomethacin (1 mg/kg) significantly reverted all these indexes compared to FCA control ($P < 0.05$).

3.7. Cytokines Levels in Plasma. Plasma levels of inflammatory cytokines TNF-α and IL-6 in untreated arthritic rats were significantly higher than those of treatment groups ($P < 0.05$). Both doses of SR fraction 50 and 100 mg/kg markedly inhibited the production of TNF-α and IL-6 in arthritic rats (Figure 3).

3.8. Histopathological Examination. Histopathological results are shown in Figure 4. In arthritic group soft tissue swelling around joints were seen with varying degrees of inflammatory cells infiltration, synovial hyperplasia, and cartilage destruction in the joint. Histological images of tibiotarsal joints were improved in arthritic animals treated with SR fraction (50 and 100 mg/kg), as evidence by marked reduction in synovial hyperplasia and inflammatory cell infiltration, which reveals the protective effect of SR fraction in arthritis.

4. Discussion

Arthritis is an immune-mediated destruction of joints, characterised by pain, swelling, tenderness, and difficulty in movement. The events that underline the progression of

Table 5: Effect of saponin rich (SR) fraction of *Achyranthes aspera* on levels of tissue marker enzymes in arthritic rats serum.

Treatment	Dose (mg/kg)	AST (U/L)	ALT (U/L)	ALP (U/L)
Control	—	152.64 ± 11.48	141.85 ± 9.40	118.47 ± 6.05
FCA control	—	220.01 ± 11.32#	217.90 ± 13.86#	205.25 ± 6.75#
Indo	1	159.22 ± 7.06**	149.48 ± 6.95***	136.98 ± 8.05***
SR fraction	50	173.43 ± 15.72*	178.16 ± 6.26*	163.34 ± 10.19**
	100	164.74 ± 6.68**	163.16 ± 10.08**	155.31 ± 9.89**

Values are presented as mean ± SEM, $n = 6$.
$^{*}P < 0.05$, $^{**}P < 0.01$, and $^{***}P < 0.001$ compared with the FCA control group.
$^{\#}P < 0.05$ compared with vehicle control.

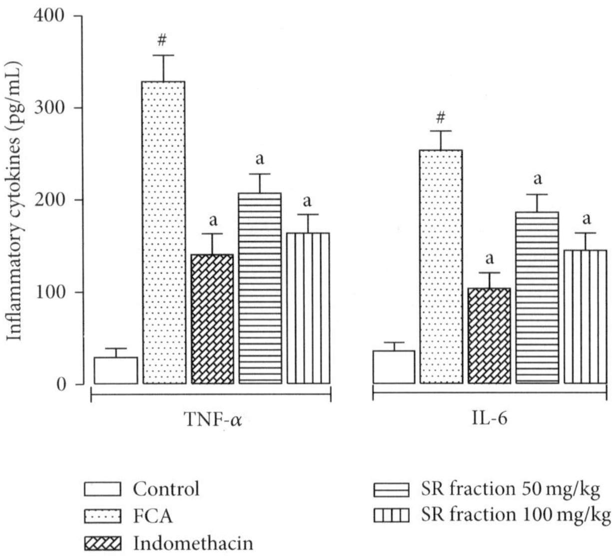

Figure 3: Effect of saponin rich (SR) fraction on inflammatory cytokines, namely, TNF-α and IL-6 levels in plasma samples. Values are presented as mean ± SEM, $n = 6$. $^{a}P < 0.05$ compared with the FCA control group. $^{\#}P < 0.05$ compared with vehicle control.

arthritis are mediated by several chemotactic factors such as interleukins (IL-1, IL-6, and IL-10), tumor necrosis factor (TNF-α), interferons (INF-γ) plus leukocytes, and adhesion factors [17]. The current lines of therapy typically involve the use of immunosuppressants which are accompanied by a range of adverse events, particularly after long-term treatment. The animal model that closely resembles human osteoarthritis is adjuvant-induced arthritis in rats [18]. Subcutaneous administration of killed *Mycobacterium* H37Ra causes activation of immune response, leading to leukocyte accumulation in the joints that subsequently causes pain and inflammation [19]. NSAIDs are effective in alleviating the joint pain and swelling associated with synovial fluid accumulation. However, they are not particularly effective in circumventing the disease progression. Here, we have chosen Indomethacin as the standard treatment because of its clinical effectiveness in human arthritis. In this study, we challenged the rats with 0.1 mL of Freund's complete adjuvant and assessed the progression of arthritis at various stages, in terms of paw volume and tibiotarsal joint thickness. Although significant increase in the paw volume and tibiotarsal thickness was evident only on Day 14, indicating synovial fluid accumulation, the increase was moderately less for indomethacin and SR treated groups (100 mg/kg) on day 14, as compared to negative control group. The effect was observed in the SR (50 mg/kg) group only on day 28.

Pain is an important parameter to assess the effect of joint destruction on motility. Hyperalgesia is important indicator of arthritic development, which can be assessed by the direct measurement of pain and its effects on motility. In this study, SR fraction (100 mg/kg) significantly improved the pain threshold in hyperalgesic rats on day 28. The effect of SR (100 mg/kg) on stair climbing was more pronounced from day 21 onwards, whereas significant increase in motility score was evident only on day 28. Indomethacin consistently showed improved motility and stair climbing score from day 14 onwards; however effects on pain score were evident only after day 20. This suggests that the anti-inflammatory action was more pronounced than effects on pain, which might be attributed to alleviation of proinflammatory cytokines. The findings are further supported by the significant inhibitory effect of SR fractions (50 mg/kg and 100 mg/kg) on the levels of TNF-α and IL-6 in the plasma of FCA-challenged rats.

Although the immune factors are responsible for triggering the pathogenic events that lead to arthritis, oxidative events do play a role in the disease progression. According to Halliwel, lipid peroxidation, caused as a result of immunological response, eventually causes increased oxidation that further worsens the condition [20]. The increased oxidative stress produces a decrease in the levels of the inherent antioxidant enzymes glutathione peroxidise, catalase, and superoxide dismutase [21]. With a decrease in antioxidant defence, there is a concurrent increase in the levels of reactive oxygen species and nitric oxide (NO), as a consequence of increased lipid peroxidation indicated by increased MDA [22]. Treatment with SR fraction significantly restored the antioxidant status by decreasing NO and MDA levels and elevating the levels of SOD, catalase, and GSH enzymes.

Clinically, arthritis has been known to result in increased levels of WBCs particularly leucocytes accompanied by enlargement in spleen [23]. The spleen has been reported to be involved in the storage and recruitment of leucocytes across the site of inflammation. Administration of FCA led to increase in the total blood leucocyte count suggesting the involvement of WBCs in response to antigen-mediated arthritic insult. These changes were significantly reversed by SR treated fractions (50 and 100 mg/kg). Treatment with

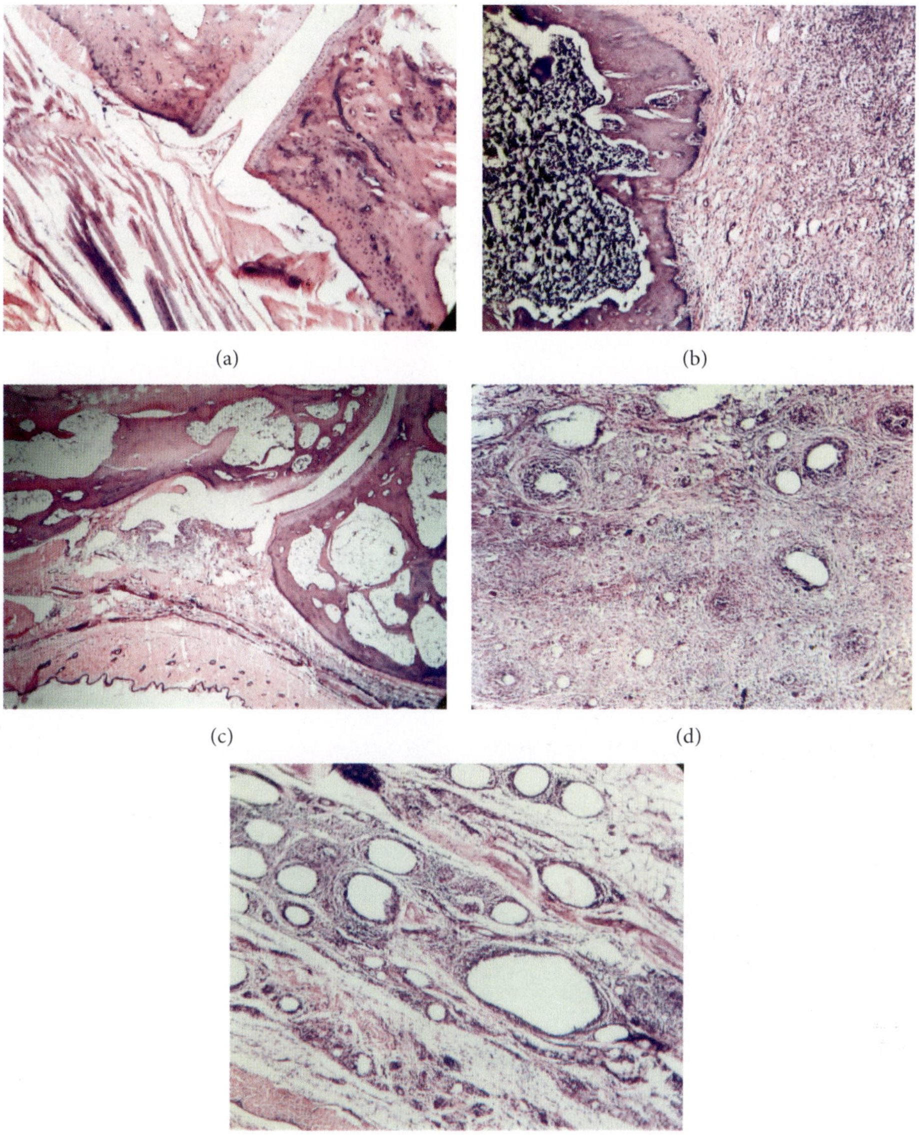

FIGURE 4: Effect of saponin rich (SR) fraction on histopathological changes of tibiotarsal joints in arthritic rats. All images of one of six in each group. (a) Vehicle control, (b) adjuvant-induced arthritic control, (c) indomethacin (1 mg/kg), (d) saponin rich fraction (50 mg/kg), and (e) saponin rich fraction (100 mg/kg).

SR fraction (50 and 100 mg/kg) also resulted in significant decrease in the weight of the spleen.

Histopathological analysis of FCA induced arthritic rats showed a mild degree of infiltration of inflammatory cells, synovial hyperplasia, and cartilage destruction in the joint. Treatment with SR (50 and 100 mg/kg) significantly improved the histology of tibiotarsal joint, resulting in decreased evidence of destruction and inflammation.

The results of the present study reveal a significant potential of SR fraction of *Achyranthes aspera* in slowing down the arthritic progression and reversing the pathological changes resulting from arthritic development. This effect can be attributed to a decrease in the level of cytokines, TNF-α, and other proinflammatory factors. At the same time, it may be suggested that improvement in oxidative stress may be as a result of direct antioxidant effect of SR fraction coupled with an improvement in the body's natural antioxidant enzyme mediated defence.

Conflict of Interests

The authors declare that there is no conflict of interests regarding the publication of this paper.

Acknowledgments

The authors are grateful to Dr. Ganesh Iyer for identification of plant material. The authors also wish to thank Ms. Amrita

Chaudhary who contributed in this study. The authors want to thank the financial support from the University Grant Commission (UGC), New Delhi, India (no. F 5-63/2007).

References

[1] F. M. Brennan and I. B. McInnes, "Evidence that cytokines play a role in rheumatoid arthritis," *Journal of Clinical Investigation*, vol. 118, no. 11, pp. 3537–3545, 2008.

[2] S. Amdekar, P. Roy, V. Singh, A. Kumar, R. Singh, and P. Sharma, "*Lactobacillus casei* and *Lactobacillus acidophilus* attenuates the severity of experimental arthritis by regulating biochemical parameters," *Biomedicine and Preventive Nutrition*, vol. 3, no. 4, pp. 351–356, 2013.

[3] X.-X. Zhang, Y. Ito, J.-R. Liang, J.-L. Liu, J. He, and W.-J. Sun, "Therapeutic effects of total steroid saponin extracts from the rhizome of *Dioscorea zingiberensis* C.H. Wright in Freund's complete adjuvant induced arthritis in rats," *International Immunopharmacology*, vol. 23, no. 2, pp. 407–416, 2014.

[4] A. Chakraborty, A. Brantner, T. Mukainaka et al., "Cancer chemopreventive activity of *Achyranthes aspera* leaves on Epstein-Barr virus activation and two-stage mouse skin carcinogenesis," *Cancer Letters*, vol. 177, no. 1, pp. 1–5, 2002.

[5] A. J. Khandagle, V. S. Tare, K. D. Raut, and R. A. Morey, "Bioactivity of essential oils of *Zingiber officinalis* and *Achyranthes aspera* against mosquitoes," *Parasitology Research*, vol. 109, no. 2, pp. 339–343, 2011.

[6] C. C. Barua, A. Talukdar, S. A. Begum et al., "Antinociceptive activity of methanolic extract of leaves of *Achyranthes aspera* Linn. (Amaranthaceae) in animal models of nociception," *Indian Journal of Experimental Biology*, vol. 48, no. 8, pp. 817–821, 2010.

[7] A. B. Gokhale, A. S. Damre, K. R. Kulkarni, and M. N. Saraf, "Preliminary evaluation of anti-inflammatory and anti-arthritic activity of *S. lappa, A. speciosa* and *A. aspera*," *Phytomedicine*, vol. 9, no. 5, pp. 433–437, 2002.

[8] T. N. Misra, R. S. Singh, H. S. Pandey, C. Prasad, and B. P. Singh, "Antifungal essential oil and a long chain alcohol from *Achyranthes aspera*," *Phytochemistry*, vol. 31, no. 5, pp. 1811–1812, 1992.

[9] R. Y. Vasudeva, G. R. Duddukuri, B. G. Sunil, and R. R. Athota, "Immunomodulatory activity of *Achyranthes aspera* on the elicitation of antigen-specific murine antibody response," *Pharmaceutical Biology*, vol. 40, no. 3, pp. 175–178, 2002.

[10] V. P. Kamboj and B. N. Dhawan, "Research on plants for fertility regulation in India," *Journal of Ethnopharmacology*, vol. 6, no. 2, pp. 191–226, 1982.

[11] A. Pakrashi and N. Bhattacharya, "Abortifacient principle of *Achyranthes aspera* Linn," *Indian Journal of Experimental Biology*, vol. 15, no. 10, pp. 856–858, 1977.

[12] C. C. Barua, A. Talukdar, S. A. Begum, P. Borah, and M. Lahkar, "Anxiolytic activity of methanol leaf extract of *Achyranthes aspera* Linn in mice using experimental models of anxiety," *Indian Journal of Pharmacology*, vol. 44, no. 1, pp. 63–67, 2012.

[13] P. Kothavade, N. Gawali, D. Thanekar, and A. Juvekar, "Triterpenoid saponin rich fraction of *Achyranthes aspera* Linn. attenuates inflammation and oxidative stress induced by carrageenan in experimental rats," *Cytokine*, vol. 70, no. 1, p. 42, 2014.

[14] J. Zuo, Y. Xia, X. Li, and J. Chen, "Therapeutic effects of dichloromethane fraction of *Securidaca inappendiculata* on adjuvant-induced arthritis in rat," *Journal of Ethnopharmacology*, vol. 153, no. 2, pp. 352–358, 2014.

[15] J. E. Baggott, S. L. Morgan, and W. J. Koopman, "The effect of methotrexate and 7-hydroxymethotrexate on rat adjuvant arthritis and on urinary aminoimidazole carboxamide excretion," *Arthritis and Rheumatism*, vol. 41, no. 8, pp. 1407–1410, 1998.

[16] V. D. Wahane and V. L. Kumar, "Atorvastatin ameliorates inflammatory hyperalgesia in rat model of monoarticular arthritis," *Pharmacological Research*, vol. 61, no. 4, pp. 329–333, 2010.

[17] S. L. Kunkel, N. Lukacs, T. Kasama, and R. M. Strieter, "The role of chemokines in inflammatory joint disease," *Journal of Leukocyte Biology*, vol. 59, no. 1, pp. 6–12, 1996.

[18] Y. Hu, W. Cheng, W. Cai, Y. Yue, J. Li, and P. Zhang, "Advances in research on animal models of rheumatoid arthritis," *Clinical Rheumatology*, vol. 32, no. 2, pp. 161–165, 2013.

[19] S. M. Nanjundaiah, J. P. Stains, and K. D. Moudgil, "Kinetics and interplay of mediators of inflammation-induced bone damage in the course of adjuvant arthritis," *International Journal of Immunopathology and Pharmacology*, vol. 26, no. 1, pp. 37–48, 2013.

[20] B. Halliwell, "Oxidants and human disease: some new concepts," *The FASEB Journal*, vol. 1, no. 5, pp. 358–364, 1987.

[21] A. Seven, S. Güzel, M. Aslan, and V. Hamuryudan, "Lipid, protein, DNA oxidation and antioxidant status in rheumatoid arthritis," *Clinical Biochemistry*, vol. 41, no. 7-8, pp. 538–543, 2008.

[22] M. M. N. Wendt, A. B. de Sá-Nakanishi, C. V. de Castro Ghizoni et al., "Oxidative state and oxidative metabolism in the brain of rats with adjuvant-induced arthritis," *Experimental and Molecular Pathology*, vol. 98, no. 3, pp. 549–557, 2015.

[23] R. Khurana and S. M. Berney, "Clinical aspects of rheumatoid arthritis," *Pathophysiology*, vol. 12, no. 3, pp. 153–165, 2005.

21

Mechanism of Xinfeng Capsule on Adjuvant-Induced Arthritis via Analysis of Urinary Metabolomic Profiles

Hui Jiang,[1,2] Jian Liu,[1] Ting Wang,[3] Jia-rong Gao,[1] Yue Sun,[1] Chuan-bing Huang,[1] Mei Meng,[1] and Xiu-juan Qin[3]

[1]*Department of Pharmacy, The First Affiliated Hospital of Anhui University of Chinese Medicine, 117 Meishan Road, Hefei 230031, China*
[2]*College of Basic Medicine, Anhui Medical University, 81 Meishan Road, Hefei 230022, China*
[3]*College of Pharmacy, Anhui University of Chinese Medicine, 103 Meishan Road, Hefei 230038, China*

Correspondence should be addressed to Jian Liu; liujianahzy@126.com

Academic Editor: Rizgar Mageed

We aimed to explore the potential effects of Xinfeng capsule (XFC) on urine metabolic profiling in adjuvant-induced arthritis (AA) rats by using gas chromatography time-of-flight mass spectrometry (GC-TOF/MS). GC-TOF/MS technology was combined with multivariate statistical approaches, such as principal component analysis (PCA), partial least squares discriminant analysis (PLS-DA), and orthogonal projections to latent structures discriminant analysis (OPLS-DA). These methods were used to distinguish the healthy group, untreated group, and XFC treated group and elucidate potential biomarkers. Nine potential biomarkers such as hippuric acid, adenine, and L-dopa were identified as potential biomarkers, indicating that purine metabolism, fat metabolism, amino acid metabolism, and energy metabolism were disturbed in AA rats. This study demonstrated that XFC is efficacious for RA and explained its potential metabolomics mechanism.

1. Introduction

Rheumatoid arthritis (RA) is a common chronic systematic autoimmune disease that is characterized by inflammation of synovial tissue. It is often recurrent and protracted, painful, and results in stiff and damaged bone and cartilage. RA has a high morbidity and disability rate and seriously affects patient's quality of life [1, 2].

Under the guidance of the Xin'an medical theory, Xinfeng capsule (XFC, Anhui medicine system Z20050062) is a Traditional Chinese Medicine (TCM) prescription with a long history used in the clinic for the treatment of RA [3–5], which has been registered in China with patent certificates (ZL 201310011369.8 and ZL201410101266.5). XFC is composed of *Coix seed* (Yiyiren), *Scolopendra* (Wugong), *Astragalus* (Huangqi), and *Tripterygium wilfordii* (Leigongteng). Methods of extraction and preparation of the XFC formulation were studied in our previous experiments; they showed that the extraction method was appropriate, simple, and feasible; quality control data were available. A proper chemical profile HPTLC for the evaluation of *Coix seed*, *Scolopendra*, *Astragalus*, and *Tripterygium wilfordii* were already studied [6]. In our previous study, XFC had a good effect on relieving the degree of joint pain, alleviating morning stiffness and enhancing grip strength in RA, without obvious adverse reactions [7, 8]. However, the metabolomics mechanism of Xinfeng Capsule that cure RA is unclear.

Metabolomics is a technology in which all endogenous metabolites are analyzed via high-throughput detection and data processing to obtain potential biomarkers [9]. This technology can elucidate the status of an organism at a specific time and under a specific environment [10]. Metabolomics has comprehensive analysis and can dynamically operate, which is conducive to the study of TCM that have complex mixtures of metabolites and compounds [11]. Therefore, metabolomics can be used to explore the relationship between changes in the physiological state of a biological system and potential biomarkers [12].

In this study, we used a metabolomic approach based on gas chromatography time-of-flight mass spectrometry

(GC-TOF/MS) technology to find potential endogenous biomarkers in urine. We aimed to explore the therapeutic effects and metabolic mechanism of XFC in a model of RA.

2. Materials and Methods

2.1. Experimental Animal. The protocol was approved by the Committee on the Ethics of Animal Experiments of Anhui University of Chinese medicine (Permit Number: 2012AH-038-01). All surgery was performed under sodium pentobarbital anesthesia, and all efforts were made to minimize suffering. Adult male Sprague-Dawley (SD) rats (180–200 g) of specified pathogen free (SPF) were purchased from Anhui Medical University Laboratory Animal Center. All animals were placed in standard cages under controlled temperature (around 22°C) and relative humidity (40%–60%) conditions, with the same amount of food and water at a regular daily time.

2.2. Drugs and Reagents. Internal standard: L-2-Chlorophenylalanine (CAS: 103616-89-3) was purchased from Shanghai Heng Bo Biological Technology Co., China. N,O-bis-trimethylsilyl-trifluoroacetamide (BSTFA) with 1% trimethylchlorosilane (TMCS) was purchased from REGIS Technologies Inc., USA. Urease from Canavalia ensiformis (Jack bean), Type III, powder, was purchased from Sigma company. Paraformaldehyde solution was purchased from Sinopharm Chemical Reagent Co. Ltd. XFC was provided by the First Affiliated Hospital of Anhui University of Chinese Medicine (Batch number: 2012100407, Hefei, China).

2.3. Instruments and Equipment. Instruments and equipment are as follows: GC chromatograph: Agilent 7890A, Agilent, USA; Mass spectrometer: LECO Chroma TOF PEGASUS 4D, LECO, USA; GL-20A Automatic high speed refrigerated centrifuge (Hunan Instruments Plant centrifuge plant); −80°C Ultra-Low Temperature Freezer-Uplight type (Sanyo company); 37°C incubator (Hubei Huangshi Medical Instruments Factory).

2.4. Induction, Treatment, and Measurement of Adjuvant-Induced Arthritis (AA). SD rats were adaptively fed for one week. All rats were divided randomly into three groups: healthy group, untreated group, and XFC treated group, with 8 rats in each group. The untreated group and XFC treated group were established with a single intracutaneous injection of 0.1 mL of complete Freund's adjuvant (CFA) into the right hind metatarsal footpad [13]. The healthy group was given liquid paraffin for comparison at the same time. From day 19 after injection of CFA, XFC (3 g/kg) were given by gavage once a day for 30 days in the XFC treated group. Rats in the healthy and untreated groups were given 0.9% saline. Urine was collected 12 h after the last administration and kept at −80°C. Two different clinical parameters, paw swelling and arthritis index (AI), were used to assess the therapeutic effects of XFC on AA rats. The volume of the left hind paw was measured with a PV-200 volume meter (Chengdu Taimeng Technology Co., Chengdu, China) before immunization (normal value, day 0) and after the last administration (day 30). Secondary paw swelling (E) was calculated with the formula $E(\%) = (V_t - V_0)/V_0 \times 100\%$, where V_0 and V_t represent the volume of the paw before modeling and after modeling, respectively [14]. For evaluation of AA, the arthritis severity was recorded on a four-point scale, where 0 indicates no swelling; 1 point indicates mind swelling; 2 points indicate slight swelling of wrist or ankle joints; 3 points indicate severe swelling of the entire joint and paw; and 4 points indicate ankylosis or deformed paws [15].

2.5. Histological Examination. All rats were sacrificed at 12 hours after the last administration. The knee was removed and placed in 4% paraformaldehyde solution. Histological changes were observed after pathological HE staining using conventional optical microscopes. Two blinded observers evaluated cartilage and bone destruction by cellular infiltration, synovial proliferation, pannus formation, and cartilage erosion, using the following scoring system: cellular infiltration: Grade 0, no changes; Grade 1, few focal infiltrates; Grade 2, extensive focal infiltrates; and Grade 3, extensive infiltrates invading the capsule with aggregate formation; synovial proliferation: Grade 0, proliferation was absent; Grade 1, proliferation was mild with two to four layers of reactive synoviocytes; Grade 2, proliferation was moderate with four plus layers of reactive synoviocytes, increased mitotic activity, and mild or absent synovial cell invasion of adjacent bone and connective tissue; and Grade 3, proliferation was severe and characterized by invasion and effacement of joint space and adjacent cartilage, bone, and connective tissue; pannus formation: Grade 0, no changes; Grade 1, pannus formation at up to two sites; Grade 2, pannus formation at up to four sites, with infiltration or flat overgrowth of joint surface; and Grade 3, pannus formation at more than four sites or extensive pannus formation at two sites; cartilage erosion: Grade 0, no changes; Grade 1, superficial, localized cartilage degradation in more than one region; Grade 2, localized deep cartilage degradation; and Grade 3, extensive deep cartilage degradation at several locations [16].

2.6. Sample Preparation. Urine samples were thawed at room temperature and vortexed for 15 s, after which 100 μL of the urine was transferred into 1.5 mL Eppendorf tubes and subsequently 10 μL of urease suspension (160 mg/mL in water) was added and vortexed for 10 s. Up to 900 μL of a mixture of methanol and chloroform (3/1, vol/vol) and 50 μL of L-2-Chlorophenylalanine (0.2 mg/mL) as internal standards were added to each sample and vortexed for 10 min and subsequently centrifuged at 12,000 rpm for 10 min at 4°C. Transfer the supernatant (approximately 0.35 mL) into new 2 mL GC-TOF/MS glass vials. The collected supernatant fluid was concentrated to complete dryness in a vacuum concentrator without heating. 80 μL methoxymethyl amine salt was added, which aimed to dry up metabolites at 37°C for 2 h in an oven after mixing and sealing. The dried samples were then derivatized with the addition of 100 μL bis-(trimethylsilyl)-trifluoroacetamide with 1% trimethylchlorosilane into each vial. The mixture was left to react for 1 h in an oven at 70°C. After incubation, the samples were again vortexed for 1 min in preparation for GC-TOF/MS analysis.

TABLE 1: Effects of XFC on paw swelling and arthritis index in AA rats.

Group	Paw swelling (%)		Arthritis index	
	Day 0	Day 30	Day 0	Day 30
Healthy	34.79 ± 10.56	42.21 ± 10.32	0.00 ± 0.00	0.00 ± 0.00
Untreated	61.19 ± 12.92**	78.15 ± 12.28**	7.50 ± 1.60**	8.63 ± 2.07**
XFC treated	64.67 ± 11.99**	56.78 ± 17.67##	7.75 ± 1.83**	5.38 ± 1.59**##

Note: day 0 shows paw swelling and arthritis index before intragastric administration of XFC; day 30 shows paw swelling and arthritis index on day 30 after intragastric administration of XFC. Data represent the mean ± SD ($n = 8$). ** $p < 0.01$ compared with healthy group; ## $p < 0.01$ compared with untreated group.

2.7. GC-TOF/MS Analysis. GC-TOF/MS analysis was performed using an Agilent 7890 gas chromatograph system coupled with a Pegasus HT time-of-flight mass spectrometer. The system utilized a DB-5MScapillary column coated with 5% diphenyl cross-linked with 95% dimethyl polysiloxane (30 m × 250 μm inner diameter, 0.25 μm film thickness; J&W Scientific, Folsom, CA, USA). A 1 μL aliquot of the analyte was injected in splitless mode. Helium was used as the carrier gas, the front inlet purge flow was 3 mL/min, and the gas flow rate through the column was 20 mL/min. The initial temperature was kept at 50°C for 1 min, then raised to 330°C at a rate of 10°C/min, and then kept for 5 min at 330°C. The injection, transfer line, and ion source temperatures were 280, 280, and 220°C, respectively. The energy was −70 eV in electron impact mode. The mass spectrometry data were acquired in full-scan mode with the m/z range of 85–600 at a rate of 20 spectra per second after a solvent delay of 366 s.

2.8. Data Analysis. Chroma TOF4.3X software of LECO Corporation and LECO-Fiehn Rtx5 database were used for raw peaks exacting, the data baselines filtering and calibration of the baseline, peak alignment, deconvolution analysis, peak identification, and integration of the peak area [17]. The resulting normalized peak intensities were analyzed by PCA, PLS-DA, and OPLS using the DEMO (Umetrics AB, Umea, Sweden). Data was processed by Spss 17.0 version (Spss, Inc., Chicago, IL), and statistical analyses were handled using Student's t-test.

3. Results

3.1. Effects of XFC on Secondary Paw Swelling and Arthritis Index (AI). Before intragastric administration of XFC, compared with the healthy group, rats in the untreated group had significantly more secondary paw swelling and higher arthritis index ($p < 0.01$). The secondary paw swelling and arthritis index in the XFC treated group were similar to those of untreated group. After intragastric administration of XFC for 30 days, the AA rats had little secondary paw swelling and a lower arthritis index in the XFC treated group, compared with the untreated group ($p < 0.01$). This result indicated that XFC could inhibit secondary inflammation in AA rats (Table 1).

3.2. Impact of XFC on Histopathology. Under HE staining, the healthy group had normally arranged synovial cells, no synovial hyperplasia, no inflammatory cell infiltration, and no cartilage erosion. The untreated group had local thickening of the surrounding synovium tissue, inflammatory cell infiltration accompanied by spalling pannus formation, joint-space narrowing, and some cartilage erosion. The XFC treated group had less pathological tissue injury than that of the untreated group to varying degrees (Figures 1 and 2).

3.3. Total Ion Chromatogram of Urine Samples. The GC-TOF/MS TIC chromatograms of urine samples from the healthy group, untreated group, and XFC treated group are shown in Figure 3. Based on LECO-Fiehn Rtx5 database, approximately 1166 metabolites were identified. After using Chroma TOF4.3X software to correct the blank value, eliminate noise, and correct an internal standard, 914 metabolites were identified. The horizontal axis represents the time at which metabolites occur; each peak represents the relative the metabolite. In order to illustrate the differences of the metabolic profiles, GC-TOF/MS spectra were further pretreated and a pattern recognition analysis was carried out.

3.4. Principal Component Analysis (PCA) of Urine Samples. PCA, the most-commonly used algorithm in metabolomic studies, was employed to process the GC-TOF/MS data using the software developed in SIMCA-P (Umetrics, Umea, Sweden). The simultaneous comparison of a large number of complex variables was facilitated by a dimensional reduction via three-dimensional mapping procedures and the output displayed with score plots, which represented the distribution of samples in multivariate space [18]. In PCA score plots (Figure 4), the urine samples from each group did not completely separate, which will need further analysis.

3.5. Partial Least Squares Discriminant Analysis (PLS-DA) of Urine Samples. Because PCA failed to completely separate, PLS-DA analysis was performed to achieve greater separation between the groups and enhance the identification of metabolites. PLS-DA used Ctr (mean-centered scaling) to process the data scale conversion mode, where the x- and y-axes represent the first and second principle components. The leave-one-out cross-validation method was used to assess the actual performance of the established model [19]. R^2 is the fraction of the Sum of Squares (SS) explained by the model, which represents model fitness; Q^2 is the fraction of Y variation predicted by the X model in that component, which represents predictive ability. These were obtained after using

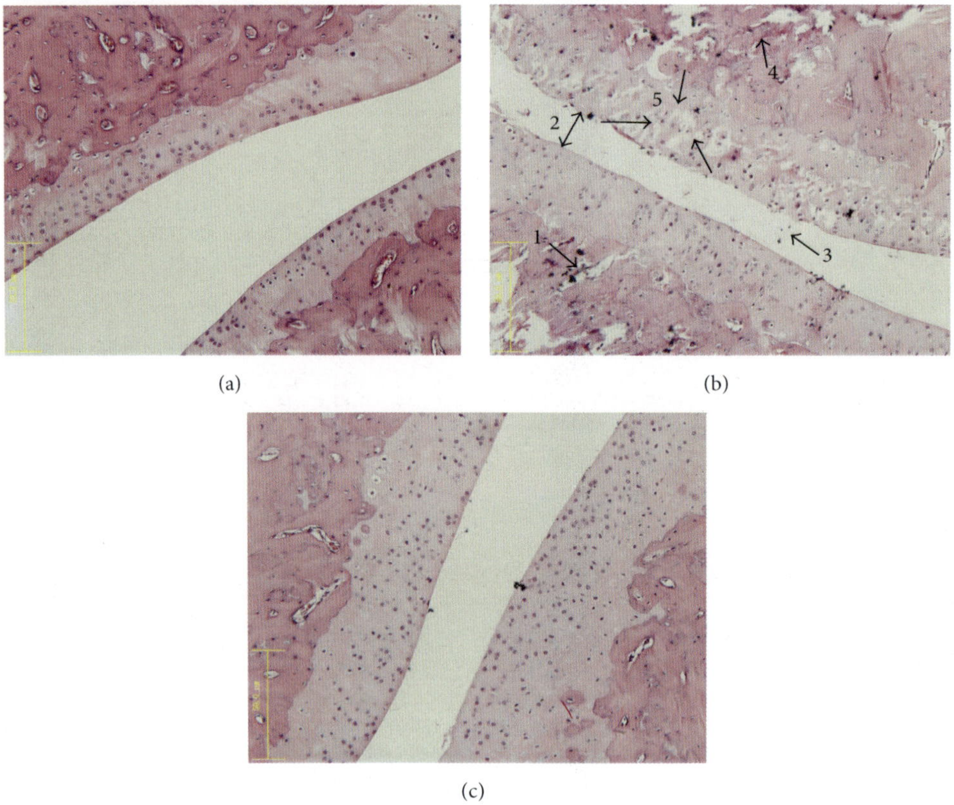

FIGURE 1: Effects of XFC on histopathologic changes of the AA rats. Photomicrographs of representative histopathologic specimens of left hind joints in SD rats taken from healthy group (a), untreated group (b), and XFC treated group (c). 1: inflammatory cell infiltration; 2: joint-space narrowing; 3: neutrophils infiltration; 4: pannus formation; 5: cartilage erosion. Original magnification 400x.

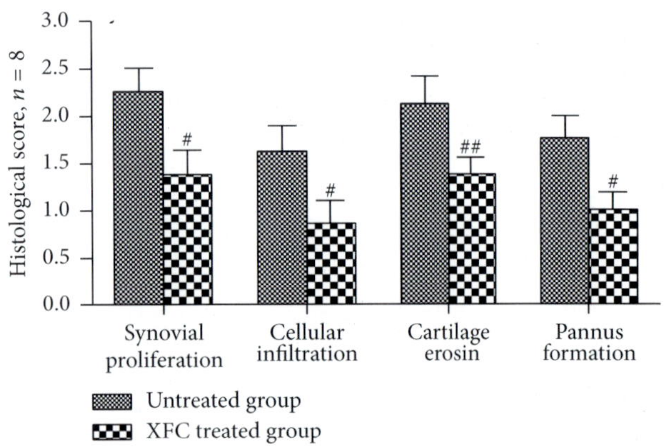

FIGURE 2: Histological score of the AA rats, $^{\#}p < 0.05$, $^{\#\#}p < 0.01$ compared with untreated group.

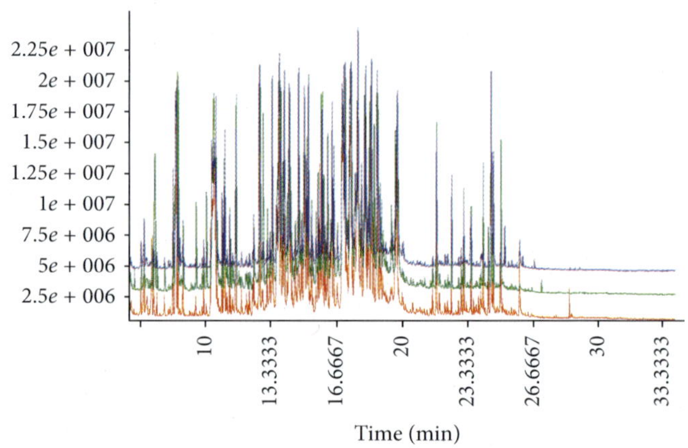

FIGURE 3: TIC chromatogram of urine samples in AA rats; the brown line represents healthy group; the green line represents untreated group; the blue line represents XFC treated group.

cross validation to evaluate validity of the model. After PLS-DA analysis, the healthy, untreated, and XFC treated groups completely separated. $R^2Y = 0.997$ and $Q^2Y = 0.553$, which indicate that the model has a perfect fitting and has reliable predictive ability. After the randomization ($n = 200$), we obtained $R^2 = 0.803$ and $Q^2 = -0.156$, indicating that both of these PLS-RA models demonstrated good performances [20]. The results are shown in Figure 5.

3.6. Orthogonal Partial Least-Squares Discriminant Analysis (OPLS-DA) of Urine Samples. OPLS-DA is a model for orthogonal correction in which the orthogonal signal correction can be filtered out with uncorrelated orthogonal variable information. This method retains only correlated orthogonal variable information and improves the accuracy

TABLE 2: Potential biomarkers selected and change of trend in each group.

Number	VarID	Compound	RT	VIP	$p_{H\text{-}U}$	$p_{U\text{-}X}$	$p_{X\text{-}H}$
1	251	2,2-Dimethylsuccinic acid	11.0616	2.70266	0.011313387	0.03490986	0.249996112
2	314	Tartronic acid	11.8754	2.94527	0.024742601	0.15475148	0.010899989
3	636	Dehydroshikimic acid	16.7414	3.05951	0.032774968	0.1022563	0.077357634
4	646	Hippuric acid	16.9083	3.21815	0.01018095	0.19488332	0.049258272
5	684	Adenine	17.5117	2.73672	0.021520896	0.59814266	0.035198717
6	697	Phenaceturic acid	17.7171	4.18817	0.016864462	0.02460963	0.503834004
7	807	L-dopa	19.405	1.31514	0.026524125	0.0252176	0.771814517
8	865	1,4-Dihydroxy-2-naphthoic acid	20.474	3.69942	0.003037716	0.00524929	0.612627294
9	1110	Melibiose	25.9579	2.33593	0.040379626	0.0682718	0.501486543

Note: VarID represents urine screening 1166 peak to the serial number of compound; RT represents retention time of compound. A variable importance in the projection (VIP) was obtained from OPLS-DA model with a threshold of 1.0; $p_{H\text{-}U}$ represents p value by healthy group versus untreated group; $p_{U\text{-}X}$ represents p value by untreated group versus XFC treated group; $p_{X\text{-}H}$ represents p value by XFC treated group versus healthy group.

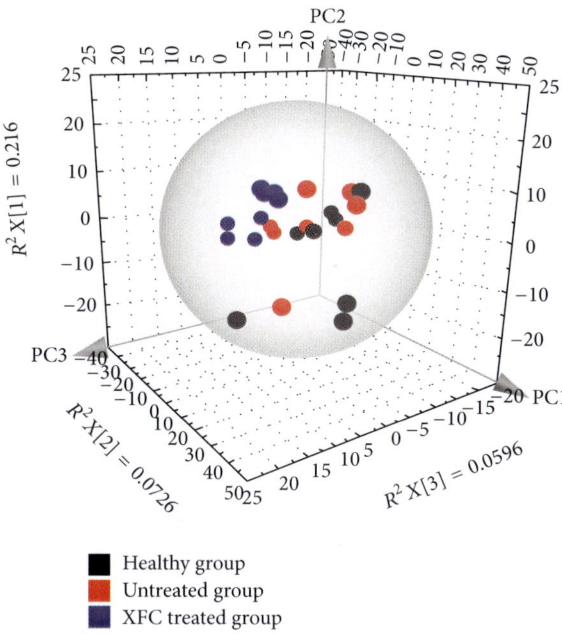

FIGURE 4: PCA score plots of adjuvant-induced arthritis in rats urine metabolic profiling of healthy group, untreated group, and XFC treated group using GC-TOF/MS.

of discrimination. OPLS-DA was performed using SIMCA-P software, which maximizes the internal differences of the model between different groups [21]. OPLS-DA used Ctr (mean-centered scaling) to process the data scale conversion mode where the X- and Y-axes represent first and second principle components, respectively. After OPLS-DA analysis, the urine metabolomes in each group were clustered. This result suggests that the metabolic pattern in AA rats was significantly altered and that XFC intervention can affect the metabolism of AA rats. The results are shown in Figures 6(a) and 6(b).

We obtained a load diagram from OPLS-DA. Each dot represents a metabolite. Dots near the center represent small difference in model classification, and dots far away from the center were considered to contribute more to the model classification. Red dots represent the nine potential biomarkers in our test. Results are shown in Figure 6(c).

3.7. Potential Biomarkers from Urine Samples. OPLS-DA filtered out unrelated orthogonal signals, so more reliable potential biomarkers were obtained. VIP is a parameter which summarizes the importance of the X-variables, both for the X and Y models, is called the variable influence on projection, which estimates the importance of each variable in the projection used in a OPLS-DA model. A variable with a VIP score close to or greater than 1 can be considered important in a given model. The VIP value and Student's t-test of the p value were used to reflect the importance of the metabolites. Variables with VIP > 1 and $p < 0.05$ were selected as potential biomarkers for further statistical analysis using SPSS version 17.0 (Spss Inc., Chicago, IL, USA). Nine potential biomarkers were observed as compared with that of healthy group ($p < 0.05$), which were correlated with adjuvant-induced arthritis. After the treatment of XFC, the levels of the 2,2-dimethylsuccinic acid, phenaceturic acid, L-dopa, and 1,4-dihydroxy-2-naphthoic acid were changed significantly ($p < 0.05$). The levels of dehydroshikimic acid, tartronic acid, adenine, hippuric acid, and melibiose were trends that have tendency toward healthy group, but there was no significant difference. Results are shown in Table 2.

To better visualize the changes in the potential biomarkers, box plots were created using straightforward statistical graphics to describe the distribution of several sets of quantitative data and compare their differences. The height of the box represents the interquartile range, the horizontal line represents the median, and the extensions up and down at the ends of the thread represent the maximum and the minimum, shown in Figure 7.

3.8. Correlation Network Analysis of Potential Biomarkers. To illustrate the links in the potential biomarker metabolic pathways, we used pathophysiology, biochemistry, physiology, and the Human Metabolome Database to provide quantitative and metabolic information on organism metabolites. We also referred to the relevant literature.

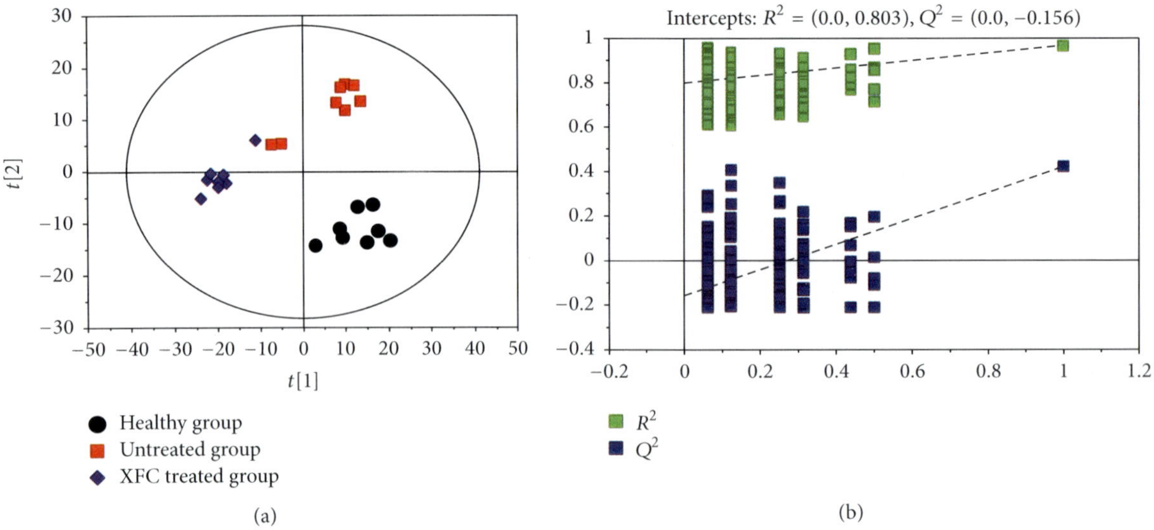

FIGURE 5: PLS-DA based on the adjuvant-induced arthritis date of urine. (a) shows the separation for the PLS-DA scores of healthy, untreated, and XFC treated groups. (b) represents validation of PLS-DA model (using 200 random permutations).

The nine potential biomarkers are involved in purine metabolism, fat metabolism, amino acid metabolism, and energy metabolism. Therefore, we constructed a network of metabolic pathways of potential biomarkers, shown in Figure 8.

4. Discussion

AA, a T-cell-mediated chronic inflammatory stress, is a well-established in vivo model that has been used in numerous studies to investigate the pathogenesis of RA and for identification of potential therapeutic targets [22]. After intragastric administration of XFC for 30 days, there was significantly less joint swelling in AA rats ($p < 0.01$) and less histological damage, compared with model rats. Therefore, XFC has a moderate therapeutic effect on AA rats.

Metabolomics focuses on changes in biological fluids to indicate changes in a biological system [23]. In recent years, metabolomics has been used to analyze biological differences in metabolic profiles to identify potential biomarkers. These differences can elucidate the overall function of organisms at specific times and in specific environments. GC-TOF/MS, liquid chromatography-mass spectrometry, and nuclear magnetic resonance are commonly used in metabolomics [24–26]. GC-TOF/MS is a variety of features including simplicity, reproducibility, high separation efficiency, high sensitivity, standard spectral library, and quantifiable metabolites in metabolomics [27]. We used GC-TOF/MS and found nine potential biomarkers. The biomarkers are mainly involved in the glucose, fat, amino acid, and energy metabolism pathways. After intragastric administration of XFC, the levels of the 2,2-dimethylsuccinic acid, phenaceturic acid, L-dopa, and 1,4-dihydroxy-2-naphthoic acid were changed significantly in the XFC treated group ($p < 0.05$). The levels of dehydroshikimic acid, hippuric acid, and melibiose are trends that have tendency toward healthy group, but there was no significant difference.

Studies have shown that free radical oxidative damage plays an important role in the pathogenesis of RA [28]. Endogenous or exogenous stimuli can result in metabolic abnormalities, which can produce excessive reactive oxygen species. When the amino acid supply is inadequate, a reduction in antioxidant enzymes results in disordered balance between prooxidant/antioxidants [29]. This imbalance eventually leaves the body in a state of oxidative stress. Reactive oxygen species can damage DNA, lipids, proteins, and other biological molecules, which can result in energy metabolism disorders. However, energy consumption will also produce acidic substances and excessive active oxygen radicals, which further aggravate tissue damage and cause inflammation. Therefore, oxidative stress and inflammation play a key role in RA [30].

Metabolomic analysis of changes in the urine of AA rats improves our understanding of significant metabolic variations during RA. Hippuric acid and phenaceturic acid are secondary metabolites of fatty acids. During RA, excessive oxygen free radicals are produced in the mitochondria, which accelerate fat mobilization and eventually significantly increase the levels of fatty acid secondary metabolites. We found higher levels of hippuric acid and phenaceturic acid in the urine of AA rats, which implies that RA is associated with lipid metabolism dysfunction [31, 32]. The XFC treated group had significantly lower level of phenaceturic acid than that of the untreated group. Hippuric acid content has no significant difference in the XFC treated group but has a tendency towards healthy group. This result implies that XFC can regulate fat metabolism and reduce oxygen free radical generation in the mitochondria.

L-dopa is a tyrosine oxidation product that is generated from tyrosine hydroxylase. Tyrosine is the major metabolite of phenylalanine, which are both amino acids. During RA,

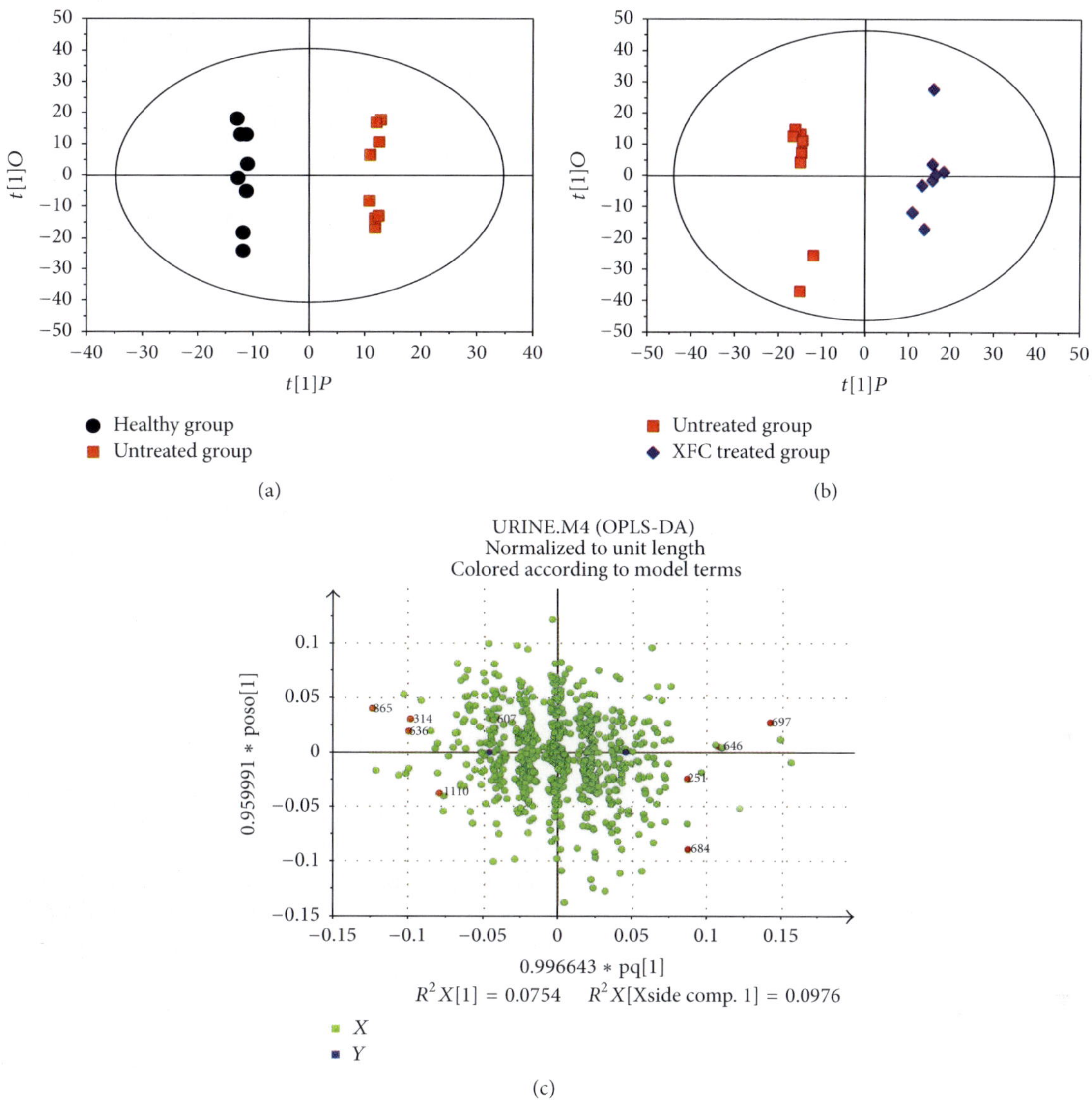

FIGURE 6: OPLS-DA of urine metabolic profiling of healthy group versus untreated group (a); OPLS-DA of urine metabolic profiling of untreated group versus XFC treated group (b); OPLS-DA variable loading plot (c).

excessive oxidative stress and inflammation inhibit amino acid intake or slow their synthesis, which affects the generation of articular cartilage protein [31–33]. The untreated group had lower levels of L-dopa compared with the healthy group, which indicates that amino acid metabolism was disrupted. The XFC treated group had higher levels of L-dopa compared with the untreated group, which implies that XFC can regulate amino acid metabolism and improve joint damage.

Lower levels of tartronic acid and higher levels of 2,2-dimethylsuccinic acid were observed in the untreated group, which indicates dysfunction of the tricarboxylic acid cycle (TCA) probably because of disturbed metabolism in the chondrocytes and cartilage. 2,2-Dimethylsuccinic acid is a succinic methylated product and succinic acid is an important metabolic intermediate in the TCA. The TCA is the final metabolic pathway for the three major nutrients, which are carbohydrates, lipids, and amino acids. The XFC treated group had significantly reduced levels of 2,2-dimethylsuccinic acid compared with the untreated group. These changes suggest that XFC has a regulatory role on the TCA.

1,4-Dihydroxy-2-naphthoic acid is an aromatic amino acid that is the product of various enzymes and is involved in ubiquinone and other terpenoid and quinone biosyntheses. 1,4-Dihydroxy-2-naphthoic acid was lower in the untreated group, probably because there were too many oxygen free radicals, which resulted in increased ubiquinone production and strengthened oxidative phosphorylation. These changes resulted in more ATP [34]. The XFC treated group had higher 1,4-dihydroxy-2-naphthoic acid levels compared with the untreated group, indicating improved energy metabolism.

Melibiose is composed of a galactose and glucose. Not only can a stachyose be decomposed into a melibiose but also

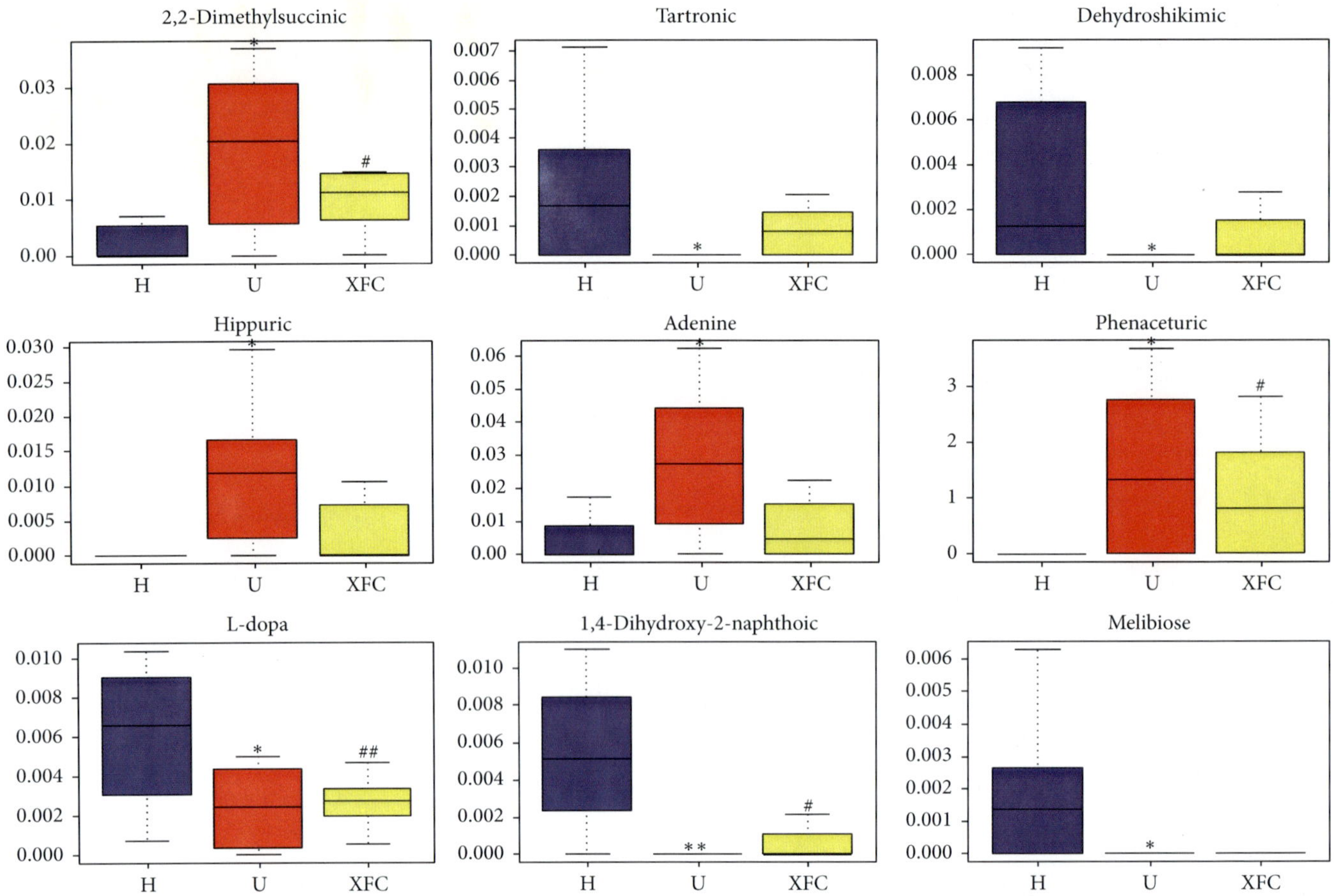

Figure 7: Box plots of data in urine samples from healthy group (H), untreated group (U), and XFC treated group (XFC). $^{*}p < 0.05$ and $^{**}p < 0.01$ compared with healthy group; $^{\#}p < 0.05$ compared with untreated group; $^{\#\#}p < 0.01$ compared with untreated group.

it generates manninotriose enhanced immune substances [35], which improve immunity to fight inflammation consistent with prophase study [36]. During RA, abnormalities in galactose metabolism lead to lower levels of melibiose and manninotriose. The XFC group had higher melibiose levels, which suggest that XFC can adjust disordered galactose metabolism and the immune system to reduce inflammation. We found lower concentrations of dehydroshikimic acid in the urine of AA rats as compared with normal controls. Abnormalities in urinary dehydroshikimic acid are generally believed to be associated with disorder of glycolytic pathway and pentose phosphate pathway. Shikimic acid has anti-inflammatory, analgesic, and antiviral effects in accord with reference [37]. The levels of melibiose and dehydroshikimic acid have no significant difference in the XFC treated group but have a tendency towards healthy group, which suggested that XFC maybe achieve a certain effect to regulate the disorder of glycometabolism and reinforced the anti-inflammatory capacity.

Tartronic acid is converted to β-alanine that is a component of coenzyme A, which plays an important role in the TCA. Adenine can generate uric acid during RA; the elevated levels of adenine lead to high levels of uric acid, which aggravates cartilage damage. In addition, adenine participating cofactors include nicotinamide adenine dinucleotide (NAD) and flavin adenine dinucleotide (FAD). These compounds are progressively oxidized by the respiratory chain to generate ATP. We hypothesize that oxidative stress leads to reduction of functional capacity of mitochondria, which leads to an energy metabolism disorder [34]. Our results show that the levels of tartronic acid and adenine had no significant difference in XFC treated group, implying that XFC did not regulate them for treatment.

5. Conclusions

We used a GC-TOF/MS metabolomics method to comprehensively and efficiently elucidate changes in the metabolites AA rats. Using a variety of multivariate statistical methods such as PCA, PLS-DA, and OPLS-DA, nine potential biomarkers were identified. These biomarkers are mainly associated with purine metabolism, fat metabolism, amino acid metabolism, and energy metabolism.

After administration of XFC, the levels of the 2,2-dimethylsuccinic acid, phenaceturic acid, L-dopa, and 1,4-dihydroxy-2-naphthoic acid were changed significantly ($p < 0.05$). The levels of dehydroshikimic acid, hippuric acid, and melibiose had no significant difference, but there are trends

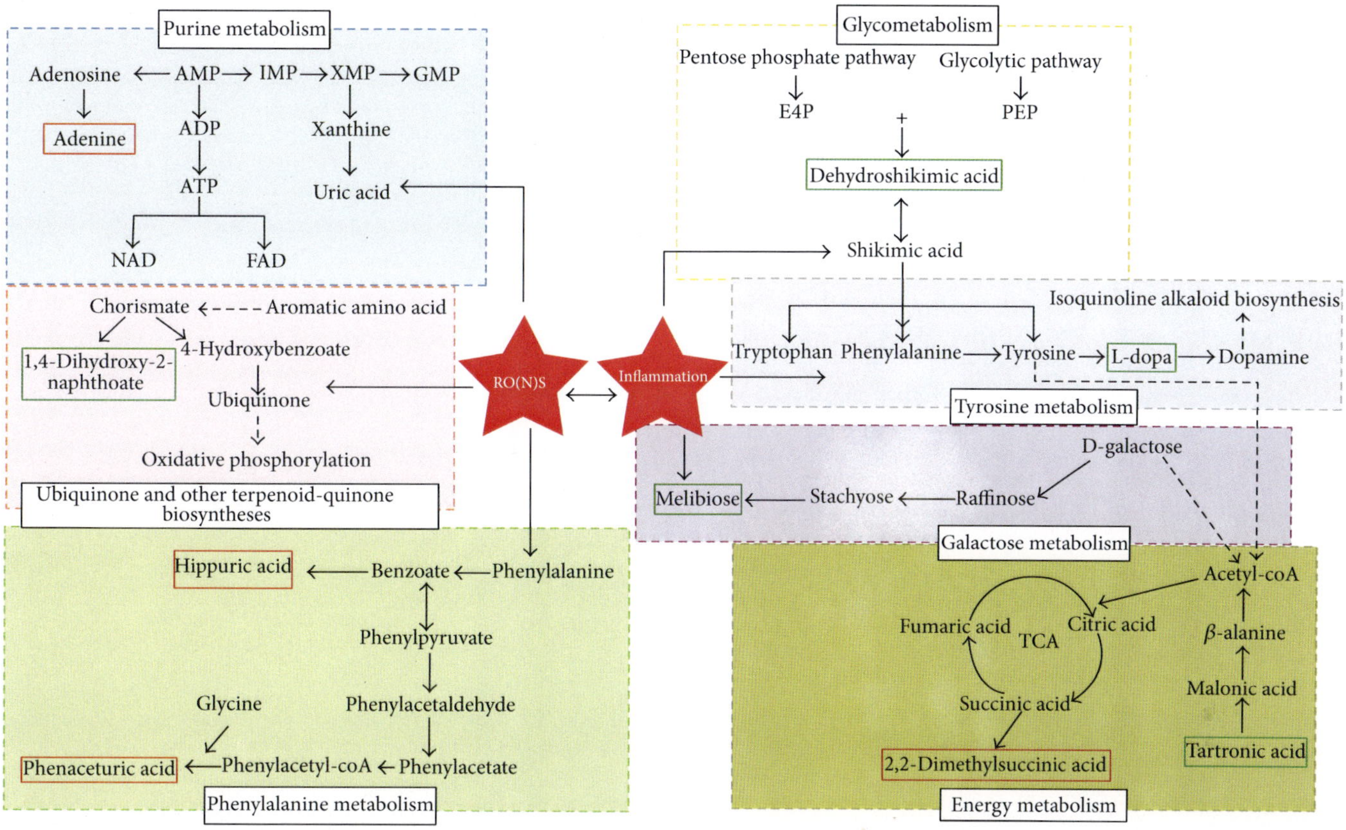

FIGURE 8: Correlation networks of all the potential biomarkers in response to RA. Nine potential biomarkers were used to explain the possible metabolic pathways. Metabolites with red box were significantly increased in untreated group compared to healthy group. Metabolites with blue box were significantly decreased in untreated group compared to healthy group.

that have tendency toward healthy group. These findings show that GC-TOF/MS-based urine metabolic profiling can provide reliable results and be used in modern TCM research. This technique has potential application in identification effective compounds to treat RA.

Conflict of Interests

The authors declare that there is no conflict of interests regarding the publication of this paper.

Acknowledgments

This study was financially supported by National Sci-tech Support Plan (2012BAI26B03). The authors are grateful to Dr. Junliang Deng (Biotree Bio-technology Co., Ltd., Shanghai, China) for providing help in data analysis.

References

[1] L. A. Criswell, "Gene discovery in rheumatoid arthritis highlights the CD40/NF-κB signaling pathway in disease pathogenesis," *Immunological Reviews*, vol. 233, no. 1, pp. 55–61, 2010.

[2] G. J. Tobón, P. Youinou, and A. Saraux, "The environment, geo-epidemiology, and autoimmune disease: rheumatoid arthritis," *Journal of Autoimmunity*, vol. 35, no. 1, pp. 10–14, 2010.

[3] J. Liu and R.-L. Liu, "The potential role of Chinese medicine in ameliorating extra-articular manifestations of rheumatoid arthritis," *Chinese Journal of Integrative Medicine*, vol. 17, no. 10, pp. 735–737, 2011.

[4] Y.-X. Cao, J. Liu, and Y. Zhu, "Effect of Xinfeng capsule on the cardiac function in patients with rheumatoid arthritis," *Chinese Journal of Integrative Medicine*, vol. 17, no. 10, pp. 738–743, 2011.

[5] Y. Sun, J. Liu, L. Wan, F. Wang, and Y. Qi, "Xinfeng Capsule increases peripheral blood BTLA expression of CD19(+) and CD24(+) B cells and relieves oxidative stress damage to improve cardiac function of patients with rheumatoid arthritis," *Xi Bao Yu Fen Zi Mian Yi Xue Za Zhi*, vol. 31, no. 1, pp. 93–96, 2015.

[6] F. Wang, M. Meng, L. Chen, X. Y. Wang, and Q. Sun, "Development and validation of a high-performance thin-layer chromatographic fingerprint method for the evaluation of QiYi capsules with the reference of myotonin," *Journal of Planar Chromatography*, vol. 27, no. 3, pp. 199–203, 2014.

[7] C.-B. Huang, J. Liu, X. Chen et al., "Treatment of rheumatoid arthritis by xinfeng capsule: an efficacy observation," *Zhongguo Zhong Xi Yi Jie He Za Zhi*, vol. 33, no. 12, pp. 1599–1602, 2013.

[8] J. Liu, C.-B. Huang, Y. Wang et al., "Chinese herbal medicine Xinfeng Capsule in treatment of rheumatoid arthritis: study protocol of a multicenter randomized controlled trial," *Journal of Integrative Medicine*, vol. 11, no. 6, pp. 428–434, 2013.

[9] S. Seijo, J. J. Lozano, C. Alonso et al., "Metabolomics discloses potential biomarkers for the noninvasive diagnosis of idiopathic

portal hypertension," *The American Journal of Gastroenterology*, vol. 108, no. 6, pp. 926–932, 2013.

[10] Y. Gu, C. Lu, Q. Zha et al., "Plasma metabonomics study of rheumatoid arthritis and its Chinese medicine subtypes by using liquid chromatography and gas chromatography coupled with mass spectrometry," *Molecular BioSystems*, vol. 8, no. 5, pp. 1535–1543, 2012.

[11] X. S. Zhangjie Huang, M. Wang, and M. Wu, "Research progress of metabolomics technology in the field of traditional Chinese medicine," *Journal of Chinese Medicinal Materials*, vol. 36, pp. 2055–2058, 2013.

[12] R. K. Madsen, T. Lundstedt, J. Gabrielsson et al., "Diagnostic properties of metabolic perturbations in rheumatoid arthritis," *Arthritis Research and Therapy*, vol. 13, article R19, 2011.

[13] L. Liu, Z. J. Zheng, and Z. H. Fang, "Experimental study on effect of xinfeng capsule in treating rats' adjuvant arthritis on ultrastructure of synoviocyte and splenic lymphocyte," *Chinese Journal of Integrated Traditional and Western Medicine*, vol. 21, no. 12, pp. 917–919, 2001.

[14] L. J. Wan, J. Liu, C. Huang, Y. Wang, and L. Zheng, "Effect of Xinfeng capsule on pulmonary function in a adjuvant arthritis rat model," *Journal of Traditional Chinese Medicine*, vol. 34, no. 1, pp. 76–85, 2014.

[15] C. Hughes, J. A. Wolos, E. H. Giannini, and R. Hirsch, "Induction of T helper cell hyporesponsiveness in an experimental model of autoimmunity by using nonmitogenic anti-CD3 monoclonal antibody," *The Journal of Immunology*, vol. 153, no. 7, pp. 3319–3325, 1994.

[16] C. Schramm, J. Kriegsmann, M. Protschka et al., "Susceptibility to collagen-induced arthritis is modulated by TGFbeta responsiveness of T cells," *Arthritis Research & Therapy*, vol. 6, no. 2, pp. R114–R119, 2004.

[17] T. Kind, G. Wohlgemuth, D. Y. Lee et al., "FiehnLib: mass spectral and retention index libraries for metabolomics based on quadrupole and time-of-flight gas chromatography/mass spectrometry," *Analytical Chemistry*, vol. 81, no. 24, pp. 10038–10048, 2009.

[18] J. Trygg, E. Holmes, and T. Lundstedt, "Chemometrics in metabonomics," *Journal of Proteome Research*, vol. 6, no. 2, pp. 469–479, 2007.

[19] S. Mahadevan, S. L. Shah, T. J. Marrie, and C. M. Slupsky, "Analysis of metabolomic data using support vector machines," *Analytical Chemistry*, vol. 80, no. 19, pp. 7562–7570, 2008.

[20] Y. Ni, M. Su, J. Lin et al., "Metabolic profiling reveals disorder of amino acid metabolism in four brain regions from a rat model of chronic unpredictable mild stress," *FEBS Letters*, vol. 582, no. 17, pp. 2627–2636, 2008.

[21] C. L. Gavaghan, I. D. Wilson, and J. K. Nicholson, "Physiological variation in metabolic phenotyping and functional genomic studies: use of orthogonal signal correction and PLS-DA," *FEBS Letters*, vol. 530, no. 1–3, pp. 191–196, 2002.

[22] R. K. Zong and J. Liu, "Effects of Xinfeng Capsule on the expression of platelet derived growth factor in synovium of adjuvant arthritis rats," *Chinese Journal of Integrative Medicine*, vol. 20, no. 9, pp. 688–694, 2014.

[23] J. K. Nicholson and I. D. Wilson, "Opinion: understanding 'global' systems biology: metabonomics and the continuum of metabolism," *Nature Reviews Drug Discovery*, vol. 2, no. 8, pp. 668–676, 2003.

[24] P. Yin, X. Zhao, Q. Li, J. Wang, J. Li, and G. Xu, "Metabonomics study of intestinal fistulas based on ultraperformance liquid chromatography coupled with Q-TOF mass spectrometry (UPLC/Q-TOF MS)," *Journal of Proteome Research*, vol. 5, no. 9, pp. 2135–2143, 2006.

[25] P. Yin, D. Wan, C. Zhao et al., "A metabonomic study of hepatitis B-induced liver cirrhosis and hepatocellular carcinoma by using RP-LC and HILIC coupled with mass spectrometry," *Molecular BioSystems*, vol. 5, no. 8, pp. 868–876, 2009.

[26] S. Bijlsma, I. Bobeldijk, E. R. Verheij et al., "Large-scale human metabolomics studies: a strategy for data (pre-) processing and validation," *Analytical Chemistry*, vol. 78, no. 2, pp. 567–574, 2006.

[27] H. Wu, T. Liu, C. Ma et al., "GC/MS-based metabolomic approach to validate the role of urinary sarcosine and target biomarkers for human prostate cancer by microwave-assisted derivatization," *Analytical and Bioanalytical Chemistry*, vol. 401, no. 2, pp. 635–646, 2011.

[28] R. Mishra, A. Singh, V. Chandra et al., "A comparative analysis of serological parameters and oxidative stress in osteoarthritis and Rheumatoid arthritis," *Rheumatology International*, vol. 32, no. 8, pp. 2377–2382, 2012.

[29] A. Kamanli, M. Naziroğlu, N. Aydilek, and C. Hacievliyagil, "Plasma lipid peroxidation and antioxidant levels in patients with rheumatoid arthritis," *Cell Biochemistry and Function*, vol. 22, no. 1, pp. 53–57, 2004.

[30] C. A. Hitchon and H. S. El-Gabalawy, "Oxidation in rheumatoid arthritis," *Arthritis Research and Therapy*, vol. 6, no. 6, pp. 265–278, 2004.

[31] H. Zhang, P. Fu, B. Ke et al., "Metabolomic analysis of biochemical changes in the plasma and urine of collagen-induced arthritis in rats after treatment with Huang-Lian-Jie-Du-Tang," *Journal of Ethnopharmacology*, vol. 154, no. 1, pp. 55–64, 2014.

[32] L. Bazzichi, M. L. Ciompi, L. Betti et al., "Impaired glutathione reductase activity and levels of collagenase and elastase in synovial fluid in rheumatoid arthritis," *Clinical and Experimental Rheumatology*, vol. 20, no. 6, pp. 761–766, 2002.

[33] E. Lubberts, L. A. B. Joosten, F. A. J. van de Loo, P. Schwarzenberger, J. Kolls, and W. B. van den Berg, "Overexpression of IL-17 in the knee joint of collagen type II immunized mice promotes collagen arthritis and aggravates joint destruction," *Inflammation Research*, vol. 51, no. 2, pp. 102–104, 2002.

[34] D. Curti, E. Izzo, L. Brambilla, G. Facchetti, G. Sangiovanni, and G. Brambilla, "Effect of a ubiquinone-like molecule on oxidative energy metabolism in rat cortical synaptosomes at different ages," *Neurochemical Research*, vol. 20, no. 9, pp. 1001–1006, 1995.

[35] Y. Qian, X. Zhao, J. L. Song et al., "Inhibitory effects of resistant starch (RS3) as a carrier for stachyose on dextran sulfate sodium-induced ulcerative colitis in C57BL/6 mice," *Experimental and Therapeutic Medicine*, vol. 6, no. 5, pp. 1312–1316, 2013.

[36] Y. X. Cao, J. Liu, and Y. Zhu, "Effect of Xinfeng capsule on the cardiac function in patients with rheumatoid arthritis," *Chinese Journal of Integrative Medicine*, vol. 17, pp. 738–743, 2011.

[37] J. Xing, C. You, K. Dong et al., "Ameliorative effects of 3,4-oxo-isopropylidene-shikimic acid on experimental colitis and their mechanisms in rats," *International Immunopharmacology*, vol. 15, no. 3, pp. 524–531, 2013.

22

Celiac Disease in Adult Patients: Specific Autoantibodies in the Diagnosis, Monitoring, and Screening

Evagelia Trigoni,[1] Alexandra Tsirogianni,[1] Elena Pipi,[2] Gerassimos Mantzaris,[3] and Chryssa Papasteriades[1]

[1] *Department of Immunology-Histocompatibility, "Evangelismos" General Hospital, 10676 Athens, Greece*
[2] *Department of Dermatology, University of Lübeck, 23562 Lübeck, Germany*
[3] *Department of Gastroenterology, "Evangelismos" General Hospital, 10676 Athens, Greece*

Correspondence should be addressed to Alexandra Tsirogianni; alextsir@gmail.com

Academic Editor: Alina Popp

The increasing prevalence of celiac disease (CD), especially in adults, its atypical clinical presentation, and the strict, lifelong adherence to gluten-free diet (GFD) as the only option for healthy state create an imperative need for noninvasive methods that can effectively diagnose CD and monitor GFD. *Aim.* Evaluation of anti-endomysium (EmA) and anti-tissue transglutaminase IgA (tTG-A) antibodies in CD diagnosis, GFD monitoring, and first degree relatives screening in CD adult patients. *Methods.* 70 newly diagnosed Greek adult patients, 70 controls, and 47 first degree relatives were tested for the presence of EmA and tTG-A. The CD patients were monitored during a 3-year period. *Results.* EmA predictive ability for CD diagnosis was slightly better compared to tTG-A ($P = 0.043$). EmA could assess compliance with GFD already from the beginning of the diet, while both EmA and tTG-A had an equal ability to discriminate between strictly and partially compliant patients after the first semester and so on. Screening of first degree relatives resulted in the identification of 2 undiagnosed CD cases. *Conclusions.* Both EmA and tTG-A are suitable markers in the CD diagnosis, in the screening of CD among first degree relatives, having also an equal performance in the long term monitoring.

1. Introduction

Celiac disease (CD) (*coeliac*, from Greek *κοιλιακός* koiliakos, "abdominal") was first described in the second century AD by the Greek physician Aretaeus of Cappadocia as a malabsorptive syndrome with chronic diarrhea [1]. Nowadays it is well known that CD is an immune-mediated systemic disorder elicited by gluten and related prolamins in genetically susceptible individuals and characterized by the presence of a variable combination of gluten dependent clinical manifestations, CD-specific antibodies, HLA-DQ2 or HLA-DQ8 haplotypes, and enteropathy. The typical but not pathognomonic lesions of the small intestinal mucosa resolve with the removal of gluten from the diet [2].

The autoantigen which is also the molecule recognized by anti-endomysium antibodies (EmA) has been identified as the enzyme "tissue transglutaminase" (tTG) [3, 4]. tTG induces the deamidation of gluten peptides and the formation of novel epitopes that, in association with HLA II antigens, induce the antibody response to gliadin and tTG antigens, resulting in the damage of the small intestinal mucosa [5, 6]. Anti-tissue transglutaminase antibodies recognize the same antigen as EmA, from which they differ in terms of detection method. EmA are tested by the indirect immunofluorescence method (IF) and directed against "reticulin-like" fibres in connective tissue around smooth muscle fibres in the oesophagus, liver, stomach, and bladder of monkeys, in the sections of the jejunum and kidneys of rats and in sections of the human umbilical cord (HUC). However, commercially primate GIT tissue is used in almost all (but not exclusively) centers. For the determination of anti-tissue transglutaminase IgA and IgG antibodies, ELISA with human extractive or recombinant transglutaminase is recommended. Both EmA and anti-tissue transglutaminase antibodies are very specific and sensitive [7–9].

Adult patients with CD rarely present with malabsorption related symptoms. Far more commonly they describe non-specific or subtle gastrointestinal symptoms or they present with extraintestinal manifestations (atypical or silent form); thus they may initially be overlooked [10, 11].

The increasing prevalence of CD, especially in adults, its atypical clinical presentation, and also the lifelong adherence to a gluten-free diet (GFD) as the only option for healthy state create an imperative need for proper immunological tests that can easily, timely, and effectively diagnose CD and monitor GFD [12–16].

2. Aim

The aim of the present retrospective study was (a) to evaluate the efficacy of specific autoantibodies in the diagnosis and monitoring of celiac disease in Greek adult patients, where the prevalent diet is the Mediterranean one, mostly based on whole grains and (b) to assess the frequency of undetected celiac disease among the first degree relatives of CD patients.

3. Materials and Methods

3.1. Patients and Controls. This long term study which took place in the Department of Immunology-Histocompatibility of "Evangelismos" General Hospital of Athens with the cooperation of the Celiac Disease Clinic of the same hospital included the following groups of individuals.

(a) 70 Greek adult patients, 50 women and 20 men with mean age 39 ± 11.1 years (range: 19–66) who were newly diagnosed with CD. The monitoring of the patients took place on the moment of the diagnosis when they had a regular unrestricted diet and consequently at 6, 12, 24, and 36 months after the initiation of GFD. 51 of the 70 patients (72.9%) followed a strict GFD while the remaining 19 (27.1%) had a partial compliance with GFD.

(b) 47 first degree relatives (10 parents, 8 siblings, and 29 offspring) of the aforementioned patients, 23 men and 24 women with mean age 24 ± 15.5 years (range: 1–59). In all these family members on gluten-containing diet, the serological tests were performed only once.

(c) 70 individuals who constituted the control group. 30 of them were patients with inflammatory and noninflammatory diseases of the intestine (8 with Crohn's disease, 7 with ulcerative colitis, 6 irritable bowel syndrome, and 9 with microscopic colitis), 20 women and 10 men with mean age 41 ± 11.3 years (range 21–55) and the remaining 40 were healthy blood donors, 22 women and 18 men with mean age 38 ± 12.1 years (range: 18–58). The control group was serologically tested also once.

No individual in this study had IgA deficiency.

3.2. Methods. The antibodies studied were as follows. (a) Anti-endomysium (EmA) which were determined semi-quantitative by the technique of indirect immunofluorescence (IIF) using a commercial kit INOVA (NOVA Lite Monkey Oesophagus IFA Kit/Slides, USA) on a 5-μm-thin cryostat section of distal monkey oesophagus as antigen substrate. Patient samples were tested in dilutions ranging from 1 : 5 to 1 : 2560. The antibody titre was defined as the highest sample dilution yielding fluorescence. Titre below 1 : 5 was considered negative. (b) Anti-tissue transglutaminase class IgA (tTG-A) which were assayed using a commercial anti-tTG type IgA ELISA test kit (QUANTA LiteTM, INOVA Diagnostics, USA). The cut-off value provided was 25 U. ELISA was performed in duplicate according to the manufacturer's instruction. Serum samples were kept frozen at −80°C until assays were performed.

The final diagnosis of CD as well as the inflammatory and noninflammatory diseases of the intestine in all these patients was based on currently accepted criteria [17, 18], after thorough clinical and laboratory investigation, including endoscopy and biopsies from the upper and lower gastrointestinal tract. Histological damage observed in the intestinal biopsy samples in CD patients was graded according to Marsh's classification [18]. Moreover, all patients in the study underwent clinical evaluation at each follow-up visit and experienced dietitians assessed their compliance to the GFD, through a standard questionnaire.

3.3. Statistics. EmA were expressed using the negative logarithms of measured values while for the comparison of proportions chi-square and Fisher's exact tests were used. Differences in changes of EmA and tTG-A during the follow-up period in total and between the two studied groups were evaluated using repeated measurements analysis of variance (ANOVA) and Bonferroni correction was used. tTG-A was log-transformed for the analysis of variance due to its skewed distribution. Receiver operating characteristic (ROC) analysis was used and area under the curve (AUC), optimal sensitivity, and specificity were determined. All P values reported are two tailed. Statistical significance was set at 0.05 and analyses were conducted using SPSS statistical software (version 18.0).

4. Results

4.1. Evaluation of EmA and tTG-A in CD Diagnosis. The frequency of autoantibodies tested in the control group and in CD patients at the time of diagnosis before they started GFD is presented in Table 1.

All CD patients but 3 presented with positive EmA while increased values of tTG-A were detected in 66 out of the 70 CD patients. Two of the three EmA negative patients were also tTG-A negative while the third one had increased values of tTG-A (155 U). In these three EmA negative patients the small intestinal biopsy showed Marsh I type lesions.

In the control group, however, none had positive EmA whereas 3 individuals showed borderline values of tTG-A (30 U, 32 U, and 28 U, resp.). Two of them were diagnosed

Table 1: Frequency of specific antibodies tested.

	Patients				P Pearson's χ^2 test
	CD patients		Controls		
	N	%	N	%	
tTG-A					
Negative	4	5.7	67	95.7	**<0.001**
Positive	66	94.3	3	4.3	
EmA					
Negative	3	4.3	70	100.0	**<0.001**
Positive	67	95.7	0	0.0	

Table 2: Evaluation of autoantibodies tested in CD diagnosis.

	Se (%) (95% CI)	Sp (%) (95% CI)	PPV (%) (95% CI)	NPV (%) (95% CI)
tTG-A	94.3 (86.0–98.4)	95.7 (88.0–99.1)	95.7 (87.8–99.1)	94.4 (86.2–98.4)
EmA	95.7 (88.0–99.1)	100.0 (94.9–100.0)	100.0 (94.6–100.0)	95.9 (88.5–99.1)

with Crohn's disease and the third one with irritable bowel syndrome.

According to the antibodies frequencies found in the studied groups, sensitivity (Se), specificity (Sp), positive (PPV) and negative predictive value (NPV), and the intervals for CD were calculated (Table 2).

As presented in Table 2, EmA showed higher specificity (100.0%), sensitivity (95.7%), PPV (100.0%), and NPV (95.9%) than tTG-A in the diagnosis of celiac disease. Furthermore, their predictive ability for CD diagnosis for CD was slightly better in comparison to the one of tTG-A ($P = 0.043$).

4.2. Changes of EmA and tTG-A over Time after Initiation of GFD. The serological changes over time in all the patients, both strictly and partially compliant, are illustrated in Figure 1 which describes the proportions of positive samples at all follow-up time points. There was a significant change in the proportions of the positive samples over time for both strictly ($P < 0.001$) and partially ($P = 0.037$) compliant patients concerning EmA but for tTG-A the change was significant only for those who had a strict diet ($P < 0.001$).

Compared to partially compliant patients, strict compliance was associated with significantly lower proportions of positive EmA and tTG-A results in the first, second, and third year of the followup ($P < 0.001$). The strictly compliant patients' EmA presented a sharper decline of positive samples proportion ($P = 0.014$) than tTG-A, in the first six months. This decline also continued through the first and second year assessment. On the other hand, for the strictly compliant patients, tTG-A showed a less prominent decrease of positive samples in the first semester ($P = 0.268$) which, however, became significant, continuous, and progressive over time ($P < 0.001$).

More specifically, at the time of diagnosis 96.1% and 94.1% of the fifty-one patients who then started a strict GFD had positive EmA and tTG-A, respectively, while after 6 months of strict GFD 60.8% and 80.4% of them were still positive compared with 27.5% and 51% after 1 year of diet. After 3 years only 3 of the patients (5.9%) had antibody titres over the cut-off level for EmA, while 10 (19.6%) remained with tTG-A positive.

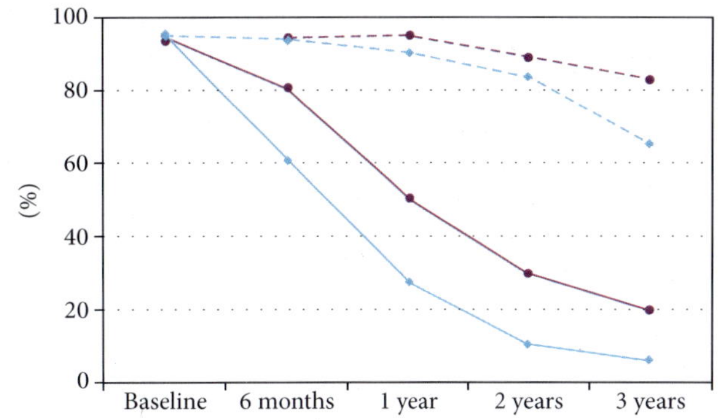

Figure 1: Changes in the percentage of positive samples for EmA and tTG-A over time in strictly compliant and partially compliant patients.

4.3. Predictive Capacity of EmA and tTG-A for the Compliance with GFD. The ability of EmA and tTG-A to discriminate the degree of adherence to GFD at the follow-up time points, 6 months, 1, 2, and 3 years was assessed by ROC analysis and is shown in Figures 2(a), 2(b), 2(c), and 2(d), respectively.

We concluded that EmA can assess the degree of compliance with GFD in the first semester from the beginning of the diet, while both EmA and tTG-A have an equal ability to discriminate between strictly and partially compliant patients in the first, second, and third year.

4.4. Prevalence of Celiac Disease among the First Degree Relatives. Forty-seven family members of 28 patients with CD underwent serological testing for EmA and tTG-A. Two family members (2/47) (4.2%) had positive EmA while in 5 of them (5/47) (10.6%) increased values of tTG-A were detected.

More specifically, positive EmA was detected in 2 first degree relatives (4.2%), in dilutions 1 : 40 and 1 : 20, respectively, 1 12-year-old girl whose father had CD and 1 18-year-old boy with CD mother. The CD in these family members was confirmed by intestinal biopsy. The two EmA positive individuals also showed high levels of tTG-A (55.0 U and 65.0 U, resp.). However, there were 3 more individuals with tTG-A positive (40.0 U, 60.2 U, and 63.0 U) who were not diagnosed with celiac disease. In these individuals CD diagnosis was excluded by an intestinal biopsy and the fact that they were EmA negative.

5. Discussion

Celiac disease in adults presents with a variety of atypical symptoms so there is a need for sensitive and specific

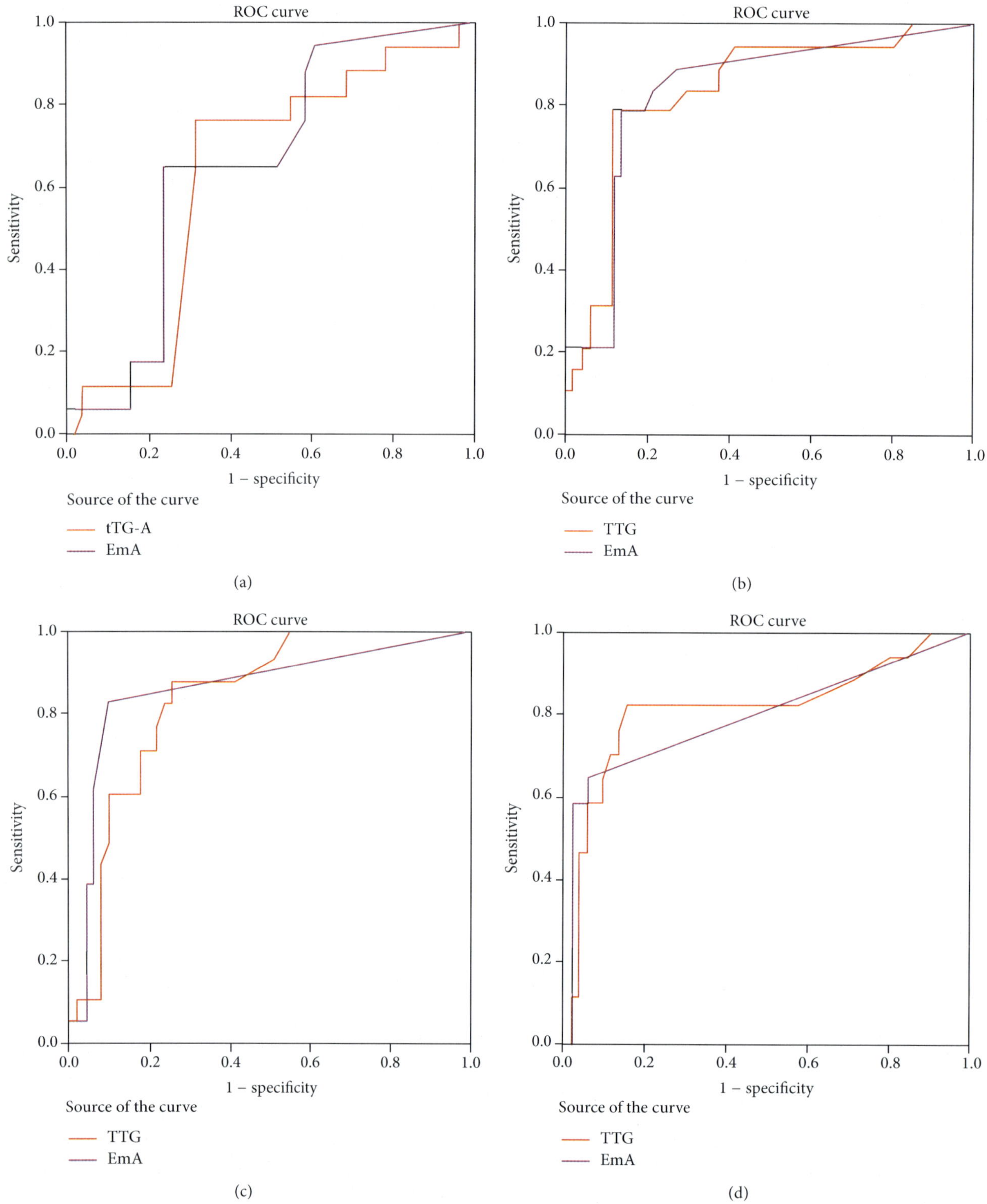

FIGURE 2: EmA and tTG-A ROC analysis (a) at 6 months after the initiation of GFD, (b) at 1 year after the initiation of GFD, (c) at 2 years after the initiation of GFD, and (d) at 3 years after the initiation of GFD.

serological tests for its accurate and early diagnosis [10]. The only effective treatment for CD is a strict gluten free diet for life [19]. Long term compliance with the GFD is essential to prevent the complications of CD and improve the quality of life [20]. Thus, reliable but also easy applicable markers are needed to monitor patient compliance with these dietary restrictions.

In the present study, which is the first study for celiac disease in Greek adults, the aim was to detect and investigate the specific autoantibodies in the diagnosis, monitoring, and the prognosis of celiac disease.

This study confirms the excellent specificity and sensitivity of EmA (100% and 95.7%, resp.) in CD diagnosis, which is also reported by previous studies [9, 21–27]. We could also recapitulate the high specificity (95.7%) and sensitivity (94.3%) of tTG-A [22, 28–31]. In addition, it was found that EmA predictive value for CD diagnosis was statistically significantly higher compared to tTG-A ($P = 0.043$).

All the three EmA negative patients were relatives of celiac disease patients. At the time of diagnosis two of them had no other clinical symptoms or signs of celiac disease except for mild anaemia which was due to iron deficiency. The third one, however, underwent a thorough endoscopy in order to investigate the cause because of an upper digestive tract bleeding.

Despite the indisputable role of EmA and tTG-A in the diagnosis of CD, the available literature is controversial on their value for assessing compliance with the diet. While some studies have not found the rate of fall of antibody concentration to be a reliable marker of strict adherence to the GFD [32–35], others have found that normalized markers can be useful to confirm GFD, but without concluding which one is the most appropriate [36–40]. In our study fifty-one of the seventeen patients (72.9%) followed a strict GFD while the remaining nineteen (27.1%) had a partial compliance. The serum concentrations of antibodies decreased over time which was inversely correlated with patients' degree of compliance with the diet. Among partially compliant patients, although antibody concentrations also declined, the trends were significantly less pronounced compared with strictly compliant cases.

It was also noticed that, during the first year of a strict compliance with GFD, EmA titres fell more rapidly than tTG-A, whereas in the third year more patients remained having tTG-A positive than EmA despite the fact that they are on a strict GFD. On the other hand, the 19 patients with a partial compliance with GFD presented with a persistence of abnormally elevated antibody concentration that could help in identifying patients with dietary lapses. We propose that EmA can assess the degree of compliance with GFD in the first semester from the beginning of the diet, while both EmA and tTG-A have an equal ability to discriminate between strictly and partially compliant patients in the long term monitoring.

In this study three individuals from the control group as well as three asymptomatic first degree relatives had increased values of tTG-A without having CD. Low levels of tTG-A have been described in a number of conditions unrelated to CD, such as other autoimmune diseases, IBD, infections, tumors, myocardial damage, and liver disorders. These antibodies are not associated with EmA reaction, which explains why EmA has higher reliability for the diagnosis of CD [41–43].

It is well known that CD presents more often among the first degree relatives. In detail, the prevalence of CD among the first degree relatives varies from 2.8% to 8.2% [44–48]. The differences could be partially explained by study methodological differences and the variability of the genetic background of the studied population. In the present study the prevalence of CD among the first degree relatives was 4.2% which is in agreement with the available literature. It is worthwhile mentioning that this prevalence dramatically increases when considering families with two or more cases of CD [49–51].

6. Conclusions

The use of serologic markers in celiac is a noninvasive, easily applicable, direct, and reliable practise than can be used for the diagnosis and monitoring of the disease. More specifically, both EmA and the tTG-A are suitable markers in the diagnostic approach of CD. Regarding the ability to discriminate between strictly and partially compliant patients, EmA can assess the degree of compliance with GFD earlier, while both EmA and tTG-A have equal performance in the long term monitoring. We finally recommend the screening for EmA and tTG-A among the first degree relatives.

Conflict of Interests

Dr. Gerassimos Mantzaris has received advisory board fees from Centocor, MSD, AbbVie, and Danon; lecture fees from Ferring International, MSD, AbbVie, FALK Pharma, and Angelini; Research support from AstraZeneca, AbbVie, MSD, Menarini, and Genesis. The rest of the authors declare no conflict of interests regarding the publication of this paper.

References

[1] W. F. Paveley, "From aretaeus to crosby: a history of coeliac disease," *British Medical Journal*, vol. 297, no. 6664, pp. 1646–1649, 1988.

[2] S. Husby, S. Koletzko, and I. R. Korponay-Szabó, "European society for pediatric gastroenterology, hepatology, and nutrition guidelines for the diagnosis of coeliac disease," *Journal of Pediatric Gastroenterology and Nutrition*, vol. 54, no. 1, pp. 136–160, 2012.

[3] W. Dieterich, T. Ehnis, M. Bauer et al., "Identification of tissue transglutaminase as the autoantigen of celiac disease," *Nature Medicine*, vol. 3, no. 7, pp. 797–801, 1997.

[4] D. Schuppan, W. Dieterich, T. Ehnis et al., "Identification of the autoantigen of celiac disease," *Annals of the New York Academy of Sciences*, vol. 859, pp. 121–126, 1998.

[5] J. M. Tjon, J. Van Bergen, and F. Koning, "Celiac disease: how complicated can it get?" *Immunogenetics*, vol. 62, no. 10, pp. 641–651, 2010.

[6] P. Rallabhandi, "Gluten and celiac disease—an immunological perspective," *Journal of AOAC International*, vol. 95, no. 2, pp. 349–355, 2012.

[7] T. P. Chorzelski, J. Sulej, and H. Tchorzewska, "IgA class endomysium antibodies in dermatitis herpetiformis and coeliac disease," *Annals of the New York Academy of Sciences*, vol. 420, pp. 325–334, 1983.

[8] P. Collin, K. Kaukinen, H. Vogelsang et al., "Antiendomysial and anti-human recombinant tissue transglutaminase antibodies in the diagnosis of coeliac disease: a biopsy-proven European multicentre study," *European Journal of Gastroenterology & Hepatology*, vol. 17, no. 1, pp. 85–91, 2005.

[9] A. Rostom, C. Dubé, A. Cranney et al., "The diagnostic accuracy of serologic tests for celiac disease: a systematic review," *Gastroenterology*, vol. 128, no. 4, supplement 1, pp. S38–S46, 2005.

[10] A. D. Hopper, M. Hadjivassiliou, S. Butt, and D. S. Sanders, "Adult coeliac disease," *British Medical Journal*, vol. 335, no. 7619, pp. 558–562, 2007.

[11] E. Lionetti and C. Catassi, "New clues in celiac disease epidemiology, pathogenesis, clinical manifestations, and treatment," *International Reviews of Immunology*, vol. 30, no. 4, pp. 219–231, 2011.

[12] K. Mustalahti, C. Catassi, A. Reunanen et al., "The prevalence of celiac disease in Europe: results of a centralized, international mass screening project," *Annals of Medicine*, vol. 42, no. 8, pp. 587–595, 2010.

[13] A. Fasano, I. Berti, T. Gerarduzzi et al., "Prevalence of Celiac disease in at-risk and not-at-risk groups in the United States: a large multicenter study," *Archives of Internal Medicine*, vol. 163, no. 3, pp. 286–292, 2003.

[14] H. B. Cook, M. J. Burt, J. A. Collett, M. R. Whitehead, C. M. Frampton, and B. A. Chapman, "Adult coeliac disease: prevalence and clinical significance," *Journal of Gastroenterology and Hepatology*, vol. 15, no. 9, pp. 1032–1036, 2000.

[15] S. Lohi, K. Mustalahti, K. Kaukinen et al., "Increasing prevalence of coeliac disease over time," *Alimentary Pharmacology and Therapeutics*, vol. 26, no. 9, pp. 1217–1225, 2007.

[16] A. Rubio-Tapia, R. A. Kyle, E. L. Kaplan et al., "Increased prevalence and mortality in undiagnosed celiac disease," *Gastroenterology*, vol. 137, no. 1, pp. 88–93, 2009.

[17] "Inflammatory bowel disease: a global perspective," World Gastroenterology Organization. Global Guidelines, 2009.

[18] "Celiac disease World Gastroenterology Organisation Practice Guidelines," 2007.

[19] S. Rshtak and J. A. Murray, "Review article: celiac disease, new approaches to therapy," *Alimentary Pharmacology & Therapeutics*, vol. 35, no. 7, pp. 768–781, 2012.

[20] M. L. Haines, R. P. Anderson, and P. R. Gibson, "Systematic review: the evidence base for long-term management of coeliac disease," *Alimentary Pharmacology and Therapeutics*, vol. 28, no. 9, pp. 1042–1066, 2008.

[21] R. J. Lock, M. C. L. Pitcher, and D. J. Unsworth, "IgA anti-tissue transglutaminase as a diagnostic marker of gluten sensitive enteropathy," *Journal of Clinical Pathology*, vol. 52, no. 4, pp. 274–277, 1999.

[22] A. Carroccio, G. Vitale, L. Di Prima et al., "Comparison of anti-transglutaminase ELISAs and an anti-endomysial antibody assay in the diagnosis of celiac disease: a prospective study," *Clinical Chemistry*, vol. 48, no. 9, pp. 1546–1550, 2002.

[23] A. Picarelli, M. Di Tola, L. Sabbatella et al., "Identification of a new coeliac disease subgroup: antiendomysial and anti-transglutaminase antibodies of IgG class in the absence of selective IgA deficiency," *Journal of Internal Medicine*, vol. 249, no. 2, pp. 181–188, 2001.

[24] F. Biagi, D. Pezzimenti, J. Campanella, G. B. Vadacca, and G. R. Corazza, "Endomysial and tissue transglutaminase antibodies in coeliac sera: a comparison not influenced by previous serological testing," *Scandinavian Journal of Gastroenterology*, vol. 36, no. 9, pp. 955–958, 2001.

[25] A. V. M. Dahele, M. C. Aldhous, K. Humphreys, and S. Ghosh, "Serum IgA tissue transglutaminase antibodies in coeliac disease and other gastrointestinal diseases," *The Quarterly Journal of Medicine Association of Physicians of Great Britain and Ireland*, vol. 94, no. 4, pp. 195–205, 2001.

[26] A. Tsirogianni, E. Trigoni, I. Kakkas et al., "Specificity, sencitivity and predictive value of specific autoantibodies in coeliac disease," in *Proceedings of the 14th European Immunology Meeting (EFIS '00)*, pp. 127–132, Monduzzi Editore, 2001.

[27] G. Mantzaris, A. Tsirogianni, E. Perivolioti et al., "Sensitivity and specificity of serum IgA class endomysial antibody in the diagnosis of coeliac disease," *Hellenic Journal of Gastroenterology*, vol. 8, no. 4, pp. 308–311, 1996.

[28] M. Sardy, U. Odenthal, S. Karpati, M. Paulsson, and N. Smyth, "Recombinant human tissue transglutaminase ELISA for the diagnosis of gluten-sensitiv enteropathy," *Clinical Chemistry*, vol. 45, no. 12, pp. 2142–2149, 1999.

[29] D. Sblattero, I. Berti, C. Trevisiol et al., "Human recombinant tissue transglutaminase ELISA: an innovative diagnostic assay for celiac disease," *American Journal of Gastroenterology*, vol. 95, no. 5, pp. 1253–1257, 2000.

[30] F. Leon, C. Camarero, R. R. Pena et al., "Anti-transglutaminase IgA ELISA: clinical potential and drawbacks in celiac disease diagnosis," *Scandinavian Journal of Gastroenterology*, vol. 36, no. 8, pp. 849–853, 2001.

[31] N. R. Lewis and B. B. Scott, "Systematic review: the use of serology to exclude or diagnose coeliac disease (a comparison of the endomysial and tissue transglutaminase antibody tests)," *Alimentary Pharmacology and Therapeutics*, vol. 24, no. 1, pp. 47–54, 2006.

[32] K. Kaukinen, S. Sulkanen, M. Mäki, and P. Collin, "IgA-class transglutaminase antibodies in evaluating the efficacy of gluten-free diet in coeliac disease," *European Journal of Gastroenterology and Hepatology*, vol. 14, no. 3, pp. 311–315, 2002.

[33] K. Vahedi, F. Mascart, J. Mary et al., "Reliability of antitransglutaminase antibodies as predictors of gluten-free diet compliance in adult celiac disease," *American Journal of Gastroenterology*, vol. 98, no. 5, pp. 1079–1087, 2003.

[34] D. A. Leffler, J. B. Edwards George, M. Dennis, E. F. Cook, D. Schuppan, and C. P. Kelly, "A prospective comparative study of five measures of gluten-free diet adherence in adults with coeliac disease," *Alimentary Pharmacology and Therapeutics*, vol. 26, no. 9, pp. 1227–1235, 2007.

[35] S. Martini, G. Mengozzi, G. Aimo, L. Giorda, R. Pagni, and C. S. Guidetti, "Comparative evaluation of serologic tests for celiac disease diagnosis and follow-up," *Clinical Chemistry*, vol. 48, no. 6, part 1, pp. 960–963, 2002.

[36] A. Bürgin-Wolff, I. Dahlbom, F. Hadziselimovic, and C. J. Petersson, "Antibodies against human tissue transglutaminase and endomysium in diagnosing and monitoring coeliac disease," *Scandinavian Journal of Gastroenterology*, vol. 37, no. 6, pp. 685–691, 2002.

[37] E. Fabiani and C. Catassi, "The serum IgA class anti-tissue transglutaminase antibodies in the diagnosis and follow up of coeliac disease. Results of an international multi-centre study. International Working Group on Eu-tTG," *European Journal of Gastroenterology & Hepatology*, vol. 13, no. 6, pp. 659–665, 2001.

[38] E. Sugai, F. Nachman, H. Váquez et al., "Dynamics of celiac disease-specific serology after initiation of a gluten-free diet and use in the assessment of compliance with treatment," *Digestive and Liver Disease*, vol. 42, no. 5, pp. 352–358, 2010.

[39] C. R. Dipper, S. Maitra, R. Thomas et al., "Anti-tissue transglutaminase antibodies in the follow-up of adult coeliac disease," *Alimentary Pharmacology and Therapeutics*, vol. 30, no. 3, pp. 236–244, 2009.

[40] F. Nachman, E. Sugai, H. Vázquez et al., "Serological tests for celiac disease as indicators of long-term compliance with the gluten-free diet," *European Journal of Gastroenterology and Hepatology*, vol. 23, no. 6, pp. 473–480, 2011.

[41] M. Di Tola, L. Sabbatella, M. C. Anania et al., "Anti-tissue transglutaminase antibodies in inflammatory bowel disease: new evidence," *Clinical Chemistry and Laboratory Medicine*, vol. 42, no. 10, pp. 1092–1097, 2004.

[42] F. Ferrara, S. Quaglia, I. Caputo et al., "Anti-transglutaminase antibodies in non-coeliac children suffering from infectious diseases," *Clinical and Experimental Immunology*, vol. 159, no. 2, pp. 217–223, 2010.

[43] N. Bizzaro, M. Tampoia, D. Villalta et al., "Low specificity of anti-tissue transglutaminase antibodies in patients with primary biliary cirrhosis," *Journal of Clinical Laboratory Analysis*, vol. 20, no. 5, pp. 184–189, 2006.

[44] J. C. Vitoria, A. Arrieta, I. Astigarraga, D. Garcia-Masdevall, and J. Rodriguez- Soriano, "Use of serological markers as a screening test in family members of patients with celiac disease," *Journal of Pediatric Gastroenterology and Nutrition*, vol. 19, no. 3, pp. 304–309, 1994.

[45] P. L. de Almeida, L. Gandolfi, I. C. Modelli, R. D. C. Martins, R. C. De Almeida, and R. Pratesi, "Prevalence of celiac disease among first degree relatives of Brazilian celiac patients," *Arquivos de Gastroenterologia*, vol. 45, no. 1, pp. 69–72, 2008.

[46] R. Grover, A. S. Puri, N. Aggarwal, and P. Sakhuja, "Familial prevalence among first-degree relatives of celiac disease in North India," *Digestive and Liver Disease*, vol. 39, no. 10, pp. 903–907, 2007.

[47] Y. Doğan, S. Yildirmaz, and I. H. Ozercan, "Prevalence of celiac disease among first degree relatives of patients with celiac disease," *Journal of Pediatric Gastroenterology and Nutrition*, vol. 55, no. 2, pp. 205–208, 2012.

[48] F. Biagi, J. Campanella, P. I. Bianchi et al., "The incidence of coeliac disease in adult first degree relatives," *Digestive and Liver Disease*, vol. 40, no. 2, pp. 97–100, 2008.

[49] K. Mustalahti, S. Sulkanen, P. Holopainen et al., "Coeliac disease among healthy members of multiple case coeliac disease families," *Scandinavian Journal of Gastroenterology*, vol. 37, no. 2, pp. 161–165, 2002.

[50] A. H. Gudjónsdóttir, S. Nilsson, J. Ek, B. Kristiansson, and H. Ascher, "The risk of celiac disease in 107 families with at least two affected siblings," *Journal of Pediatric Gastroenterology and Nutrition*, vol. 38, no. 3, pp. 338–342, 2004.

[51] L. Book, J. J. Zone, and S. L. Neuhausen, "Prevalence of celiac disease among relatives of sib pairs with celiac disease in U.S. Families," *American Journal of Gastroenterology*, vol. 98, no. 2, pp. 377–381, 2003.

Risk Factors and Adverse Events Poorly Predict Infections and Hypogammaglobulinemia in Granulomatosis with Polyangiitis Patients Receiving Rituximab

Emilio Besada

Bone and Joint Research Group, Institute of Clinical Medicine, UiT The Arctic University of Norway, 9037 Tromsø, Norway

Correspondence should be addressed to Emilio Besada; emilio.besada@uit.no

Academic Editor: Corrado Betterle

Background. 29 GPA patients from the Northern Norway vasculitis disease registry received rituximab (RTX) induction and maintenance. 24% and 31% had, respectively, severe and chronic infections while 45% had hypogammaglobulinemia and 28% discontinued RTX due to hypogammaglobulinemia. The aim of the study was to examine how known predictors and adverse events interacted with adverse events using structural statistical methods. *Methods.* Five predictors (age, cyclophosphamide, total Ig and CD4/CD8 ratio prior RTX, and type of RTX maintenance regimen) and 4 adverse events (severe and chronic infections, hypogammaglobulinemia, and RTX discontinuation) were modeled in principal component and redundancy analyses. *Results.* The 5 predictors explained 51% of the variance of the GPA cohort. Models including cyclophosphamide exposure and total Ig level predicted best adverse events. However total Ig level has low R squared. The 2 best combinations of adverse events explained 13% of the variance of the predictors and adverse events. Only chronic infections were associated with combination of all adverse events ($P = 0.014$). Hypogammaglobulinemia did not seem associated with the other adverse events. *Conclusions.* Traditional risk factors for infections and hypogammaglobulinemia seemed to poorly predict adverse events in our GPA cohort.

1. Introduction

Granulomatosis with polyangiitis (GPA) is an ANCA-associated vasculitis (AAV) that affects small- and medium-sized vessels. It frequently involves the upper and lower respiratory tracts and the kidneys. GPA was a uniformly fatal disease prior to the use of cyclophosphamide [1]. The current standard of care of AAV that includes remission induction with high dose of glucocorticoids and cyclophosphamide [2], followed by lower dose of glucocorticoids with either azathioprine or methotrexate for remission maintenance [3, 4], is challenged by rituximab (RTX).

Rituximab is a chimeric monoclonal antibody against CD20 that depletes B-cells. The mechanisms of B-cells depletion include antibody-dependent, cell-mediated, and complement-mediated cytotoxicity with subsequent apoptosis [5]. RTX was effective in randomized controlled trials (RCT) both in induction [6, 7] and in maintenance of remission [8] in AAV and GPA. RTX did not increase the risk of adverse events [6–8] and did not seem to decrease the risk of severe infection during induction compared with CYC [9] in RCT. In 2 retrospective studies, 24% and 41% of GPA patients had severe infections while receiving RTX maintenance [10, 11]. Older age, the cumulative dose of CYC, kidney involvement, low CD4 cell count, and decrease of total Ig after the first 2 g of RTX seemed to increase the risk of severe infection [10]. The risk of hypogammaglobulinemia seemed to be associated with CYC use [12–14] and with the type of RTX maintenance regimen [14] independently of the RTX cumulative dose [13, 14]. However the impact of hypogammaglobulinemia on GPA patients seems to differ in terms of infections and RTX discontinuation between study cohorts [11–14].

In order to predict the risk of adverse events such as infections and hypogammaglobulinemia, we analyzed how patients' characteristics, known predictors, and adverse events interacted with adverse events using structural statistical methods.

2. Subjects and Methods

2.1. Patients' Characteristics of the Tromsø Cohort at RTX Initiation. 29 GPA patients from the Northern Norway vasculitis disease registry received RTX induction and maintenance between April 2004 and 30 September 2011. All patients gave informed written consent at inclusion in accordance with the Declaration of Helsinki. Patients' characteristics are previously published [14]. To summarize, the patients (48% women) with a median age of 50 years at baseline had renal (59%), pulmonary (66%), and orbital-subglottic (62%) involvements. They were 90% ANCA positive (86% PR3-ANCA) at diagnosis. At RTX initiation, patients had median disease duration of 57 months and had received a median total CYC cumulative dose of 17 g (range 0–250).

2.2. Treatment Regimen. RTX treatment was initiated as two 1 g infusions 2 weeks apart with coadministration of methylprednisolone 125 mg, paracetamol 1000 mg, and either cetirizine 10 mg or Polaramine 4 mg (rheumatoid arthritis protocol). Due to the observed RTX efficacy and the relapsing nature of GPA, RTX was then readministered preemptively either as a 2 g infusion (1 g twice during a fortnight) annually or as a 1 g infusion biannually (1 g every 6 months).

Patients received a median cumulative RTX dose of 9 g (range 5–13) during a median of 49 months (range 19–88) after RTX initiation. During maintenance, 41% received the regimen of 1 g biannually, 21% received the regimen of 2 g annually, and 38% alternated between regimens.

RTX was added to other immunosuppressive drugs (IDs) (other than prednisolone) in 93% of the patients during a median duration of 24 months (range 1–54). The timing and pace of ID discontinuation were at the discretion of the treating physician, whereas the daily prednisolone dose was tapered from a median of 22.5 mg at baseline and discontinued in a controlled manner. At the last visit, 59% were still treated with long-term preemptive RTX and 90% had discontinued other IDs.

2.3. Predictors and Adverse Events Definitions. The 5 chosen predictors of adverse events were age, CYC cumulative dose, total Ig and CD4/CD8 ratio prior RTX, and type of RTX maintenance regimen defined as gram per RTX round (Gpr). These predictors were previously associated with infections and hypogammaglobulinemia [10, 14]. Gpr was calculated as Gpr = (total cumulative RTX dose − 2)/(number of rounds − 1). Patients with Gpr = 1 received the regimen of 1 g biannually, patients with Gpr = 2 received the regimen of 2 g annually, and patients with $1 < \text{Gpr} < 2$ alternated between the two regimens.

Infections were defined either as severe or as chronic. Severe infections included all infections that required either intravenous antibiotics or hospitalization. Chronic infections are symptomatic localized infections lasting over 3 months or more that required multiple antibiotic courses. They are also referred to in the literature as recurrent infections secondary to hypogammaglobulinemia [11].

Hypogammaglobulinemia and hypogammaglobulinemia leading to RTX discontinuation [14] were defined as total Ig level less than 6 g/L during RTX maintenance. The 2 definitions of hypogammaglobulinemia were necessary to include not only patients with severe hypogammaglobulinemia who discontinued RTX maintenance, but also patients with total Ig level under 6 g/L who had either a transitory decrease of Ig or a more benign course [11].

2.4. Statistical Analysis. All statistical analysis was done with R (R Project for Statistical Computing, https://www.r-project.org/) with focus on structural methods.

Correspondence analysis (CA) of adverse events during RTX maintenance included all categorical variables: gender, organ involvement, use of concomitant immunosuppressive drugs, type of RTX regimen, age defined in 3 categories (under 40, between 40 and 55, and over 55 years), low and high levels of each immunoglobulin type prior RTX (cut-offs were determined with generalized additive modeling [see Supplementary file and Figure S1 in Supplementary Material available online at http://dx.doi.org/10.1155/2016/8095695]), inverted and normal ratio CD4/CD8 (using cut-off of 1), and low and high cumulative dose of CYC (using median as cut-off).

Principal component analysis (PCA) of the 5 predictors from standardized data determined the variance and significance of each predictor in the Tromsø study cohort. Multivariable analysis with logistic regression using the five predictors individually and in pairs as well as the 2 best PCA dimensions determined the best model explaining the different adverse events. Vectors analysis with biplot after range standardization identified how predictors and adverse outcomes interacted together.

Finally, we determined how the best 2 linear combinations of adverse events explained both predictors and adverse events individually with redundancy analysis (RDA).

3. Results

3.1. Correspondence Analysis of Adverse Events during RTX Maintenance. Seven patients (24%) had severe infections and 9 (31%) had chronic infections in the Tromsø cohort study, while 8 patients (28%) discontinued RTX due to hypogammaglobulinemia and 13 (45%) had total Ig under 6 g/L during RTX maintenance.

In the CA, the presence and absence of adverse events were grouped in the opposite ends of the map, except for chronic infections that remained close to the centroid (Figure 1). The 2 types of hypogammaglobulinemia and severe infection were utterly separated. Being a woman, being younger than 55 years, being without kidney and lung involvement, being with orbital-subglottic involvement, being previously treated with lower CYC cumulative dose, and receiving the RTX regimen of 2 g annually were factors protective against adverse events (Figure 1). On the other hand, being a man, being older than 55 years, being with kidney and without orbital-subglottic involvements, being with ratio CD4/CD8 < 1, being previously treated with higher CYC cumulative dose, and receiving RTX maintenance regimen other than 2 g annually increased the risk of adverse events (Figure 1). Being a man and having lower levels of IgG and IgA prior RTX (resp., lower than

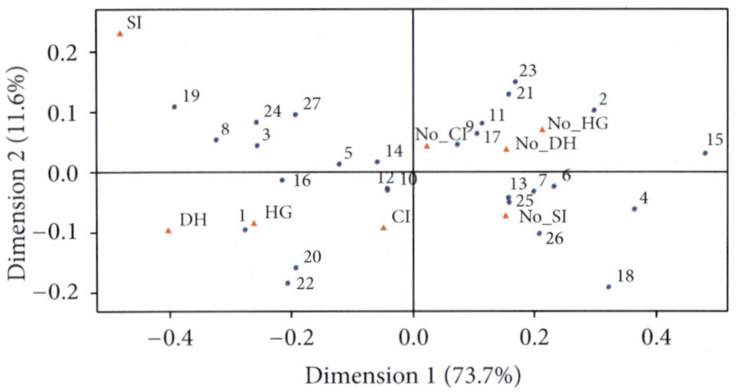

Figure 1: Correspondence analysis of adverse events during RTX maintenance. CI: chronic infection; DH: hypogammaglobulinemia leading to RTX discontinuation; HG: hypogammaglobulinemia with total Ig < 6 g/L; SI: severe infection. No_CI: absence of chronic infection; No_DH: absence of hypogammaglobulinemia leading to RTX discontinuation; No_HG: absence of hypogammaglobulinemia with total Ig < 6 g/L; No_SI: absence of severe infection. 1: men; 2: women; 3: kidney involvement; 4: no kidney involvement; 5: lung involvement; 6: no lung involvement; 7: orbital and subglottic involvement; 8: no orbital and subglottic involvement; 9: use of MTX during RTX; 10: no MTX use; 11: use of AZA during RTX; 12: no use of AZA; 13: use of MMF during RTX; 14: no use of MMF; 15: RTX maintenance with the 2 g annually regimen; 16: other maintenance regimes; 17: age under 40 y at baseline; 18: age between 40 and 55; 19: age over 55 years; 20: low IgG level prior RTX; 21: high IgG prior RTX; 22: low IgA level prior RTX; 23: high IgA prior RTX; 24: inverted CD4/CD8 ratio prior RTX; 25: normal ratio prior RTX; 26: low CYC cumulative dose; 27: high CYC cumulative dose.

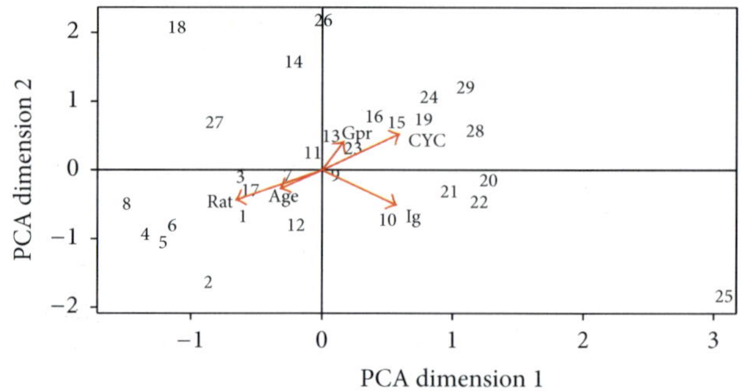

Predictors	Dimension 1	Dimension 2	R squared
Age	**<0.001**	**<0.001**	0.647
CYC	**<0.001**	**<0.001**	0.593
Gpr	**<0.001**	**0.001**	0.632
Ig	0.166	0.538	0.085
Ratio	**<0.001**	**<0.001**	0.575

Figure 2: Principal component analysis of the five predictors during RTX maintenance. Data is standardized. P values and R squared of each predictor are presented in the included table. 1–29: patients' study number; age; CYC: cyclophosphamide cumulative dose; Gpr: gram of RTX per round; Ig: total level of immunoglobulin prior rituximab; Rat: ratio CD4/CD8 prior rituximab.

7.5 and 1.6 g/L) seemed to be more closely associated with hypogammaglobulinemia than severe infections (Figure 1).

3.2. Principal Component Analysis of the 5 Predictors. PCA identified one outlier in the study cohort (Figure 2). The outlier represented an older patient who had received 250 g of CYC prior RTX. The best linear combination of the five predictors explained 51% of the variance of the study cohort. All predictors, except for total Ig levels prior RTX, were significant in the PCA (Figure 2).

3.3. Multivariable Analysis of Adverse Events

3.3.1. Severe Infection. The pair of CYC cumulative dose and age was the strongest predictor of severe infection in the study cohort. Being 10 years older or receiving 10 more grams of CYC more than doubled the risk of severe infection although it was only significant for the CYC cumulative dose (P = 0.011) (Figure S2 and Table S1).

3.3.2. Chronic Infection. The strongest predictor of chronic infection was the ratio CD4/CD8 prior RTX. Every increase of 0.2 in ratio prior to RTX increased the risk of chronic infection by 14% although this was not found significant (P = 0.210) (Table S2).

3.3.3. Hypogammaglobulinemia Defined as Total Ig < 6 g/L. The pair of CYC cumulative dose and total Ig level prior RTX was the strongest predictor of hypogammaglobulinemia in the study cohort. Receiving 10 more grams of CYC and decrease of 1 g/L of total Ig level increased the risk of hypogammaglobulinemia, respectively, by 51% and 67%, although this was only found significant for total Ig level prior RTX (P = 0.044) (Figure S3 and Table S3).

3.3.4. Hypogammaglobulinemia Leading to Discontinuation. The strongest predictor in the univariable analysis was the cumulative dose of CYC although it was not significant (P = 0.137) (Table S4). The best model predicting discontinuation due to hypogammaglobulinemia included the cumulative dose of CYC and the level of total Ig prior RTX (Figure S4). The risk of discontinuation due to hypogammaglobulinemia increased by 54% for each decrease of 1 g/L of total Ig and by 30% for every 10 g increase of CYC cumulative dose, although none were significant (Table S4).

3.4. Analysis of Outcomes Using PCA of the 5 Predictors Using Range Standardization. The vectors of severe infection, hypogammaglobulinemia, and RTX discontinuation due to hypogammaglobulinemia had the same direction in the PCA (Figure 3). The 2 first vectors were almost superposed while the vector of RTX discontinuation due to hypogammaglobulinemia was lying towards the chronic infection vector (Figure 3). Being older, receiving a higher dose of CYC, lower ratio and total Ig level prior RTX, and the regimen of 1 g biannually seemed to increase the risk of severe infection and of hypogammaglobulinemia (Figure 3).

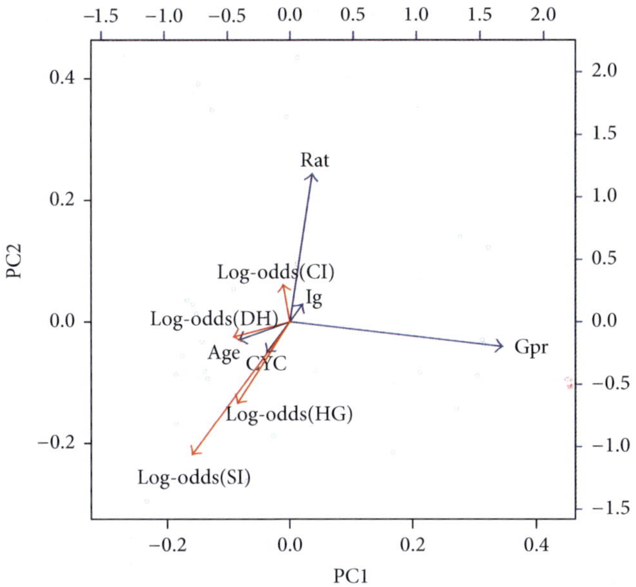

FIGURE 3: Two-dimensional biplot of adverse events using the principal component analysis of the five predictors. CI: chronic infection; CYC: cyclophosphamide cumulative dose; DH: discontinuation due to hypogammaglobulinemia; Gpr: gram of RTX per round; HG: hypogammaglobulinemia defined as total Ig < 6 g/L; Ig: total level of immunoglobulin prior rituximab; Rat: ratio CD4/CD8 prior rituximab; SI: severe infection.

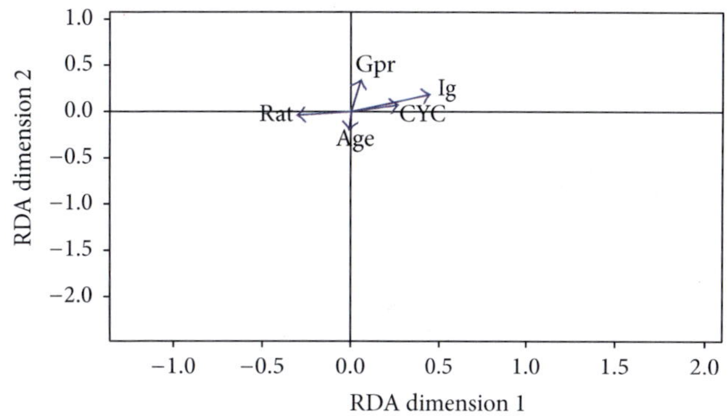

Predictors	Dimension 1	Dimension 2	R squared
Age	0.951	0.271	0.045
CYC	0.165	0.691	0.078
Gpr	0.759	0.059	0.156
Ig	**0.014**	0.268	0.248
Ratio	0.094	0.835	0.105

FIGURE 4: Redundancy analysis of the five predictors using the two best combinations of outcomes. P values and R squared of each predictor are presented in the included table. Age: age in years at rituximab initiation; CYC: cyclophosphamide cumulative dose; Gpr: gram of RTX per round; Ig: total level of immunoglobulin prior rituximab; Rat: ratio CD4/CD8 prior rituximab; severe I: severe infection.

3.5. Redundancy Analysis of Predictors and Adverse Events Using the Best Linear Combination of Adverse Events. Severe and chronic infections, hypogammaglobulinemia, and discontinuation due to hypogammaglobulinemia explained together an average of 12.6% of the variance of the 5 predictors (Figure 4). The adverse events only explained significantly the variance of the total Ig prior to RTX (Figure 4). Of interest, the vectors of total CYC cumulative dose and of total Ig level prior RTX had the same direction in the RDA.

The 2 best combinations of adverse events explained an average of 12.5% of the variance of the 4 adverse events (Figure 5). Only the risk of chronic infection was found significant in the RDA. Vector of hypogammaglobulinemia defined as total Ig < 6 g/L had a different direction compared with the other outcomes (Figure 5).

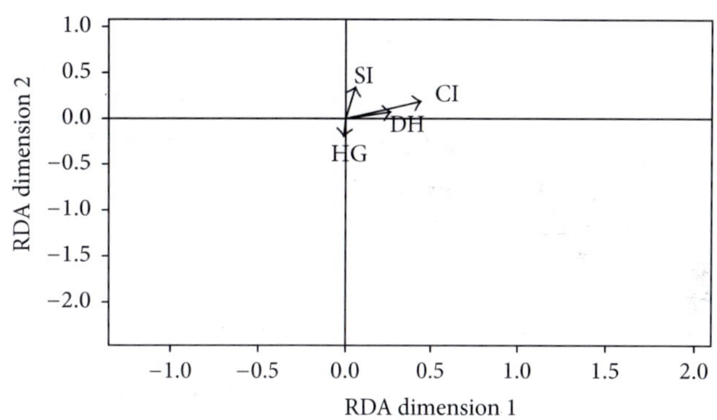

Outcomes	Dimension 1	Dimension 2	R squared
Hypo < 6 g/L	0.951	0.271	0.045
Hypo-D	0.165	0.691	0.078
Severe I	0.759	0.059	0.133
Chronic I	**0.014**	0.268	0.242

FIGURE 5: Redundancy analysis of the outcomes using the two best combinations of outcomes. P values and R squared of each outcome are presented in the included table. CI: chronic infection; DH: discontinuation due to hypogammaglobulinemia; HG: hypogammaglobulinemia defined as total Ig < 6 g/L; SI: severe infection.

4. Discussion

The 5-predictor model explained 51% of the variance of the cohort although this was not significant for total Ig levels prior RTX. CYC and total Ig level prior RTX were important predictors of the different adverse events, apart from chronic infection. However the 2 best combinations of adverse events explained 13% of the variance of both the predictors and the adverse events, only being significant for total Ig level prior RTX and chronic infection, respectively.

Total Ig level prior RTX seemed to be the most important predictor of adverse events during RTX maintenance. However predicting adverse events using total Ig level could be problematic due to the inherent large prediction interval associated with low R squared, as observed in our cohort. Total CYC cumulative dose was a significant predictor of severe infections and possibly of hypogammaglobulinemia. It seemed more reliable in detecting patients at risk of adverse events since it had a smaller prediction interval. Nevertheless the total cumulative dose of CYC and the total Ig level prior RTX were closely related in terms of combination of adverse events.

The type of RTX maintenance regimen was not a strong predictor of adverse events; however it is a modifiable factor, like the total cumulative dose of CYC. Categorical variables such as gender and organ involvement were not used in modeling the outcomes and could still be of importance when predicting adverse events during RTX maintenance.

Chronic infections seemed to be more associated with severe infection and discontinuation due to hypogammaglobulinemia than with predictors. The 5 predictors did not manage to model the risk of chronic infection, while chronic infection was significantly associated with adverse events in the outcome analysis.

Hypogammaglobulinemia, discontinuation due to hypogammaglobulinemia, and severe infections seemed closely related in the study cohort whereas hypogammaglobulinemia was not associated with discontinuation of RTX and severe infection in the outcome analysis. Hypogammaglobulinemia defined as low levels of either IgG or total Ig levels could lack specificity when compared with severe infections and discontinuation due to hypogammaglobulinemia, since half of the patients receiving RTX had erratic IgG concentration-time profile in one study [15]. Another possible explanation is the timing of the different adverse events since transitory hypogammaglobulinemia could occur early during RTX treatment [15], while hypogammaglobulinemia leading to RTX discontinuation usually occurred later [14].

In our cohort of GPA patients, outcome was poorly associated with predictors and with individual adverse events making it difficult for physicians to stratify patients' risk individually. To make risk stratification more complicated, some adverse events either lacked specificity or were unrelated to predictors. When physicians are not able to predict adverse events, modifiable factors such as limiting the cumulative dose of CYC and limiting the number of times B-cells are depleted are of importance when treating GPA patients. More studies are clearly needed to clarify not only the timing, but also the dosage of RTX therapy, since lower RTX doses at induction [16, 17] and during maintenance [8] are also effective in AAV/GPA.

5. Principal Findings from the Structural Statistical Analysis

The 5 predictors explained 51% of the variance of the GPA cohort from Tromsø.

Total Ig was a strong predictor of adverse events, but it was not reliable due to a large prediction interval.

The best 2 combinations of outcomes explained only 13% of the variance of all 5 predictors and of all 4 adverse events.

Vectors of total cumulative dose of CYC and of total Ig level prior RTX had the same direction in the outcome analysis indicating that the 2 predictors were closely related.

Vectors of discontinuation of RTX due to hypogammaglobulinemia and of severe infection have the same direction in the outcome analysis. These 2 adverse events were closely related, contrary to hypogammaglobulinemia defined as total Ig < 6 g/L.

There were no predictors for chronic infection. Chronic infection is only significantly associated with adverse events.

Conflict of Interests

The author declares no conflict of interests.

References

[1] C. Mukhtyar, L. Guillevin, M. C. Cid et al., "EULAR recommendations for the management of primary small and medium vessel vasculitis," *Annals of the Rheumatic Diseases*, vol. 68, no. 3, pp. 310–317, 2009.

[2] A. S. Fauci and S. M. Wolff, "Wegener's granulomatosis: studies in eighteen patients and a review of the literature," *Medicine*, vol. 52, no. 6, pp. 535–561, 1973.

[3] D. Jayne, N. Rasmussen, K. Andrassy et al., "A randomized trial of maintenance therapy for vasculitis associated with antineutrophil cytoplasmic autoantibodies," *The New England Journal of Medicine*, vol. 349, no. 1, pp. 36–44, 2003.

[4] C. Pagnoux, A. Mahr, M. A. Hamidou et al., "Azathioprine or methotrexate maintenance for ANCA-associated vasculitis," *The New England Journal of Medicine*, vol. 359, no. 26, pp. 2790–2803, 2008.

[5] M. J. Leandro and I. de la Torre, "Translational mini-review series on B cell directed therapies: the pathogenic role of B cells in autoantibody-associated autoimmune diseases—lessons from B cell-depletion therapy," *Clinical and Experimental Immunology*, vol. 157, no. 2, pp. 191–197, 2009.

[6] R. B. Jones, J. W. Cohen Tervaert, T. Hauser et al., "Rituximab versus cyclophosphamide in ANCA-associated renal vasculitis," *The New England Journal of Medicine*, vol. 363, no. 3, pp. 211–220, 2010.

[7] J. H. Stone, P. A. Merkel, R. Spiera et al., "Rituximab versus cyclophosphamide for ANCA-associated vasculitis," *The New England Journal of Medicine*, vol. 363, no. 3, pp. 221–232, 2010.

[8] L. Guillevin, C. Pagnoux, A. Karras et al., "Rituximab versus azathioprine for maintenance in ANCA-associated vasculitis," *The New England Journal of Medicine*, vol. 371, no. 19, pp. 1771–1780, 2014.

[9] J. C. Nossent, "Rituximab or cyclophosphamide in ANCA-associated renal vasculitis," *The New England Journal of Medicine*, vol. 363, no. 21, pp. 2072–2074, 2010.

[10] E. Besada, W. Koldingsnes, and J. C. Nossent, "Long-term efficacy and safety of pre-emptive maintenance therapy with rituximab in granulomatosis with polyangiitis: results from a single centre," *Rheumatology*, vol. 52, no. 11, Article ID ket257, pp. 2041–2047, 2013.

[11] F. Alberici, R. M. Smith, R. B. Jones et al., "Long-term follow-up of patients who received repeat-dose rituximab as maintenance therapy for ANCA-associated vasculitis," *Rheumatology*, vol. 54, no. 7, pp. 1153–1160, 2015.

[12] H. Marco, R. M. Smith, R. B. Jones et al., "The effect of rituximab therapy on immunoglobulin levels in patients with multisystem autoimmune disease," *BMC Musculoskeletal Disorders*, vol. 15, article 178, 2014.

[13] N. Venhoff, N. M. Effelsberg, U. Salzer et al., "Impact of rituximab on immunoglobulin concentrations and B cell numbers

after cyclophosphamide treatment in patients with ANCA-associated vasculitides," *PLoS ONE*, vol. 7, no. 5, Article ID e37626, 2012.

[14] E. Besada, W. Koldingsnes, and J. C. Nossent, "Serum immunoglobulin levels and risk factors for hypogammaglobulinemia during long-term maintenance therapy with rituximab in patients with granulomatosis with polyangiitis," *Rheumatology*, vol. 53, pp. 1818–1824, 2014.

[15] D. M. Roberts, R. B. Jones, R. M. Smith et al., "Rituximab-associated hypogammaglobulinemia: incidence, predictors and outcomes in patients with multi-system autoimmune disease," *Journal of Autoimmunity*, vol. 57, pp. 60–65, 2015.

[16] T. Turner-Stokes, E. Sandhu, R. J. Pepper et al., "Induction treatment of ANCA-associated vasculitis with a single dose of rituximab," *Rheumatology*, vol. 53, no. 8, pp. 1395–1403, 2014.

[17] P. Moog, M. Probst, C. Kuechle, C. Hauser, U. Heemann, and K. Thuermel, "Single-dose rituximab for remission induction and maintenance therapy in ANCA-associated vasculitis: a retrospective analysis of 17 patients," *Scandinavian Journal of Rheumatology*, vol. 43, no. 6, pp. 519–523, 2014.

24

Intravenous Immunoglobulin Treatment in Chronic Neurological Diseases: Do We Have Maintenance Dose Right?

Ondrej Dolezal

NHS Scotland, Dumfries and Galloway Royal Infirmary, Bankend Road, Dumfries DG14AP, UK

Correspondence should be addressed to Ondrej Dolezal; odol.cuni.cz@gmail.com

Academic Editor: Ricard Cervera

Objectives. We tried to define, on individual basis, minimal effective maintenance dose of intravenous immunoglobulins (IVIG) in 26 patients with chronic neurological conditions requiring long-term IVIG treatment. *Methods.* Clinical criteria were reviewed in individual cases (Phase 1) followed by titration phase (Phase 2, 12 months) and posttitration/follow-up phase (Phase 3, 3 months). Objective neurological examination and patient self-reports were used for clinical follow-up. *Results.* 69.2% of patients reported condition as stable, 26.9% as better, and 3.9% as mildly worse. Original mean monthly dose was 1 g/kg; over the period of 12 months we reduced dose of IVIG to mean dose 0.67 g/kg (range 0.3–2.5 g/kg, $P < 0.0001$) which meant reduction by 36.4%. We identified 4 nonresponders and diagnosis in one case was reclassified to degenerative disease. In follow-up phase we reduced dose further to 0.60 g/kg. Cumulative monthly dose dropped from 2040 g to 1298 g and to 991 g, respectively. Financial expenses were reduced significantly (by −36.4% during titration phase and by −51.4% during follow-up phase) (comparing with baseline) ($P < 0.0001$). *Conclusion.* Individual dose titration leads to significant maintenance IVIG dose reduction with preserved clinical efficacy. Maintenance dose below 1 g/kg (in our study around 0.7 g/kg) has acceptable risk/benefit ratio.

1. Introduction

Human intravenous immunoglobulins (IVIG) are used in various neurological diseases, especially myasthenia gravis (MG), chronic inflammatory demyelinating polyneuropathy (CIDP), and multifocal motor neuropathy (MMN), and less commonly in paraneoplastic polyneuropathy (PNP), polyneuropathy associated with paraproteinaemia (PAP), and stiff-man syndrome (SMS).

Clinical effects and mechanism of IVIG action remain unclear. In diseases mediated primarily by antibodies, effect of IVIG is based on their neutralising features (forming immunocomplexes, facilitating phagocytosis, etc.). Other effects such as stabilising "information network" within immune system by providing physiological immunoglobulin spectrum, downregulation of endogenous immunoglobulin production, neutralising autoantibodies, opsonization, facilitation of endogenous immunoglobulin catabolism, complement interactions, and T and B cell suppression were mentioned [1–7]. Mechanisms influencing oligodendroglia and remyelination seem to be even more complicated [8–10]; however, these concepts are mostly theoretical and experimental ("in vitro") with lack of reliable biomarker available for clinical practice. There is currently range of recommendations available about dosing regimens and frequency of maintenance treatment administration (between 0.6 and 2 gm/kg in regular intervals (3–8 weeks, over one or two days)) [11–16]. Most commonly used maintenance dose is 1 g/kg every 3–6 weeks [17, 18]. Some authors were mentioning since 1990s the need of better definition of effective dose based on frequent follow-up and individualised approach [19–21]. There seems to be simple way of how to achieve this: (1) following strict diagnostic criteria (reducing probability of misdiagnosis), (2) regular and frequent clinical follow-up, and (3) readjusting of dose according to clinical progression/development. This approach can lead to lower frequency of side effect, better tolerability/efficacy, and significant financial savings.

2. Methods

In our study we observed group of patients ($N = 26$) with various neurological conditions (see Table 1) for 15 months.

Table 1: Demographics and diagnoses ($N = 26$).

	Number of pts.
CIDP	13
Multifocal motor neuropathy	4
Myasthenia gravis	3
Stiff-man syndrome	1
Paraprotein assoc. neuropathy	1
Paraneoplastic neuropathy	4
Gender (M/F)	11/15
Mean age (yrs)	62.3
Mean weight (kg)	78.5

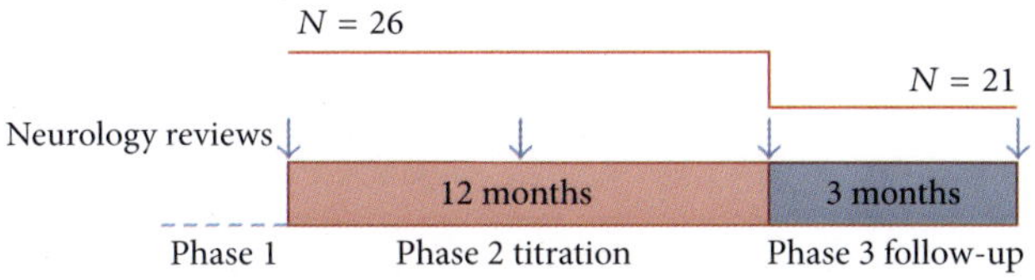

Figure 1: Study design (number of patients, phases).

They were treated by IVIG for more than 3 months at the beginning of observation (range 3–58 months). They all provided oral agreement with IVIG treatment. Patients were on no concomitant immunosuppressive treatment. Aim of our study was to establish minimal effective dose and lowest tolerable infusion frequency without compromising clinical efficacy. At the beginning of our study maintenance dose used in patients was 1 g/kg administered every 4 weeks (as per guidelines of joint task force of the European Federation of Neurological Societies (EFNS) and Peripheral Nerve Society (PNS)) [22–24], and infusion was administered over two consecutive days. That required member of junior medical staff (clerking connected with admission) and there were additional expenses connected with admission. Our study was divided into three separate phases (see Figure 1). In the first phase (Phase 1) general review of currently treated patients was performed; diagnosis and diagnostic criteria (including available test results, lumbar puncture, nerve conduction studies (NCS), etc.) were reviewed as well. All patients were offered to switch to "one-day" infusion (preventing hospital admission). At that point monthly dose never dropped under minimal recommended dose of 0.6 g/kg. This dose allowed us to prevent two-day administration and avoid admission (maximal daily dose administered in one day was 50 g). Intervals were set to 2–6 weeks (on the basis of individual patient experience). Second phase lasted for 12 months and during that period dose and intervals between infusions were changed according to clinical need (titration period). Patients were instructed to report any changes in clinical condition to trained staff and dose was readjusted when needed (month-to-month basis). Infusion room staff (two staff nurses) regularly took part in specialised clinic alongside neurology consultant to provide them with appropriate clinical training. Third phase (lasted 3 months) included another detailed clinical review and further dose adjustments; if clinical condition deteriorated introducing of steroid treatment was considered. Nonresponders were identified. For clinical evaluation subjective information from patients (quality of life, severity of sensory and motor symptoms, etc.) and detailed neurological examination (muscle strength, reflexes, etc.) were used. No serum biomarkers were monitored. Electrophysiology and other diagnostic tests were repeated only if diagnostic doubts were present. For statistical analysis we used Statistica software (StatSoft Inc.) to obtain descriptive statistics and to establish level of significance; t-test was used.

3. Results

All 26 patients agreed on new administration protocol; one patient after two infusions expressed wish to continue with two-day administration (admission). Admission was therefore not needed in 96.1% of patients. If we would use recommended maintenance dose of IVIG (1 g/kg), monthly dose would be 2040 g. Intervals range between infusions was between 2 and 6 weeks and all doses were recalculated to monthly format. Thanks to frequent clinical reviews and appropriate staff training we were able to reduce amount of IVIG to mean dose 0.67 g/kg/month (range 0.3–2.5 g/kg, $P < 0.0001$). So at the end of the second phase (approximately after 12 months) cumulative monthly dose was reduced to 1298 g per month (−36.4% reduction, $P < 0.000005$). Majority of patients were not reporting any significant clinical progression during second phase (69.2% reported their condition as stable, 26.9% as better, and 3.9% as mildly worse) and this agreed with objective examination. 5 patients discontinued treatment at the end of titration period (second phase). Two patients with paraneoplastic polyneuropathy (anti-Hu positive) and one patient with paraprotein mediated polyneuropathy and one with myasthenia gravis discontinued treatment for infectivity (clinical progression or lack of improvement (nonresponders) despite escalation of treatment to maximal dose). One patient was reclassified from multifocal motor neuropathy to degenerative anterior horn cell degeneration/motor neuron disease on the basis of clinical picture and follow-up neurophysiology. Deescalation protocol clearly failed in one patient (CIDP patient) who remained on 2.5 g/kg every month (administered over two days) despite steroids added to treatment regimen. 21 patients entered final observational period and at the end of observation (after further 3 months) mean monthly dose was reduced further to 0.60 g/kg and cumulative monthly dose dropped to 991 gm/month (Figure 2).

Pharmacoeconomic results were surprisingly encouraging as financial expenses were significantly reduced (savings regarding hospital admission are not included in calculation) by 36.4% ($P < 0.0001$) at the end of titration phase. Further decrease to by −51.4% from baseline ($P < 0.0001$) was found at the end of the observation.

From general point of view treatment was well tolerated; during five IVIG administrations some side effects were observed (temporary abdominal discomfort and headaches) (once during the study); in one patient treatment led to

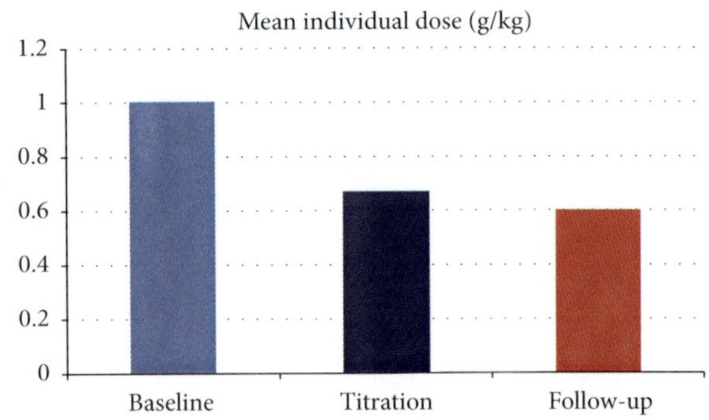

Figure 2: Individual mean dose reduction (g/kg).

chronic eczema reactivation but settled on different IVIG preparation.

3.1. CIDP Subgroup. Majority of our patients suffered from CIDP (13 subjects). Their results were copying overall results when mean monthly dose was reduced from 1 g/kg to 0.70 g/kg ($P = \text{NS}$) at the end of titration phase and to 0.55 g/kg ($P < 0.0001$) at the end of observation. Clinically patients remained stable or improved (nine and three, resp.) and only one patient deteriorated (deescalation failed; see above).

4. Discussion

IVIG are the oldest and most commonly used biological treatment. Currently health services worldwide are under pressure regarding maintaining quality of care and quality of patients' life and simultaneously controlling care costs and expenses. Dosage of IVIG is based on clinical studies mostly from 1990s and EFNS guidelines mentioned possibility of dose reduction (maintenance dose defined between 0.6 and 1 gm/kg per 3–8 weeks and 0.4 and 1.2 g/kg per 2–6 weeks) [17, 25]. Our results proved that investing time and resources to frequent follow-up in patient with chronic autoimmune conditions and adjusting doses (or timely discontinuation in nonresponders) according to clinical outcome are not only leading to significant cost/benefit ratio improvement but also leading to better tolerability of treatment. At least some of the serious side effects (procoagulation and high viscosity state connected with higher risk of cardiovascular, renal events, anaemia, etc.) seem to be dose dependent [26–29]. In our observation we were reducing dose significantly initially however still within recommended guidelines. We duly titrated dose up if needed (range of dose at the end of titrating Phase 2 was 0.3–2.5 g/kg/month). Critics can argue that reduction of IVIG dose was reached by discontinuation of treatment in resistant cases; however all 26 patients were involved in calculation of average dose at the end of titration phase (Phase 2) when mean dose was already reduced to 0.67 g/kg/month. Another criticism could be heterogeneity of the sample. When we analysed subgroup of CIDP patients we found similar findings to other conditions, not statistically different to other diagnoses.

Discontinuation of treatment took place in 5 patients and their condition remained stable in the following three months during Phase 3. Remarkably, but not surprisingly, nonresponders were recruited from the group of paraprotein mediated and paraneoplastic polyneuropathy [30]. Next step could be considering home IVIG treatment as already piloted in some places [31], which would seem to be appropriate for rural and isolated areas. Subcutaneous administration looks as feasible option as well especially in CIDP patients [32, 33].

5. Conclusion

We succeeded in reducing IVIG dose and avoiding hospital admissions in vast majority of our patients. We believe that maintenance dose significantly lower than of 1 gm/kg, administered every 4–6 weeks, could be sufficient when titration process is conducted carefully. Lower dose of IVIG is providing healthy balance between tolerability, admission need, and financial cost.

Abbreviations

IVIG: Intravenous immunoglobulins
MG: Myasthenia
CIDP: Chronic inflammatory demyelinating polyneuropathy
MMN: Multifocal motor neuropathy
PNP: Paraneoplastic polyneuropathy
PAP: Polyneuropathy associated with paraproteinaemia
SMS: Stiff-man syndrome
NCS: Nerve conduction studies
EFNS: European Federation of Neurological Societies
PNS: Peripheral Nerve Society.

Conflict of Interests

The author declares that there is no conflict of interests regarding the publication of this paper.

Acknowledgments

The author would like to thank the pharmacists, especially Lynn Kean and Mandy MacIntosh, for helping with data collection. Thanks are due to Rhona and Joanna, the nurses, for providing essential link between patients and Neurology Department and naturally to the patients. Special thanks are due to Elissa Bastow and Liz Clark for support and to managers of Dumfries and Galloway Royal Infirmary who provided resources for frequent patients' reviews.

References

[1] N. Kondo, K. Kasahara, T. Kameyama et al., "Intravenous immunoglobulins suppress immunoglobulin productions by suppressing Ca^{2+}-dependent signal transduction through FCγ receptors in B lymphocytes," *Scandinavian Journal of Immunology*, vol. 40, no. 1, pp. 37–42, 1994.

[2] M. D. Kazatchkine, G. Dietrich, V. Hurez et al., "V region-mediated selection of autoreactive repertoires by intravenous immunoglobulin (i.v.Ig)," *Immunological Reviews*, vol. 139, pp. 79–107, 1994.

[3] M. D. Kazatchkine and S. V. Kaveri, "Immunomodulation of autoimmune and inflammatory diseases with intravenous immune globulin," *The New England Journal of Medicine*, vol. 345, no. 10, pp. 747–755, 2001.

[4] S. Lacroix-Desmazes, S. V. Kaveri, L. Mouthon et al., "Self-reactive antibodies (natural autoantibodies) in healthy individuals," *Journal of Immunological Methods*, vol. 216, no. 1-2, pp. 117–137, 1998.

[5] O. Aktas, S. Waiczies, U. Grieger, U. Wendling, R. Zschenderlein, and F. Zipp, "Polyspecific immunoglobulins (IVIg) suppress proliferation of human (auto)antigen-specific T cells without inducing apoptosis," *Journal of Neuroimmunology*, vol. 114, no. 1-2, pp. 160–167, 2001.

[6] P. L. Masson, "Elimination of infectious antigens and increase of IgG catabolism as possible modes of action of IVIg," *Journal of Autoimmunity*, vol. 6, no. 6, pp. 683–689, 1993.

[7] C. Ritter, D. Forster, P. Albrecht, H. P. Hartung, B. C. Kieseier, and H. C. Lehmann, "IVIG regulates BAFF expression in patients with chronic inflammatory demyelinating polyneuropathy (CIDP)," *Journal of Neuroimmunology*, vol. 274, no. (1-2), pp. 225–229, 2014.

[8] K. Asakura, D. J. Miller, K. Murray, R. Bansal, S. E. Pfeiffer, and M. Rodriguez, "Monoclonal autoantibody SCH94.03, which promotes central nervous system remyelination, recognizes an antigen on the surface of oligodendrocytes," *Journal of Neuroscience Research*, vol. 43, no. 3, pp. 273–281, 1996.

[9] K. Asakura, R. J. Pogulis, L. R. Pease, and M. Rodriguez, "A monoclonal autoantibody which promotes central nervous system remyelination is highly polyreactive to multiple known and novel antigens," *Journal of Neuroimmunology*, vol. 65, no. 1, pp. 11–19, 1996.

[10] M. Stangel, A. Compston, and N. J. Scolding, "Oligodendroglia are protected from antibody-mediated complement injury by normal immunoglobulins ("IVIg")," *Journal of Neuroimmunology*, vol. 103, no. 2, pp. 195–201, 2000.

[11] P. J. Dyck, W. J. Litchy, K. M. Kratz et al., "A plasma exchange versus immune globulin infusion trial in chronic inflammatory demyelinating polyradiculoneuropathy," *Annals of Neurology*, vol. 36, no. 6, pp. 838–845, 1994.

[12] F. Eftimov, J. B. Winer, M. Vermeulen, R. de Haan, and I. N. van Schaik, "Intravenous immunoglobulin for chronic inflammatory demyelinating polyradiculoneuropathy," *The Cochrane Database of Systematic Reviews*, no. 1, Article ID CD001797, 2009.

[13] A. F. Hahn, C. F. Bolton, D. Zochodne, and T. E. Feasby, "Intravenous immunoglobulin treatment in chronic inflammatory demyelinating polyneuropathy. A double-blind, placebo-controlled, cross-over study," *Brain*, vol. 119, no. 4, pp. 1067–1077, 1996.

[14] J. R. Mendell, R. J. Barohn, M. L. Freimer, and tal, "Randomized controlled trial of IVIg in untreated chronic inflammatory demyelinating polyradiculoneuropathy," *Neurology*, vol. 56, no. 4, pp. 445–449, 2001.

[15] M. Jinka and V. Chaudhry, "Treatment of multifocal motor neuropathy," *Current Treatment Options in Neurology*, vol. 16, no. 2, article 269, 2014.

[16] M. Vermeulen, "Is intravenous administration of immunoglobulins a first-choice method in autoimmune diseases?" *Nederlands Tijdschrift voor Geneeskunde*, vol. 137, no. 39, pp. 1955–1958, 1993.

[17] R. A. C. Hughes, P. Donofrio, V. Bril et al., "Intravenous immune globulin (10% caprylate-chromatography purified) for the treatment of chronic inflammatory demyelinating polyradiculoneuropathy (ICE study): a randomised placebo-controlled trial," *The Lancet Neurology*, vol. 7, no. 2, pp. 136–144, 2008.

[18] J.-M. Léger, J. L. De Bleecker, C. Sommer et al., "Efficacy and safety of Privigen in patients with chronic inflammatory demyelinating polyneuropathy: results of a prospective, single-arm, open-label Phase III study (the PRIMA study)," *Journal of the Peripheral Nervous System*, vol. 18, no. 2, pp. 130–140, 2013.

[19] A. Baumann, C. W. Hess, and M. Sturzenegger, "IVIg dose increase in multifocal motor neuropathy," *Journal of Neurology*, vol. 256, no. 4, pp. 608–614, 2009.

[20] R. Broyles, L. Rodden, P. Riley, and M. Berger, "Variability in intravenous immunoglobulin G regimens for autoimmune neuromuscular disorders," *Postgraduate Medicine*, vol. 125, no. 2, pp. 65–72, 2013.

[21] P. Gajdos, "Intravenous immune globulin in myasthenia gravis," *Clinical and Experimental Immunology, Supplement*, vol. 97, supplement 1, pp. 49–51, 1994.

[22] Joint Task Force of the EFNS and the PNS, "European Federation of Neurological Societies/Peripheral Nerve Society guideline on management of multifocal motor neuropathy. Report of a joint task force of the European Federation of Neurological Societies and the Peripheral Nerve Society—first revision," *Journal of the Peripheral Nervous System*, vol. 15, no. 4, pp. 295–301, 2010.

[23] R. Hadden, "European federation of neurological societies/peripheral nerve society guideline on management of paraproteinemic demyelinating neuropathies. Report of a joint task force of the European federation of neurological societies and the peripheral nerve society-First revision," *Journal of the Peripheral Nervous System*, vol. 15, no. 3, pp. 185–195, 2010.

[24] "European Federation of Neurological Societies/Peripheral Nerve Society Guideline on management of chronic inflammatory demyelinating polyradiculoneuropathy: report of a joint task force of the European Federation of Neurological Societies and the Peripheral Nerve Society—First Revision," *Journal of the Peripheral Nervous System*, vol. 15, no. 1, pp. 1–9, 2010.

[25] K. Kuitwaard and P. A. van Doorn, "Newer therapeutic options for chronic inflammatory demyelinating polyradiculoneuropathy," *Drugs*, vol. 69, no. 8, pp. 987–1001, 2009.

[26] P. D. Donofrio, V. Bril, M. C. Dalakas et al., "Safety and tolerability of immune globulin intravenous in chronic inflammatory demyelinating polyradiculoneuropathy," *Archives of Neurology*, vol. 67, no. 9, pp. 1082–1088, 2010.

[27] L. H. Markvardsen, I. Christiansen, T. Harbo, and J. Jakobsen, "Hemolytic anemia following high dose intravenous immunoglobulin in patients with chronic neurological disorders," *European Journal of Neurology*, vol. 21, no. 1, pp. 147–152, 2014.

[28] D. Paran, Y. Herishanu, O. Elkayam, L. Shopin, and R. Ben-Ami, "Venous and arterial thrombosis following administration of intravenous immunoglobulins," *Blood Coagulation & Fibrinolysis*, vol. 16, no. 5, pp. 313–318, 2005.

[29] A. S. Wolberg, R. H. Kon, D. M. Monroe, and M. Hoffman, "Coagulation factor XI is a contaminant in intravenous

immunoglobulin preparations," *The American Journal of Hematology*, vol. 65, no. 1, pp. 30–34, 2000.

[30] M. Uchuya, F. Graus, F. Vega, R. René, and J.-Y. Delattre, "Intravenous immunoglobulin treatment in paraneoplastic neurological syndromes with antineuronal autoantibodies," *Journal of Neurology Neurosurgery & Psychiatry*, vol. 60, no. 4, pp. 388–392, 1996.

[31] H. D. Katzberg, V. Rasutis, and V. Bril, "Home IVIG for CIDP: a focus on patient centred care," *The Canadian Journal of Neurological Sciences*, vol. 40, no. 3, pp. 384–388, 2013.

[32] F. Eftimov, M. Vermeulen, R. J. de Haan, L. H. van den Berg, and I. N. van Schaik, "Subcutaneous immunoglobulin therapy for multifocal motor neuropathy," *Journal of the Peripheral Nervous System*, vol. 14, no. 2, pp. 93–100, 2009.

[33] L. H. Markvardsen, J.-C. Debost, T. Harbo et al., "Subcutaneous immunoglobulin in responders to intravenous therapy with chronic inflammatory demyelinating polyradiculoneuropathy," *European Journal of Neurology*, vol. 20, no. 5, pp. 836–842, 2013.

Frequency and Type of Hepatic and Gastrointestinal Involvement in Juvenile Systemic Lupus Erythematosus

Leila Tahernia,[1,2] Hosein Alimadadi,[3,4] Fatemeh Tahghighi,[2,3] Zahra Amini,[2] and Vahid Ziaee[2,3,5]

[1]*Growth and Development Research Center, Tehran University of Medical Sciences, Tehran, Iran*
[2]*Children's Medical Center, Pediatrics Center of Excellence, Tehran, Iran*
[3]*Department of Pediatrics, Tehran University of Medical Sciences, Tehran, Iran*
[4]*Pediatric Gastroenterology and Hepatology Research Center, Tehran University of Medical Sciences, Tehran, Iran*
[5]*Pediatric Rheumatology Research Group, Rheumatology Research Center, Tehran University of Medical Sciences, Tehran, Iran*

Correspondence should be addressed to Vahid Ziaee; ziaee@tums.ac.ir

Academic Editor: Ricard Cervera

Background. Systemic lupus erythematosus (SLE) is a frequent rheumatology disorder among children. Since hepatic involvement is a common systemic manifestation in lupus, the frequency and type of hepatic involvement were determined in pediatric cases of SLE admitted to Children's Medical Hospital from 2005 to 2014. *Methods and Patients.* In this observational case-series study, 138 pediatric cases of SLE were admitted in Children's Medical Center (a pediatric rheumatology referral center in Tehran, Iran) enrolled from 2005 to 2014 and the outcomes, frequency, and type of hepatic involvement were assessed among them. *Results.* Hepatic involvement was reported in 48.55% of total SLE patients. Aspartate aminotransferase (AST), alanine aminotransferase (ALT), and both enzymes higher than normal upper limits were detected in 8.7%, 5%, and 34.7% of lupus patients, respectively. Increased level of liver enzymes was categorized as less than 100, between 100 and 1000, and more than 1000 levels in 23.1%, 23.1%, and 2.1% of cases. The only gastrointestinal involvement in lupus patients contributing to hepatic involvement was gastrointestinal bleeding. Rising in liver enzymes was detected mostly in lupus patients without gastrointestinal bleeding (52.2% without versus 25.8% with gastrointestinal bleeding, $P = 0.007$). *Conclusion.* Approximately half of the pediatric patients suffering from SLE have hepatic involvement. No significant correlation was observed between various organs involvement and abnormal level of liver enzymes.

1. Introduction

Since systemic lupus erythematous (SLE) is an autoimmune multisystem disease, early diagnosis before the involvement of major organs is crucial. Involvement of kidney, central nervous system, and liver would result in numerous problems such as dialysis and cirrhosis [1, 2]. The liver involvement may be life-threatening [3]. Hepatic involvement in lupus could be the result of various factors including lupus hepatitis, medications during management of SLE (NSAIDs, Aspirin, immune-suppressors, hydroxyzine, hydroxychloroquine), fatty liver (due to corticosteroids), associated autoimmune hepatitis, primary biliary cirrhosis, cholangitis, and viral hepatitis [4].

In previous studies, the hepatic involvement and increase in liver enzymes in lupus patients had been reported mainly due to medications in the management of patients [5]. Since hepatic involvement could be primary or secondary in SLE, lupus hepatitis could be considered only after ruling out secondary causes and other etiological factors [6–9]. However, the majority of studies had assessed secondary causes of hepatic involvement in SLE [6, 9]. Primary hepatic involvement had rarely been studied in lupus [7, 8]. Moreover, most studies had been conducted mainly in the adult population [6, 7, 9]. Hepatic involvement in lupus is a challenging issue in rheumatology specially difference between lupoid (or autoimmune) hepatitis and overlap SLE with autoimmune liver diseases [10, 11].

Hepatic involvement in lupus is associated with higher mortality rate in children [12]. SLE disease is multisystem and rapidly progressive in childhood cases; so, a study on hepatic and gastrointestinal involvement in pediatric cases may be helpful in reduction of lupus burden especially with the absence of this involvements in diagnostic criteria. Accordingly, in this study frequency and type of hepatic involvement were evaluated among childhood-onset SLE admitted in a pediatric rheumatology referral center in Iran since 2005 to 2014.

2. Methods and Materials

In this observational study which was performed as a case-series, 138 consecutive pediatric cases of SLE admitted in Children's Medical Center, Pediatric Center of Excellence, Tehran, Iran, were enrolled by a census manner from 2005 to 2014. The outcomes, frequency, and type of hepatic involvement were assessed as the main purpose of this study, but other gastrointestinal (abdominal pain, gastrointestinal bleeding, pancreatitis, gastritis, esophagitis, cholestasis, etc.) and major organ involvements (cardiac, cerebral, renal, etc.) were evaluated as minor objectives. Lupus cases were diagnosed based on the presence of 4 of 11 American College of Rheumatology (ACR) criteria. ACR SLE classification criteria were revised and validated by Systemic Lupus International Collaborating Clinics (SLICC) group in 2012. According to SLICC, a person is classified as having SLE in presence of biopsy-proven lupus nephritis with ANA or anti-ds-DNA antibodies or 4 of diagnostic criteria, including at least one clinical and one immunologic criterion 2 [13].

Hepatic involvement due to underlying lupus disease was considered as lupus hepatopathy after ruling out all other medical problems that could result in the elevated level of aspartate aminotransferase (AST) and alanine aminotransferase (ALT), with normal level of alkaline phosphatase (ALP) and ultrasound assessment. Gastrointestinal endoscopic study was performed in all patients with gastrointestinal bleeding. Cholestasis was detected by the increased level of alkaline phosphatase (ALP) and gamma-glutamyltransferase (GGT). Liver ultrasound study was carried out in all patients in order to rule out local liver problems such as hepatic steatosis, granuloma, and cholestasis. Improvement in liver enzymes by medication withdrawal was considered as drug-induced hepatotoxicity.

All data were extracted from clinical records of lupus patients in hospital archives. Medical information was inserted in related forms.

Data analysis was performed on 138 childhood-onset SLE cases by SPSS (version 13.0). Chi-Square, Fisher, and Independent-Sample T tests were used for analyzing data. They were considered statistically significant at P values less than 0.05.

3. Results

Mean age at diagnosis was 8.45 ± 3.9 years. Patients were prominently female (79%). Jaundice, cholestasis, and hepatomegaly were considered in 3.6%, 0.7%, and 28.2%, respectively. Hepatic involvement was detected in 48.55% including one patient with increased hepatic enzymes induced by medications (prescribed for lupus disease). Splenomegaly was realized in 15.2% of lupus patients. The abnormal level of liver enzymes was observed in total 48.55% including 8.7%, 5%, and 34.7% abnormal AST, ALT, and both, respectively. The increased level of liver enzymes was categorized into three levels, including liver enzymes less than 100 (23.1%), between 100 and 1000 (23.1%), and more than 1000 (2.1%).

No major and minor organ involvement and lupus signs and symptoms were associated positively with SLE hepatic involvement in this study ($P > 0.05$). The only negative relation was realized between gastrointestinal bleeding and increased level of liver enzymes in lupus patients. Abnormal level of liver enzymes was reported 52.2% and 25.8% in those without and with gastrointestinal bleeding ($P = 0.007$).

Comorbidity was observed in 21.7% of lupus patients (Table 1). The abdominal pain was reported in 37%. Location of abdominal pain in lupus patients was detected mainly in epigastric (25%) following right upper quadrant area. The ascites, pleural effusion, anorexia, weight loss, and nausea/vomiting were present in 16.6%, 12.3%, 10.1%, 17.3%, 13.7%, and 11.6%, respectively. Gastroesophageal endoscopic study was performed in 14 lupus patients with gastrointestinal bleeding (10.14%). Abnormal level of liver enzymes was detected in 5 patients with gastrointestinal bleeding (3.6%). Endoscopic results were positive in all five cases including one patient with peptic ulcer, two cases with gastritis, and two esophagitis cases.

One patient with SLE was presented with pancreatitis in the first admission (0.7%) and one of them has macrophage activation syndrome as first presentation of SLE (0.7%). The prothrombin time test (PT) result and partial thromboplastin time (PTT) were abnormal in 14.5% and 2.9%, respectively. Abnormal PT was corrected with vitamin K injection without any signs and symptoms of liver encephalopathy. Hypoalbuminemia and low total protein were realized in 20.3% and 11.6%, respectively.

Prevalence of positive lupus classification criteria has been reported in Table 2. Skin and renal involvement were the most common clinical involvement in our patients. Anti ds-DNA as a specific immunologic criteria was positive in 63% of patients. The complement (C3, C4, and CH50) test was low in 31.1%.

Table 1: Comorbidity in children with systemic lupus erythematosus.

Comorbidity	Frequency
Hypertension	14 (10.1%)
Hypothyroidism	4 (2.9%)
JIA	3 (2.17%)
Diabetes	2 (1.44%)
Myopathy	1 (0.7%)
Sjogren	1 (0.7%)
ITP	1 (0.7%)
Macrophage activation syndrome	1 (0.7%)
Scleroderma	1 (0.7%)

TABLE 2: Frequency of clinical and immunologic criteria in lupus patients.

Clinical criteria	Positive (%)	Immunologic criteria	Positive (%)
Acute cutaneous lupus	57.2%	Positive	93.5%
Chronic cutaneous lupus	5.1%	Positive anti-ds-DNA	63%
Oral or nasal ulcers	23.2%	Positive anti-SM	2.1%
Nonscarring alopecia	2.9%	Positive APL-Ab	8%
Synovitis	39.8%	Low complement	31.2%
Serositis	18.1%	Coombs	14.5%
Renal	51.5%		
Neurologic	33.3%		
Hemolytic anemia	2.9%		
Leukopenia	30.5%		
Thrombocytopenia	21%		

ANA: antinuclear antibody; anti-ds-DNA: double-stranded DNA antibody; anti-SM: anti-Smith antibody; APL-Ab: antiphospholipid antibody.

4. Discussion

Liver enzyme abnormalities have been described in various studies in up to 60% of patients with SLE at some point during the course of their disease [7, 14]. Patients with SLE and elevated liver enzymes can interfere with complicated differential diagnosis. In order to ascribe the elevated level of liver enzymes to SLE disease, different factors and liver involving diseases have to be ruled out such as drug hepatotoxicity, autoimmune hepatitis, viral hepatitis, and fatty liver [7, 10, 11].

Assessment of these factors requires the full evaluation of SLE associated diseases which could result in elevated level of liver enzymes including lupus hepatitis and overlap syndrome [10, 11]. Accurate clinical evaluation, serological tests, and often liver biopsy would be crucial in order to prove the abnormal level of liver enzymes as a component of SLE disease. SLE by itself is not usually associated with a significant liver disease. Liver involvement in lupus is often asymptomatic which is referred to as "lupus hepatitis." It is characterized by a mild increase in serum transaminase levels. In 28–42% of patients, no obvious causes of liver dysfunction were found, and it was thought to be due to lupus itself [10, 11]. Lupus hepatitis usually responds to SLE treatment and has a benign course with no complication and liver enzymes return to normal in lupus-induced hepatitis by steroid therapy [3, 4, 15]. This result was observed in our study as well.

It is still a controversial issue, but a great deal of evidence exists in the literature in favor of this hypothesis that lupus itself is not associated with a severe and progressive liver injury. However, several authors have mentioned SLE as a trigger of subclinical liver involvement [11]. Asymptomatic elevated level of liver enzymes is frequently associated with lupus exacerbation.

Moreover, sometimes there are overlapping profiles with other autoimmune diseases, such as autoimmune hepatitis, acute hemolytic anemia, and primary biliary cirrhosis which could result in higher levels of hepatic enzymes. If there is autoimmune evidence in some organs such as thyroid, hematologic, central nervous system, or joints and raising of liver transaminase, SLE should be considered as the first diagnosis [8, 14]. Isolated autoimmune liver involvement is compatible with autoimmune hepatitis, but these patients should be followed up for complete SLE criteria for several years. These are accompanied by changes in immunological liver markers and autoantibodies that help to establish an accurate diagnosis. Positive anti-smooth-muscle (sm) antibodies and anti-liver-kidney antibody (LKM) are expected in primary autoimmune hepatitis [16]. In a study in pediatrics and adult SLE, the rate of on autoimmune hepatitis was more common in children (9.8% compared with 1.3% in adult patients) [17].

Another cause that must be considered as a contributing factor in lupus hepatitis is drug-induced liver toxicity. It is also common in SLE and may be ascribed to chronic consumption or high doses of medicines used to control autoimmune disorders such as immunosuppressants, anti-inflammatory drugs (steroidal and nonsteroidal), and disease-modifying antirheumatic drugs (DMARDS). Increased rate of drug-induced hepatotoxicity was reported in lupus patients [7, 14]. All medication that was being prescribed in lupus could result in elevated liver enzymes but this complication is uncommon in some drug such as monoclonal antibodies (rituximab, belimumab) and antimalarial antibodies [11]. In a study by Huang et al., 35 cases of drug-induced hepatotoxicity were reported among 1533 SLE patients [18], but in another study, by Takahashi et al., liver involvement by drug-induced injury was reported in 31% of total 123 SLE patients [7]. At the moment, it is impossible to know with certainty whether this high incidence could be the result of chronic lupus drug use, relatively high doses of medicine, and different drugs commonly prescribed to treat this disease, or the presence of any kind of susceptibility that makes these patients prone to drug-induced hepatotoxicity. Drug-induced hepatitis in lupus patients was mainly as lobular, portal, or periportal involvement. In our study, hepatic involvement due to medications was not as high as these studies. It was reported in 2.1% of patients during follow-ups.

SLE patients have elevated levels of systemic oxidative stress that could be obvious in lupus patients with the elevated liver enzyme [19]. The spectrum of liver disease in SLE was assessed in a study by Piga et al. in 2010. Liver enzyme abnormalities were observed in 18.6% of patients. They concluded that liver hepatitis is generally subclinical with a fluctuating course and responds greatly to moderate to high doses of prednisone without progression to end-stage liver disease [20].

In our study, totally 48.55% of childhood lupus cases had hepatic involvement. No significant association was observed between various organs involvement and abnormal level of liver enzymes in children with lupus in our study. But elevated liver enzymes were detected mostly in lupus patients without gastrointestinal bleeding (52.2% without versus 25.8% with gastrointestinal bleeding). In other studies, hepatic dysfunction was reported approximately between 23% and 60% of total SLE patients [3, 4]. According to these studies, hepatomegaly and splenomegaly were reported in one-third and one-tenth of patients, respectively. Jaundice was considered in one-quarter of all cases. Hepatic dysfunction was usually mild and nonspecific similar to results in our study.

Different types of hepatic involvement in various studies included lupus hepatitis, Budd-Chiari syndrome, regenerative nodular hyperplasia, autoimmune hepatitis, drug-induced hepatitis, and primary biliary cirrhosis [8, 11].

Hepatic involvement was mild and asymptomatic in our subjects, except in four lupus cases with overlapping autoimmune hepatitis. They were presenting with increased levels of alkaline phosphatase and gamma-glutamyltranspeptidase as well as specific autoimmune hepatitis antibodies. In these cases, liver enzymes did not reach the normal level after initiation of standard SLE treatment.

In a study in Japan, the hepatic dysfunction was seen at the time of lupus diagnosis in 45% [7]. In this study, neurological involvement was more common among lupus patients with hepatitis rather than those without hepatitis [7]. However, in our study, there was no significant correlation between hepatic and neurological involvement.

The jaundice was not a common finding related to lupus hepatitis and it was considered as an indicator of hemolysis. The rate of jaundice in SLE patients was reported to be 24% in Runyon et al.'s study [14]. In our study, hemolytic anemia (positive coombs test and elevated retic count) was reported in 2.9% of lupus patients, although there is positive coombs test in 14.5% of patients.

Hepatic involvement including hyperbilirubinemia and increased liver transaminases can be the only presentation or one of the main symptoms in neonatal lupus erythematosus (NLE) but the mechanism of NLE is different with SLE [21].

Pancreatitis was observed in one of our SLE patients. Acute pancreatitis is not common in SLE patients especially as a first presentation of SLE but it is associated with sever and fatal coarse of SLE [22, 23]. Prevalence of pancreatitis has been reported 0.9% in juvenile SLE [23]. Another cause of hepatitis in SLE patients is macrophage activation syndrome [24].

Treatment of underlying disease also resulted in subsequent alleviation of abdominal pain and anorexia in all subjects of our study.

Liver biopsy was not performed in all our lupus cases because of later normalization of liver enzymes following initiation of standard treatment of SLE and ethical concern. This was a limitation of this study.

5. Conclusion

Approximately half of pediatric subjects with SLE have hepatic involvement. No significant correlation was observed between various organs involvement and abnormal level of liver enzymes. But, it was reported more frequently in lupus patients without gastrointestinal bleeding (about one-third of patients with gastrointestinal bleeding had abnormal level of liver enzymes). Serum transaminases should be routinely checked out in lupus patients in order to rule out other accompanying liver problems, particularly in patients with higher level of liver enzymes.

Disclosure

This study was a part of a dissertation (of Dr. L. Tahernia) and was approved by vice-chancellor for Research of School of Medicine, Tehran University of Medical Sciences.

Conflicts of Interest

The authors have no financial or other conflicts of interest to disclose.

References

[1] M. Schneider, "Pitfalls in lupus," *Autoimmunity Reviews*, vol. 15, no. 11, pp. 1089–1093, 2016.

[2] A. Kuhn, G. Bonsmann, H-J. Anders, P. Herzer, K. Tenbrock, and M. Schneider, "The diagnosis and treatment of systemic lupus erythematosus," *Deutsches Ärzteblatt International*, vol. 112, no. 25, pp. 423–432, 2015.

[3] M. H. Miller, M. B. Urowitz, D. D. Gladman, and L. M. Blendis, "The liver in systemic lupus erythematous," *The Quarterly Journal of Medicine*, vol. 53, pp. 401–409, 2005.

[4] T. Gibson and AR. Myers, "Subclinical liver disease in systemic lupus erythematous," *The Journal of Rheumatology*, vol. 8, pp. 752–759, 1995.

[5] B. I. Hoffman and W. A. Katz, "The gastrointestinal manifestations of sytemic lupus erythematosus: a review of the literature," *Seminars in Arthritis and Rheumatism*, vol. 9, no. 4, pp. 237–247, 1980.

[6] V. R. Chowdhary, C. S. Crowson, J. J. Poterucha, and K. G. Moder, "Liver involvement in systemic lupus erythematosus: case review of 40 patients," *The Journal of Rheumatology*, vol. 35, no. 11, pp. 2159–2164, 2008.

[7] A. Takahashi, K. Abe, R. Saito et al., "Liver dysfunction in patients with systemic lupus erythematosus," *Internal Medicine*, vol. 52, no. 13, pp. 1461–1465, 2013.

[8] B. Van Hoek, "The spectrum of liver disease in systemic lupus erythematosus," *The Netherlands Journal of Medicine*, vol. 48, no. 6, pp. 244–253, 1996.

[9] T. Matsumoto, T. Yoshimine, K. Shimouchi et al., "The Liver in systemic lupus erythematosus; pathologic analysis of 52 cases and review of Autopsy," *Human Pathology*, vol. 23, no. 10, pp. 1151–1158, 1992.

[10] A. Adiga and K. Nugent, "Lupus Hepatitis and Autoimmune Hepatitis (Lupoid Hepatitis)," *The American Journal of the Medical Sciences*, vol. 353, no. 4, pp. 329–335, 2017.

[11] F. Bessone, N. Poles, and M. G. Roma, "Challenge of liver disease in systemic lupus erythematosus: clues for diagnosis and hints for pathogenesis," *World Journal of Hepatology*, vol. 6, no. 6, pp. 394–409, 2014.

[12] F. Tavangar-Rad, V. Ziaee, M.-H. Moradinejad, and F. Tahghighi, "Morbidity and mortality in Iranian children with juvenile systemic lupus erythematosus," *Iranian Journal of Pediatrics*, vol. 24, no. 4, pp. 365–370, 2014.

[13] M. Petri, A. M. Orbai, and G. S. Alarcón, "Derivation and validation of the systemic lupus international collaborating clinics classification criteria for systemic lupus erythematosus," *Arthritis & Rheumatology*, vol. 64, no. 8, pp. 2677–2686, 2012.

[14] B. A. Runyon, D. R. LaBrecque, and S. Anuras, "The spectrum of liver disease in systemic lupus erythematosus. Report of 33 histologically-proved cases and review of the literature," *American Journal of Medicine*, vol. 69, no. 2, pp. 187–194, 1980.

[15] R. H. Zheng, J. H. Wang, and S. B. Wang, "Clinical and immunopathological features of patients with lupus hepatitis," *Chinese Medical Journal*, vol. 126, pp. 260–266, 2013.

[16] M. E. J. Deen, G. Porta, F. J. Fiorot, L. M. A. Campos, A. M. E. Sallum, and C. A. A. da Silva, "Autoimmune hepatitis and juvenile systemic lupus erythematosus," *Lupus*, vol. 18, no. 8, pp. 747–751, 2009.

[17] K. S. Irving, D. Sen, H. Tahir, C. Pilkington, and D. A. Isenberg, "A comparison of autoimmune liver disease in juvenile and adult populations with systemic lupus erythematosus—A retrospective review of cases," *Rheumatology*, vol. 46, no. 7, pp. 1171–1173, 2007.

[18] D. Huang, E. Aghdassi, J. Su et al., "Prevalence and risk factors for liver biochemical abnormalities in Canadian patients with systemic lupus erythematosus," *The Journal of Rheumatology*, vol. 39, no. 2, pp. 254–261, 2012.

[19] M. A. Lozovoy, A. N. Simão, C. Panis et al., "Oxidative stress is associated with liver damage, inflammatory status, and corticosteroid therapy in patients with systemic lupus erythematosus," *Lupus*, vol. 20, no. 12, pp. 1250–1259, 2011.

[20] M. Piga, A. Vacca, G. Porru, A. Cauli, and A. Mathieu, "Liver involvement in systemic lupus erythematosus: incidence, clinical course and outcome of lupus hepatitis," *Clinical and Experimental Rheumatology*, vol. 28, no. 4, pp. 504–510, 2010.

[21] R. Assari, V. Ziaee, M.-H. Moradinejad, and A. Mirmohammadsadeghi, "Neonatal lupus erythematosus following rheumatoid arthritis: case report and literature review," *Iranian Journal of Pediatrics*, vol. 24, no. 4, pp. 445–448, 2014.

[22] V. Pascul-Ramos, A. Duarte-Rojo, A. R. Villa, and etal., "Systemic lupus erythematosus as a cause and prognostic factor of acute pancreatitis," *The Journal of Rheumatology*, vol. 31, pp. 707–712, 2004.

[23] Q. Wang, M. Shen, X. Leng, X. Zeng, F. Zhang, and J. Qian, "Prevalence, severity, and clinical features of acute and chronic pancreatitis in patients with systemic lupus erythematosus," *Rheumatology International*, vol. 36, no. 10, pp. 1413–1419, 2016.

[24] P. E. Gavand, I. Serio, L. Arnaud et al., "Clinical spectrum and therapeutic management of systemic lupus erythematosus-associated macrophage activation syndrome: a study of 103 episodes in 89 adult patients," *Autoimmunity Reviews*, vol. 16, no. 7, pp. 743–749, 2017.

26

An Update in Guillain-Barré Syndrome

J. B. Winer

Queen Elizabeth Hospital, B15 2TH Birmingham, UK

Correspondence should be addressed to J. B. Winer; j.b.winer@bham.ac.uk

Academic Editor: Cristoforo Comi

Guillain-Barré syndrome (GBS) was first described in 1916 (Guillain G, 1916) and is approaching its 100th anniversary. Our knowledge of the syndrome has hugely expanded since that time. Once originally considered to be only demyelinating in pathology we now recognise both axonal and demyelinating subtypes. Numerous triggering or antecedent events including infections are recognised and GBS is considered an immunological response to these. GBS is now considered to be a clinical syndrome of an acute inflammatory neuropathy encompassing a number of subtypes with evidence of different immunological mechanisms. Some of these are clearly understood while others remain to be fully elucidated. Complement fixing antibodies against peripheral nerve gangliosides alone and in combination are increasingly recognised as an important mechanism of nerve damage. New antibodies against other nerve antigens such as neurofascin have been recently described. Research databases have been set up to look at factors associated with prognosis and the influence of intravenous immunoglobulin (IvIg) pharmacokinetics in therapy. Exciting new studies are in progress to examine a possible role for complement inhibition in the treatment of the syndrome.

1. Introduction

Our understanding of the Guillain-Barré syndrome has improved greatly over the last decade with a much clearer idea of the clinical subtypes of the syndrome and the pathogenesis of some of the rarer variants. 2016 will mark the centenary of the original description by Guillain, Barré and Strohl [1]. They described a rapidly progressive motor disorder associated with absent reflexes and a raised CSF protein in the absence of the expected cerebrospinal fluid (CSF) pleocytosis that characterised poliomyelitis. It became clear, over the ensuing years, that the syndrome varied in severity so that in its severest form it could lead to respiratory paralysis and death [2]. Acute inflammatory demyelinating polyradiculoneuropathy (AIDP) is the most frequent subtype in the Western world with a primarily demyelinating pathology and various degrees of secondary axonal damage. Acute motor axonal neuropathy (AMAN) [3] is the next most frequent and appears to be a primary axonal disorder affecting just motor nerves. Axonal variants involving both sensory and motor nerves are much rarer Acute Motor and Sensory Axonal Neuropathy (AMSAN) [3]. Miller Fisher syndrome is generally considered to be allied to GBS although it has a uniquely tight association with anti-GQ1b antibodies.

2. Clinical Features

GBS has an incidence of about 1/100,000 across several studies [4, 5] in a number of countries. It increases in incidence with age and there is a small predominance of males [5].

Sensory symptoms in the legs usually mark the onset of the disease followed by rapidly progressive distal weakness that soon spreads proximally. Lumbar pain is common and may represent inflammation in the nerve roots and may coincide with the breakdown in the nerve CSF barrier that allows protein to leak into the CSF. The weakness of GBS is typically "pyramidal in distribution" with ankle dorsiflexion and knee and hip flexion often severely affected and likewise the weakness in the arms is usually more severe in shoulder abduction and elbow extension. While sensory symptoms are common sensory signs are usually minor and may be limited to loss of vibration and proprioception. The significance of reduced or absent reflexes with no objective large fibre sensory loss and yet complete paralysis leads to a frequent misdiagnosis of hysteria.

Respiratory involvement may be sudden and unexpected but usually the vital capacity falls steadily and intubation and ventilation are required at level of approximately 1 litre [6]. A small number of patients develop unusual signs such as papilloedema [7] thought to be secondary to cerebral oedema and hyponatraemia [8]. Mild autonomic disturbance is seen in three quarters of patients but a few develop severe bradyarrhythmias which are recognised as a cause of infrequent death from the syndrome. Mortality in most population studies is between 5 and 10 percent [9]. The disease is monophasic with weakness reaching its most severity in 4 weeks followed by a plateau phase and then recovery. 60% of patients are able to walk unaided by 12 [10] months and the rest are left with various degrees of residual symptoms.

Three quarters of patients give a history of a preceding illness usually respiratory or gastrointestinal which may be so mild as to be completely asymptomatic. The neuropathy typically begins 7–10 days after any triggering infection. Numerous other antecedent events are described including surgery and immunisation. Most recent epidemiological surveys show the risk of immunisation triggering GBS to be very low [11]. It is estimated that the risk of contracting GBS from current influenza vaccines is significantly lower than the risk of getting GBS from influenza itself. Serological studies have shown that *Campylobacter jejuni*, Epstein Bar virus, and Cytomegalovirus are the most frequent antecedent infections. Patients sometimes continue to secrete *C. jejuni* in their stool for up to 3 months following the onset of GBS [12]. Persistent infection with CMV or EBV is very rare. A number of reports associate GBS with mycoplasma pneumonia, influenza, and varicella [13].

3. Pathology

Autopsy studies in GBS are rare because few patients die. Early studies reported oedema of the peripheral nerves with sparse inflammatory infiltrate [2]. Classic studies by Asbury and colleagues emphasised the importance of perivascular lymphocytes which resembled the findings in the animal model experimental allergic neuritis [14]. They postulated an immunological basis for the demyelination involving these lymphocytes and strongly influenced thinking about the cause of GBS. Electron microscopic studies of nerve biopsy have demonstrated macrophage associate demyelination. Macrophages appeared to invade the Schwann cell basement membrane and phagocytose myelin debris [14, 15].

Pathological studies in AMAN show a relative paucity of inflammatory infiltrate with axonal destruction but this time macrophages were situated between axons and the myelin especially in the region of the node of Ranvier [16].

The pathological studies suggest that the macrophage is the instrument of nerve damage but may well be targeted to either the myelin or axon by antibodies. In AMSAN pathological changes are similar but involve both motor and ventral nerve roots [17].

4. Immunology

The recognition that there was an association between GBS and a variety of triggering infections strongly suggested that there must be an immunological cause for the syndrome. This was supported by the nature of the pathological changes with macrophage targeted, demyelination in at least AIP which could be used to support an antibody mediated disorder. The efficacy of plasma exchange in shortening the time taken to recover also argued for a serum factor mediating the disease. In the 1960's Melnick [18] was one of the first to publish data suggesting complement fixing antibodies in the acute phase of GBS. These studies were difficult to replicate but sensitive C1 esterase assays supported complement consumption and a role for complement in the disorder [19]. In rabbits immunisation with galactocerebroside can produce a demyelinating neuropathy, suggesting that antibodies against myelin antigens are capable of causing neuropathy [20]. The pathology of the human disease resembled the experimental model experimental allergic neuritis produced by immunising susceptible species with peripheral nerve in adjuvant. EAN can be elicited using individual proteins from myelin such as P0 and P2 and T cell lines reacting with P2 can transfer the disease [21, 22].

This stimulated numerous studies attempting to find antibodies to P2, P0, and other protein antigens in GBS but these were largely negative [23]. Antibodies recognising lipids were identified in the 1980's and increasingly recognised in certain subgroups of GBS [24]. The identification of antibodies against one of these gangliosides, GQ1b in 95% of patients with Miller Fisher Syndrome [25, 26], supported a role for such antibodies in the pathogenesis of this syndrome thought to be very closely related to GBS. Similar antibodies were also found in GBS with ophthalmoplegia and in Bickerstaff's encephalitis [27, 28]. In vitro studies of mouse hemidiaphragm preparations showed that antiGq1b monoclonals immunostained the neuromuscular junction where they fixed complement and bound in identical ways to patient serum [29]. Antiganglioside antibodies were found to be associated with AMAN [30] and were implicated in animal models of the disease in rabbits [31]. Furthermore, patients immunised with gangliosides [32] were known to develop neuropathies in certain circumstances adding to the body of evidence supporting a pathology for GBS which involved complement fixing antibodies against human gangliosides.

Although the evidence in support of antiganglioside antibodies as a cause of MFS and AMAN was strong the most common form of GBS on Western countries (AIDP) was only rarely associated with ganglioside antibodies using conventional techniques [33]. The frequency of antiganglioside antibodies increases if antibodies against complexes of more than one ganglioside are considered although there are as yet few published studies [34, 35]. These are eagerly awaited.

Antibodies against gangliosides are usually found to be of the IgG1 or IgG3 subtype that conventionally require T cell help in their production. T cells infiltrate the pathological lesion in GBS nerve and so it seems likely that they play a part in mediating antibody production. Several studies have identified raised concentrations of activated T cells in the peripheral blood among patients with GBS [36] as well as changes in regulatory T cells [37] and raised levels of T cell derived cytokines [38]. The early studies looking at T cell reactivity against protein antigens such as the P2 Protein which were implicated in EAN proved to be negative. **ϒδ** T cells that are capable of recognising nonprotein antigens such as gangliosides have been isolated from GBS nerve but may be isolated from patients with vasculitis [39]. It is possible that such T cells may play a role but strong evidence is lacking. **Yδ** T cells are restricted by CD1 which is upregulated in nerve from patients with GBS [40] but no clear CD1 polymorphism is linked to GBS [41].

The clinical features of GBS are very variable and attempts have been made to correlate this with the distribution of gangliosides in different nerves [42]. There is more GQ1b in the ocular nerves which might explain the ophthalmoplegia in Miller Fisher syndrome. Similarly ventral nerve roots contain more GM1 than dorsal roots. The actual densities and accessibilities of the gangliosides in different tissues may be more important and there are studies suggesting that access to gangliosides by antibodies may differ [43].

C. jejuni is the best studied triggering agent for GBS and has been shown to have ganglioside like structures in the lipopolysaccharide coat of the bacterium [44–46]. Similar examples of molecular mimicry are seen with other organisms that rigger GBS such as *Haemophilus* [47] and *Cytomegalovirus* [48]. It therefore seems plausible to hypothesise that infection with one of these agents leads to antibody production which cross-reacts with gangliosides and other glycolipids leading to myelin destruction. This could occur by complement activation or by antibodies targeting macrophages via the fc receptor and leading to both conduction failure and demyelination.

For such specific antibodies to mediate disease they would need to pass through the blood nerve barrier. Studies in EAN suggest that activated T cells may open up the barrier to allow the antineural antibodies to mediate nerve damage [49, 50]. It is of course possible that breakdown in the blood nerve barrier is a nonspecific event that allows antigen specific antibodies to penetrate and mediate disease. Matrix metalloproteinases have been implicated in mediating barrier breakdown [51]. There may be specific factors about the triggering infection that increase the likelihood of immune sensitivity to a specific agent. Certain serotypes of *C. jejuni* appear more likely to produce these autoreactive antibodies perhaps by containing more neuritogenic epitopes [52, 53]. The risk of GBS after *C. jejuni* enteritis is estimated to be about 1 in 1000. This risk must be influenced by immunological genetic factors. Studies of HLA associations with GBS are generally weak [54, 55]. Only a very small number of familial cases of GBS have been described [56, 57].

Although antiganglioside antibodies are the most commonly reported antibody in GBS there are other reports of antibodies that might be pathogenic in a small number of patients. Antibodies against a protein in the node of Ranvier "neurofascin" have received recent attention with serum of 4% of patients with AIDP being positive in one recent study [58].

5. Neurophysiology

Neurophysiology is extremely useful in the diagnosis and definition of the subtype of GBS. Assessment early in the course of the syndrome frequently shows small action potentials, prolonged distal motor latency, delayed F waves, and conduction block [59]. Occasionally the first study is normal and a repeat study is required to document a peripheral nerve disorder. Axonal forms of the disease are characterised by reduced motor and/or sensory action potentials with denervation potentials once the acute stage of the disease is over. Neurophysiological studies carried out as part of the European IvIg and steroid trial found 69% of the studies to be consistent with AIDP with only 3% suggesting axonal pathology on studies carried out within 3 weeks of onset. Twenty-three percent of studies were equivocal at this early stage and may have gone on to be predominantly axonal [60].

6. Management

Supportive aspects of management have been the major factor in improving mortality in GBS with the advent of good ITU care and modern methods of ventilation. Infection, emboli, and autonomic instability are the major causes of death. Passive movement of limbs and active physiotherapy once the initial acute stage is over appear to be beneficial although it has never been subject to a controlled clinical trial.

Active immune modulation with IvIg [61] or plasma exchange [62] is the mainstay of treatment with IvIg being preferred in most circumstances due to ease of availability and greater safety in patients with unstable blood pressure and pulse. IvIg is usually given at a dose of 0.4 gm/kg for 5 days although the optimum dose has never been established. Recent studies suggest that metabolism of IvIg is faster in patients with a worse prognosis and there are studies in place to see whether a higher dose of IvIg would benefit some patients [63].

Patients that either fail to improve or exhibit a deterioration are often given a further course of IvIg although trials have yet to justify such an approach. The combination of IvIg with either steroids or plasma exchange seems to confer little benefit [64].

Better treatments of GBS are clearly needed to reduce the proportion of patients that are left disabled. Complement inhibitors such as eculizumab have been shown to be effective in animal models of Miller Fisher syndrome [65] and to be safe in man [66] but have yet to be the subject of a controlled trial. Since much of the damage to nerves occurs early in the course of the disease it may be more effective to look at chemicals capable of improving nerve regrowth and regeneration. Such neuroprotective drugs would clearly be of value in a number of diseases with a common end point of axonal damage.

Conflict of Interests

The author declares that there is no conflict of interests regarding the publication of this paper.

References

[1] G. Guillain, J. Barré, and A. Strohl, "Sur un syndrome de radiculo-nevrite avec hyperalbuminose du liquide cephalo-rachidien sans reaction cellulaire. Remarques sur les characteres

clinique et graphique des reflexes tendinaux," *Bulletins et Memories de la Societe Medicale des Hopitaux de Paris*, vol. 40, pp. 1462–1470, 1916.

[2] W. K. J. Haymaker, "The Landry-Guillain-Barré syndrome: a clinicopathologicic report of fifty fatal cases and a critique of the literature," *Medicine*, vol. 28, pp. 59–141, 1949.

[3] J. W. Griffin, C. Y. Li, T. W. Ho et al., "Guillain-Barré syndrome in northern China. The spectrum of neuropathological changes in clinically defined cases," *Brain*, vol. 118, no. 3, pp. 577–595, 1995.

[4] A. McGrogan, G. C. Madle, H. E. Seaman, and C. S. De Vries, "The epidemiology of Guillain-Barré syndrome worldwide: a systematic literature review," *Neuroepidemiology*, vol. 32, no. 2, pp. 150–163, 2009.

[5] J. J. Sejvar, A. L. Baughman, M. Wise, and O. W. Morgan, "Population incidence of Guillain-Barré syndrome: a systematic review and meta-analysis," *Neuroepidemiology*, vol. 36, no. 2, pp. 123–133, 2011.

[6] N. D. Lawn, D. D. Fletcher, R. D. Henderson, T. D. Wolter, and E. F. M. Wijdicks, "Anticipating mechanical ventilation in Guillain-Barré syndrome," *Archives of Neurology*, vol. 58, no. 6, pp. 893–898, 2001.

[7] A. C. Reid and I. T. Draper, "Pathogenesis of papilloedema and raised intracranial pressure in Guillain-Barré syndrome," *British Medical Journal*, vol. 281, no. 6252, pp. 1393–1394, 1980.

[8] B. M. Colls, "Guillain-Barré syndrome and hyponatraemia," *Internal Medicine Journal*, vol. 34, no. 4, p. 218, 2004.

[9] N. Souayah, A. Nasar, M. F. K. Suri, and A. I. Qureshi, "National trends in hospital outcomes among patients with Guillain-é syndrome requiring mechanical ventilation," *Journal of Clinical Neuromuscular Disease*, vol. 10, no. 1, pp. 24–28, 2008.

[10] J. B. Winer, R. A. C. Hughes, and C. Osmond, "A prospective study of acute idiopathic neuropathy. I. Clinical features and their prognostic value," *Journal of Neurology Neurosurgery & Psychiatry*, vol. 51, no. 5, pp. 605–612, 1988.

[11] C. Bardage, I. Persson, A. Ortqvist, U. Bergman, J. F. Ludvigsson, and F. Granath, "Neurological and autoimmune disorders after vaccination against pandemic influenza A (H1N1) with a monovalent adjuvanted vaccine: population based cohort study in Stockholm, Sweden," *BMJ*, vol. 343, p. d5956, 2011.

[12] E. A. Goddard, A. J. Lastovica, and A. C. Argent, "Campylobacter 0:41 isolation in Guillain-Barré syndrome," *Archives of Disease in Childhood*, vol. 76, no. 6, pp. 526–528, 1997.

[13] F. Cresswell, J. Eadie, N. Longley, and D. Macallan, "Severe Guillain-Barré syndrome following primary infection with varicella zoster virus in an adult," *International Journal of Infectious Diseases*, vol. 14, no. 2, pp. e161–e163, 2010.

[14] A. K. Asbury, B. G. Arnason, and R. D. Adams, "The inflammatory lesion in idiopathic polyneuritis. Its role in pathogenesis," *Medicine*, vol. 48, no. 3, pp. 173–215, 1969.

[15] J. W. Prineas, "Acute idiopathic polyneuritis. An electron microscope study," *Laboratory Investigation*, vol. 26, no. 2, pp. 133–147, 1972.

[16] J. W. Griffin, C. Y. Li, C. Macko et al., "Early nodal changes in the acute motor axonal neuropathy pattern of the Guillain-Barré syndrome," *Journal of Neurocytology*, vol. 25, no. 1, pp. 33–51, 1996.

[17] J. W. Griffin, C. Y. Li, T. W. Ho et al., "Pathology of the motor-sensory axonal guillain-barré syndrome," *Annals of Neurology*, vol. 39, no. 1, pp. 17–28, 1996.

[18] S. C. Melnick, "Thirty-eight cases of the Guillain-Barré syndrome: an immunological study," *British Medical Journal*, vol. 1, no. 5327, pp. 368–373, 1963.

[19] C. L. Koski, R. Humphrey, and M. L. Shin, "Anti-peripheral myelin antibody in patients with demyelinating neuropathy: quantitative and kinetic determination of serum antibody by complement component 1 fixation," *Proceedings of the National Academy of Sciences of the United States of America*, vol. 82, no. 3, pp. 905–909, 1985.

[20] T. Saida, K. Saida, D. H. Silberberg, and M. J. Brown, "Experimental allergic neuritis induced by galactocerebroside," *Annals of Neurology*, vol. 9, pp. 87–101, 1981.

[21] H.-P. Hartung, B. Schafer, W. Fierz, K. Heininger, and K. V. Toyka, "Ciclosporin A prevents P2 T cell line-mediated experimental autoimmune neuritis (AT-EAN) in rat," *Neuroscience Letters*, vol. 83, no. 1-2, pp. 195–200, 1987.

[22] J. Zhu, S.-H. Pelidou, G. Deretzi et al., "P0 glycoprotein peptides 56–71 and 180–199 dose-dependently induce acute and chronic experimental autoimmune neuritis in Lewis rats associated with epitope spreading," *Journal of Neuroimmunology*, vol. 114, no. 1, pp. 90–106, 2001, [erratum appears in *Journal of Neuroimmunology*, vol. 119, no. 1, p. 150, 2001].

[23] R. A. C. Hughes, I. A. Gray, and N. A. Gregson, "Immune responses to myelin antigens in Guillain-Barré syndrome," *Journal of Neuroimmunology*, vol. 6, no. 5, pp. 303–312, 1984.

[24] R. H. Quarles, A. A. Ilyas, and H. J. Willison, "Antibodies to glycolipids in demyelinating diseases of the human peripheral nervous system," *Chemistry and Physics of Lipids*, vol. 42, no. 1–3, pp. 235–248, 1986.

[25] A. Chiba, S. Kusunoki, T. Shimizu, and I. Kanazawa, "Serum IgG antibody to ganglioside GQ1b is a possible marker of Miller Fisher syndrome," *Annals of Neurology*, vol. 31, no. 6, pp. 677–679, 1992.

[26] H. J. Willison, J. Veitch, G. Paterson, and P. G. E. Kennedy, "Miller Fisher syndrome is associated with serum antibodies to GQ1b ganglioside," *Journal of Neurology Neurosurgery & Psychiatry*, vol. 56, no. 2, pp. 204–206, 1993.

[27] M. Odaka, N. Yuki, and K. Hirata, "Anti-GQ1b IgG antibody syndrome: clinical and immunological range," *Journal of Neurology Neurosurgery & Psychiatry*, vol. 70, no. 1, pp. 50–55, 2001.

[28] M. Odaka, N. Yuki, M. Yamada et al., "Bickerstaff's brainstem encephalitis: clinical features of 62 cases and a subgroup associated with Guillain-Barré syndrome," *Brain*, vol. 126, no. 10, pp. 2279–2290, 2003.

[29] G. M. O'Hanlon, J. J. Plomp, M. Chakrabarti et al., "Anti-GQ1b ganglioside antibodies mediate complement-dependent destruction of the motor nerve terminal," *Brain*, vol. 124, no. 5, pp. 893–906, 2001.

[30] T. W. Ho, H. J. Willison, I. Nachamkin et al., "Anti-GD1a antibody is associated with axonal but not demyelinating forms of Guillain-Barré syndrome," *Annals of Neurology*, vol. 45, pp. 168–173, 1999.

[31] N. Yuki, M. Yamada, M. Koga et al., "Animal model of axonal Guillain-Barré syndrome induced by sensitization with GM1 ganglioside," *Annals of Neurology*, vol. 49, no. 6, pp. 712–720, 2001.

[32] V. Govoni, E. Granieri, M. R. Tola et al., "Exogenous gangliosides and Guillain-Barré syndrome. An observational study in the Local Health District of Ferrara, Italy," *Brain*, vol. 120, no. 7, pp. 1123–1130, 1997.

[33] H. J. Willison and C. S. Goodyear, "Glycolipid antigens and autoantibodies in autoimmune neuropathies," *Trends in Immunology*, vol. 34, no. 9, pp. 453–459, 2013.

[34] K. Kaida and S. Kusunoki, "Antibodies to gangliosides and ganglioside complexes in Guillain-Barré syndrome and Fisher syndrome: mini-review," *Journal of Neuroimmunology*, vol. 223, no. 1-2, pp. 5–12, 2010.

[35] S. Kusunoki, K.-I. Kaida, and M. Ueda, "Antibodies against gangliosides and ganglioside complexes in Guillain-Barré syndrome: new aspects of research," *Biochimica et Biophysica Acta*, vol. 1780, no. 3, pp. 441–444, 2008.

[36] W. Hu, A. Janke, S. Ortler et al., "Expression of CD28-related costimulatory molecule and its ligand in inflammatory neuropathies," *Neurology*, vol. 68, no. 4, pp. 277–282, 2007.

[37] L.-J. Chi, H.-B. Wang, Y. Zhang, and W.-Z. Wang, "Abnormality of circulating $CD4^{+}CD25^{+}$ regulatory T cell in patients with Guillain-Barré syndrome," *Journal of Neuroimmunology*, vol. 192, no. 1-2, pp. 206–214, 2007.

[38] K. K. Nyati, K. N. Prasad, A. Verma, and V. K. Paliwal, "Correlation of matrix metalloproteinases-2 and -9 with proinflammatory cytokines in Guillain-Barré syndrome," *Journal of Neuroscience Research*, vol. 88, no. 16, pp. 3540–3546, 2010.

[39] A. Ben-Smith, J. S. H. Gaston, P. C. Barber, and J. B. Winer, "Isolation and characterisation of T lymphocytes from sural nerve biopsies in patients with Guillain-Barré syndrome and chronic inflammatory demyelinating polyneuropathy," *Journal of Neurology Neurosurgery & Psychiatry*, vol. 61, no. 4, pp. 362–368, 1996.

[40] A. Khalili-Shiraz, N. Gregson, and R. Hughes, "CD 1 expression in human peripheral nerve of GBS patients," *Biochemical Society Transactions*, vol. 25, no. 2, p. 172, 1997.

[41] M. L. Kuijf, K. Geleijns, N. Ennaji, W. van Rijs, P. A. van Doorn, and B. C. Jacobs, "Susceptibility to Guillain-Barré syndrome is not associated with CD1A and CD1E gene polymorphisms," *Journal of Neuroimmunology*, vol. 205, no. 1-2, pp. 110–112, 2008.

[42] A. Chiba, S. Kusunoki, H. Obata, R. Machinami, and I. Kanazawa, "Ganglioside composition of the human cranial nerves, with special reference to pathophysiology of Miller Fisher syndrome," *Brain Research*, vol. 745, no. 1-2, pp. 32–36, 1997.

[43] Y. Gong, Y. Tagawa, M. P. T. Lunn et al., "Localization of major gangliosides in the PNS: implications for immune neuropathies," *Brain*, vol. 125, no. 11, pp. 2491–2506, 2002.

[44] C. W. Ang, H. P. Endtz, B. C. Jacobs et al., "Campylobacter jejuni lipopolysaccharides from Guillain-Barré syndrome patients induce IgG anti-GM1 antibodies in rabbits," *Journal of Neuroimmunology*, vol. 104, no. 2, pp. 133–138, 2000.

[45] K. A. Sheikh, I. Nachamkin, T. W. Ho et al., "Campylobacter jejuni lipopolysaccharides in Guillain-Barré syndrome: molecular mimicry and host susceptibility," *Neurology*, vol. 51, no. 2, pp. 371–378, 1998.

[46] N. Yuki, "Molecular mimicry between gangliosides and lipopolysaccharides of Campylobacter jejuni isolated from patients with Guillain-Barré syndrome and Miller Fisher syndrome," *Journal of Infectious Diseases*, vol. 176, no. 6, pp. S150–S153, 1997.

[47] M. Mori, S. Kuwabara, M. Miyake et al., "Haemophilus influenzae has a GM1 ganglioside-like structure and elicits Guillain-Barré syndrome," *Neurology*, vol. 52, no. 6, pp. 1282–1284, 1999.

[48] A. Khalili-Shirazi, N. Gregson, I. Gray, J. Rees, J. Winer, and R. Hughes, "Antiganglioside antibodies in Guillain-Barré syndrome after a recent cytomegalovirus infection," *Journal of Neurology Neurosurgery & Psychiatry*, vol. 66, no. 3, pp. 376–379, 1999.

[49] J. M. Spies, J. D. Pollard, J. G. Bonner, K. W. Westland, and J. G. McLeod, "Synergy between antibody and P2-reactive T cells in experimental allergic neuritis," *Journal of Neuroimmunology*, vol. 57, no. 1-2, pp. 77–84, 1995.

[50] K. W. Westland, J. D. Pollard, S. Sander, J. G. Bonner, C. Linington, and J. G. McLeod, "Activated non-neural specific T cells open the blood-brain barrier to circulating antibodies," *Brain*, vol. 122, no. 7, pp. 1283–1291, 1999.

[51] A. Créange, T. Sharshar, T. Planchenault et al., "Matrix metalloproteinase-9 is increased and correlates with severity in Guillain-Barré syndrome," *Neurology*, vol. 53, no. 8, pp. 1683–1691, 1999.

[52] M. Koga, M. Gilbert, J. Li et al., "Antecedent infections in Fisher syndrome: a common pathogenesis of molecular mimicry," *Neurology*, vol. 64, no. 9, pp. 1605–1611, 2005.

[53] N. Yuki, T. Taki, M. Takahashi et al., "Penner's serotype 4 of Campylobacter jejuni has a lipopolysaccharide that bears a GM1 ganglioside epitope as well as one that bears a GD1a epitope," *Infection and Immunity*, vol. 62, no. 5, pp. 2101–2103, 1994.

[54] J. B. Winer, D. Briggs, K. Welsh, and R. A. C. Hughes, "HLA antigens in the Guillain-Barré syndrome," *Journal of Neuroimmunology*, vol. 18, no. 1, pp. 13–16, 1988.

[55] J. H. Rees, R. W. Vaugham, E. Kondeatis, and R. A. C. Hughes, "HLA-class II alleles in Guillain-Barré syndrome and miller fisher syndrome and their association with preceding Campylobacter jejuni infection," *Journal of Neuroimmunology*, vol. 62, no. 1, pp. 53–57, 1995.

[56] G. A. MacGregor, "Familial Guillain-Barré syndrome," *The Lancet*, vol. 2, no. 7425, p. 1296, 1965.

[57] M. Saunders and M. Rake, "Familial Guillain-Barré syndrome," *The Lancet*, vol. 286, no. 7422, pp. 1106–1107, 1965.

[58] J. K. Ng, J. Malotka, N. Kawakami et al., "Neurofascin as a target for autoantibodies in peripheral neuropathies," *Neurology*, vol. 79, pp. 2241–2248, 2012.

[59] D. R. Cornblath, "Electrophysiology in Guillain-Barré syndrome," *Annals of Neurology*, vol. 27, pp. S17–S20, 1990.

[60] R. D. M. Hadden, D. R. Cornblath, R. A. C. Hughes et al., "Electrophysiological classification of Guillain-Barré syndrome: clinical associations and outcome," *Annals of Neurology*, vol. 44, no. 5, pp. 780–788, 1998.

[61] R. A. Hughes, J. C. Raphaël, A. V. Swan, and P. A. van Doorn, "Intravenous immunoglobulin for Guillain-Barré syndrome," *Cochrane Database of Systematic Reviews*, no. 1, Article ID CD002063, 2006.

[62] J. C. Raphaël, S. Chevret, R. A. Hughes, and D. Annane, "Plasma exchange for Guillain-Barré syndrome," *Cochrane Database of Systematic Reviews*, no. 2, Article ID CD001798, 2001.

[63] K. Kuitwaard, J. De Gelder, A. P. Tio-Gillen et al., "Pharmacokinetics of intravenous immunoglobulin and outcome in Guillain-Barré syndrome," *Annals of Neurology*, vol. 66, no. 5, pp. 597–603, 2009.

[64] Anonymous, "Randomised trial of plasma exchange, intravenous immunoglobulin, and combined treatments in Guillain-Barré syndrome," *The Lancet*, vol. 349, no. 9047, pp. 225–230, 1997.

27

Anal Involvement in Pemphigus Vularis

Somayeh Khezri,[1] Hamid-Reza Mahmoudi,[1] Seyedeh Nina Masoom,[1] Maryam Daneshpazhooh,[1] Kamran Balighi,[1] S. Hamed Hosseini,[2] and Cheyda Chams-Davatchi[1]

[1] *Autoimmune Bullous Diseases Research Center, Department of Dermatology, Tehran University of Medical Sciences, Razi Hospital, Vahdate-Eslami Square, Tehran 11996, Iran*

[2] *Knowledge Utilization Research Center, School of Public Health, Tehran University of Medical Sciences, Tehran 1417613151, Iran*

Correspondence should be addressed to Maryam Daneshpazhooh; maryamdanesh.pj@gmail.com

Academic Editor: Paulo Ricardo Criado

Background. Pemphigus vulgaris (PV) is an autoimmune blistering disease of the skin and mucosa. Anal mucosa may be involved in PV, but the frequency and clinical profile are not fully ascertained. *Objective.* The aim was to investigate the involvement of the anal area in newly diagnosed PV patients. *Patients and Methods.* A total of 168 consecutive newly diagnosed PV patients were enrolled. Anal symptoms and signs, involvement of other body sites, and severity of disease were recorded. *Results.* A total of 47 out of 168 patients (27.9%) had involvement of the anal area. Anal involvement was significantly associated with PV lesions in ophthalmic ($P = 0.03$), nasal ($P = 0.02$), and genital mucosa ($P < 0.001$) but not the oral cavity ($P = 0.24$). There was a significant association between number of involved mucosal sites and anal involvement ($P < 0.001$). Anal involvement was associated with oral severity ($P = 0.02$). Constipation was the most frequent symptom (73.8%) followed by pain on defecation (50%). Seventeen patients (36%) were symptom-free. Erosion was the most frequent sign (91.5%). *Conclusion.* Anal involvement in PV seems to be more frequent than previously assumed. Routine anal examination is recommended even in asymptomatic patients as anal involvement appears to correlate with the severity of PV.

1. Introduction

Pemphigus vulgaris (PV) is a rare, autoimmune, potentially fatal mucocutaneous bullous disease in which pathogenic autoantibodies are directed against the keratinocyte cell surface molecules desmoglein 3 (Dsg3) and to a lesser extent Dsg1 [1]. The incidence of this disease varies from 0.16 to 1.62 cases per 100,000 with increased incidence in Jews, Indians, and middle easterners [2]. PV is characterized by bullae that typically begin in the oral cavity and may spread to involve the skin. Other mucosal surfaces including conjunctiva, nasal mucosa, pharynx, larynx, epiglottis, esophagus, cervix, vagina, and penile mucosa may also be affected in the course of disease [3–8]. Anal involvement may also be seen in PV but its frequency and clinical profile are not fully ascertained yet [9–12]. The aim of this study was to investigate the involvement of the anal area in newly diagnosed PV patients presenting to the Autoimmune Bullous Diseases Research Center (ABDRC), Tehran, Iran, during a 15-month period.

2. Patients and Methods

This prospective study included 168 consecutive patients newly diagnosed with PV, attending the ABDRC, between October 2009 and January 2011. The diagnosis of PV was based on the presence of clinical features of the disease, including mucocutaneous bullae and erosions along with histopathological (suprabasal cleft and acantholysis) and direct immunofluorescence (lattice-like intercellular epidermal IgG and/or C3 deposits) findings of the biopsy material [13]. Only patients with new-onset untreated disease were enrolled in this study and all subjects underwent physical examination of the anal area. Anoscopy was not performed.

The following information was collected on each patient: (1) age at onset of PV and gender; (2) anal symptoms and signs; (3) nonanal involvement; (4) severity of disease. The severity of skin and mucosal disease was rated based on a grading system proposed by Harman et al. [14] as follows: oral grading: Grade 0, without any lesion; Grade I, minor activity

TABLE 1: Characteristics of pemphigus vulgaris patients with or without anal involvement.

	Total (n = 168)	Patients with anal involvement (n = 47)	Patients without anal involvement (n = 121)	P value for differences between patients with and without anal involvement
Age y; mean ± SD	44 ± 12.6	45 ± 13.3	44 ± 12.3	0.6
M : F ratio	1 : 1.21	1 : 0.96	1 : 1.33	0.4
Phenotype-n (%)				
Mucosal	8 (4.8)	2 (4.3)	4 (3.3)	
Mucocutaneous	141 (84)	43 (91.5)	98 (81)	0.08
Cutaneous	19 (11.2)	2 (4.3)	19 (15.7)	
Number (%) of patients with				
Oral involvement	137 (81.5)	41 (87.2)	96 (79.3)	0.24
Genital involvement	44 (26.2)	23 (48)	20 (16.5)	<0.001
Nasal mucosal involvement	38 (22.6)	17 (34)	22 (18)	0.02
Ophthalmic involvement	36 (21.4)	15 (32)	20 (16.5)	0.03

SD: standard deviation; M: male; F: female; P value less than 0.05 was considered significant.

(up to three lesions); Grade II, moderate activity (more than three but less than 10 erosions or generalized desquamative gingivitis); Grade III, severe (more than 10 discrete erosions or extensive, confluent erosions, or generalized desquamative gingivitis with discrete erosions at other oral sites). Skin grading: Grade 0, without any lesions; Grade I, minor activity (less than five discrete lesions); Grade II, moderate activity (more than five but less than 20 discrete lesions); Grade III, severe (more than 20 discrete lesions or extensive, confluent areas of eroded skin). Only lesions within 2 cm or less from the anal orifice were considered as anal involvement.

Statistical analysis was performed by Student's t-test for differences in means of ages of patients with or without anal lesions. The chi-square test was used to analyze differences between involvement of different anatomical sites in patients with or without anal involvement. P value <0.05 was considered significant. Fisher's exact test was used wherever necessary.

3. Results

A total of 168 newly diagnosed PV patients were examined, 92 patients (54.8%) were female, and 76 patients (45.2%) were male (M : F ratio = 1 : 1.21). Age distribution of PV was from 19 to 72 years with a mean ± SD of 44 ± 12.6 years. A total of 47 out of 168 patients (27.9%) had involvement of the anal area. The lesions were confined to the stratified epithelium of the anal region.

Table 1 shows characteristics of patients with or without anal involvement. Twenty-three of 47 patients with anal involvement were female (48.9%) and 24 patients (51.1%) were male (M : F ratio= 1 : 0.96). Forty-one (87.2%) out of 47 patients with anal involvement had concomitant oral lesions, while this figure was 79.3% (96 out of 121) for patients without anal involvement. The difference was not significant (P = 0.24). On the other hand, anal involvement was significantly associated with PV lesions in other mucosal sites including ophthalmic (P = 0.03), nasal (P = 0.02), and genital mucosa (P < 0.001).

Focusing on severity of oral disease, 54 cases (32.1%) were grade II followed by grade I (51 cases, 30.4%), grade III (32 cases, 19%), and grade 0 (31 cases, 18.5%). Significant association between severity of oral disease and anal involvement was seen (P = 0.02). Skin grading was as follows: 6 cases (3.6%) were grade 0, grade I (39 cases, 23.2%), grade II (56 cases, 33.3%), and grade III (67 cases, 39.9%). There was no association between anal involvement and severity of skin disease (P = 0.06).

Two of our patients (4.3%) showed anal lesions in the absence of involvement of other mucosal surfaces; 16 patients (34%) had involvement in one other mucosal site in addition to anal area, and 29 out of 47 patients with anal lesions (62%) showed involvement of PV in at least two other mucosal sites. There was a significant association between the number of involved mucosal sites and anal involvement (P < 0.001).

Table 2 shows clinical signs and symptoms reported by patients. Thirty out of 47 patients with anal lesions (64%) complained of anorectal symptoms, while 17 patients (36%) were symptom-free. Constipation was the presenting symptom in the majority of cases (73.8%) followed by pain on defecation (50%). Erosion was found in 43 patients (91.5%) and was the most common anal sign with a mean of 1.3 anal erosions per patient.

4. Discussion

Our study shows greater frequency of anal involvement in PV patients than previous reports (27.9%). Although anal area is a well-known site of involvement in PV, the frequency of this involvement is not fully investigated and figures vary widely (2% [2], 9.3% [10, 11], and 16.5% [15]). There are several reasons for the underestimation of the incidence of anal PV: firstly there may be underreporting of cases, because patients are uncomfortable discussing anal symptoms and may attribute them to other causes such as fissures or hemorrhoids [10, 11]; secondly physicians may not routinely examine the anal area, and at last a significant number of lesions may be asymptomatic or subtle. We performed anal

TABLE 2: Symptoms and signs in patients with pemphigus vulgaris.

	Number (%) among total patients	% among patients with anal involvement
Symptoms		
Spontaneous pain	10 (6)	23.8
Bleeding	16 (9.5)	38
Pain on defecation	21 (12.5)	50
Constipation	31 (18.5)	73.8
Total	**42 (25)**	
Signs related to PV		
Erosion	43 (25.6)	91.5
Leukoedema	16 (9)	34
Perianal involvement	8 (4.8)	17
Pseudofissure	7 (4.2)	15
Ulcer	6 (3.5)	12.8
Vegetant	2 (1.2)	4.3
Bullae	1 (0.6)	2.1
Total	**47 (27.9)**	
Signs unrelated to PV		
Hemorrhoid	17 (10)	16 (34%)*
Prolapse	1 (0.6)	0**

*One of the patients shows hemorrhoid in absence of other anal pathology in physical examination.
**One patient showed prolapse in examination without any other anal pathology.

examination regardless of patients' symptoms and severity of disease.

In this study the presence of anal involvement correlated with the severity of mucosal disease as well as with the number of other involved mucosal sites. To our knowledge no study had ascertained anal involvement with the severity of PV. Most of our patients with anal involvement (62%) showed involvement of multiple other mucosal sites. The few patients described in the literature also tended to have involvement of PV at multiple sites, especially the oral mucosa. Epstein et al. reported a patient with widespread involvement at multiple mucosal and cutaneous sites [16]. Malik et al. [17] reported 16 patients with anal involvement and suggested that anal involvement generally occurs in the setting of extensive involvement of PV at other sites. Hotz et al. [15] studied 103 PV patients; seventeen of them had anal involvement. Signs in eleven patients included 9 cases of erosions, one pseudofissure, and one bulla. Regarding the association of anal involvement with the severity of PV, the inclusion of involvement of other mucosa including anal mucosa in any future criteria of severity of PV may be justified.

As expected, erosions were the most common anal sign. Pseudofissure—a linear erosion or ulcer not in a typical site for anal fissure (12 o'clock)—was also a frequent, noticeable finding. Hemorrhoids were found in 17 patients (10%) in anal examination. Interestingly, 16 out of 17 patients with hemorrhoids had anal PV; all of these 16 patients had erosions as the anal sign in their examination. Hemorrhoids are subject to repeated trauma during defecation, and it seems that they could be considered a vulnerable site for erosions in PV. Seventeen patients (10%) showed leukoedema described as pearly white appearance of the mucosa surrounding anal erosions. This has been previously described by Hotz et al. [15].

In conclusion, anal involvement in PV seems to be more frequent than previously assumed. Although most patients with anal lesions were symptomatic and had defecation problems, routine anal examination is recommended even in asymptomatic patients as it appears to correlate with the severity of PV.

Conflict of Interests

The authors declare that they have no conflict of interests.

Authors' Contribution

Somayeh Khezri and Hamid-Reza Mahmoudi made equal contribution to this research.

References

[1] J.-C. Bystryn and J. L. Rudolph, "Pemphigus," *The Lancet*, vol. 366, no. 9479, pp. 61–73, 2005.

[2] C. Chams-Davatchi, M. Valikhani, M. Daneshpazhooh et al., "Pemphigus: analysis of 1209 cases," *International Journal of Dermatology*, vol. 44, no. 6, pp. 470–476, 2005.

[3] M. Akhyani, C. Chams-Davatchi, Z. Naraghi et al., "Cervicovaginal involvement in pemphigus vulgaris: a clinical study of 77 cases," *British Journal of Dermatology*, vol. 158, no. 3, pp. 478–482, 2008.

[4] E. K. Hale and J.-C. Bystryn, "Laryngeal and nasal involvement in pemphigus vulgaris," *Journal of the American Academy of Dermatology*, vol. 44, no. 4, pp. 609–611, 2001.

[5] E. Hodak, I. Kremer, M. David et al., "Conjunctival involvement in pemphigus vulgaris: a clinical, histopathological and immunofluorescence study," *British Journal of Dermatology*, vol. 123, no. 5, pp. 615–620, 1990.

[6] G. M. Palleschi, E. M. Cipollini, and T. Lotti, "Development of oesophageal involvement in a subject with pemphigus vulgaris: a case report and review of the literature," *Journal of the European Academy of Dermatology and Venereology*, vol. 16, no. 4, pp. 405–408, 2002.

[7] N. Sami and A. R. Ahmed, "Penile pemphigus," *Archives of Dermatology*, vol. 137, no. 6, pp. 756–758, 2001.

[8] N. Schlesinger, M. Katz, and A. Ingber, "Nail involvement in pemphigus vulgaris," *British Journal of Dermatology*, vol. 146, no. 5, pp. 836–839, 2002.

[9] B. Haskell and H. Rovner, "Pemphigus of the anal canal," *Diseases of the Colon and Rectum*, vol. 1, no. 6, pp. 439–442, 1958.

[10] S. Brenner, E. Tur, J. Shapiro et al., "Pemphigus vulgaris: environmentalfactors. Occupational, behavioral, medical, and qualitative food frequency questionnaire," *International Journal of Dermatology*, vol. 40, no. 9, pp. 562–569, 2001.

[11] S. Brenner, E. Tur, J. Shapiro et al., "Erratum: pemphigus vulgaris: environmental factors. Occupational, behavioral, medical, and qualitative food frequency questionnaire," *International Journal of Dermatology*, vol. 42, no. 9, p. 760, 2003.

[12] D. D. Stone, "Rectal lesions and toxic dilatation of the colon in a case of pemphigus vulgaris," *The American Journal of Digestive Diseases*, vol. 16, no. 2, pp. 163–166, 1971.

[13] S. Ikeda, S. Imamura, I. Hashimoto, S. Morioka, M. Sakuma, and H. Ogawa, "History of the establishment and revision of diagnostic criteria, severity index and therapeutic guidelines for pemphigus in Japan," *Archives of Dermatological Research*, vol. 295, supplement 1, pp. S12–S16, 2003.

[14] K. E. Harman, P. T. Seed, M. J. Gratian, B. S. Bhogal, S. J. Challacombe, and M. M. Black, "The severity of cutaneous and oral pemphigus is related to desmoglein 1 and 3 antibody levels," *British Journal of Dermatology*, vol. 144, no. 4, pp. 775–780, 2001.

[15] C. Hotz, A. Zaleski, M. Alexandre, C. Le Roux, F. Pascal, S. Doan et al., "Les atteintes annales dans les pemphigus vulgaires: incidence, description et evolution des lesions," *Annales de Dermatologie et de Vénéréologie*, vol. 135, supplement 2, p. A67, 2008.

[16] J. H. Epstein, G. M. Feigen, and N. N. Epstein, "Pemphigus vulgaris with lesions of the rectal mucosa," *AMA Archives of Dermatology*, vol. 78, no. 1, pp. 36–38, 1958.

[17] M. Malik, A.-E. El Tal, and A. R. Ahmed, "Anal involvement in pemphigus vulgaris," *Diseases of the Colon and Rectum*, vol. 49, no. 4, pp. 500–506, 2006.

28

Clinical and Immunologic Profiles in Incomplete Lupus Erythematosus and Improvement with Hydroxychloroquine Treatment

Nancy J. Olsen,[1] Carl McAloose,[1] Jamie Carter,[1] Bobby Kwanghoon Han,[2] Indu Raman,[3] Quan-Zhen Li,[3] and Duanping Liao[4]

[1] *Division of Rheumatology, Department of Medicine, Penn State MS Hershey Medical Center, Hershey, PA, USA*
[2] *Division of Rheumatology, Department of Medicine, University of Washington, Seattle, WA, USA*
[3] *Department of Immunology, University of Texas Southwestern Medical Center, Dallas, TX, USA*
[4] *Department of Public Health Sciences, Penn State University, College of Medicine, Hershey, PA, USA*

Correspondence should be addressed to Nancy J. Olsen; nolsen@hmc.psu.edu

Academic Editor: Ricard Cervera

Objective. The study goals were to evaluate performance of SLE classification criteria, to define patients with incomplete lupus erythematosus (ILE), and to probe for features in these patients that might be useful as indicators of disease status and hydroxychloroquine response. *Methods*. Patients with ILE ($N = 70$) and SLE ($N = 32$) defined by the 1997 American College of Rheumatology criteria were reclassified using the 2012 Systemic Lupus International Collaborating Clinics criteria. Disease activity, patient reported outcomes, and levels of Type I interferon- (IFN-) inducible genes, autoantibodies, and cytokines were measured. Subgroups treated with hydroxychloroquine (HCQ) were compared to patients not on this drug. *Results*. The classification sets were correlated ($R^2 = 0.87$). ILE patients were older ($P = 0.0043$) with lower disease activity scores ($P < 0.001$) and greater dissatisfaction with health status ($P = 0.034$) than SLE patients. ILE was associated with lower levels of macrophage-derived cytokines and levels of expressed Type I IFN-inducible genes. Treatment of ILE with HCQ was associated with better self-reported health status scores and lower expression levels of Type I IFN-inducible genes than ILE patients not on HCQ. *Conclusion*. The 2012 SLICC SLE classification criteria will be useful to define ILE in trials. Patients with ILE have better health status and immune profiles when treated with HCQ.

1. Background

A significant number of individuals seeking care in rheumatology clinics have some findings suggestive of SLE but do not have 4 of the defined classification criteria. Some of these individuals are identified through anti-nuclear antibody (ANA) screening that was carried out for nonspecific symptoms. Others have cutaneous complaints and are seen by dermatologists. A patient with significant ANA positivity and a photosensitive malar rash, for example, does not fit classification criteria for SLE, but the findings may be of concern and warrant further evaluations or treatment. This is especially true for young females, who are in the highest risk group for development of SLE. Such a patient may be considered to have incomplete lupus or ILE. This terminology has been used for many years and has implications for lupus risk [1, 2]. Patients with ILE are often treated with low doses of prednisone or with hydroxychloroquine and monitored for development of further lupus manifestations. At least one study from a university-based dermatology clinic suggests that some patients who present with an incomplete and largely cutaneous symptom complex do progress to SLE but have a low risk of developing organ-damaging manifestations [3]. But concerns also have been raised about whether overuse of the ILE terminology is inappropriate in view of the fact that many will never develop SLE or another significant illness [4, 5]. Determining which ILE patients are at greatest risk has some urgency, as it will open possibilities for interventional trials to modify disease and reduce progression to SLE.

The goals of the current study were to characterize patients with ILE who were seen in an academic rheumatology clinic and to evaluate approaches to classification and outcome assessment that could be applicable to clinical trial interventions. Effects of one potential intervention, hydroxychloroquine (HCQ), on clinical and immune parameters were determined. The results suggest that this treatment has benefits in ILE and potential to modulate long-term outcome in these patients.

2. Methods

2.1. Subjects. Patients with lupus syndromes were identified during routine care in the clinics of the rheumatology division. SLE was defined using the 1997 ACR criteria [6]. ILE was defined as any individual who had accumulated 1 to 3 of the ACR criteria. Each individual was then reclassified using the 2012 SLICC set of criteria [7]. Individuals with ANA as the only criterion also had other clinical or immunologic findings suggestive of autoimmunity and disease risk such as positivity for Ro/SSA or other autoantibodies, presence of Raynaud's, or strong history of autoimmune disease in one or more first degree relatives. Most of these individuals were being followed regularly in the outpatient clinics because of these ongoing concerns. Some results were also compared to 13 healthy control (HC) subjects. The research protocol followed Declaration of Helsinki principles and was approved by the Penn State Hershey Institutional Review Board. All patients provided written informed consent prior to any study-related activities.

2.2. Blood Samples. Peripheral blood samples were drawn for collection of serum, stored as frozen aliquots at −80°C, and drawn separately into PAXgene tubes that were also frozen and used for later isolation of RNA.

2.3. ANA and Autoantibody Profiles. The ANA was performed as part of usual clinical care and carried out in the hospital laboratory using the indirect immunofluorescence assay (IFA) on Hep-2 cells that was used to score the classification criteria; titers of 1 : 80 or greater were considered positive. Other autoantibodies used for classification (double-stranded DNA, Sm, anti-phospholipid) were measured in the clinical laboratory as part of standard care and were obtained by chart review. Each ILE and SLE patient also had measurement of ANA carried out in the research laboratory on serum samples using an immunoassay (Inova, San Diego CA) and results were expressed as Elisa Units (EU) using standards provided with the kit, as described previously [8]. Values that are greater than 20 U in this assay are considered positive.

2.4. Self-Assessment Questionnaire. Ten questions from the Multi-Dimensional Health Assessment Questionnaire (MDHAQ) regarding ability to perform daily activities were scored on a scale of 0–3 and expressed as an average [9]. Fatigue and pain in the past week as well as global health status were rated on 10 cm continuous visual analog scales. Two additional questions were as follows.

(1) In general would you say that your health is (scores shown in parentheses):

Excellent (score = 1)

Very good (2)

Good (3)

Fair (4)

Poor (5)

(2) Compared to one year ago, how would you rate your health in general now?

Much better than one year ago (score = 1)

Somewhat better than one year ago (2)

About the same as one year ago (3)

Somewhat worse than one year ago (4)

Much worse than one year ago (5)

2.5. Immunoassays. Commercial Elisa kits were used for serum measurements of C reactive protein (CRP) (Abnova, Taipei, Taiwan), anti-C1q (Novus Biologicals, Littleton CO), soluble CD27 (sCD27; eBioscience, San Diego, CA), antithyroglobulin (Novus), and IgM-rheumatoid factor (IgM-RF; Alpha Diagnostics, San Antonio, TX).

2.6. Cytokines. Levels of cytokines were measured in serum samples using the Bio-Rad Human 27-Plex array (Bio-Rad, Hercules, CA, USA) which uses a magnetic bead-based technique [10]. Results are expressed as the mean of two replicates in pg/mL using standard curves provided by the manufacturer for each cytokine.

2.7. Gene Expression. Total RNA was purified from PAXgene tubes and quantitated with a NanoDrop 2000 (Thermo Scientific, Wilmington, DE, USA). Preparation of cDNA was done using the High Capacity RNA-to-cDNA Kit (Applied Biosystems/Life Technologies, Carlsbad, CA, USA) with 100 to 200 ng RNA per synthesis reaction. RT-PCR analysis was performed for selected genes using TaqMan Gene Expression Assays (Life Technologies) with GAPDH as the housekeeping control gene with an ABI-7300 Real-Time PCR instrument. Expression values are normalized to GAPDH levels using the following formula: $2^{(\text{GAPDH Ct} - \text{Test gene CT})}$ as previously described [11].

2.8. Statistical Analyses. Data are shown as mean values and standard errors of the means. Correlations between pairs of continuous variables were done using Pearson's r. Dichotomized variables were compared between subject groups using Fisher's Exact Chi-Square Test. Bonferroni correction was applied in some of the analyses. All P values

TABLE 1: Characteristics of ILE and SLE study groups.

Feature	ILE (N = 70)	SLE (N = 32)	P
Age (years)	45.3 ± 1.6	37.3 ± 2.1	0.005
Female/male	66/4	31/1	1.0
ACR criteria	2.0 ± 0.1	5.3 ± 0.2	4×10^{-29}
SLEDAI score	1.31 ± 0.21	4.00 ± 0.60	< 0.001
ANA (EU)	63.41 ± 5.77	81.32 ± 10.44	0.30
Fatigue (mm)	5.46 ± 0.38	5.59 ± 0.61	0.85
Pain (mm)	3.65 ± 0.35	4.23 ± 0.46	0.33
mHAQ (0–3)	1.40 ± 0.05	1.52 ± 0.09	0.22
Health status (1–5)	2.84 ± 0.11	3.55 ± 0.17	0.0005
Rate current health (1–5)	3.24 ± 0.13	2.71 ± 0.23	0.034
Hydroxychloroquine	15 (21%)	21 (65%)	<0.0001
Cyclophosphamide	0 (0%)	1 (3%)	0.31

P values are calculated by t-test or Fisher's Exact Test for dichotomized variables.

were from 2-sided tests and values of <0.05 were considered significant. Analyses and graphics were carried out using SAS version 9.3 software (SAS Institute Inc., Cary, NC, USA) and Prism version 6.0 (Graph Pad, San Diego, CA, USA).

3. Results

3.1. Classification, Demographics, and Health Status of ILE versus SLE. More than 94% of patients were female (Table 1), greater than 80% were Caucasian, and more than 90% were non-Hispanic, with no significant differences between the ILE and SLE groups (data not shown). Mean age was greater in ILE (45.3 ± 1.6 years (mean ± SEM)) than in SLE (37.3 ± 2.1 years; P = 0.005). The range of ages was also greater for ILE (18–74 years) than for SLE (20–60 years); 41% of ILE patients were older than 50 years while only 15% of SLE patients were in that age range (P = 0.0029). The HC group (N = 13) was predominantly female (92%) and had an average age of 32 years; this was not significantly different from the mean age of SLE patients but was less than the mean value for the ILE group ($P \leq 0.01$).

The number of ACR criteria satisfied was significantly different between ILE and SLE (Table 1), consistent with the way the groups were defined. Disease activity measured by SLEDAI was low in both groups; only four patients had scores > 6. However the mean value was significantly higher in SLE than ILE (P = 0.003; Table 1). ANA levels measured by Elisa were not significantly different in ILE than in SLE (63.41 ± 5.8 EU versus 81.3 ± 10.44 EU; P = 0.11). Measures of fatigue, pain, and difficulty scored on the MHAQ were not significantly different in the two groups (Table 1). Self-assessed health status was significantly better in ILE (2.84 ± 0.11) than in SLE (3.55 ± 0.17; P = 0.0005). However when asked to rate their current health status compared to a year previously, the ILE patients had a significantly higher average score (3.24 ± 0.13), corresponding to slightly worse than the descriptor "about the same," than those with SLE, in whom the average score was significantly better (2.71 ± 0.23; P = 0.034). The most commonly used lupus specific medication

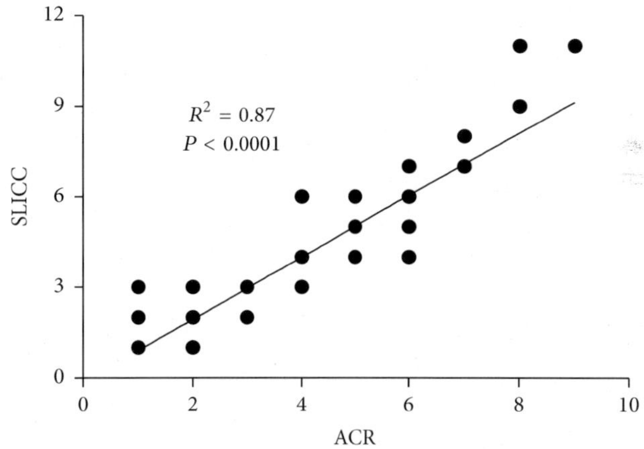

FIGURE 1: Correlation between two classification SLE criteria, the 1997 ACR and 2012 SLICC sets, in 102 patients with either ILE or SLE. Values on each axis correspond to numbers of criteria in each of the sets. Significance determined using Pearson's R.

was hydroxychloroquine, taken by 21% of ILE and 65% of SLE patients (P < 0.0001). For the complete group of patients, including both ILE and SLE, those who were currently taking HCQ rated their health status as better than those who were not on this medication (2.53 ± 0.20 versus 3.30 ± 0.11; P = 0.0005).

All enrolled individuals were classified first with the 1997 ACR criteria and then with the 2012 SLICC criteria. The two datasets were highly correlated (R^2 = 0.87; P < 0.0001; Figure 1). The same levels of correlation and significance were obtained when the 19 individuals who had only ANA positivity (1 criterion) in both sets of criteria were removed. Two of these 19 patients had more than one of the SLICC criteria. Only one individual changed from SLE, with 4 of the ACR criteria, to ILE with only 3 of the SLICC criteria. Significant differences in the prevalence of specific features in ILE compared to SLE were examined for the two sets of classification criteria. When corrected for multiple comparisons, 6 of the 11 ACR criteria were significantly

TABLE 2: ACR classification criteria in ILE and SLE patients.

Criterion	ILE ($N = 70$)	SLE ($N = 32$)	P	P_{corr}
Malar rash	11 (16)	19 (59)	<0.0001	**
Discoid rash	1 (1)	5 (16)	0.0111	NS
Photosensitivity	16 (23)	24 (75)	<0.0001	**
Oral ulcers	9 (13)	21 (66)	<0.0001	**
Arthritis	14 (20)	14 (44)	0.0172	NS
Serositis	6 (9)	15 (47)	<0.0001	**
Renal	0 (0)	4 (13)	0.0085	N/A
Neuro	0 (0)	3 (9)	0.0289	N/A
Heme	5 (7)	16 (50)	<0.0001	**
Immunologic	8 (11)	17 (53)	<0.0001	**
ANA	68 (97)	32 (100)	1.00	N/A

Values represent number of individuals (percent).
P values are calculated by Fisher's Exact Test.
Pcorr are values after Bonferroni correction of multiple (8) comparisons:
** P value less than 0.00125.
NS: not statistically significant; N/A–cell = zero; no statistical test was done.

TABLE 3: SLICC 2012 classification criteria in ILE and SLE patients.

Criterion	ILE ($N = 71$)	SLE ($N = 31$)	P	P_{corr}
		Clinical		
Acute cutaneous	16 (22.5)	20 (64.5)	<0.0001	**
Chronic cutaneous	1 (1.4)	5 (16.1)	0.0095	NS
Oral ulcers	9 (12.7)	21 (67.7)	<0.0001	**
Alopecia	1 (1.4)	0 (0)	1.00	N/A
Synovitis	14 (19.7)	16 (51.6)	0.0019	**
Serositis	7 (9.9)	15 (48.4)	0.0001	**
Renal	0 (0)	4 (12.9)	0.0074	N/A
Neurologic	0 (0)	3 (9.7)	0.0262	N/A
Hemolytic	1 (1.4)	2 (6.5)	0.2185	NS
Leukopenia	4 (5.6)	11 (35.5)	0.0003	**
Thrombocytopenia	2 (2.8)	3 (9.7)	0.1630	NS
		Immunologic		
ANA	70 (98.6)	31 (100)	1.0	N/A
dsDNA	3 (4.2)	13 (41.9)	<0.0001	**
Sm	1 (1.4)	7 (22.6)	0.0009	*
APL	4 (5.6)	5 (16.1)	0.1261	NS
Complement	6 (8.5)	10 (32.3)	0.0057	NS
Coombs	0 (0)	0 (0)	N/A	N/A

See Table 2 footnotes. P corr significance level after Bonferroni correction for multiple (13) comparisons: * P value less than 0.0038; ** P value less than 0.00077.

higher in SLE than in ILE (Table 2). These were malar rash, photosensitivity, oral ulcers, serositis, hematologic disorder, and immunologic disorder ($P_{corr} < 0.01$ for each). The SLICC criteria yielded similar findings, with 6 of the 17 criteria being significantly higher in SLE than in ILE: acute cutaneous, oral ulcers, serositis, leukopenia, and antibodies to Sm and dsDNA (Table 3; $P_{corr} \leq 0.05$ for each). None of the ILE patients had renal or neurologic criteria using either classification set. Viewed qualitatively, the criteria with significant differences between ILE and SLE are in similar categories, involving skin, mucosa, serosa, hematologic abnormalities, and autoantibodies. These results confirm that the SLICC classification matches closely the previous ACR version when ILE patients are included in the analysis and suggest that classification using the 2012 SLICC criteria will not reduce prevalence of the ILE designation, as has been suggested [12].

3.2. Gene Expression and Immune Variables in ILE and SLE. Expression of the Type I IFN gene signature that is elevated in SLE was probed by measuring expression levels of three specificities, MX1, OAS1, and IFI27. Each of these three genes was expressed at a higher level in SLE group than in ILE (Figure 2(a)). Differences were significant for OAS1 (P =

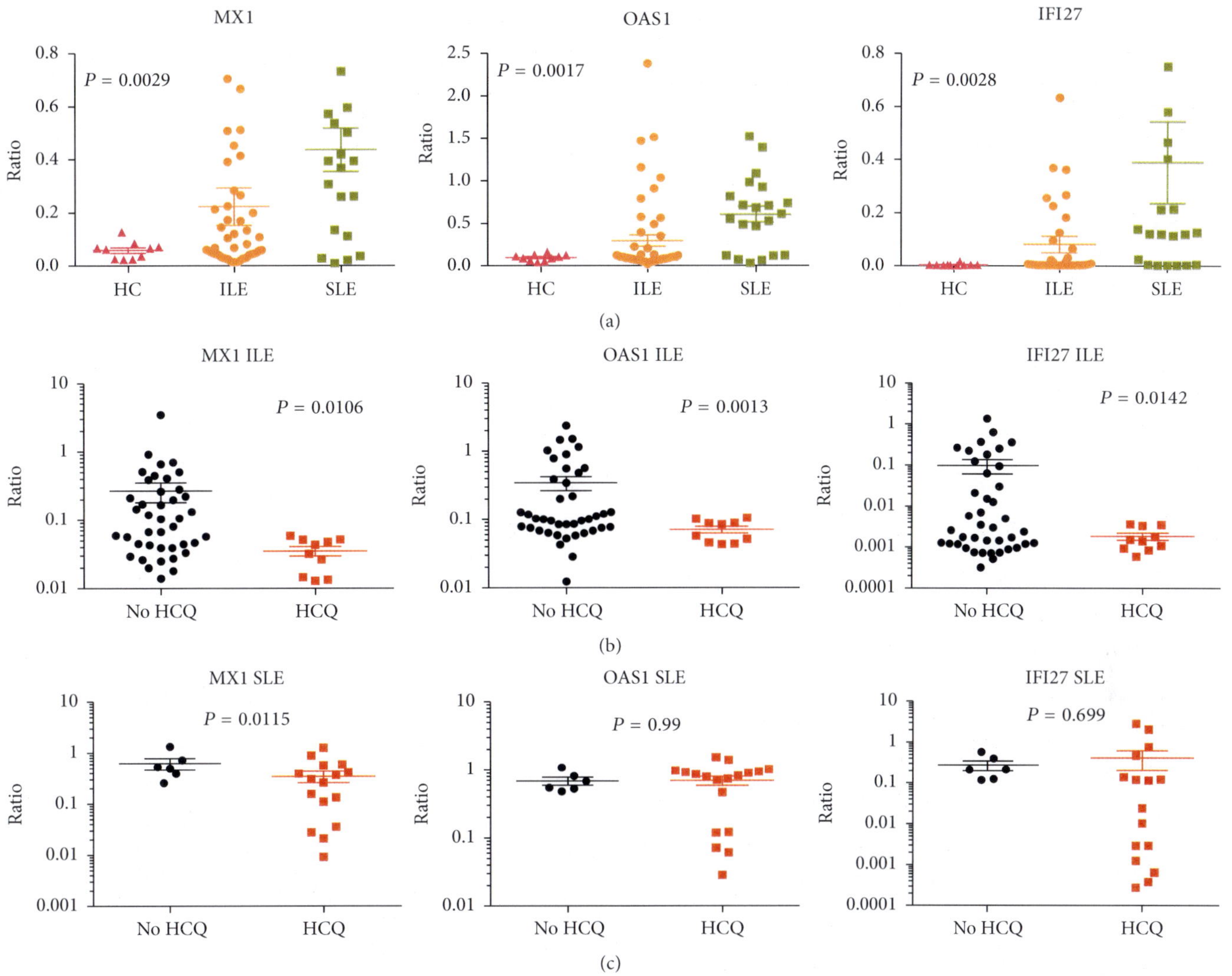

FIGURE 2: Expression levels of three specificities in the Type I IFN signature, MX1, OAS1, and IFI27, measured by RT-PCR, are shown in patients with ILE and SLE: (a) HC, ILE, and SLE groups; (b) ILE patients grouped by HCQ use; (c) SLE patients grouped by HCQ use. Values are expressed as a ratio relative to GAPDH, as described in the methods section. Individual data points are shown, with mean and SEM values also indicated. For 3-group comparisons in (a), 1-way ANOVA was used to calculate significance. HCQ and non-HCQ groups were compared in (b) and (c) using Student's t-test.

0.0108) and IFI27 ($P = 0.0061$) but not for MX1 ($P = 0.0846$). Both IFI27 and OAS-1 were significantly correlated with the number of ACR criteria ($P = 0.0021$ and $P = 0.047$, resp.). The specificity most closely related to SLE was IFI27, confirming our previous findings [13].

A panel of immune parameters was measured in ILE and SLE (Table 4(a)). Two of these were autoantibodies associated with diagnoses other than SLE that ILE patients might differentiate into IgM-RF for rheumatoid arthritis and antithyroglobulin (TG) for autoimmune thyroid disease. Other markers were CRP for inflammation and cardiovascular risk, sCD27 associated with lymphocyte activation in autoimmune diseases, and anti-C1q associated with nephritis in SLE [14]. Only anti-C1q was significantly lower in ILE than in SLE ($P = 0.045$), consistent with the association of this specificity with nephritis, which is absent in the ILE patients.

Levels of anti-C1q also showed significant correlation with the number of ACR criteria and with SLEDAI score ($P < 0.0001$ for each).

3.3. Cytokines and Chemokines. Measurement of soluble mediators including cytokines and chemokines on a multiplex array was carried out to evaluate ILE/SLE differences as well as effects of HCQ in ILE. Five cytokines, IL-9, IP10, MCP-1, MIP1 alpha, and TNF alpha, were significantly higher in SLE than in ILE (Table 5(a)). In addition, IL-13 showed a statistically significant but relatively low level of correlation with the number of SLE criteria ($R^2 = 0.15$; $P = 0.020$).

3.4. Effects of HCQ Treatment in ILE. Use of HCQ in early disease stages has been proposed as a preventive strategy in

Table 4: Autoantibodies and immunologic measures in ILE and SLE patients.

(a)

Variable	ILE	SLE	P
ANA (EU)	63.41 ± 5.77	81.30 ± 10.44	0.11
CRP (mg/L)	7.77 ± 0.672	6.18 ± 1.11	0.21
Clq (U/ml)	3.53 ± 0.91	15.69 ± 5.77	0.045
IgM-RF (IU/ml)	32.34 ± 5.42	22.93 ± 2.70	0.37
Anti-TG (IU/ml)	45.40 ± 4.50	47.12 ± 7.98	0.048
sCD27 (U/ml)	16.07 ± 3.28	43.06 ± 19.70	0.19

(b)

Variable	ILE		SLE		P_1	P_2
	No HCQ	HCQ	No HCQ	HCQ		
ANA	64.18 ± 6.74	60.36 ± 6.74	94.53 ± 19.16	74.40 ± 12.44	0.74	0.37
CRP	7.91 ± 0.75	7.19 ± 0.75	4.49 ± 1.33	8.78 ± 1.63	0.67	0.06
Clq	4.18 ± 1.12	0.99 ± 0.57	8.81 ± 6.51	14.51 ± 8.68	0.013	0.66
IgM-RF	33.90 ± 6.60	26.43 ± 7.54	22.85 ± 0.76	23.05 ± 7.06	0.59	0.97
Anti-TG	45.46 ± 5.43	45.17 ± 6.15	66.38 ± 29.06	41.17 ± 5.22	0.98	0.17
sCD27	14.91 ± 3.22	20.73 ± 10.43	35.34 ± 30.75	45.20 ± 24.46	0.48	0.81

P values are calculated by t-test.
P_1 compares ILE patients in non-HCQ and HCQ groups.
P_2 compares SLE patients in non-HCQ and HCQ groups.

Table 5: Cytokine array results in ILE and SLE patients.

(a)

Cytokine	ILE	SLE	P^{**}
IL-9	27.54 ± 2.64*	54.66 ± 23.21	0.05
IP10	903.3 ± 72.62	2090 ± 939	0.028
MCP-1	45.68 ± 4.32	78.87 ± 15.92	0.006
MIP1α	10.86 ± 4.01	364.5 ± 355.3	0.032
TNFα	52.06 ± 5.58	100.3 ± 36.83	0.048

(b)

Cytokine	ILE		SLE		P_1	P_2
	No HCQ	HCQ	No HCQ	HCQ		
IL-9	29.56 ± 3.14	18.67 ± 1.88	82.67 ± 48.74	29.76 ± 4.75	0.00046	0.31
IP10	946.6 ± 87.75	730.3 ± 78.62	3286 ± 1961	1027 ± 207	0.0744	0.29
MCP-1	43.50 ± 4.88	53.96 ± 9.28	94.03 ± 29.39	67.50 ± 17.84	0.3302	0.46
MIP1α	12.26 ± 4.84	4.32 ± 0.60	721.8 ± 709.8	7.29 ± 1.5	0.46	0.38
TNFα	52.12 ± 6.23	51.83 ± 13.26	164.5 ± 73.8	43.23 ± 5.13	0.98	0.14

*Values shown represent mean fluorescence intensity ± SEM.
**P values are calculated by t-test.
P_1 compares ILE patients in non-HCQ and HCQ groups.
P_2 compares SLE patients in non-HCQ and HCQ groups.

SLE [15]. To develop insights into this approach, the SLE and ILE patients were further examined in subgroups defined by current HCQ usage. The ILE subgroup treated with HCQ rated their overall disease compared to a year ago significantly better than ILE patients who were not on HCQ ($P = 0.0005$) and also had lower modified health assessment questionnaire scores ($P = 0.0146$).

The HCQ-ILE group also had significantly lower expression levels of all three of the measured Type I IFN-inducible genes ($P \leq 0.01$; Figure 2(b)), suggesting that treatment with HCQ has quenching effects on the IFN signature. The SLE patients in HCQ and non-HCQ subgroups did not show significant differences in IFN-inducible gene expression, but it was clear that the lowest levels for all 3 genes were in the SLE-HCQ patients (Figure 2(c)).

For the immune assays, the mean anti-Clq level was significantly lower in the ILE-HCQ group compared to the ILE patients who were not on this drug (0.99 ± 0.57 versus

4.18 ± 1.12; $P = 0.013$; Table 4(b)). In the cytokine array, analysis of HCQ-defined ILE subgroups showed only IL-9 to be significantly different in HCQ versus non-HCQ treated patients (18.67 ± 1.88 versus 29.56 ± 3.14; $P = 0.00046$; Table 5(b)).

4. Discussion

Approaches to classifying ILE and to assessing risks of SLE in this population are needed, to perform approaches to clinical care and to understand the pathogenesis of lupus syndromes. Tools will be necessary to organize intervention trials in the ILE population that may be designed to develop insights into SLE prevention. The results of the present study indicate that the 2012 SLICC classification criteria can be used to define the ILE population for clinical trials. In terms of looking for early disease candidates for such trials, these criteria are more sensitive than the ACR criteria, in both adult and pediatric populations [7, 12, 16], offering potential benefits in screening for patients at risk. Furthermore, the greater number of criteria, 17 versus 11, offers more range of possible change as an outcome measure. One previous report had suggested that the new criteria might result in a reduction in the frequency of an ILE classification result [12], but that does not appear likely. Approximately half of the ILE patients in this study were greater than 50 years of age, representing a lower risk group for development of lupus. For a trial to test prevention strategies, it will be important to focus on younger patients.

The general distributions of specific categories in the two sets of criteria that appear in ILE and SLE were very similar. One change in the 2012 criteria is the loss of photosensitivity as a separately scored point. Photosensitivity is a frequent feature of patients with unclassifiable lupus-like syndromes, present in more than 20% of these patients [17], but the loss of this as a separate criterion did not appear to have a great impact on the ILE scores in the present study. Another change in the 2012 criteria is the addition of low complement as scored item. In the present study, 6 of the ILE patients (8.9%) had low complement levels, and none of these individuals had positivity for any of the autoantibodies that would have been scored under the ACR immunologic category (anti-dsDNA, anti-Sm, and antiphospholipid). In some of these ILE patients, loss of scoring for photosensitivity was counterbalanced by the addition of hypocomplementemia, resulting in no change in the overall score. As in most of the other reports, renal and neurologic criteria were rare or absent in ILE [18] and the more specific antibodies such as dsDNA were also significantly less prevalent than in SLE.

Relatively simple demographics and clinically available variables can be very useful in assessing SLE risk [19]. Female gender, age less than 40 years, and high levels of ANA positivity are readily identifiable variables which can identify a subgroup of ILE patients at risk for development of SLE [20]. However, biomarkers that would assist with early diagnosis of SLE or that would aid in assessment of risk prediction are needed to help guide referral practices of primary care physicians, counsel individual patients in clinical practice, and design trials that would target those patients who are at greatest risk for progression [21]. In clinical care, repeated and inconclusive evaluations may go on for many years. In one cohort, 56% of patients identified as "potential" SLE remained in that category after a mean of 6.3 years of followup [17]. This long period of diagnostic uncertainty may explain the somewhat surprising finding of the self-assessment responses in the ILE group reported here, showing that these patients thought that they were actually worse than they had been a year previously, even though a diagnosis of a more serious illness, SLE, had not been made.

Biomarkers of SLE risk include the Type I IFN signature, which is elevated in about half of ILE patients [13]. The present study confirms previous results showing that IFI27 is one specificity of this signature which is less likely to be elevated in ILE than SLE, suggesting potential utility as an indicator of lupus risk. Other useful markers of risk or disease progression in ILE patients will likely include soluble mediators and autoantibodies [20, 22, 23]. Candidate autoantibody specificities investigated in the present study include C1q, levels of which were associated with number of criteria and SLEDAI score. This observation is consistent with the association of anti-C1q with nephritis, which is not present in ILE [14], and suggests that the presence of an elevated anti-C1q in a patient with ILE might raise concerns for SLE or more specifically, nephritis. Few ILE patients in this study had significant levels of C1q, so sensitivity for detection of impending nephritis may be low, and it remains undetermined whether anti-C1q is, like anti-dsDNA, a demonstrated predictor of SLE risk [17].

Five cytokines were significantly lower in ILE than in SLE patients. Three of these, IP10, MCP-1, and MIP1α are chemokines that are associated with Type I IFN and have been reported to be elevated in individuals who later develop SLE [22, 24]. Another, TNFα, has been shown to have a central role in mediating cutaneous inflammation in lupus syndromes [25]. IL-9 is a Th2 or Th9-derived cytokine that has also been implicated in the pathogenesis of SLE [26], possibly by expanding the Th17 cell population [27].

The ILE population showed significant differences in subsets defined by the use of HCQ, with patients on this responding more positively about their health status than ILE patients not on HCQ. The Type I IFN-inducible genes were also significantly lower in the HCQ-ILE subset, consistent with in vitro studies demonstrating that HCQ blocks production of Type I IFN by dendritic cells from patients with SLE [28]. A subset of SLE patients treated with HCQ also showed low levels of the IFN genes, although differences with the non-HCQ group were not statistically significant in the small sample tested. The lack of effect of HCQ on expression of Type I IFN-inducible genes in some SLE patients is consistent with the concept proposed elsewhere that once the immune response is amplified, which would be anticipated in SLE more than in ILE, it becomes difficult to arrest the abnormalities [29]. The finding of clinical benefit and decreased expression of the Type I IFN signature is also consistent with other reports showing a correlation between disease activity in SLE patients and circulating IFN-a levels [30]. Significant efforts are being made to develop anti-IFN therapeutics for SLE [31]. The potential for HCQ to modulate this signature may contribute substantially to its therapeutic effects, especially in early stages of disease.

The limitations of this study include the small sample size and the cross-sectional design. Longitudinal studies of ILE patients in larger cohorts will be required to determine whether any of the mediators or expressed genes identified in the present study can be used to reliably identify those patients who are at risk for progressive disease. The definition of ILE used here was intentionally broad, in order to be exploratory and hypothesis-generating. Trials to evaluate preventive strategies will need to focus on higher risk younger patients, with at least 2 SLICC criteria.

5. Conclusions

The 2012 SLICC SLE classification criteria will be useful in defining patients with ILE syndromes in longitudinal observational or interventional trials. Patients with ILE have self-assessment metrics suggesting the perception that they are not doing well over time, reflecting burdens of illness and anxiety that may be underrecognized by providers. The use of HCQ in ILE may prevent progression to SLE by modulation of Type I IFN pathways. Longitudinal, controlled studies of this intervention will be of interest.

Disclosure

The Pennsylvania Department of Health specifically disclaims responsibility for any analyses, interpretations, or conclusions.

Competing Interests

The authors declare that there is no conflict of interests regarding the publication of this paper.

Acknowledgments

This study was supported in part by a grant from the National Institutes of Health, U34 AR067392, and by a grant from the Pennsylvania Department of Health using Tobacco CURE Funds. The assistance of Fan He for data entry is appreciated.

References

[1] J. M. Greer and R. S. Panush, "Incomplete lupus erythematosus," *Archives of Internal Medicine*, vol. 149, no. 11, pp. 2473–2476, 1989.

[2] L. M. Vilá, A. M. Mayor, A. H. Valentín, M. García-Soberal, and S. Vilá, "Clinical outcome and predictors of disease evolution in patients with incomplete lupus erythematosus," *Lupus*, vol. 9, no. 2, pp. 110–115, 2000.

[3] I. T. Wieczorek, K. J. Propert, J. Okawa, and V. P. Werth, "Systemic symptoms in the progression of cutaneous to systemic lupus erythematosus," *JAMA Dermatology*, vol. 150, no. 3, pp. 291–296, 2014.

[4] M. F. Ugarte-Gil and G. S. Alarcón, "Incomplete systemic lupus erythematosus: early diagnosis or overdiagnosis?" *Arthritis Care & Research*, vol. 68, no. 3, pp. 285–287, 2016.

[5] K. H. Costenbader and P. H. Schur, "We need better classification and terminology for 'people at high risk of or in the process of developing lupus'," *Arthritis Care and Research*, vol. 67, no. 5, pp. 593–596, 2015.

[6] M. C. Hochberg, "Updating the American College of Rheumatology revised criteria for the classification of systemic lupus erythematosus," *Arthritis and Rheumatism*, vol. 40, no. 9, p. 1725, 1997.

[7] M. Petri, A.-M. Orbai, G. S. Alarcón et al., "Derivation and validation of the systemic lupus international collaborating clinics classification criteria for systemic lupus erythematosus," *Arthritis and Rheumatism*, vol. 64, no. 8, pp. 2677–2686, 2012.

[8] A. E. Wandstrat, F. Carr-Johnson, V. Branch et al., "Autoantibody profiling to identify individuals at risk for systemic lupus erythematosus," *Journal of Autoimmunity*, vol. 27, no. 3, pp. 153–160, 2006.

[9] T. Pincus, "A multidimensional health assessment questionnaire (MDHAQ) for all patients with rheumatic diseases to complete at all visits in standard clinical care," *Bulletin of the NYU Hospital for Joint Diseases*, vol. 65, no. 2, pp. 150–160, 2007.

[10] H. Zhu, W. Mi, H. Luo et al., "Whole-genome transcription and DNA methylation analysis of peripheral blood mononuclear cells identified aberrant gene regulation pathways in systemic lupus erythematosus," *Arthritis Research & Therapy*, vol. 18, no. 1, article 162, 2016.

[11] N. J. Olsen, C. F. Spurlock III, and T. M. Aune, "Methotrexate induces production of IL-1 and IL-6 in the monocytic cell line U937," *Arthritis Research and Therapy*, vol. 16, no. 1, article R17, 2014.

[12] L. Inês, C. Silva, M. Galindo et al., "Classification of systemic lupus erythematosus: Systemic Lupus International Collaborating Clinics versus American College of Rheumatology criteria. A comparative study of 2,055 patients from a real-life, international systemic lupus erythematosus cohort," *Arthritis Care and Research*, vol. 67, no. 8, pp. 1180–1185, 2015.

[13] Q.-Z. Li, J. Zhou, Y. Lian et al., "Interferon signature gene expression is correlated with autoantibody profiles in patients with incomplete lupus syndromes," *Clinical and Experimental Immunology*, vol. 159, no. 3, pp. 281–291, 2010.

[14] A.-M. Orbai, L. Truedsson, G. Sturfelt et al., "Anti-C1q antibodies in systemic lupus erythematosus," *Lupus*, vol. 24, no. 1, pp. 42–49, 2015.

[15] M. Y. Choi, M. R. Barber, C. E. Barber, A. E. Clarke, and M. J. Fritzler, "Preventing the development of SLE: identifying risk factors and proposing pathways for clinical care," *Lupus*, vol. 25, no. 8, pp. 838–849, 2016.

[16] A. R. Fonseca, M. I. C. Gaspar-Elsas, M. G. P. Land, and S. K. F. de Oliveira, "Comparison between three systems of classification criteria in juvenile systemic lupus erythematous," *Rheumatology*, vol. 54, no. 2, pp. 241–247, 2015.

[17] M. Al Daabil, E. M. Massarotti, A. Fine et al., "Development of SLE among "potential SLE" patients seen in consultation: long-term follow-up," *International Journal of Clinical Practice*, vol. 68, no. 12, pp. 1508–1513, 2014.

[18] N. J. Olsen, M. Yousif, A. Mutwally, M. Cory, N. Elmagboul, and D. R. Karp, "Organ damage in high-risk patients with systemic and incomplete lupus syndromes," *Rheumatology International*, vol. 33, no. 10, pp. 2585–2590, 2013.

[19] G. K. Bertsias, C. Pamfil, A. Fanouriakis, and D. T. Boumpas, "Diagnostic criteria for systemic lupus erythematosus: has the time come?" *Nature Reviews Rheumatology*, vol. 9, no. 11, pp. 687–694, 2013.

[20] N. J. Olsen, Q.-Z. Li, J. Quan, L. Wang, A. Mutwally, and D. R. Karp, "Autoantibody profiling to follow evolution of lupus syndromes," *Arthritis Research and Therapy*, vol. 14, no. 4, article no. R174, 2012.

[21] J. M. Ahearn, C.-C. Liu, A. H. Kao, and S. Manzi, "Biomarkers for systemic lupus erythematosus," *Translational Research*, vol. 159, no. 4, pp. 326–342, 2012.

[22] R. Lu, M. E. Munroe, J. M. Guthridge et al., "Dysregulation of innate and adaptive serum mediators precedes systemic lupus erythematosus classification and improves prognostic accuracy of autoantibodies," *Journal of Autoimmunity*, vol. 74, pp. 182–193, 2016.

[23] I. R. Cohen, C. Putterman, N. Jordan et al., "SLE-key rule-out serologic test for SLE using the immunarray ICHIP," *Annals of the Rheumatic Diseases*, vol. 74, 2015.

[24] C. Eriksson and S. Rantapää-Dahlqvist, "Cytokines in relation to autoantibodies before onset of symptoms for systemic lupus erythematosus," *Lupus*, vol. 23, no. 7, pp. 691–696, 2014.

[25] E. S. Robinson and V. P. Werth, "The role of cytokines in the pathogenesis of cutaneous lupus erythematosus," *Cytokine*, vol. 73, no. 2, pp. 326–334, 2015.

[26] H.-F. Pan, R.-X. Leng, X.-P. Li, S. G. Zheng, and D.-Q. Ye, "Targeting T-helper 9 cells and interleukin-9 in autoimmune diseases," *Cytokine and Growth Factor Reviews*, vol. 24, no. 6, pp. 515–522, 2013.

[27] K. E. Graeber and N. J. Olsen, "Th17 cell cytokine secretion profile in host defense and autoimmunity," *Inflammation Research* vol. 61, no. 2, pp. 87–96, 2012.

[28] K. Sacre, L. A. Criswell, and J. M. McCune, "Hydroxychloroquine is associated with impaired interferon-alpha and tumor necrosis factor-alpha production by plasmacytoid dendritic cells in systemic lupus erythematosus," *Arthritis Research and Therapy*, vol. 14, no. 3, article R155, 2012.

[29] R. M. Clancy, A. J. Markham, and J. P. Buyon, "Endosomal Toll-like receptors in clinically overt and silent autoimmunity," *Immunological Reviews*, vol. 269, no. 1, pp. 76–84, 2016.

[30] R. Willis, A. M. Seif, G. McGwin Jr. et al., "Effect of hydroxychloroquine treatment on pro-inflammatory cytokines and disease activity in SLE patients: data from LUMINA (LXXV), a multiethnic US cohort," *Lupus*, vol. 21, no. 8, pp. 830–835, 2012.

[31] K. C. Kalunian, "Interferon-targeted therapy in systemic lupus erythematosus: is this an alternative to targeting B and T cells?" *Lupus*, vol. 25, no. 10, pp. 1097–1101, 2016.

Evaluation of a Multiplex ELISA for Autoantibody Profiling in Patients with Autoimmune Connective Tissue Diseases

Alejandro Caro Pérez,[1] Sarita Kumble,[2] Krishnanand D. Kumble,[2] M. Consuelo Alonso Cañizal,[1] Luis M. Jiménez Jiménez,[3] Lorena Alonso Díez,[1] and Pilar Durán Parejo[3]

[1] *Gennova Research, Gennova Scientific S.L. Seville, Spain*
[2] *Pictor Limited, Auckland, New Zealand*
[3] *Department of Metabolopathy, Hospital Virgen del Rocio, Seville, Spain*

Correspondence should be addressed to Alejandro Caro Pérez; alejandro.caro.perez@gmail.com

Academic Editor: Ricard Cervera

The performance of immunoassays for the detection of autoantibodies is of critical importance in the diagnosis and assessment of patients with autoimmune connective tissue diseases (ACTD). Our objective was to compare the features of two multiplexed assays—INNO-LIA ANA and Gennova-PictArray ENA ELISA—for measurement of multiple autoantibodies and their utility as a clinical tool in ACTD diagnosis. The antigens included SS-A/Ro (60 and 52), SSB/La, Sm, Sm/RNP, CENP-B, Jo-1, and Scl-70. Stored sera from 85 ACTD patients and 80 controls consisting of patients with vasculitis, rheumatoid arthritis and infectious diseases, as well as healthy subjects were analyzed jointly with clinical and laboratory data. Agreement between the two methods varied between 58 and 99% (Cohen's kappa: 0.21–0.71) mostly for SSA and SSB. The frequency of specific autoantibodies measured using the two methods was more variable for SSA, SSB, and RNP/Sm. There were a higher number of ambiguous results when using INNO-LIA. The optimized cut-off values of the Gennova-PictArray resulted in over 99% specificities in samples obtained from the control group. Sensitivity patterns were more accurate in Gennova-PictArray than in INNO-LIA, as suggested in previously reported studies. A third method could be applied to determine which of the two methods is more accurate.

1. Introduction

The detection of antinuclear antibodies (ANA) has long been an important tool in the early diagnosis of autoimmune connective tissue diseases [1]. The antigens used in their detection are purified by the saline extraction of animal origin nuclei, being termed as extractable nuclear antigens (ENA). The correct use and interpretation of serologic testing for diagnosing autoimmune diseases present a challenge to clinicians for several reasons: (a) the sensitivity and specificity of most laboratory tests for autoimmune disease are significantly less than 100% and (b) detection of autoantibodies using different techniques such as indirect immunofluorescence or multiplex bead assays give different results [2]. Multiplex microarray-based ELISA assays have been reported to provide concordant results when compared with ELISA-based tests [3] with the added advantage offered by multiplexing reduced labor and provision of the complete autoantibody profile with a single test.

Autoantibodies play a role as biomarkers assisting in diagnosis and monitoring of disease activity, predicting disease onset, classifying disease subsets, and defining prognosis [4]. Their detection with high sensitivity and specificity is therefore of the highest importance. Despite various testing methods now being used for autoantibody profiling, new techniques continue to be developed and reported to facilitate diagnosis and therapeutic monitoring in CTD patients [5]. It is critical to evaluate the new methods with those being used in testing laboratories in order to assess their performance as well as to identify deficiencies of methods that are in current use. In this paper, we provide an overview of a new methodology based on ELISA called Gennova-PictArray, in comparison with INNO-LIA based in Western blot immunoassays.

TABLE 1: Source and composition of antigens in INNO-LIA and Gennova-PictArrays.

	INNO-LIA ANA	Gennova-PictArray ENA ELISA
RNP/Sm	Recombinant	Native
Ro60	Native	Native
Ro52	Recombinant	Recombinant
SSB	Recombinant	Native
Jo1	Recombinant	Native
Sm antigen	Modified peptide	Native
Scl70	Recombinant	Native
CENP-B	Recombinant	Recombinant

2. Materials and Methods

2.1. Patients. The study included 85 serum samples submitted to our reference laboratory for autoimmune testing from patients with ACTD. Patients were recruited through input clinical diagnosis according to criteria of SLE diagnosis issued in 1997 by American College of Rheumatology [6]. Samples were tested using Gennova-PictArrays and INNO-LIA and the results used for comparative analysis.

The study also included 80 serum samples from a control group to determine the clinical specificity of both tests. The control group consisted of samples from patients with vasculitis, rheumatoid arthritis, infectious diseases, and healthy subjects. Vasculitis is an accompanying or atypical symptom for a number of rheumatic diseases such as rheumatoid arthritis, systemic lupus erythematosus, and dermatomyositis. Infectious diseases are characterized by a high titre of serum antibodies which may result in false positive results in tests measuring serum antibodies to autoantigens.

2.2. Autoantibody Profiling Methods. The most commonly measured ENA specificities are anti-SS-A/Ro (60 and 52), anti-SSB/La, anti-Sm, anti-Sm/RNP, anti-CENP-B, anti-Jo-1, and anti-Scl-70 [7]. Table 1 lists the source and nature of the antigens in the two assay systems being evaluated. Only antigens common in both test kits were compared in this study.

2.2.1. Line Blot Immunoassay (INNO-LIA). INNO-LIA (Innogenetics NV, Belgium) is a qualitative line blot for identifying the reactivity of serum antibodies to specific antigens coated as discrete lines on a nylon membrane with a plastic backing. Briefly, the strips are incubated in buffer containing blocking protein, followed by incubation with prediluted serum samples. Autoantibodies present in the sample bind to specific antigens deposited on the membrane, which are identified by alkaline phosphatase conjugated anti-human-IgG antibodies showing blue stained bands on the strips. The results are interpreted by comparing the intensity of the reaction with control lines and measured by image analysis. The strips can be scanned and analyzed using software [8]. LIA strips are easy to use, require less processing time, and has a similar sensitivity and specificity to ELISA.

2.2.2. Multiplex Microarray ELISA (Gennova-PictArray). Microarrays are prepared by depositing 300 μL antigen spots along with a number of control spots included to ensure that the test has been performed correctly. The spots are deposited at the bottom of sixteen specially designed nanowell slides containing a protein binding membrane. The array layout has been shown in Figure 1. After spot deposition, nonspecific binding of serum antibodies to the membrane is reduced by incubation with a protein blocker. The microarray panel consisted of the most commonly detected antigens following positive outcome from ANA testing by immunofluorescence assays.

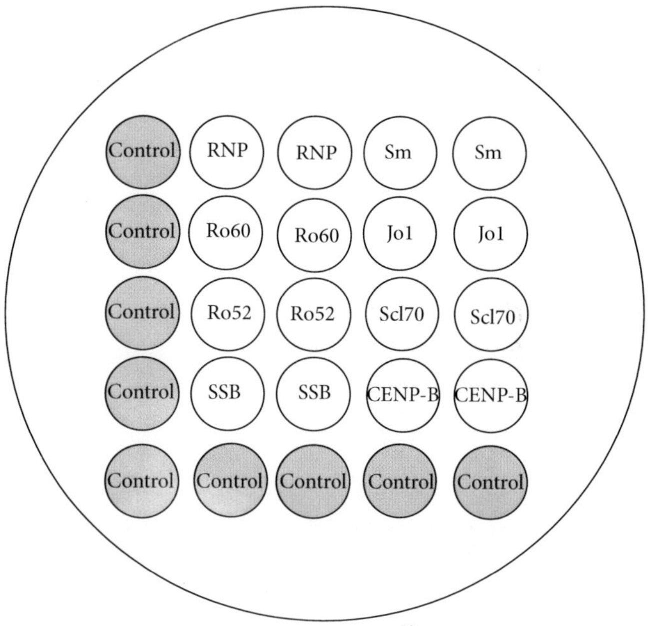

FIGURE 1: Gennova-PictArray layout for ENA panel including assay controls: RNP/Sm, SSA (Ro60), SSA (Ro52), SSB, Sm Antigen, Jo1, Scl70, and CENP-B.

Diluted serum samples were added to the wells and after incubating at 37°C, the nonbound material was washed followed by sequential incubation with biotin-conjugated anti-human IgG and horseradish peroxidase-conjugated Streptavidin. The amount of IgG bound to antigens was measured by adding diaminobenzidine (DAB) to each well. The peroxidase reaction is stopped by a single wash to remove excess substrate and the wells dried. The colour intensity is proportional to the amount of autoantigens present in

TABLE 2: The frequency (%) of positive autoantibodies using immunological assays in the connective tissue disease group ($n = 85$).

	INNO-LIA positives (%)	Gennova-PictArray positives (%)
RNP/Sm	1 (0,85)	8 (6,8)
Ro60	12 (10,2)	48 (40,8)
Ro52	37 (31,45)	49 (41,65)
SSB	28 (23,8)	18 (15,3)
Jo1	1 (0,85)	1 (0,85)
Sm antigen	6 (5,1)	2 (1,7)
Scl70	1 (0,85)	2 (1,7)
CENP-B	1 (0,85)	2 (1,7)
Total no. of positives	**87**	**130**

the original serum sample. The intensity of spots images was analysed by Pictorial Software which was developed to analyze spot intensities for Gennova-PictArrays.

The method offers the advantages of enabling automated sample processing using off-the-shelf ELISA processors, consistent performance, cost-effectiveness, and precision in measurement of antibody levels.

2.3. Interpretation of Results. For INNO-LIA results, are reported as negative (<67% of control line), equivocal (between 67% and 100% of control line), or positive (>100% of control line) according to the manufacturer's recommendations.

Gennova-PictArray results were quantified and reported as IU/mL. This unit reports the fold difference in signal for the patient sample as compared to samples that are negative for the antibodies. The units are interpreted with the following ranges: negative (0–0.8 IU/mL), weak positive (0.9–1.3 IU/mL) or ambiguous result, positive (1.4–25 IU/mL), and strong positive (>25.1 IU/mL).

2.4. Statistical Analysis. The analysis was performed using SPSS statistics, version 19.0 (International Business Machines, USA). Agreement between the INNO-LIA and Gennova-PictArrays was assessed using Kappa coefficient as previously described [9, 10]. A recommended interpretation of kappa values is 0.01–0.2 indicating poor agreement, 0.21–0.4 is fair, 0.41–0.6 is moderate, 0.61–0.8 is substantial agreement, and 0.81–0.99 is almost perfect agreement [11].

3. Results

3.1. Agreement between Autoantibody Assays. The frequency of autoantibodies detected by the two immunoassays is summarized in Table 2. Comparison of the two techniques showed a higher frequency of discrepant results for autoantibodies to SSA, SSB, and RNP/Sm. The rest of the antigens showed concordant results between the two techniques.

There were a higher number of ambiguous results when using INNO-LIA (Table 3). Of all the antigens that gave ambiguous results autoantibodies binding to Ro60 antigen, in serum tested using the INNO-LIA assay resulted in 20 of 85 samples giving ambiguous results, one ambiguous result for

TABLE 3: The number of ambiguous (+/−) results using immunological assays in the connective tissue disease group.

	INNO-LIA	Gennova-PictArray
RNP/Sm	7	2
Ro60	20	1
Ro52	6	7
SSB	7	9
Jo1	0	2
Sm antigen	1	4
Scl70	0	3
CENP-B	0	3
Total	**41**	**31**

Ro60 autoantibody reactivity was obtained with Gennova-PictArray.

As seen in Table 4, the specificity of antibody binding to all antigens in the array but Ro52 was 100% (Ro52 gave a 98.8% specificity).

The agreement between the two assays for autoantibody detection is summarized in Table 5. The observed agreement was consistently ≥90% for anti-RNP/Sm, anti-Sm Antigen, anti-Scl70, and anti-CENP-B. In contrast, the observed agreement for the detection of anti-Ro60, anti-Ro52, and anti-SSB was between 51 and 88%.

The estimated Kappa coefficient for specific agreement between the different assays was "fair" for anti-RNP/Sm, anti-Ro60, and anti-Sm Antigen; "substantial" for anti-Ro52, anti-SSB, anti-Scl70, and anti-CENP-B; and "undefined" for anti-Jo1, due to the high proportion of negative results with INNO-LIA and Gennova-PictArrays.

4. Discussion

Quantification of autoantibodies is essential for the diagnosis of autoimmune diseases such as ACTD. Clinicians can use these results as guidance for classifying patients and/or for assessing their response to specific therapies, especially in cases where development of targeted biological therapies is possible [12–14].

There are many factors involved in the measurement of autoantibodies. Patients with ACTD have a high concentration of serum antibodies to autoantigens. New assays need

TABLE 4: Prevalence of autoantibodies detected by Gennova-PictArray in different control groups.

	RA ($n = 7$)	V ($n = 8$)	ID ($n = 35$)	HC ($n = 30$)	Total ($n = 80$)
	No. of pos	No. of pos	No. of pos	No. of pos	Specificity
RNP/Sm	0	0	0	0	**100**
Ro60	0	0	0	0	**100**
Ro52	0	0	0	1	**98.8**
SSB	0	0	0	0	**100**
Jo1	0	0	0	0	**100**
Sm antigen	0	0	0	0	**100**
Scl70	0	0	0	0	**100**
CENP-B	0	0	0	0	**100**
				Average (%)	**99.8**

RA: rheumatoid arthritis; V: vasculitis; ID: infectious disease; HC: healthy control.

TABLE 5: Results for connective tissue diseases group. Concordance between INNO-LIA and Gennova-PictArray.

	INNO-LIA compared with Gennova-PictArray	
	Kappa (CI)	Agree (%)
RNP/Sm	0,21 (−0,36–0,77)	92
Ro60	0,22 (0,03–0,42)	58
Ro52	0,63 (0,47–0,79)	81
SSB	0,71 (0,54–0,88)	88
Jo1	not defined	—
Sm Antigen	0,22 (−0,38–0,82)	93
Scl70	0,66 (0–1,32)	99
CENP-B	0,66 (0–1,32)	99

Kappa coefficient (0.01–0.2 indicates poor agreement, 0.21–0.4 is fair, 0.41–0.6 is moderate, and 0.61–0.8 is substantial agreement, 0.81–0.99 is almost perfect agreement).

to be developed for measuring newly reported biomarkers for the diagnosis and pathogenesis of this disease [15–17]. Biomarkers can show a different pattern of expression during the evolution of disease [18]. In this variable context, the measurement of a panel of autoantibodies has become an important tool of assessment of ACTD patient status in clinical practice [1, 6].

Recent technologies have provided a new approach for autoantibody quantification based on multiplex testing which represents an advantage compared to earlier methods such as line blot assays and conventional one well-one test microtiter ELISA [5, 19]. These multiplex assays have made it possible to simultaneously detect multiple biomarkers using a single platform and a single serum sample. In this study we have compared two immunoassays for the measurement of autoantibodies to ENA in a cohort of ACTD patients. Our results show different levels of clinical sensitivity for the detection of the most frequently detected autoantibodies in ACTD patients.

Gennova-PictArrays enable the testing of eight antigens in parallel from individual serum samples with high specificity (99.8%). This method provides significant savings in time, avoiding the conventional first screening and post-confirmation algorithm currently being used in most clinical testing laboratories for ACTD sample testing. Gennova-PictArrays require only 50 μL of a 200-fold diluted sample and follows the same steps as a traditional ELISA assay. Together with low setup costs and a fast sample processing time, Gennova-PictArrays provide an affordable alternative to currently available multiplex testing systems. These cost-saving features enable small laboratories with limited budgets to use this technology without a large capital outlay and training of laboratory technicians. Gennova-PictArrays have demonstrated an excellent analytical specificity and sensitivity when compared with established ELISA assays [20]. Moreover, when compared with a line immunoassay, Gennova-PictArray represents the quantitative advantage for clinical management of patients.

The lack of a substantial agreement between techniques and the differences in sensitivities for detection of autoantibodies was relevant in SSA and SSB, the most frequent biomarkers in ACTD according to other studies [21]. This highlights the importance of careful selection of a methodology for the correct diagnostic and consequent classification and treatment of ACTD patients, especially in light of the fact that there is no existence of internationally accepted reference standards for quantification of autoantibodies. It is important to note that differences in antibody binding to antigens can also result from variability in the source and composition of antigens used for autoantibody detection (all but one of the antigens used in INNO-LIA were recombinantly produced while most of the antigens were purified from native sources for Gennova-PictArrays) [20, 22, 23].

Ambiguous results from a diagnostic test leads to uncertain diagnosis and are generally disregarded by clinicians in making treatment decisions. The decrease in the number of ambiguous results by Gennova-PictArray as compared to INNO-LIA assay (36.5% versus 48.2%) may help clinicians make better clinical decisions when using Gennova-PictArray technology.

The results of this study indicate that microarray assays are superior to line immunoassays since selection of assay methodology by a laboratory depends upon several factors such as differences in protocol time, simplicity of use, and cost. It is important to note that clinical service laboratories select tests which can provide results with reliability and confidence to assure correct results, avoiding platforms which require a second test to confirm results [24].

For future analysis of microarray technique, longitudinal cohort studies may be performed which provide new information about ACTD. To determine which method is more accurate, a third method or "positive" reference samples from patients with confirmed Sjogren Syndrome should be tested. This was an exploratory study to assess the use of microarrays in autoimmune diagnostic testing from a clinical angle.

In conclusion, the optimized cut-off values of the Gennova-PictArray resulted in high specificities in samples obtained from healthy donors and other controls (average of 99.8%). Sensitivity patterns were more accurate in Gennova-PictArray than in the line immunoassay, in accordance with the high degree of variability found in other studies. A poor agreement between techniques was observed. The most significant discordance (58–88%) occurred with autoantibodies to SSA and SSB which are the most prevalent specificities identified in ENA profiling and most frequently detected in patients with ACTD [25]. Prospective studies are required to evaluate the significance of a change in level of autoantibodies and to determine the stability of autoantibody profiles over time.

Conflict of Interests

The authors declare that there is no conflict of interests regarding the publication of this paper.

Acknowledgments

The authors are grateful for the support of FISEVI, the Andalusian Public Health & Research Foundation to the Departments of Infectious disease, Immunology, and Metabolopathy at the Hospital "Virgen del Rocío" of Seville, Spain. This study was also supported by Pictor Limited and Gennova Scientific companies.

References

[1] D. E. Habash-Bseiso, S. H. Yale, I. Glurich, and J. W. Goldberg, "Serologic testing in connective tissue diseases," *Clinical Medicine and Research*, vol. 3, no. 3, pp. 190–193, 2005.

[2] S. E. Self, "Autoantibody testing for autoimmune disease," *Clinics in Chest Medicine*, vol. 31, no. 3, pp. 415–422, 2010.

[3] J. G. Hanly, L. Su, V. Farewell, and M. J. Fritzler, "Comparison between multiplex assays for autoantibody detection in systemic lupus erythematosus," *Journal of Immunological Methods*, vol. 358, no. 1-2, pp. 75–80, 2010.

[4] K. G. Moder, "Use and interpretation of rheumatologic tests: a guide for clinicians," *Mayo Clinic Proceedings*, vol. 71, no. 4, pp. 391–396, 1996.

[5] Y. Kumar, A. Bhatia, and R. W. Minz, "Antinuclear antibodies and their detection methods in diagnosis of connective tissue diseases: a journey revisited," *Diagnostic Pathology*, vol. 4, no. 1, article 1, 2009.

[6] M. C. Hochberg, "Updating the American College of Rheumatology revised criteria for the classification of systemic lupus erythematosus," *Arthritis and Rheumatism*, vol. 40, no. 9, p. 1725, 1997.

[7] E. Fishbein, D. Alarcon-Segovia, and J. M. Vega, "Antibodies to histones in systemic lupus erythematosus," *Clinical and Experimental Immunology*, vol. 36, no. 1, pp. 145–150, 1979.

[8] J. Damoiseaux, K. Boesten, J. Giesen, J. Austen, and J. W. C. Tervaert, "Evaluation of a novel line-blot immunoassay for the detection of antibodies to extractable nuclear antigens," *Annals of the New York Academy of Sciences*, vol. 1050, pp. 340–347, 2005.

[9] M. G. Kendall, *Rank Correlation Methods*, Charles Griffin & Co., London, UK, 1955.

[10] J. L. Fleiss, J. C. Nee, and J. R. Landis, "Large sample variance of kappa in the case of different sets of raters," *Psychological Bulletin*, vol. 86, no. 5, pp. 974–977, 1979.

[11] N. J. Blackman and J. J. Koval, "Interval estimation for Cohen's kappa as a measure of agreement," *Statistics in Medicine*, vol. 19, no. 5, pp. 723–741, 2000.

[12] P. K. Chugh and B. S. Kalra, "Belimumab: targeted therapy for lupus," *International Journal of Rheumatic Diseases*, vol. 16, no. 1, pp. 4–13, 2013.

[13] S. L. Gurevitz, J. A. Snyder, E. K. Wessel, J. Frey, and B. A. Williamson, "Systemic lupus erythematosus: a review of the disease and treatment options," *The Consultant Pharmacist*, vol. 28, pp. 110–121, 2013.

[14] R. Vij and M. E. Strek, "Diagnosis and treatment of connective tissue disease-associated interstitial lung disease," *Chest*, vol. 143, no. 3, pp. 814–824, 2013.

[15] E. Binder and M. Edelbauer, "Use of biomarkers in the management of children with lupus," *Current Rheumatology Reports*, vol. 15, no. 3, p. 312, 2013.

[16] M. Hamburger, S. Hodes, and P. Barland, "The incidence and clinical significance of antibodies to extractable nuclear antigens," *American Journal of the Medical Sciences*, vol. 273, no. 1, pp. 21–28, 1977.

[17] Y. Zafrir, B. Gilburd, M. G. Carrasco et al., "Evaluation of an automated chemiluminescent immunoassay kit for antinuclear antibodies in autoimmune diseases," *Immunologic Research*, vol. 56, no. 2-3, pp. 451–456, 2013.

[18] A. G. Juby, P. Davis, J. E. McElhaney, and S. Gravenstein, "Prevalence of selected autoantibodies in different elderly subpopulations," *British Journal of Rheumatology*, vol. 33, no. 12, pp. 1121–1124, 1994.

[19] J. G. Hanly, K. Thompson, G. McCurdy, L. Fougere, C. Theriault, and K. Wilton, "Measurement of autoantibodies using multiplex methodology in patients with systemic lupus erythematosus," *Journal of Immunological Methods*, vol. 352, no. 1-2, pp. 147–152, 2010.

[20] S. Kumble, L. Choi, C. Lopez-Muedano, and K. D. Kumble, "Microarray ELISA for autoantibody screening in connective tissue diseases," *Journal of Clinical and Diagnostic Research*, vol. 6, no. 2, pp. 200–206, 2012.

[21] L. Meheus, W. J. Van Venrooij, A. Wiik et al., "Multicenter validation of recombinant, natural and synthetic antigens used in a single multiparameter assay for the detection of specific anti- nuclear autoantibodies in connective tissue disorders," *Clinical and Experimental Rheumatology*, vol. 17, no. 2, pp. 205–214, 1999.

[22] C. Galperin, R. L. Coppel, and M. E. Gershwin, "Use of recombinant proteins in the diagnosis of autoimmune connective tissue diseases," *International Archives of Allergy and Immunology*, vol. 111, no. 4, pp. 337–347, 1996.

[23] C. Bordet, "Test performance of Inno-Lia Ana update in detection of the main autoantibodies involved in connective diseases," *Annales de Biologie Clinique*, vol. 59, no. 6, pp. 767–768, 2001.

[24] C. J. Froelich, J. Wallman, J. L. Skosey, and M. Teodorescu, "Clinical value of an integrated ELISA system for the detection of 6 autoantibodies (ssDNA, dsDNA, Sm, RNP/Sm, SSA, and SSB)," *Journal of Rheumatology*, vol. 17, no. 2, pp. 192–200, 1990.

[25] C. Defendenti, F. Atzeni, M. F. Spina et al., "Clinical and laboratory aspects of Ro/SSA-52 autoantibodies," *Autoimmunity Reviews*, vol. 10, no. 3, pp. 150–154, 2011.

Hepatic but Not CNS-Expressed Human C-Reactive Protein Inhibits Experimental Autoimmune Encephalomyelitis in Transgenic Mice

Tyler T Wright,[1] Rachel V. Jimenez,[1] Todd E. Morgan,[2] Namrata Bali,[2] Xiaogang Hou,[2] Mark A. McCrory,[3] Caleb E. Finch,[2] and Alexander J. Szalai[1]

[1]*Department of Medicine, The University of Alabama Birmingham, Birmingham, AL 35294, USA*
[2]*Davis School of Gerontology and Department of Biological Sciences, The University of Southern California, Los Angeles, CA 90089, USA*
[3]*Department of Pathology, The University of Alabama Birmingham, Birmingham, AL 35294, USA*

Correspondence should be addressed to Alexander J. Szalai; alexszalai@uab.edu

Academic Editor: Ricard Cervera

We recently demonstrated that human C-reactive protein (CRP), expressed hepatically in transgenic mice (CRPtg), improved the outcome of experimental autoimmune encephalomyelitis (EAE), a murine model of multiple sclerosis (MS). The liver is the primary site of CRP synthesis in humans and in CRPtg mice but is also expressed by both at low levels in the CNS. To determine if CNS expression of human CRP is sufficient to impact EAE, we generated neuronal CRP transgenic mice (nCRPtg) wherein human CRP expression is driven by the neuron-specific Ca^{2+}/calmodulin-dependent protein kinase IIα (CaMKIIα) gene promoter. We found that hepatically expressed/blood-borne CRP, but not CNS expressed CRP, lessened EAE severity. These outcomes indicate that the protective actions of human CRP in EAE are manifested in the periphery and not in the CNS and reveal a previously unappreciated site specificity for the beneficial actions of CRP in CNS disease.

1. Introduction

C-reactive protein (CRP) is a blood-borne acute phase reactant produced primarily by hepatocytes [1]. It binds ligands expressed on bacteria and damaged tissues and subsequently promotes inflammatory and immune processes via activation or inhibition of complement or by engagement of various Fc receptors [2, 3]. Growing evidence indicates that blood-borne CRP can cross the blood-brain and blood-spinal cord barriers, and thus CRP can be found in the cerebrospinal fluid (CSF) [4, 5] and is deposited in the diseased CNS [6–8]. The source of CRP might also be local however, as CRP production by multiple CNS-resident cells including neurons, microglia, and astrocytes has been reported [9–11]. Regardless of its origin (hepatic versus local), the presence of CRP in the CNS is associated with numerous diseases including Alzheimer's disease [8, 9, 12], amyotrophic lateral sclerosis [13], and multiple sclerosis (MS) [12, 14].

Our laboratory has used transgenic mice expressing human CRP in the liver (CRPtg) [15] to demonstrate that blood-borne human CRP ameliorates experimental autoimmune encephalomyelitis (EAE), a rodent model of MS [16]. We observed delayed onset and milder clinical symptoms of EAE in CRPtg compared to wildtype mice, an outcome we attribute to human CRP-mediated suppression of encephalitogenic T cells [16]. This scenario is consistent with the protective effect of hepatically derived/blood-borne human CRP that we have documented in other mouse models of autoimmunity [17]. Additional EAE studies showed that human CRP's ability to ameliorate disease in CRPtg depends on its ability to engage the inhibitory type IIB Fc gamma receptor (FcγRIIB) [18], a finding which may

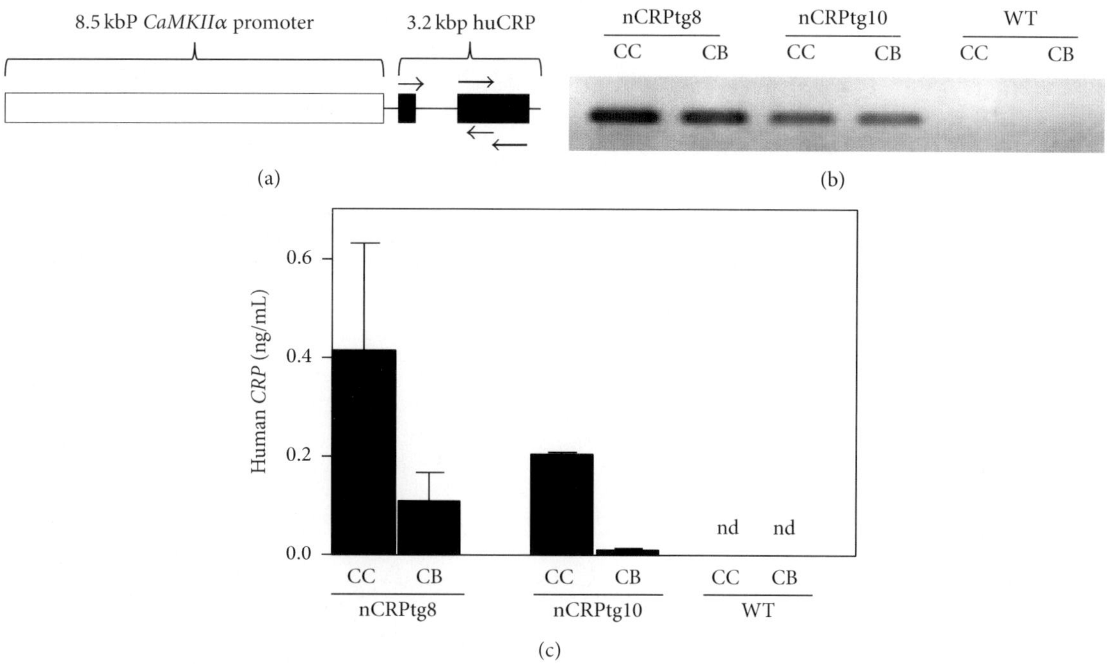

FIGURE 1: The nCRPtg construct and generation of nCRPtg mice. (a) The transgene comprises the protein coding region of the human *CRP* gene (huCRP; black boxes) fused to the mouse Ca^{2+}/calmodulin-dependent protein kinase α (*CaMKIIα*) gene promoter (open box). Small arrows indicate the approximate positions and directions of elongation of the intron-flanking sense and antisense primers used to ensure proper *CRP* mRNA processing, and the large arrows show the location of primers used to genotype mice. Horizontal dimension is not to scale. (b) Agarose gel electrophoresis of amplification products generated by human *CRP* specific qRT-PCR. mRNA for qRT-PCR was isolated from the cerebral cortex (CC) and cerebellum (CB) and qRT-PCR was performed using primers that flanked the *CRP* intron (small arrows in (a)). The size of the resulting reaction product (~290 bp) indicates excision of the intron. (c) Enzyme linked immunosorbent assay of cerebral (CC) and cerebellar (CB) homogenates from the same mice shown in (b). nd, not detected. WT, wildtype mouse.

partially explain the tonic suppressive effect of CRP on T cell-driven autoimmunity [16, 17]. It remains unknown, however, whether human CRP exerts its protective effect on EAE in the periphery or in the CNS. The present study was performed to directly address this question.

We generated mice wherein expression of a human *CRP* transgene is directed by the Ca^{2+}/calmodulin-dependent protein kinase IIα (CaMKIIα) gene promoter [19]. CaMKIIα is constitutively expressed by neurons in the brain and spinal cord [19–23]. We demonstrate that, in these neuronal CRPtg mice (nCRPtg), human *CRP* mRNA expression and protein production are restricted to the CNS and that the presence of CRP *per se* does not alter the inflammatory state of the CNS parenchyma. Unlike blood-borne human CRP of hepatic origin [16, 18], CSF-borne CRP of CNS origin did not attenuate EAE. This finding strongly suggests that CRP's beneficial actions in EAE likely are manifested in the periphery and reveals a previously unexpected site-specificity to the influence of CRP in autoimmune disease of the CNS.

2. Materials and Methods

2.1. Generation of nCRPtg Mice. To target expression of human CRP to the CNS we utilized a mouse *CaMKIIα* gene promoter construct previously employed to drive neuronal expression of other transgenes [19, 21–23]. The *CaMKIIα* promoter clone was a generous gift of Mark Mayford (The Scripps Research Institute, La Jolla, CA) and has been fully described elsewhere [19]. Briefly, a 3.2 kbp cDNA insert encoding the human *CRP* gene was digested by NotI and ligated into the unique *NotI* site of pMM403, immediately upstream of the 8.5 kbp *CaMKIIα* promoter (Figure 1(a)). The orientation of the *CRP* insert and the integrity of the resulting *CaMKIIα-CRP* construct (Figure 1(a)) were checked by linearization of the plasmid via HindIII digestion followed by direct DNA sequencing. Expression of *CaMKIIα-CRP* mRNA was verified by transient transfection of cultured mouse neuronal N2a cells (data not shown), and transgenic mice were subsequently made in the USC Cancer Center Transgenic Core Facility by injecting the linearized *CaMKIIα-CRP* construct directly into C57BL/6 pronuclei, followed by zygote transfer into pseudopregnant females. Genomic DNA isolated from the resultant pups was screened by polymerase chain reaction (PCR) to detect the transgene (Figure 1(a)). Two rounds of injections yielded five nCRPtg positive mice. CRPtg mice, also on the C57BL/6 background, have been described in detail elsewhere [15]. In CRPtg, human CRP is expressed primarily in the liver and acts as an acute phase reactant, reaching blood levels comparable to those observed in humans with inflammatory disease (up to 500 μg/mL) [15].

All mice were fed a standard mouse pellet diet (Ralston Purina Diet) *ad libitum* and maintained under standard conditions at constant humidity (60 ± 5%) and temperature (24 ± 1°C) with a 12-hour light cycle (6 a.m. to 6 p.m.). All protocols were approved by the Institutional Animal Care and Use Committee at the University of Alabama at Birmingham and were consistent with the *Guide for the Care and USE of Laboratory Animals* published by the National Institutes of Health (NIH publication 96-01, revised 1996).

2.2. In Situ Hybridization and Immunofluorescence. Anesthetized mice were perfused with cold phosphate-buffered saline (PBS) via transcardial perfusion. A small incision was made in the right atrium, a sterile syringe was inserted into the left ventricle, and PBS was slowly injected until all organs were fully perfused. Brains, spinal cords, and livers were then removed and processed. Frozen sections (10–16 μm) were used for *in situ* hybridization and immunofluorescence studies. Sense and antisense digoxigenin-labeled riboprobes specific for human *CRP* mRNA were used for hybridization [17], followed by sequential washing and immunodetection using an antibody conjugated to alkaline phosphatase. Hybridization signals were developed overnight using nitro blue tetrazolium chloride/5-bromo-4-chloro-3-indolyl phosphate (NBT/BCIP) substrate (Roche) and images were captured by standard light microscopy. For immunofluorescence, frozen sections were stained with a monoclonal antibody against human CRP directly conjugated to fluorescein isothiocyanate (FITC) (HyTest, Turku, Finland; mAb 4C28F) and counterstained with a monoclonal antibody against the nuclear antigen NeuN (a marker of neurons) directly conjugated to biotin (Millipore, Billerica, MA; mAb377). The anti-NeuN antibody was detected using a streptavidin-Texas Red conjugate (Rockland Immunochemicals, Gilbertsville, PA; catalog number S000-09). Nuclei were stained using 4′,6-diamidino-2-phenylindole (DAPI) (IHC World, Woodstock, MA). Fluorescence micrographs were captured using a Leica DMRB microscope at 40x magnification.

2.3. Quantitative Reverse Transcription PCR (qRT-PCR). To measure human *CRP* expression total RNA was extracted from perfused isolated organs using TRIZOL according to the manufacturer's instructions (Invitrogen, Grand Island, NY). RNA was then treated with DNaseI (Ambion, Grand Island, NY) and cDNA was synthesized using the iScript kit (Bio-Rad, Hercules, CA). SYBR Green Mastermix (Bio-Rad) and human *CRP* primers were used to amplify cDNA on a CFX96 thermocycler (Bio-Rad). To assess mRNA processing we used *CRP* primers that annealed to exon 1 (sense: 5′-CTCTCATGCTTTTGGCCAGAC-3′) and to exon 2 (antisense: 5′-CTACTGTGACTTCAGGAACCTC-3′) (Figure 1(a), small arrows), yielding an amplicon of 576 bp if the intron was present or 288 bp if the intron was absent (Figure 1(b)). Otherwise we used primers that amplified a 209 bp stretch of exon 2 (sense: 5′-TTTACAGTGGGTGGGTCTGAA-3′ and antisense: 5′-CCACCGAAGGAATCCTG-3′) (large arrows in Figure 1(a)). All *CRP* qRT-PCR amplification reactions were run using the following conditions: initial denaturation at 95°C for 5 min, followed by 50 cycles of amplification (95°C for 10 sec, 55°C for 30 sec, and 72°C for 30 sec) and a final elongation at 65°C for 30 sec. To ensure purity, melt curve analysis was done starting at 95°C with a temperature decrease of 0.5°C at each step. To measure expression of neuronal nitric oxide synthase (*nNOS*), inducible nitric oxide synthase (*iNOS*), endothelial nitric oxide synthase (*eNOS*), glial acidic fibrillary protein (*GFAP*), and *CD68*, we used similar protocols, differing only in primer sequences and annealing temperatures. The primer sequences and annealing temperatures are as follows: *nNOS* (sense: 5′-GGGCAAACAGTCTCCTACCA-3′ and antisense: 5′-AGGGTGTCAGTGAGGACCAC-3′, annealing temperature of 60°C); *iNOS* (sense: 5′-TGCATGGACCAGTATAAGCAAGC-3′ and antisense: 5′-GCTTCTGGTCGATGTCATGCAA-3′, annealing temperature of 60°C); *eNOS* (sense: 5′-TGTCTGCGGCGATGTCACTATG-3′ and antisense: 5′-CGAAAATGTCCTCGTGGTAGCG-3′, annealing temperature of 60°C); *GFAP* (sense: 5′-GCAGAAGCTCCAAGATGAAAC-3′ and antisense: 5′-CCTTTCTCTCCAAATCCACAC-3′, annealing temperature of 54°C); *CD68* (sense 5′-GCACAGTGGACATTCATGGC-3′ and antisense: 5′CGGTTGCAAGAGAAACATGG-3′, annealing temperature of 51.3°C). For each gene of interest mRNA expression was normalized to expression of glyceraldehyde 3-phosphate dehydrogenase (*GAPDH*), amplified using the following primers: sense: (5′- ATTCTTCCACCTTTGATGC-3′) and antisense: (5′-TGGTCCAGGGTTTCTTACT-3′). All expression data are expressed using the ΔCt method.

2.4. CSF and Blood Collection. CSF was collected using a modification of an established method [24]. Briefly, under deep anesthesia an incision was made from the occipital bone down the back of the neck, separating the musculature and exposing the meninges overlying the cisterna magna. A small capillary tube was inserted gently between the occipital protuberance and the spine of the atlas, thus penetrating the atlantooccipital membrane. CSF was slowly collected by allowing internal luminal pressure to fill the capillary; yields of 10–20 μL of clear fluid were typically obtained with no sign of blood contamination. CSF samples were stored at 4°C and analyzed within 24 hours. Heparinized blood was collected by submandibular cheek punch [25] and the plasma was stored at −20°C until analysis less than one week later. In some instances, CSF and blood were collected from mice 24 hours following i.p. administration of 25 μg of bacterial lipopolysaccharide (*E. coli* 055:B5, Sigma-Aldrich). Blood, CSF, and brain homogenate CRP levels were determined by a human CRP specific ELISA.

2.5. Induction of EAE. Myelin oligodendrocyte protein (MOG) peptide (MOG_{35-55}) was used to immunize mice as previously described [16, 18]. On day 0, mice received a subcutaneous injection of 150 μg MOG_{35-55} emulsified in incomplete Freund's adjuvant containing 500 μg heat-killed *Mycobacterium tuberculosis* (Difco, Detroit, MI). Also on day 0 and again on day 2, mice received an intraperitoneal injection of 200 ng pertussis toxin (List Biological Laboratories, Campbell, CA). Development of EAE symptoms was monitored daily using a clinical scale ranging from 0 to 6 as follows: 0, asymptomatic; 1, loss of tail tone; 2, flaccid tail; 3, incomplete paralysis of one or both hind limbs; 4, complete hind limb paralysis; 5, moribund (in which case animals were humanely euthanized); 6, dead. Mice were observed for at least 30 days. All immunized mice developed EAE, and with the day of onset considered to be the first of two consecutive days the clinical score reached or eclipsed 2. The maximum clinical score achieved by each animal during the 30-day observation period was averaged for each genotype and used to estimate disease severity, and for each genotype the daily average clinical score was plotted. The cumulative disease index (CDI) was determined by summation of clinical scores from the day of disease onset to day 30.

2.6. Statistical Analysis. All statistics are presented as means with associated standard errors. Group differences were determined by one-way analysis of variance (ANOVA) and post hoc Tukey's multiple comparison tests. In all cases, a value of $p < 0.05$ was considered significant.

3. Results and Discussion

Two of the original five transgenic mice (nCRPtg8 and nCRPtg10) were sacrificed and used to confirm that *CRP* mRNA was expressed and appropriately processed *in vivo* (Figure 1(b)) and that CRP protein was present in the CNS (Figure 1(c)). *In situ* hybridization using digoxigenin-labelled riboprobes and immunofluorescence microscopy utilizing anti-human CRP in combination with anti-NeuN antibodies confirmed that human *CRP* mRNA (Figure 2, (b), (b1), and (b2)) and CRP protein (Figure 2, (e) and (e1)) were both localized to neurons within the CNS. The remaining nCRPtg mice were mated to wildtype C57BL/6, which confirmed germline transmission of the transgene for nCRPtg13. nCRPtg13 thus served as the founder and was mated to wildtype C57BL/6 mice to produce animals for all subsequent studies. Descendants of nCRPtg13 robustly express human *CRP* mRNA in their brains and spinal cords, but not in their livers (Figure 3(a)). More importantly, human CRP protein was detected in the CSF of nCRPtg (Figure 3(b)) but not in the blood, even after LPS injection (Figures 3(b) and 3(c)). As initially reported [15], in CRPtg we observed robust human *CRP* expression in the liver (Figure 3(a)) and a large quantity of CRP protein in the blood, especially after LPS injection (Figure 3(c)). These results are consistent with the CNS as the exclusive source of human CRP in nCRPtg. No embryonic lethality, gender specificity, or unusual phenotype related to neuronal CRP has been observed to date.

To gauge whether neuronally expressed CRP altered the inflammatory environment of the CNS, we measured baseline expression of several different biomarkers of CNS inflammation. None of these markers were upregulated in the CNS of nCRPtg (Figure 4). Having verified that human *CRP* expression and CRP protein are restricted to the CNS in nCRPtg and that the presence of CRP in the CNS is not inflammatory, we tested whether CNS-expressed CRP was sufficient to influence the outcome of MOG peptide-induced EAE. As we reported previously [16, 18], we found that EAE onset was significantly delayed and EAE severity was significantly reduced in CRPtg compared to wildtype, but neuronal expression of CRP had no such impact (Figure 5 and Table 1).

Table 1: The outcome of EAE in wildtype and human CRP transgenic mice[a].

Strain (n)	Disease onset, days mean (sem)	CDI mean (sem)	Maximum score mean (sem)
Wildtype (13)	11.46 (.65)	61.65 (1.68)	3.88 (.08)
CRPtg (13)	14.77 (.61)[b]	44.58 (3.38)[c]	3.29 (.16)[ns]
nCRPtg (11)	12.09 (.51)[ns]	65.77 (1.61)[ns]	3.95 (.05)[ns]
ANOVA	$p = 0.0006$	$p < 0.0001$	$p = 0.03$

[a]Mice were immunized with MOG peptide and the day of onset of EAE as well as its incidence and severity were determined as described in Section 2. The data are pooled from two experiments.
[b]$p < 0.05$, Neuman-Kuel's multiple comparison test.
[c]$p < 0.05$, Tukey's multiple comparison test.
[ns]not significant.

Expression of human CRP in the CNS has been documented by several groups [9–11] and while local expression is low relative to that seen in the liver, it may nevertheless have important physiological and/or psychological consequences [26–28]. In this paper, we report the generation of a new transgenic mouse wherein human *CRP* is expressed by a neuron-targeting transgene. To our knowledge, this is the first human CRP transgenic animal wherein human CRP is expressed by cells other than those in the liver and the first model wherein the human CRP protein production is restricted to the CNS. Using these mice we provide important new evidence that CRP expression in the CNS *per se* does not alter the environment of the CNS, yet unlike hepatically expressed human CRP, which delays the onset and decreases the clinical severity of EAE [16, 18], CNS-specific expression of human CRP is not sufficient to modify the course of EAE.

4. Conclusion

These new findings strongly support our earlier contention that blood-borne/hepatically synthesized human CRP exerts its protective actions against EAE outside the blood-brain-barrier of CRPtg [16, 18, 29]. Our previous studies indicate that this beneficial effect is most likely the result of suppression of the encephalitogenic T cell response, which is achieved either indirectly by CRP acting on one or more FcγRIIB expressing antigen-presenting cells [16], by directly

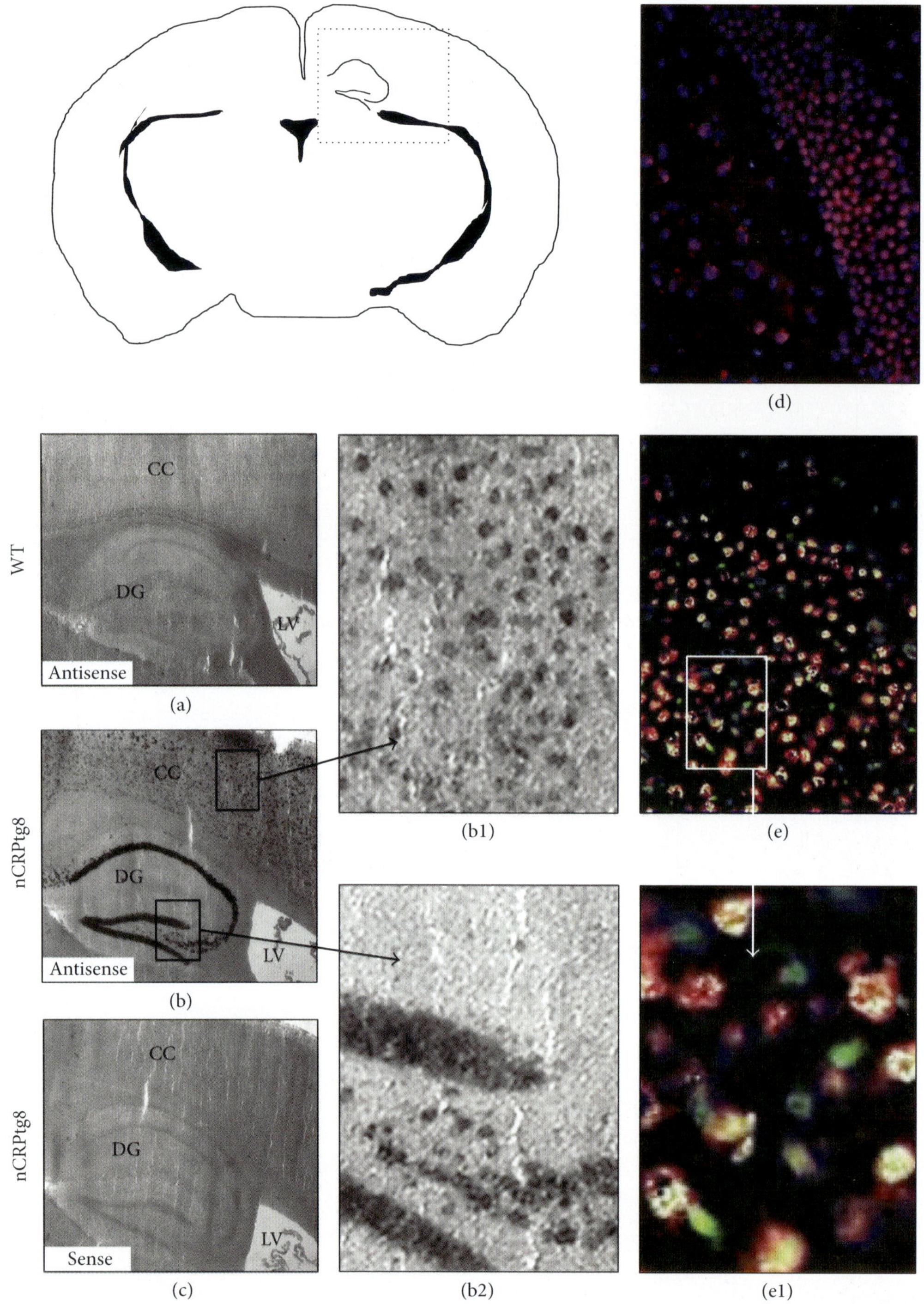

FIGURE 2: CNS-restricted expression of the *CaMKIIα*-driven human *CRP* transgene and CRP production in the CNS of nCRPtg mice. ((a)–(c)) Thin coronal sections of brains from a wildtype (WT, (a)) and a nCRPtg mouse ((b) and (c)) were incubated with a digoxigenin-labelled antisense probe to localize human *CRP* mRNA or with a similarly labeled sense probe to reveal nonspecific hybridization. Note the strong hybridization signals generated by the antisense probe in the cerebral cortex (CC) and dentate gyrus (DG) of nCRPtg mice ((b); (b1) and (b2) are tenfold magnifications of the areas indicated). LV = lateral ventricle. ((d)-(e)) Frozen sections of wild type (d) and nCRPtg brains ((e); (e1) is a tenfold magnification of the indicated area) were incubated with a FITC-conjugated anti-human CRP antibody (green) and a Texas Red-conjugated anti-NeuN antibody (red). An orange-yellow color indicates colocalization of the FITC and Texas Red signals. DAPI (blue) was also used to stain cell nuclei. The dashed box in the cartoon shows the approximate position and orientation of the thin sections shown in (a)–(e).

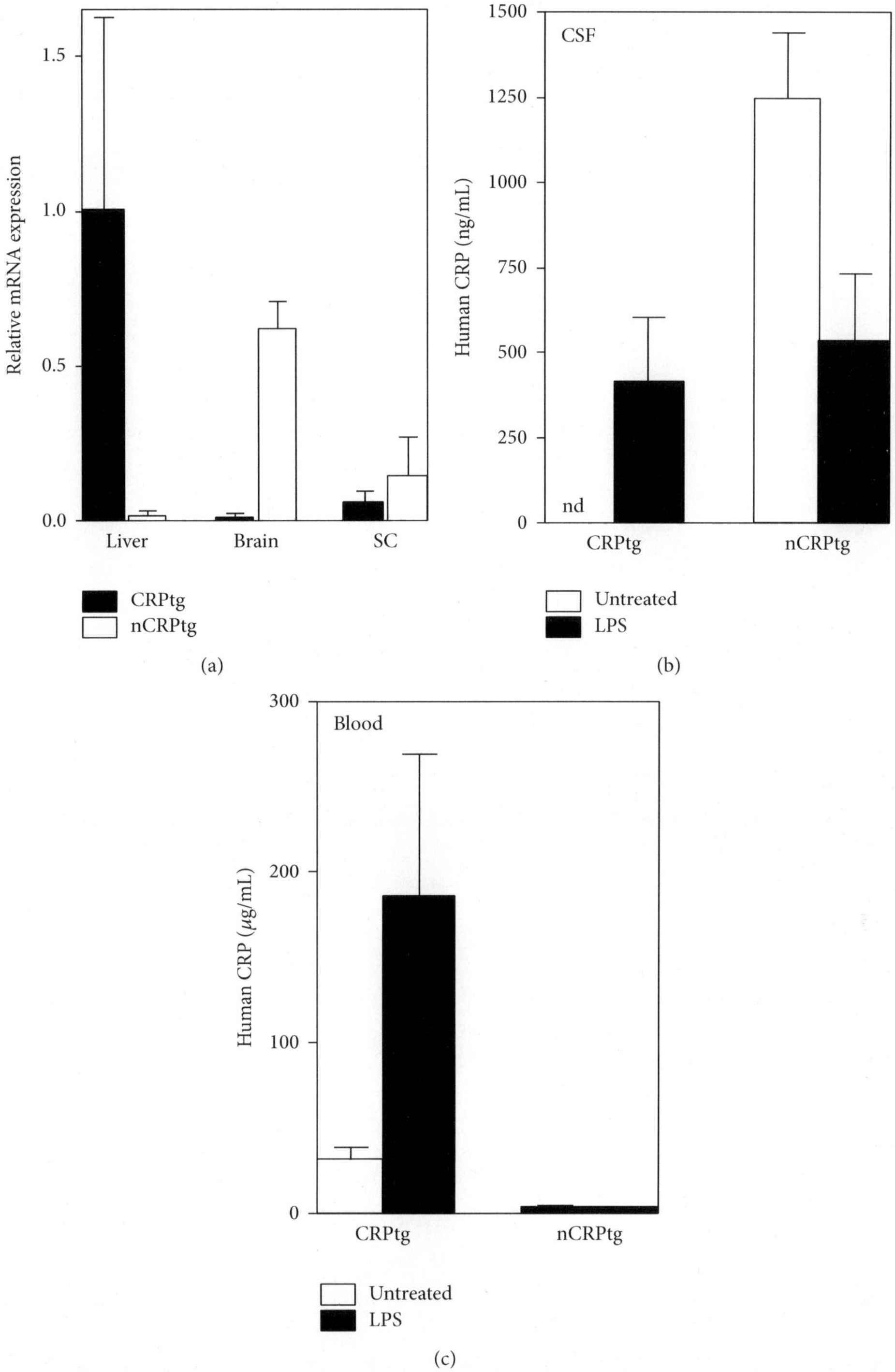

FIGURE 3: Human CRP is expressed exclusively in the CNS in nCRPtg mice. (a) qRT-PCR of mRNA isolated from livers, brains, and spinal cords (SC) of CRPtg (black bars) and nCRPtg mice (open bars). The data shown are from $n = 3$ mice of each genotype and are normalized to baseline expression of *CRP* by CRPtg livers. Robust human *CRP* mRNA is detectable in the CNS of nCRPtg and in the livers of CRPtg. (b) Human CRP protein levels in the CSF collected from CRPtg and nCRPtg mice, injected with LPS, or left untreated ($n = 3$ mice per group). Human CRP was detected in the CSF of nCRPtg but was not detected (nd) in the CSF of CRPtg. (c) as in (b), but showing blood levels of human CRP, only detectable in the plasma of CRPtg.

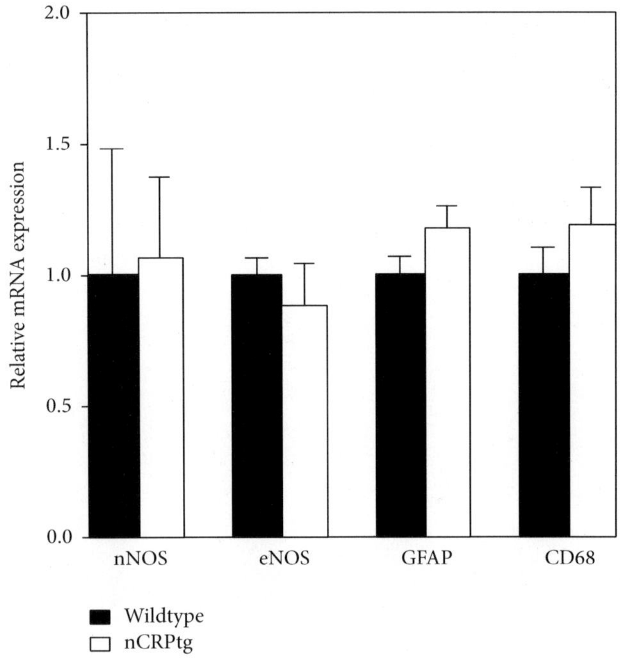

FIGURE 4: CNS-expressed human CRP does not upregulate the expression of inflammatory biomarkers in the CNS. qRT-PCR of mRNA isolated from the brains of wildtype and nCRPtg mice, $n = 3$ per genotype. Human CRP expression in nCRPtg brains does not influence the expression of endothelial or neuronal nitric oxide synthases (eNOS and nNOS, resp.), GFAP, or CD68. Inducible nitric oxide synthase (iNOS) was not detected in either genotype. Expression of each gene is normalized to expression in wildtype mice.

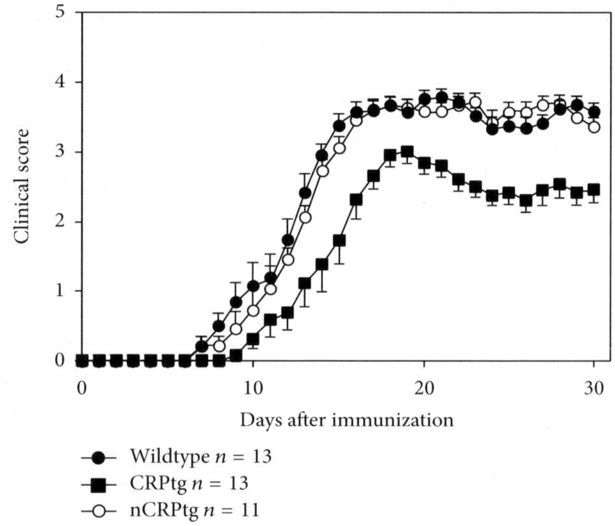

FIGURE 5: CRPtg, but not nCRPtg mice, are resistant to EAE. Wildtype, CRPtg, and nCRPtg mice were immunized with MOG peptide and symptoms of EAE were monitored over the course of 30 days. EAE onset was significantly delayed and its symptoms ameliorated in CRPtg, but not in nCRPtg (see Table 1).

binding to naïve T cells [29], or through the combination of both mechanisms. Thus when expression of human CRP is restricted to the CNS, as is the case in nCRPtg, human CRP likely has little opportunity to impact the generation of encephalitogenic T cells in the periphery, and thus it cannot act to delay EAE onset or ameliorate its symptoms. This finding provides compelling new evidence that the biological impact of CRP is site specific.

Conflict of Interests

The authors declare that there is no conflict of interests regarding the publication of this paper.

Acknowledgments

This work was supported by grants from the NIH (NINDS F31NS081903 to Tyler T Wright and NIDDK 1R01DK099092-01A1 to Alexander J. Szalai) and by Award CA 1059-A-13 from the National Multiple Sclerosis Society. The authors also wish to acknowledge the UAB High Resolution Imaging Facility (HRIF), which is supported by grants from Cancer Center Support Grant (P30 CA013148) and the Rheumatic Disease Core Center (P30 AR048311).

References

[1] J. Hurlimann, G. J. Thorbecke, and G. M. Hochwald, "The liver as the site of C-reactive protein formation," *Journal of Experimental Medicine*, vol. 123, no. 2, pp. 365–378, 1966.

[2] T. W. Du Clos, "Pentraxins: structure, function, and role in inflammation," *ISRN Inflammation*, vol. 2013, Article ID 379040, 22 pages, 2013.

[3] J. E. Volanakis, "Human C-reactive protein: expression, structure, and function," *Molecular Immunology*, vol. 38, no. 2-3, pp. 189–197, 2001.

[4] G. Rajs, Z. Finzi-Yeheskel, A. Rajs, and M. Mayer, "C-reactive protein concentrations in cerebral spinal fluid in gram-positive and gram-negative bacterial meningitis," *Clinical Chemistry*, vol. 48, no. 3, pp. 591–592, 2002.

[5] C. J. M. Sindic, D. Collet-Cassart, A. Depré, E. C. Laterre, and P. L. Masson, "C-reactive protein in serum and cerebrospinal fluid in various neurological disorders. Apparent local consumption during bacterial meningitis," *Journal of the Neurological Sciences*, vol. 63, no. 3, pp. 339–344, 1984.

[6] T. W. Du Clos, C. Mold, P. Y. Paterson, J. Alroy, and H. Gewurz, "Localization of C-reactive protein in inflammatory lesions of experimental allergic encephalomyelitis," *Clinical and Experimental Immunology*, vol. 43, no. 3, pp. 565–573, 1981.

[7] W. M. Juma, A. Lira, A. Marzuk, Z. Marzuk, A. M. Hakim, and C. S. Thompson, "C-reactive protein expression in a rodent model of chronic cerebral hypoperfusion," *Brain Research*, vol. 1414, pp. 85–93, 2011.

[8] T. Duong, M. Nikolaeva, and P. J. Acton, "C-reactive protein-like immunoreactivity in the neurofibrillary tangles of Alzheimer's disease," *Brain Research*, vol. 749, no. 1, pp. 152–156, 1997.

[9] K. Yasojima, C. Schwab, E. G. McGeer, and P. L. McGeer, "Human neurons generate C-reactive protein and amyloid P: upregulation in Alzheimer's disease," *Brain Research*, vol. 887, no. 1, pp. 80–89, 2000.

[10] R. D. Wight, C. A. Tull, M. W. Deel et al., "Resveratrol effects on astrocyte function: relevance to neurodegenerative diseases," *Biochemical and Biophysical Research Communications*, vol. 426, no. 1, pp. 112–115, 2012.

[11] S. D. Mulder, C. E. Hack, W. M. Van Der Flier, P. Scheltens, M. A. Blankenstein, and R. Veerhuis, "Evaluation of intrathecal serum amyloid P (SAP) and C-reactive protein (CRP) synthesis in Alzheimer's disease with the use of index values," *Journal of Alzheimer's Disease*, vol. 22, no. 4, pp. 1073–1079, 2010.

[12] E. G. McGeer, K. Yasojima, C. Schwab, and P. L. McGeer, "The pentraxins: possible role in Alzheimer's disease and other innate inflammatory diseases," *Neurobiology of Aging*, vol. 22, no. 6, pp. 843–848, 2001.

[13] H. Ryberg, J. An, S. Darko et al., "Discovery and verification of amyotrophic lateral sclerosis biomarkers by proteomics," *Muscle and Nerve*, vol. 42, no. 1, pp. 104–111, 2010.

[14] G. Hon, M. Hassan, S. J. Van Rensburg et al., "Immune cell membrane fatty acids and inflammatory marker, C-reactive protein, in patients with multiple sclerosis," *British Journal of Nutrition*, vol. 102, no. 9, pp. 1334–1340, 2009.

[15] G. Ciliberto, R. Arcone, E. F. Wagner, and U. Rüther, "Inducible and tissue-specific expression of human C-reactive protein in transgenic mice," *The EMBO Journal*, vol. 6, no. 13, pp. 4017–4022, 1987.

[16] A. J. Szalai, S. Nataf, X.-Z. Hu, and S. R. Barnum, "Experimental allergic encephalomyelitis is inhibited in transgenic mice expressing human C-reactive protein," *The Journal of Immunology*, vol. 168, no. 11, pp. 5792–5797, 2002.

[17] A. J. Szalai, C. T. Weaver, M. A. McCrory et al., "Delayed lupus onset in (NZB × NZW)F_1 mice expressing a human C-reactive protein transgene," *Arthritis & Rheumatism*, vol. 48, no. 6, pp. 1602–1611, 2003.

[18] X.-Z. Hu, T. T. Wright, N. R. Jones et al., "Inhibition of experimental autoimmune encephalomyelitis in human C-reactive protein transgenic mice is FcγRIIB dependent," *Autoimmune Diseases*, vol. 2011, Article ID 484936, 2011.

[19] M. Mayford, M. E. Bach, Y.-Y. Huang, L. Wang, R. D. Hawkins, and E. R. Kandel, "Control of memory formation through regulated expression of a CaMKII transgene," *Science*, vol. 274, no. 5293, pp. 1678–1683, 1996.

[20] D. Liang, X. Li, and J. Clark, "Increased expression of Ca^{2+}/calmodulin-dependent protein kinase IIα during chronic morphine exposure," *Neuroscience*, vol. 123, no. 3, pp. 769–775, 2004.

[21] X. Wang, C. Zhang, G. Szábo, and Q.-Q. Sun, "Distribution of CaMKIIα expression in the brain *in vivo*, studied by CaMKIIα-GFP mice," *Brain Research*, vol. 1518, pp. 9–25, 2013.

[22] M. Mayford, D. Baranes, K. Podsypanina, and E. R. Kandel, "The 3′-untranslated region of CaMKII alpha is a cis-acting signal for the localization and translation of mRNA in dendrites," *Proceedings of the National Academy of Sciences of the United States of America*, vol. 93, no. 23, pp. 13250–13255, 1996.

[23] N. Kojima, J. Wang, I. M. Mansu, S. G. N. Grant, M. Mayford, and E. R. Kandel, "Rescuing impairment of long-term potentiation in fyn-deficient mice by introducing Fyn transgene," *Proceedings of the National Academy of Sciences of the United States of America*, vol. 94, no. 9, pp. 4761–4765, 1997.

[24] A. R. Consiglio and A. B. Lucion, "Technique for collecting cerebrospinal fluid in the cisterna magna of non-anesthetized rats," *Brain Research Protocols*, vol. 5, no. 1, pp. 109–114, 2000.

[25] W. T. Golde, P. Gollobin, and L. L. Rodriguez, "A rapid, simple, and humane method for submandibular bleeding of mice using a lancet," *Lab Animal*, vol. 34, no. 9, pp. 39–43, 2005.

[26] C. R. W. Kuhlmann, L. Librizzi, D. Closhen et al., "Mechanisms of C-reactive protein-induced blood-brain barrier disruption," *Stroke*, vol. 40, no. 4, pp. 1458–1466, 2009.

[27] H. Hsuchou, A. J. Kastin, P. K. Mishra, and W. Pan, "C-reactive protein increases BBB permeability: implications for obesity and neuroinflammation," *Cellular Physiology and Biochemistry*, vol. 30, no. 5, pp. 1109–1119, 2012.

[28] C. Mineo, A. K. Gormley, I. S. Yuhanna et al., "FcgammaRIIB mediates C-reactive protein inhibition of endothelial NO synthase," *Circulation Research*, vol. 97, no. 11, pp. 1124–1131, 2005.

[29] L. Zhang, S. Liu, T. T. Wright et al., "C-reactive protein directly suppresses Th1 cell differentiation and alleviates experimental autoimmune encephalomyelitis," *The Journal of Immunology*, vol. 194, no. 11, pp. 5243–5252, 2015.

31

The Prevalence of *S. aureus* Skin and Soft Tissue Infections in Patients with Pemphigus

Zeinab Fagheei Aghmiyuni,[1] Ahmad Khorshidi,[1] Rezvan Moniri,[1,2] Tahereh Soori,[3] and Seyed Gholam Abbas Musavi[4]

[1]*Department of Microbiology and Immunology, Faculty of Medicine, Kashan University of Medical Sciences, Kashan, Iran*
[2]*Anatomical Sciences Research Center, Kashan University of Medical Sciences, Kashan, Iran*
[3]*Razi Hospital, Tehran University of Medical Sciences, Tehran 11996 63911, Iran*
[4]*Department of Statistics, Health Faculty, Kashan University of Medical Sciences, Kashan, Iran*

Correspondence should be addressed to Ahmad Khorshidi; khorshidimalahmadi@gmail.com

Academic Editor: Alexander Szalai

Pemphigus vulgaris are autoimmune blistering diseases that may result in significant morbidity and death. Immunosuppressive therapy of pemphigus vulgaris would predispose the patients to infections. The aim of this study was to assess the prevalence of *S. aureus* infection and *PVL* gene in patients with pemphigus admitted to dermatology clinic. *Materials and Methods*. This descriptive study was conducted on 196 pemphigus vulgaris patients (119 males, 77 females) admitted to dermatology clinic between 2014 and 2015. In this study, the diagnosis of pemphigus vulgaris was made by histology, immunofluorescence pattern of perilesional skin, and indirect immunofluorescence testing of serum. Data were collected through a questionnaire. *Results*. 59.1% of pemphigus vulgaris patients had *S. aureus* infection. 49 out of 116 were methicillin-resistant. *PVL* gene was detected in 25 out of 116 *S. aureus* positive patients. *Conclusion*. This is the first report of *S. aureus* infection in pemphigus patients in Iran. More than forty percent of isolates were methicillin-resistant *S. aureus*. *PVL* gene carried by methicillin-resistant *S. aureus* was high in this study.

1. Introduction

Pemphigus is defined as a group of life-threatening blistering disorders which results in the formation of intraepithelial blisters in mucous membranes and skin [1–3]. The four major types of pemphigus are pemphigus vulgaris, pemphigus foliaceus, IgA pemphigus, and paraneoplastic pemphigus. Incidence rates between 0.1 and 0.5 per 100,000 people per year have been described; however, higher rates have been reported in certain populations [4]. Inhabitants of India, Southeast Europe, and the Middle East have the greatest risk for pemphigus vulgaris. Pemphigus occurs in men and women with equal frequency. In most geographic locations, pemphigus vulgaris is more common than pemphigus foliaceus. However, in certain locations, such as North Africa, Turkey, and South America, the prevalence of pemphigus foliaceus goes over pemphigus vulgaris [5]. Pemphigus vulgaris and pemphigus foliaceus are potentially life-threatening disorders. First-line treatment for these diseases consists of a systemic glucocorticoid with or without an adjuvant immunosuppressant. Local skin care measures may reduce the risk for infection. The possibility of secondary infection should be considered when lesions fail to respond to therapy, and infection should be treated appropriately if it is detected [6–8]. Bacterial infection was not reported as an inducing factor of pemphigus, while septicemia of *Staphylococcus aureus* dose occurs, as a complication of immunosuppressive therapy. There are a number of possible clarifications for the association of pemphigus with bacterial infection [9, 10]. The bacteria could simply be an opportunistic infection, because pemphigus patients are treated with immunosuppressive therapy for a long time. Early recognition of concurrent pemphigus and bacterial infection, especially *S. aureus*, is extremely important because of the possible fatal consequences of the disease. The aim of this study was to assess the prevalence of *S. aureus* infection and *PVL* gene in patients with pemphigus.

2. Materials and Methods

2.1. Study Population and Strain Collection. This cross-sectional study was performed on 338 patients with skin and soft tissue infection who were admitted to Tehran dermatology service of Razi Hospital affiliated to the Tehran University of Medical Sciences. Patients with a clinical diagnosis of pemphigus with compatible histopathology and direct immune fluorescence (DIF) findings confirming the clinical diagnosis of pemphigus entered the study. The diagnosis of pemphigus vulgaris was made by histology, immunofluorescence pattern of perilesional skin, and indirect immunofluorescence testing of serum. A questionnaire was completed to collect the patient's data. Clinical *Staphylococcus aureus* samples which were collected from pemphigus patients with skin and soft tissue infection who were admitted to Tehran dermatology service of Razi Hospital affiliated to the Tehran University of Medical Sciences were taken to the microbiology lab of Kashan Medical Faculty to approve the diagnosis of *S. aureus*. Samples from the skin and soft tissue infection were collected from all patients and were cultured on sheep blood agar and mannitol salt agar incubated for 24–48 h at 37°C. The isolates confirmed to the species level by gram staining, catalase activity, DNase, slide coagulase, and free coagulation of citrated rabbit plasma in tube.

2.2. S. aureus Identification. All swabs were inoculated onto mannitol salt agar, incubated at 37°C. Any suspected colony was subcultured on tryptic soy agar and the isolates were confirmed as being *S. aureus* by colonial morphology, Gram staining, catalase activity, DNase tests, slide coagulase test, and free coagulation of citrated rabbit plasma in tube [11, 12].

2.3. Determination of Methicillin Resistance. Methicillin resistance was evaluated using two methods. The first method was disk diffusion method using Mueller Hinton agar according to the recommendations of Clinical and Laboratory Standards Institute (CLSI), 30 μg cefoxitin disk ($\leq$21 mm indicated MRSA), and 1 μg oxacillin disk ($\leq$10 mm indicated MRSA). The second method was polymerase chain reaction (PCR) for the detection of *mecA* gene (positive indicated MRSA) [13, 14].

2.4. Antimicrobial Susceptibility Testing and Determination of MDR. Antimicrobial susceptibility and resistance were determined by disk diffusion method using Mueller Hinton agar according to the recommendations of Clinical and Laboratory Standards Institute (CLSI) [13]. The following disks were used: oxacillin (1 μg), penicillin (1 μg), teicoplanin (30 μg), tetracycline (30 μg), azithromycin (15 μg), clindamycin (2 μg), cefoxitin (30 μg), ciprofloxacin (30 μg), gentamicin (10 μg), linezolid (30 μg), daptomycin (30 μg), amikacin (30 μg), and cefazolin (30 μg). The reference strain *S. aureus* ATCC 3359 was used as a control. Results were interpreted as susceptible, intermediate, or resistant according to the criteria recommended by the CLSI and the manufacturer protocols (Mast Group Ltd., Merseyside, UK). Defining of MDR in *S. aureus* isolates was done according to new standardized international document. The isolates were classified as multidrug resistant (MDR) if they were resistant to more than three classes of antimicrobial drugs [15].

2.5. Preparation of Genomic DNA. DNA was prepared by boiling. It was stored at −20°C. Aliquots of 2 μL of template DNA were used for PCR.

2.6. Detection of PVL Gene. The presence of the *lukS-PV* and *lukF-PV* genes encoding components of *PVL* was determined by a polymerase chain reaction- (PCR-) based method with the primer pair described in Lina et al. 2 Primers used in this study were as follows: **5′**ATCATTAGGTAAAATGTCTGGACATGATCCA **3′** as forward and **5′**GCATCAASTGTATTGGATAGCAAAAGC **3′** as reverse [16]. In this study *Staphylococcus aureus* strain, ATCC 49775, was used as positive control and distilled water was used as a negative control. DNA amplification was performed on an Eppendorf cycler in a final volume of 20 μL reaction containing 1.5 mM of $MgCl_2$, 250 μM dNTPmix, 1 μM of each primer (20 NM), 1 U of Taq DNA polymerase, 10 mM Tris-HCL (PH 9.0), 30 mM KCL, and 4 μM of template DNA. Amplification was carried out with first denaturation at 94°C for 5 min (first denaturation) followed by 36 cycles according to the following program: denaturation at 94°C for 45 sec, annealing at 61.3°C for 45 sec, and extension at 72°C for 45 sec, plus a final extension at 72°C for 5 min to complete partial polymerization. The PCR products were resolved by electrophoresis through a 1.5% agarose gel containing ethidium bromide (Bio-Rad, UK). The PCR purification kit (Bioneer Co., Korea) was used to purify PCR products and sequencing of forward strand was performed by the Bioneer Company (Korea). The nucleotide sequences were analyzed with Chromas 1.45 software and MEGA-4 software and BLAST in NCBI.

2.7. Statistical Analysis. The statistical analysis was performed with SPSS (version 19, Chicago, IL, USA). The chi-square test or Fisher's exact test was used to compare proportions. A p value of < 0.05 was considered significant.

3. Result

57.9% (196/338) were pemphigus patients and 42.1% (142/338) were other skin infections. 52.9% (179/338) were *Staphylococcus aureus* isolates. 116 out of 196 (59.1%) pemphigus patients had *Staphylococcus aureus* skin and soft tissue infection, 55 out of 196 (28%) had *S. epidermidis*, 3.5% had *E. coli*, 2.5% had *Pseudomonas aeruginosa*, 2% had *Klebsiella* spp., 1% had *Proteus* spp., 1% had nonhemolytic *Streptococcus*, 0.5% had Diphtheroids, 0.5% had *Citrobacter* spp., 0.5% had *Providencia* spp., 0.5% had *Enterobacter* spp., and 0.5% had *Serratia* spp. (Figure 1).

The mean age of 116 patients was 42.5±17.53 years (range: 6–88) including 54.4% male and 45.6% female. 87 out of 116 (75%) pemphigus patients with *S. aureus* skin and soft

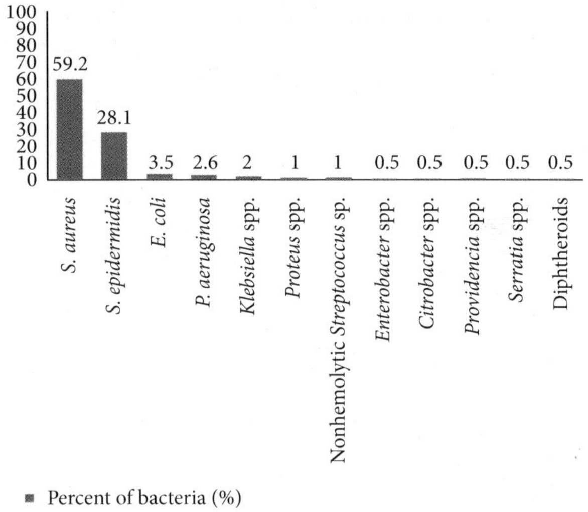

Figure 1: Etiological agents of skin and soft tissue infection of pemphigus patients.

Table 1: Demographic information of *S. aureus* infection of pemphigus patients in this study.

Characteristics	Number (%)
Age range (year)	6–88
Mean age (year) (SD)	42.5 ± 17.53
Length of stay (day) range	0–15
Mean length of stay (day) (SD)	8.3 ± 5.3
Length of stay (day)	
≤1 week	67 (57.7)
More than one week	21 (18.1)
Sex	
Male	63 (54.4)
Female	53 (45.6)
Hospitalization	
Yes	87 (75)
No	29 (25)
Nosocomial infection	
Yes	22 (18.9)
No	94 (81.1)
MRSA	49 (42.2)
MSSA	67 (57.7)
PVL gene positive	25 (18.3)
MRSA carry PVL gene	14 (28.5)
MSSA carry PVL gene	11 (16.4)

tissue were hospitalized. 22 out of 116 (18.9%) had nosocomial infection. The mean days of hospitalization were 4.5±3.9 days (Table 1).

Of the 116 *S. aureus* isolates from skin infection of pemphigus patients included in this study, 48 (41.3%) were MRSA (OR = 2.3, $p = 0.006$), 57.7% were MSSA (67/116), and 52.5% were MDR (OR = 1.8, $p = 0.036$). The prevalence rate of *PVL*-producing *S. aureus* infection in pemphigus patients was 21.5% (25/116) (Figure 2). Of these *PVL* positive *S. aureus* isolates, 14 (56%) were MRSA and 11 (44%) were MSSA (Table 2).

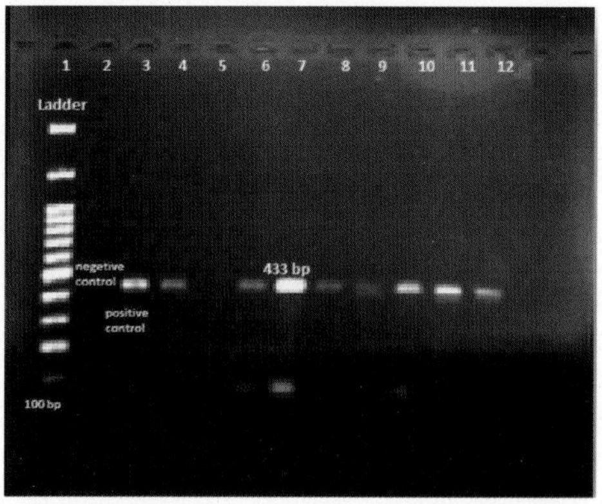

Figure 2: PCR product of *PVL gene* (agarose 1.5%). Lane Ladder: molecular size marker. Lane 3: positive control for *PVL* gene (433 bp). Lane 2: negative control. Lanes 4 and 6–12: positive isolate from patient For *PVL* gene.

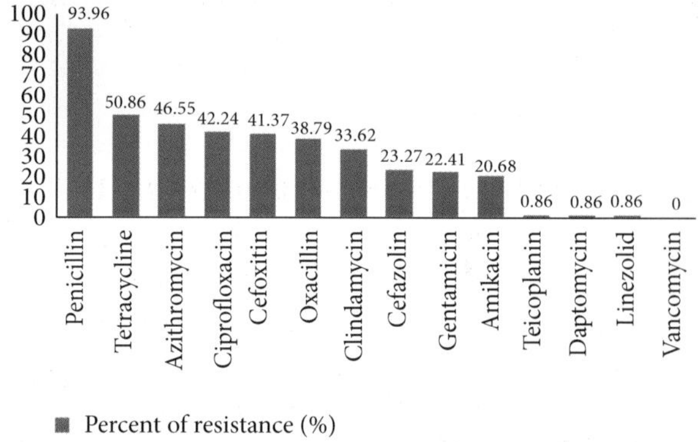

Figure 3: The frequency percent of antibiotic resistance of *S. aureus* isolated from pemphigus patients.

93.9% of the isolates were penicillin resistant; all of the strains showed sensitivity to linezolid and 99.1% of the isolates were daptomycin susceptible. All isolates were sensitive to vancomycin (Figure 3).

4. Discussion

Pemphigus is a well-known autoimmune disease [17]. Nowadays, the relationship between autoimmunity, immunodeficiency, and infection is well recognized. It is believed that autoimmunity and immunodeficiency are not separate entities; rather some connection exists between them [18, 19]. On the other hand, hospitalization in addition to immunosuppressive therapy would predispose the PV patients to infection. In some studies bacterial infections have been reported [20, 21]. Most bacterial skin infections detected in our patients were due to *Staphylococcus aureus*. In other studies in PV patients, skin infections due to *Staphylococcus aureus* have been reported as well [22]. Kanwar and Dhar reported that sepsis was the most common cause of causes of deaths in PV patients, and *S. aureus* was the responsible

TABLE 2: Factors associated with *S. aureus* skin and soft tissue infections in pemphigus patients and other skin infections.

	Pemphigus patients	Other skin infection	OR (95% CI)	*p* value
MRSA	49 (42.2)	29 (46)	2.3 (1.2–4.2)	0.006
MDR	61 (52.5)	35 (55.5)	1.8 (1.03–3.3)	0.036
PVL gene	25 (21.5)	10 (15.8)	1.1 (0.5–2.3)	0.7
Sex (male/female)	63/53	28/35	0.6 (0.36–1.15)	0.13
Nosocomial infection	22 (18.9)	17 (26.9)	2.28 (1.06–4.9)	0.032
Antibiotic usage	94 (81.03)	53 (84.1)	3.28 (1.57–6.81)	0.001
Usage of vancomycin	22 (18.9)	20 (31.7)	4.09 (1.7–9.6)	0.001
Usage of aminoglycosides	42 (36.2)	24 (38)	3.39 (1.7–6.6)	<0.001
Previous antibiotic usage	17 (14.6)	9 (14.2)	2.61 (1.08–6.29)	0.028
Corticosteroids usage	79 (68.1)	35 (55.5)	4.6 (2.5–8.7)	<0.001

pathogenic agent in 4 cases of death [23]. In our study 53.7% of pemphigus patients had *S. aureus* skin and soft tissue infections (SSTIs), and 53.6% were MRSA. To date no study has described the clinical spectrum and epidemiology of MRSA and PVL positive infections in the pemphigus patient population in Iran. Our study found association of MRSA with *S. aureus* SSTIs in pemphigus patients. This study showed that 21.5% of *S. aureus* isolates from skin or soft tissue infections of pemphigus patients had PVL positive *S. aureus*. Data from the UK in 2010 found that 20% of *S. aureus* isolates from skin or soft tissue infections contained PVL positive *S. aureus*. The result of study of Fogo et al. on PVL positive *Staphylococcus aureus* skin infections described that the prevalence of PVL is considered to be higher than 2% [24]. The study of Havaei et al. on prevalence of genes encoding bicomponent leukocidins among clinical isolates of methicillin-resistant *S. aureus* in Iran showed that 24.2% of the isolates were PVL positive and this percentage was higher than that in the European countries [25]. Indeed more than 94% of the patients were PVL positive isolates related to cutaneous samples [25]. *PVL* gene is carried by 19.2% of isolates of methicillin-resistant *S. aureus*. The study of Holems et al. on *S. aureus* isolates carrying Panton-Valentine leucocidin genes in England and Wales reported that *PVL* gene is carried by <2% of isolates of *S. aureus*, both methicillin-sensitive *S. aureus* (MSSA) and methicillin-resistant *S. aureus* (MRSA) [26]. In summary, more than fifty percent of the pemphigus patients in this study were colonized by MRSA. 3 out of 32 nosocomial MRSA cases were *PVL* gene positive. Pemphigus was significantly associated with MRSA colonization. The significant difference was seen between *S. aureus* SSTI in pemphigus patients with male gender, MDR, previous antibiotic usage, especially vancomycin and aminoglycosides, corticosteroids usage, and nosocomial infection.

5. Conclusion

This is the first report of *S. aureus* infection in pemphigus patients in Iran. Autoimmune process and immunosuppressive therapy of pemphigus would predispose the patients to infections. *S. aureus* infection in patients with pemphigus was high compared to other bacteria. *PVL* gene carried by methicillin-resistant *S. aureus* was high in this study.

Competing Interests

The authors declare that there are no competing interests regarding the publication of this paper.

Authors' Contributions

Rezvan Moniri and Ahmad Khorshidi were responsible for the study conception and design, Zeinab Fagheei Aghmiyuni, and Tahereh Soori performed data collection, and Rezvan Moniri prepared the first draft of the paper. Seyed Gholam Abbas Mousavi and Rezvan Moniri did the data analysis, made critical revisions to the paper for important intellectual content, and supervised the study.

Acknowledgments

The paper is based on the thesis of M.S. degree and was supported by Kashan University of Medical Sciences Research fund (Grant no. 93106). The authors thanks Azam Rezaee and Fatemeh Moradi for data collection.

References

[1] S. Mihai and C. Sitaru, "Immunopathology and molecular diagnosis of autoimmune bullous diseases," *Journal of Cellular and Molecular Medicine*, vol. 11, no. 3, pp. 462–481, 2007.

[2] C. Sitaru and D. Zillikens, "Mechanisms of blister induction by autoantibodies," *Experimental Dermatology*, vol. 14, no. 12, pp. 861–875, 2005.

[3] M. Hertl, R. Eming, and C. Veldman, "T cell control in autoimmune bullous skin disorders," *The Journal of Clinical Investigation*, vol. 116, no. 5, pp. 1159–1166, 2006.

[4] A. Kneisel and M. Hertl, "Autoimmune bullous skin diseases. Part 1: clinical manifestations," *Journal der Deutschen Dermatologischen Gesellschaft*, vol. 9, no. 10, pp. 844–857, 2011.

[5] N. Meyer and L. Misery, "Geoepidemiologic considerations of auto-immune pemphigus," *Autoimmunity Reviews*, vol. 9, no. 5, pp. A379–A382, 2010.

[6] J.-C. Bystryn and J. L. Rudolph, "Pemphigus," *The Lancet*, vol. 366, no. 9479, pp. 61–73, 2005.

[7] M. Hertl, "Pemphigus vulgaris," *CME Dermatology*, vol. 4, article 94, 2009.

[8] G. Caldarola, A. Kneisel, M. Hertl, and C. Feliciani, "Herpes simplex virus infection in pemphigus vulgaris: clinical and immunological considerations," *European Journal of Dermatology*, vol. 18, no. 4, pp. 440–443, 2008.

[9] S. Brenner, A. Sasson, and O. Sharon, "Pemphigus and infections," *Clinics in Dermatology*, vol. 20, no. 2, pp. 114–118, 2002.

[10] L. Sagi, Y. Sherer, H. Trau, and Y. Shoenfeld, "Pemphigus and infectious agents," *Autoimmunity Reviews*, vol. 8, no. 1, pp. 33–35, 2008.

[11] T. L. Bannerman, S. Peacock, P. Murray et al., "Staphylococcus, micrococcus, and other catalase-positive cocci," in *Manual of Clinical Microbiology*, vol. 1, pp. 390–411, 9th edition, 2006.

[12] M. Cheesbrough, *District Laboratory Practice in Tropical Countries*, Cambridge University Press, New York, NY, USA, 2006.

[13] CLSI, "Performance standards for antimicrobial susceptibility testing," 24nd Informational Supplement M100-S24, CLSI, Wayne, Pa, USA, 2014.

[14] K. Murakami, W. Minamide, K. Wada, E. Nakamura, H. Teraoka, and S. Watanabe, "Identification of methicillin-resistant strains of staphylococci by polymerase chain reaction," *Journal of Clinical Microbiology*, vol. 29, no. 10, pp. 2240–2244, 1991.

[15] A.-P. Magiorakos, A. Srinivasan, R. B. Carey et al., "Multidrug-resistant, extensively drug-resistant and pandrug-resistant bacteria: an international expert proposal for interim standard definitions for acquired resistance," *Clinical Microbiology and Infection*, vol. 18, no. 3, pp. 268–281, 2012.

[16] G. Lina, Y. Piémont, F. Godail-Gamot et al., "Involvement of Panton-Valentine leukocidin-producing Staphylococcus aureus in primary skin infections and pneumonia," *Clinical Infectious Diseases*, vol. 29, no. 5, pp. 1128–1132, 1999.

[17] M. Hertl and R. Eming, "Autoimmune skin disorders, pemphigus," in *Autoimmune Diseases of the Skin (Pathogenesis, Diagnosis, Management)*, pp. 33–63, 2011.

[18] A. P. Grammatikos and G. C. Tsokos, "Immunodeficiency and autoimmunity: lessons from systemic lupus erythematosus," *Trends in Molecular Medicine*, vol. 18, no. 2, pp. 101–108, 2012.

[19] T. P. Atkinson, "Immune deficiency and autoimmunity," *Current Opinion in Rheumatology*, vol. 24, no. 5, pp. 515–521, 2012.

[20] F. Z. Belgnaoui, K. Senouci, H. Chraibi et al., "Prédisposition aux infections des malades ayant un pemphigus: étude rétrospective de 141 cas," *La Presse Médicale*, vol. 36, no. 11, part 1, pp. 1563–1569, 2007.

[21] N. Esmaili, H. Mortazavi, P. Noormohammadpour et al., "Pemphigus vulgaris and infections: a retrospective study on 155 patients," *Autoimmune Diseases*, vol. 2013, Article ID 834295, 5 pages, 2013.

[22] N. Chmurova and D. Svecova, "Pemphigus vulgaris: a 11-year review," *Bratislava Medical Journal*, vol. 110, no. 8, pp. 500–503, 2009.

[23] A. J. Kanwar and S. Dhar, "Factors responsible for death in patients with pemphigus," *Journal of Dermatology*, vol. 21, no. 9, pp. 655–659, 1994.

[24] A. Fogo, N. Kemp, and R. Morris-Jones, "PVL positive *Staphylococcus aureus* skin infections," *British Medical Journal*, vol. 343, Article ID d5343, 2011.

[25] S. A. Havaei, S. O. Moghadam, M. R. Pourmand, and J. Faghri, "Prevalence of genes encoding bi-component leukocidins among clinical isolates of methicillin-resistant Staphylococcus aureus," *Iranian Journal of Public Health*, vol. 39, no. 1, pp. 8–14, 2010.

[26] A. Holmes, M. Ganner, S. McGuane, T. L. Pitt, B. D. Cookson, and A. M. Kearns, "*Staphylococcus aureus* isolates carrying Panton-Valentine leucocidin genes in England and Wales: frequency, characterization, and association with clinical disease," *Journal of Clinical Microbiology*, vol. 43, no. 5, pp. 2384–2390, 2005.

32

Rituximab for Remission Induction and Maintenance in Refractory Systemic Lupus Erythematosus

Fabio Bonilla-Abadía,[1] Nicolás Coronel Restrepo,[2] Gabriel J. Tobón,[1] Andrés F. Echeverri,[1] Evelyn Muñoz-Buitrón,[3] Andres Mauricio Castro,[3] Mercedes Andrade Bejarano,[4] and Carlos A. Cañas[1]

[1] *Rheumatology Unit, Fundación Valle del Lili, ICESI University, Carrera 98 18-49, Cali, Colombia*
[2] *Internal Medicine Unit, Fundación Valle del Lili, CES University, Cali, Colombia*
[3] *Clinical Research Unit, Fundación Valle del Lili, Cali, Colombia*
[4] *School of Statistics, Universidad del Valle, Cali, Colombia*

Correspondence should be addressed to Fabio Bonilla-Abadía; fbac1982@hotmail.com

Academic Editor: Juan-Manuel Anaya

Systemic lupus erythematosus (SLE) is a chronic inflammatory autoimmune disease with high morbidity if untreated. Sometimes, despite aggressive treatments, the disease remains active with cumulative organic damage. We conducted a retrospective and descriptive observational study of patients with SLE refractory to conventional treatment who were treated with rituximab (RTX) as remission induction therapy and maintenance. There was a significant reduction in the conventional immunosuppressive drug dose and the number of relapses of disease. RTX appeared to be effective and safe for the induction and maintenance of remission in patient with SLE refractory to conventional treatment.

1. Introduction

Systemic lupus erythematosus (SLE) is a chronic inflammatory autoimmune disease with no permanent cure or high morbidity if left untreated [1]. Sometimes, despite aggressive treatments with high dose of glucocorticoids and immunosuppressive drugs, the disease remains active with cumulative organic damage [2]. The disease severity appears to be higher in Hispanics compared to Caucasians. Thus, the overall survival rates vary by race and ethnic background with a 5-year survival rate of approximately 95% among whites, 90% among blacks, and 87% among Hispanics [3]. The management of patients with SLE depends on the type of organ involvement and severity of the disease. When manifestations are severe, with threatening life conditions, the treatment is based on high-dose steroids, plasmapheresis, intravenous gamma globulin, and various types of immunosuppressants such as cyclophosphamide, azathioprine, or mofetil mycophenolate [4]. Some patients remain with active disease despite full immunosuppressive drugs. Two monoclonal antibodies targeting B cells have been used successfully in refractory SLE: belimumab directed against B-cell activating factor (BAFF) [5] and Rituximab which is a genetically engineered chimeric anti-CD20 monoclonal antibody. CD20 is a B-cell surface antigen that is expressed only on pre-B and mature B cells. It is not present on stem cells and is lost before differentiation of B cells into plasma cells. Therefore, rituximab causes a selective transient depletion of the CD20+ B-cell subpopulation [6]. Rituximab (RTX) is currently approved for the management of B-cell lymphomas, rheumatoid arthritis (RA) and systemic vasculitis ANCA (antineutrophil cytoplasmic antibodies) positive [7, 8], and it is used as a single dose for SLE crisis with varying results [9–11]. There are few reports in the literature about routine and chronic use of RTX as a maintenance drug therapy in SLE [12]. Being a chronic and incurable disease with high rates of relapse, we decide to treat indefinitely a group of patients that previously had favorable response to single doses. In this study, we evaluate the efficacy and safety of RTX both as a rescue and maintenance agent in a group of patients with refractory SLE.

2. Patients and Methods

The data was taken from the electronic medical records of patients at a fourth-level center (Fundación Valle del Lili) in Cali, Colombia, throughout twelve years (from August/2001 to April/2013). Patients were eligible for the study if they had provided authorization for review of their medical records, were older than 18 years old at the time of the study, had a diagnosis of SLE based on the criteria of the American College of Rheumatology [13], and had refractory SLE to conventional treatments: hydroxychloroquine, high dose steroids, cyclophosphamide, azathioprine, and mofetil mycophenolate, which despite receiving recommended doses and validated protocols in the adequate time persisted with active disease (defined as a SLEDAI score higher than 4) [14]. Patients with active infections or cancer were excluded from the study. Medical records were reviewed and demographic and clinical data, including the number of RTX cycles, frequency and severity of relapses, glucocorticoids doses, and type and doses of conventional immune-suppressor agents, were collected. Assess of lupus activity was done with SLEDAI score [15]. Patients with refractory SLE were treated with RTX both as rescue medication for lupus flare and for maintenance (dose of 1 gr at day 0 and 1 gr at day 15 with retreatment every 9 months). Administration of acetaminophen 1 g, diphenhydramine 50 mg, and prednisone 50 mg prior to each RTX infusion was done. RTX was given as additional agent to the treatment received. We did not use the CD20+ cell counts as an indicator of the moment to retreat these patients.

2.1. Statistical Analysis. An exploratory analysis of the data was made using percentages for categorical variables and medians (interquartile range (IQR)) for continuous variables. The Wilcoxon nonparametric test was done for comparisons. Data analysis was done using STATA 1.2. software. P values less than 0.05 were considered significant for all statistical tests. The study was approved by the ethics committee of Fundación Valle del Lili research center.

3. Results

Out of 350 patients of the initial cohort, eighteen patients with refractory and active SLE were included in the analysis. Seventeen out of eighteen patients were women and all patients were Hispanic. The median age was 28.5 years (range: 22–36). At the time of inclusion, median SLEDAI score was 12.5 (range: 8–18). Median initial doses were as follow: prednisone, 25 mg/day (range: 15–20); mofetil mycophenolate, 2.0 gr/day; azathioprine, 100 mg/day (2 mg/kg/day); hydroxychloroquine, 200 mgr/day; and endovenous cyclophosphamide, 750 mgr each month. The mean follow-up was 37.5 months (range: 18–63) with a mean average of 5 RTX cycles (range: 3–8). Baseline clinical characteristics, treatment history, and refractory organ system involvement in these 18 patients at the time of their first RTX course are described in Table 1. At the end of follow-up, SLEDAI score was 0 in fourteen patients, 2 in three patients, and 4 in one patient ($P = 0.0002$)—(Table 2 and Figure 1). Median prednisone dose at the end of follow-up was 3.75 mg/day (range: 2.5–5) ($P = 0.0002$). In addition, mofetil mycophenolate and azathioprine were both discontinued in all patients ($P = 0.0071$ and $P = 0.052$, resp., compared to baseline), and hydroxychloroquine median dose decreased to 75 mgr/day. The median relapses rate at the beginning of RTX treatment was 3 per year (IQR 3–5), decreasing to 0 (IQR 0-1) at the end of follow-up.

Because the use of RTX in rescue dose in our patients with acute disease was favorable in all but one, we decided to retreat them every nine months.

Three patients presented an adverse reaction to RTX at the first course of treatment consistent with cytokine release syndrome [16]. However, the application of the drug was not suspended in these cases, and a desensitization protocol was successfully performed in the hospital.

Table 1: Baseline characteristics of the 18 systemic lupus erythematosus patients and their main refractory and active involvement.

Characteristics	Values (n = 18)
Age, years*	28.5 (22–36)
Female, Gender	17 (94.4)
Prednisone dose*	25 (15–50)
Use of Azathioprine	5 (27)
Use of Cyclophosphamide	6 (33)
Use of Mycophenolate	9 (50)
Use of Hydroxychloroquine	11 (61)
Relapses/year*	3 (3–5)
Renal criteria**	11 (61.1)
Hematological criteria***	13 (72.2)
Cardiopulmonary criteria	8 (44.4)
Musculoskeletal criteria	14 (77.8)
Low C3	13 (72.2)
Low C4	10 (55.6)
Anti-DNA positive	9 (50)

All the data correspond to n (%) with the exemption of those marked with *.
*Median IQR (interquartile range).
**Proteinuria (higher than 0.5 g/day), casts (erythrocytes, hemoglobin, granular, tubular, or mixed), hematuria, and pyuria.
***Leukopenia (less than 4.000 cells/mm^3), thrombocytopenia (less than 100.000 cells/mm^3), and hemolytic anemia.

4. Discussion

Here, we present a case series that evaluated and demonstrated safety and efficacy of RTX therapy in induction and maintenance for the treatment of SLE.

Two randomized clinical trials have been published trying to prove the clinical effectiveness of RTX in SLE

TABLE 2: SLEDAI Score in the initial and at the end of the last cycle of RTX.

(a)

Patient	SLEDAI score	
	Beginning	End
1	40	0
2	8	0
3	14	0
4	18	2
5	14	0
6	8	2
7	18	0
8	8	0
9	7	0
10	11	0
11	8	0
12	14	0
13	22	2
14	14	0
15	6	0
16	22	4
17	11	0
18	9	0

(b)

	Beginning	End	*P* value
Score	12.5 (8–18)	0 (0-0)	$P = 0.0002$

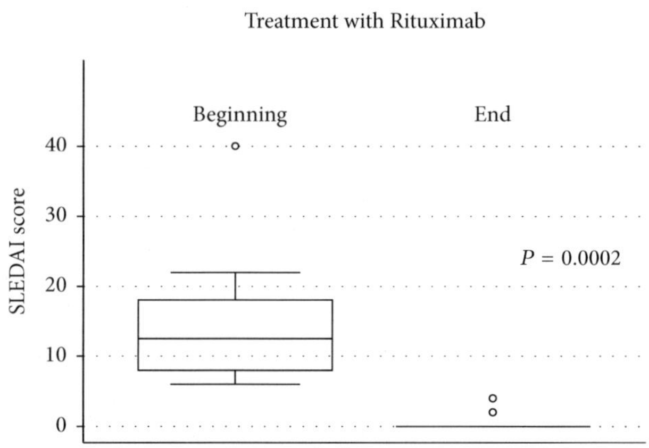

FIGURE 1: Box plot diagram of the SLEDAI score at the beginning and at the end of the last cycle of RTX.

with mixed results. The EXPLORER study [9], a case-control study conducted in 257 patients with extrarenal SLE, showed no statistical significance in reduction in disease activity between RTX and conventional immunosuppressive therapy. The LUNAR study [10] randomized 144 patients to receive either RTX or placebo, under a mofetil-mycophenolate-based immunosuppression and steroids, showing a significant improvement in the levels of C3, C4, and anti-DNA but no differences in renal response rates at week 52 of treatment. Pinto et al. [11] conducted a prospective study of a cohort of 42 patients with refractory SLE in Colombia, adding RTX as a rescue therapy in one initial dose, with 36% of the patients showing complete remission and an overall significant reduction in steroid use. The preferred scheme used for ablation of B cells with RTX was an initial dose of 1 g and then 1 g in two weeks. Subsequent doses were not indicated. The excellent clinical response in Colombian patients may be explained by racial grounds, which has been shown in the present study and in other recent publications included Latin American population [17–19]. All patients including in our series were mestizos. More studies are needed to confirm these findings.

Our scheme was done based on the protocols used in RA patients and as now it is beginning to be recommended in refractory granulomatosis with polyangiitis [20]. All patients showed to the end of the study remission criteria. This follow-up study showed that depletion of B lymphocytes with repeated RTX is effective and safe in patients with SLE. A decrease in the number of relapses by disease activity was also evident. Relapses were prevented with RTX retreatment and conventional immunosuppressive doses were decreased gradually. Adverse events related to the infusion were few and there was no contraindication for retreatment with RTX. All patients in this cohort reached remission of the disease.

One of the most interesting findings and strengths of this study is that only few reports have shown the effectiveness of RTX retreatment in SLE patients, as used in a routine way in rheumatoid arthritis patients and not only at the moment of refractory involvement. Several shortcomings are presented in our study. First of all, this is a retrospective series, and no randomized assessment was done. In addition, only 18 patients were evaluated and no B-cell count was done to define the adequate moment to retreatment.

In conclusion, RTX seems to be effective and safe for the induction and maintenance of remission in Colombian mestizo patients with SLE refractory to conventional immunosuppressive therapy. Our results provide important information for the design of future studies in order to confirm the results obtained here.

Conflict of Interests

The authors declare that there is no conflict of interests regarding the publication of this paper.

References

[1] R. Cervera, M. A. Khamashta, J. Font et al., "Morbidity and mortality in systemic lupus erythematosus during a 10-year period: a comparison of early and late manifestations in a cohort of 1.000 patients," *Medicine*, vol. 82, no. 5, pp. 299–308, 2003.

[2] G. C. Tsokos, "Mechanisms of disease: systemic lupus erythematosus," *The New England Journal of Medicine*, vol. 365, no. 22, pp. 2110–2121, 2011.

[3] G. J. Pons-Estel, G. S. Alarcón, L. Scofield, L. Reinlib, and G. S. Cooper, "Unde rsta nding the epidemiology a nd progression

of s ys temic lupus erythematosus," *Seminars in Arthritis and Rheumatism*, vol. 39, pp. 257–268, 2010.

[4] G. Bertsias, J. P. A. Ioannidis, J. Boletis et al., "EULAR recommendations for the management of SLE," *Annals of the Rheumatic Diseases*, vol. 67, no. 2, pp. 195–205, 2008.

[5] P. K. Chugh and B. S. Kalra, "Belimumab: targeted therapy for lupus," *International Journal of Rheumatic Diseases*, vol. 16, pp. 4–13, 2013.

[6] L. Lan, F. Han, and J. H. Chen, "Efficacy and safety of rituximab therapy for systemic lupus erythematosus: a systematic review and meta-analysis," *Journal of Zhejiang University-Science B*, vol. 13, pp. 731–744, 2012.

[7] J. H. Stone, P. A. Merkel, R. Spiera et al., "Rituximab versus cyclophosphamide for ANCA-associated vasculitis," *The New England Journal of Medicine*, vol. 363, no. 3, pp. 221–232, 2010.

[8] R. B. Jones, J. W. C. Tervaert, T. Hauser et al., "Rituximab versus cyclophosphamide in ANCA-associated renal vasculitis," *The New England Journal of Medicine*, vol. 363, no. 3, pp. 211–220, 2010.

[9] J. T. Merrill, C. M. Neuwelt, D. J. Wallace et al., "Efficacy and safety of rituximab in moderately-to-severely active systemic lupus erythematosus: the randomized, double-blind, phase II/III systemic lupus erythematosus evaluation of rituximab trial," *Arthritis and Rheumatism*, vol. 62, no. 1, pp. 222–233, 2010.

[10] B. H. Rovin, R. Furie, K. Latinis et al., "Efficacy and safety of rituximab in patients with active proliferative lup us nephritis: the lup us nep hritis assessme nt with rituximab study," *Arthritis & Rheumatism*, vol. 64, no. 4, pp. 1215–1226, 2012.

[11] L. F. Pinto, C. J. Velásquez, C. Prieto, L. Mestra, E. Forero, and J. D. Márquez, "Rituximab induces a rapid and sustained remission in Colombian patients with severe and refractory systemic lupus erythematosus," *Lupus*, vol. 20, no. 11, pp. 1219–1226, 2011.

[12] F. Catapano, A. N. Chaudhry, R. B. Jones, K. G. C. Smith, and D. W. Jayne, "Long-term efficacy and safety of rituximab in refractory and relapsing systemic lupus erythematosus," *Nephrology, Dialysis, Transplantation*, vol. 25, no. 11, pp. 3586–3592, 2010.

[13] E. M. Tan, A. S. Cohen, and J. F. Fries, "The 1982 revised criteria for the classification of systemic lupus erythrematosus," *Arthritis and Rheumatism*, vol. 25, no. 11, pp. 1271–1277, 1982.

[14] M. Mosca and S. Bombardieri, "Assessing remission in systemic lupus erythematosus," *Clinical and Experimental Rheumatology*, vol. 24, no. 6, supplement 43, pp. S100–S104, 2006.

[15] C. Bombardier, D. D. Gladman, M. B. Urowitz, D. Caron, and C. H. C. Chi Hsing Chang, "Derivation of the SLEDAI: a disease activity index for lupus patients," *Arthritis and Rheumatism*, vol. 35, no. 6, pp. 630–640, 1992.

[16] L. F. Ramírez, C. A. Cañas, G. J. Tobon, F. Bonilla, and C. D. Serrano, "Successful desensitizationtorituximab in four patients with autoinmune diseases," in *Proceedings of the EAACI-WAO congress*, Abstract 498, 2013.

[17] C. Galarza, D. Valencia, G. J. Tobón et al., "Should rituximab be considered as the first-choice treatment for severe autoimmune rheumatic diseases?" *Clinical Reviews in Allergy and Immunology*, vol. 34, no. 1, pp. 124–128, 2008.

[18] R. Guzman Moreno, "B-cell depletion in autoimmune diseases. Advances in autoimmunity," *Autoimmunity Reviews*, vol. 8, no. 7, pp. 585–590, 2009.

[19] C. Galarza-Maldonado, M. R. Kourilovitch, J. E. Molineros et al., "The administration of low doses of rituximab followed by hydroxychloroquine, prednisone and low doses of mycophenolate mofetil is an effective therapy in Latin American patients with active systemic lupus erythematosus," *Autoimmunity Reviews*, vol. 10, no. 2, pp. 108–111, 2010.

[20] R. Cartin-Ceba, J. M. Golbin, K. A. Keogh et al., "Rituximab for remission induction and maintenance in refractory granulomatosis with polyangiitis (Wegener's): ten year experience at asingle center," *Arthritis and Rheumatism*, vol. 64, pp. 3770–3778, 2012.

Infiltrating CD16^{+} Are Associated with a Reduction in Peripheral CD14^{+}CD16^{++} Monocytes and Severe Forms of Lupus Nephritis

Anabel Barrera García,[1] José A. Gómez-Puerta,[1,2] Luis F. Arias,[3] Catalina Burbano,[1] Mauricio Restrepo,[2] Adriana L. Vanegas,[2] Carlos H. Muñoz,[2] Mauricio Rojas,[1] Luis A. González,[2] and Gloria Vásquez[1,2]

[1] *Grupo de Inmunología Celular e Inmunogenética, GICIG, Universidad de Antioquia, Medellín, Colombia*
[2] *Grupo de Reumatología, Universidad de Antioquia, Medellín, Colombia*
[3] *Grupo de Patología Renal y Trasplante, Universidad de Antioquia, Medellín, Colombia*

Correspondence should be addressed to Gloria Vásquez; glomavas@gmail.com

Academic Editor: Ricard Cervera

Our aim was to characterize glomerular monocytes (Mo) infiltration and to correlate them with peripheral circulating Mo subsets and severity of lupus nephritis (LN). *Methods.* We evaluated 48 LN biopsy samples from a referral hospital. Recognition of Mo cells was done using microscopic view and immunohistochemistry stain with CD14 and CD16. Based on the number of cells, we classified LN samples as low degree of diffuse infiltration (<5 cells) and high degree of diffuse infiltration (≥5 cells). Immunophenotyping of peripheral Mo subsets was done using flow cytometry. *Results.* Mean age was 34.0 ± 11.7 years and the mean SLEDAI was 17.5 ± 6.9. The most common SLE manifestations were proteinuria (91%) and hypocomplementemia (75%). Severe LN was found in 70% of patients (Class III, 27%; Class IV, 43%). Severe LN patients and patients with higher grade of CD16^{+} infiltration had lower levels of nonclassical (CD14^{+}CD16^{++}) Mo in peripheral blood. *Conclusions.* Our results might suggest that those patients with more severe forms of LN had a higher grade of CD14^{+}CD16^{+} infiltration and lower peripheral levels of nonclassical (CD14^{+}CD16^{++}) Mo and might reflect a recruitment process in renal tissues. However, given the small sample, our results must be interpreted carefully.

1. Introduction

Systemic lupus erythematosus (SLE) is the most representative of autoimmune diseases being renal involvement one of the main features. Lupus nephritis (LN) is one of the hallmark features of SLE, seen in 40%–60% of patients at the moment of diagnosis, and is one of main causes of mortality among these patients [1]. Among 10 to 15% can develop an end stage renal disease during the follow-up and might require renal replacement therapies and/or kidney transplant [2, 3].

In the pathogenesis of SLE, innate immunity and immune complex had been widely evaluated but several cellular mechanisms have not been described in depth. Monocytes (Mo) are heterogeneous cells in their morphology, phenotype, and function. In humans, three different subpopulations of circulating Mo have been described. Those subsets are defined according to the expression of CD14 and CD16. In healthy subjects, 90% of Mo are CD14^{++}CD16^{-} (classic Mo); 4% have the phenotype CD14^{++}CD16^{+} (intermediate) and are also considered mature and can participate in the inflammatory response. The third subpopulation are CD14^{+}CD16^{++} (nonclassic) that in comparison with other subpopulations of Mo are low producers of IL-10 [4].

Although the role of these subpopulations is controversial, it is well known that they can recognize immune complex through CD16, additionally can differentiate to diverse types of cells such as macrophages or dendritic cells (DC), and can polarize adaptive immune responses [5].

The main modifications of subpopulations of Mo cells have not been studied extensively in SLE patients. We described recently that $CD14^{+}CD16^{++}$ Mo are decreased in patients with active SLE and display changes in the molecules associated with their functions [6]. Those findings may suggest a potential role of these subpopulations in the pathogenesis of SLE and ultimately in kidney tissue lesions in LN.

There are enough "in vitro" evidences that a subpopulation of CD16 can differentiate to DC under the presence of GM-CSF, TGF-β, and IL-10, but without complete maturation. In that way, nonclassic $CD16^{+}$ Mo might play a role as an important immunomodulator for innate and adaptive response in SLE participating in tissue damage, even before its differentiation to macrophages [7–10].

Some previous studies have investigated some subpopulations of Mo in murine models [11], but there is limited information in humans [12, 13]. This is explained in part for the differences between murine and human phagocytes, for the wide variability on Mo subpopulations, and for the lack of equivalence in translation studies among murine and humans models.

Pathogenic mechanisms of LN are not well understood. Some previous studies suggested that phagocytes $CD14^{+}CD16^{+}$ might participate in glomerular infiltration, interact with immune complex, and regulate some phases of inflammatory response including the process of antigen presentation [14].

Given the previous information and the lack of studies in patients with LN, our aim was to characterize glomerular Mo infiltration in kidney tissue and to correlate those infiltrates with peripheral blood levels of Mo, disease features, disease activity, and histological characteristics.

2. Material and Methods

2.1. Selection of Sample. We included 328 biopsy samples with diagnosis of LN by histopathology and immunofluorescence from clinical records of Pathology Department, Universidad de Antioquia. 241 out of 328 samples were done at Hospital San Vicente Fundación at Medellín, Colombia, from 2000 to 2011. Only those patients older than 18 years were included ($n = 169$). Finally, 48 tissue samples were classified as good enough to perform new analysis.

2.2. Histopathological Studies and Immunohistochemistry. Kidney biopsies were embedded in paraffin and sectioned at 4 μm; then those samples were deparaffinized in xylene and rehydrated using graded concentrations of ethanol. Samples were stained with hematoxylin and eosin and then were examined under a light microscope. Tissue histopathologic state was classified according to ISN/RPS criteria. Patients with proliferative LN were grouped such as severe LN. Activity and chronicity indices of the histological appearance also were assessed based on National Institutes of Health scores. One observer (LA) with no prior knowledge of the clinical course examined renal tissue to establish the diagnosis by using standard pathological methods. Patients with renal involvement at SLE onset or with less than 1 year of disease duration were classified as early LN.

Different antibodies were used including CD14: Thermo Scientific, Rockford, Illinois, USA, number MA5-11394, dilution 1 : 40; CD16: Thermo Scientific, number MA5-11413, dilution 1 : 200; and CD68: Dako, Carpinteria, USA, code M0876, dilution 1 : 200. Those monoclonal antibodies were incubated at room temperature during 60 minutes. Endogenous peroxidase was blocked with hydrogen peroxide. Antigen retrieval was done with heat (steam) and tris-buffer with ethylenediaminetetraacetic acid at pH 7.0 for 30 minutes. The detection system used was based on polymer (Ultravision Quanto, Thermo Fisher Scientific, Fremont, CA, USA).

Recognition of Mo cells was done using microscopic view. Positive markers were quantified using the following parameters: If the stain was positive but with <2 cells together the stain was classified as "diffuse," and the diffuse infiltrate was scored as follows: high degree of diffuse ≥5 cells or low degree of diffuse <5 cells. Whether quantification detects more than 2 cells together was classified as "aggregates." Based on the number of cell counts aggregates were classified as grade 1, less than 5 cell counts; grade 2, five to 10 cell counts; and grade 3, more than 10 cell counts.

2.3. Immunophenotyping of Monocytes Subsets. Mo subpopulations were defined as three subsets based on previous reports in classic, ($CD14^{++}CD16^{-}$), nonclassic ($CD14^{+}CD16^{++}$), and intermediate ($CD14^{++}CD16^{+}$) Mo [15]. Briefly, 25 microliters of EDTA-anticoagulated peripheral blood was stained with anti-CD14-PerCP, anti-CD16-FITC, and anti-HLA-DR-PE or the isotype controls. Samples were mixed and incubated for 20 min at room temperature in darkness. Red cells were lysed with 250 μL of OptiLyse and analyzed using the FACS Canto™ II (Becton Dickinson, San Jose, CA). Manual counting was compared with absolute counting. All patients gave informed consent for study. This study was approved by the Ethics Committee of the Universidad de Antioquia Medical Research Institute.

2.4. Statistical Analysis. Several variables were dichotomized for the analysis. Patients with proliferative LN were grouped as severe LN. Additionally patients were classified according to disease duration (early LN versus non-early) and according to degree of $CD16^{+}$ infiltration (low or high level) as we mentioned above. Values are represented as means. Differences in means in normally distributed variables were analyzed using the parametric t-test, and variables without a normal distribution were assessed using Wilcoxon's test. The analysis was made using the IBM SPSS v22 statistical package.

3. Results

A total of 48 Mestizo patients with biopsy proven LN were enrolled for the study, of which 87% were females with a mean disease duration of 2.91 ± 5.6 years. Fifty-six percent of patients had early onset LN. Median age for the whole group was 34.0±11.7 years. Proteinuria was the most frequent renal feature (91%), followed by hematuria (66%) and sterile pyuria (38%). The main clinical features are summarized in Table 1. Mean 24-hour proteinuria levels were 4.668 ± 3906 mg and mean glomerular filtration rate (GFR) was

TABLE 1: General characteristics of 48 SLE patients with biopsy proven LN.

Clinical characteristics	
Mean age (years ± SD)	34.0 ± 11.7
Gender (female)	87%
Proteinuria	43 (91.5%)
Hematuria	31 (66.0%)
Arthritis	21 (44.7%)
Pyuria	18 (38.3%)
Urinary casts	16 (34.0%)
Pleuritis	11 (23.4%)
Alopecia	9 (19.1%)
Mouth ulcers	9 (19.1%)
Malar rash	8 (17.0%)
Pericarditis	6 (12.8%)
Vasculitis	6 (12.8%)
Fever	5 (10.6%)
Headache	1 (2.1%)
Seizures	1 (2.1%)
SLEDAI (SD)	17.5 ± 6.9
Laboratory findings	
Hypocomplementemia (either C3 or C4)	38 (80.8%)
dsDNA antibodies	27 (57.4%)
Leukopenia	8 (17%)
Thrombocytopenia	8 (17%)
LN classification	
Class I	2 (4.2%)
Class II	6 (12.5%)
Class III	13 (27.0%)
Class IV	21 (43.8%)
Class V	6 (12.5%)
Mean activity index score (SD)	5.7 ± 4.9
Mean chronicity index score (SD)	1.54 ± 2.2

TABLE 2: Histopathology characteristics in 48 patients with biopsy proven LN.

Glomerular findings	
Local necrosis	9 (18.7%)
Cellular proliferation	40 (83.3%)
Karyorrhexis	12 (25.0%)
Fibrinoid exudate	1 (2.1%)
Wire loop lesions	9 (18.7%)
Hyaline thrombosis	6 (12.5%)
Basal membrane thickening	13 (27.1%)
Fibrosis	4 (8.3%)
Tubulointerstitial findings	
Inflammatory infiltrate	34 (70.8%)
Edema	1 (2.1%)
Fibrosis	18 (37.5%)
Tubular atrophy	18 (37.5%)
Artery and arterioles	
Fibrinoid exudate	1 (2.1%)
Fibrinoid/platelet thrombus	1 (2.1%)
Necrosis	1 (2.1%)
Arterial sclerosis	5 (10.4%)
Arteriolar hyalinosis	4 (8.3%)

74.2 ± 40.6 mL/min. As expected, proteinuria levels were significantly higher in patients with severe LN forms than in patients without severe forms (4.301 ± 917 vérsus 626 ± 280 mg, $p = 0.018$). No differences in GFR were found among groups.

The Mean Systemic Lupus Erythematosus Disease Activity Index (SLEDAI) score was 17.5 ± 6.9. We observed a high disease activity in most of the patients, in part explained by the specific weight of renal involvement (12 points).

3.1. Pathological Features. Proliferative glomerulonephritis (Class IV) was detected in 21 (43.8%) patients, Class III was detected in 13 (27%) of patients, and Class II and Class V LN were detected in six (12.5%) patients each. Only two patients were classified as Class I LN. We used activity and chronicity index proposed by Rovin [14] as our guide for the description of histological findings. Most common findings for acute lesion were cellular proliferation (83%) and karyorrhexis (25%). Tubular interstitial infiltrates were found in 71% of the cases. Arterial and arteriole abnormalities were found in a minority of patients.

Chronic changes were less common reported in renal biopsies. Tubular and glomerular fibrosis were found in 37% and 8% of patients, respectively. Other chronic changes were tubular atrophy in 37% of patients, basal membrane thickening in 27% of patients, arterial sclerosis in 10.4%, and arterial hyalinosis in 8.3% of patients. Histological findings are shown in Table 2.

We compared activity and chronicity indices scores among Class II and Class IV LN based on National Institutes of Health scores. Both acute and chronicity indices on kidney biopsies were significantly higher in Class IV LN than in Class III LN patients. Mean acute index was 4.1±1.7 versus 9.6±4.4, $p = 0.001$, for Classes III and IV, respectively, and mean chronicity index was 0.8 ± 2.0 versus 1.9 ± 2.0, $p = 0.032$, for Classes III and IV, respectively.

3.2. Characterization of Mo Infiltrates. Diffuse $CD16^+$ cells were found in 25 biopsies and $CD14^+$ cells in only sixteen biopsies. Representative pictures are shown in Figure 1 of the immunostainings for $CD16^+$ and CD14 cells.

Patients with higher degree of CD16 diffuse infiltrates had a higher prevalence of hypocomplementemia (100% versus 0%, $p = 0.028$), higher but not significant levels of dsDNA antibodies, and higher disease activity (SLEDAI score ≥ 10). Five patients had $CD16^+$ Mo aggregates. All patients who had grade 3 aggregates had Class IV LN in histologic classification. Grade 1 was observed in one patient with Class II and aggregates grade 2 was observed in one patient with Class III LN. With respect to $CD14^+$ Mo cells, only

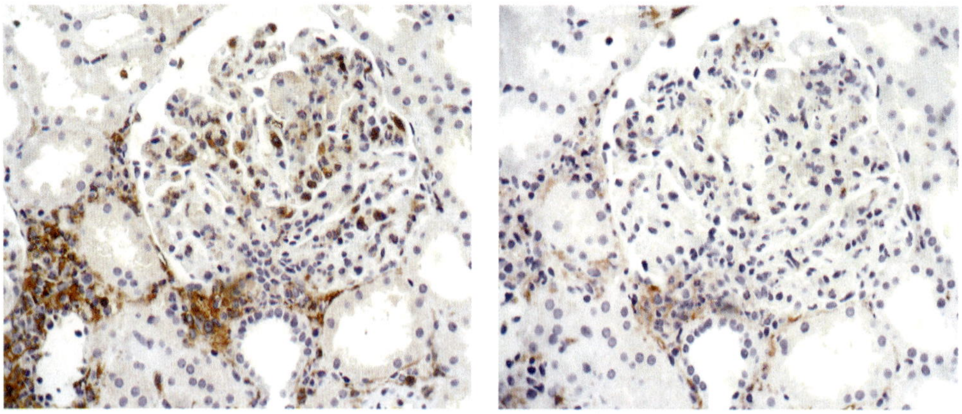

(a) (b)

FIGURE 1: (a) Immunohistochemistry for CD16: abundant CD16$^+$ cells in the glomerular tuft; these cells are also evidenced in the interstitium. (b) Immunohistochemistry for CD14: a glomerulus with few positive CD14$^+$ cells. There are also some CD14$^+$ cells in the interstitium. Both images, ×400.

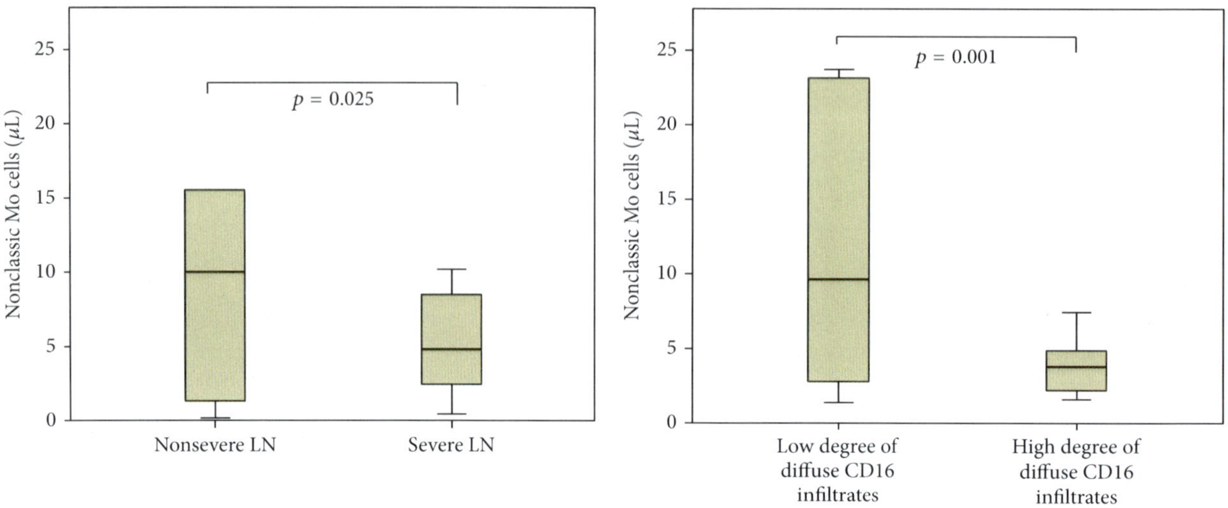

(a) (b)

FIGURE 2: Peripheral blood levels of Mo subsets according to severity of LN (a) and degree of infiltrations by CD16$^+$ cells (b).

accumulated grade 1 aggregates were observed in a patient with Class III LN.

3.3. Peripheral Mo Subsets. Mo subsets around the time of kidney biopsy were available in 21 patients. Mean levels of absolute Mo were 497.63 ± 329 cells/μL, classical Mo 459.46 ± 315.98 cells/μL, intermediate Mo 17.33 ± 16.05 cells/μL, and nonclassic Mo 10.09 ± 14.82 cells/μL. When we classified patients in severe and nonsevere forms of LN, severe forms had lower levels of nonclassic Mo in peripheral blood (7.14 ± 7.22 versus 17.47 ± 25.32 cells/μL, $p = 0.025$, Figure 2(a)). When we classified patients according to diffuse CD16$^+$ infiltrates in high or low degree, patients with higher degree of infiltrates had lower levels of nonclassical Mo in peripheral blood (37.53 ± 21.98 versus 8.39 ± 5.70 cells/μL, $p = 0.001$, Figure 2(b)). Table 3 summarizes levels of different Mo subsets according to disease duration, severity of LN, and degree of infiltration.

At the same time, patients with higher degree of CD16$^+$ infiltrates had higher but not significant activity index scores (5.46 ± 4.12 versus 4.70 ± 4.71, $p = 0.363$) and higher chronicity index scores (2.0 ± 2.72 versus 0.40 ± 0.51, $p = 0.004$). We did not find any association among subsets of Mo in peripheral blood with clinical characteristics, serological markers (including complement antibodies or anti-dsDNA) either with disease activity (SLEDAI).

4. Discussion

Mo and macrophages play an important role in murine models and human subjects with renal disease. Those cells have been involved in not only several processes such as

TABLE 3: Peripheral blood levels of Mo subsets according to disease duration, severity of LN, and degree of infiltrations by $CD16^+$ cells.

(a)

	Early onset LN	Non-early onset LN	p value
Classic ($CD14^{++}CD16^-$)	411.53 ± 377.48	465.27 ± 138.48	0.021
Intermediate ($CD14^{++}CD16^-$)	14.35 ± 15.37	22.41 ± 18.17	0.488
Nonclassic ($CD14^+CD16^{++}$)	7.51 ± 7.38	15.32 ± 20.80	0.138

(b)

	Severe LN	Nonsevere LN	p value
Classic ($CD14^{++}CD16^-$)	485.80 ± 345.81	393.63 ± 239.20	0.340
Intermediate ($CD14^{++}CD16^-$)	18.32 ± 18.11	14.84 ± 10.10	0.240
Nonclassic ($CD14^+CD16^{++}$)	7.14 ± 7.22	17.47 ± 25.32	0.025

(c)

	High degree of diffuse $CD16^+$ infiltrates (≥5 cells)	Low degree of diffuse $CD16^+$ infiltrates (<5 cells)	p value
Classic ($CD14^{++}CD16^-$)	496.35 ± 443.38	543.71 ± 368.67	0.627
Intermediate ($CD14^{++}CD16^-$)	9.65 ± 7.35	17.06 ± 18.79	0.198
Nonclassic ($CD14^+CD16^{++}$)	3.95 ± 2.32	11.70 ± 10.37	0.001

Severe LN was defined as either Class III or Class IV LN.

renal injury and fibrosis but also several repair processes. We found that patients with more severe forms of LN (proliferative forms) have a higher grade of diffuse $CD16^+$ Mo infiltrates. At the same time, severe forms had lower levels of peripheral nonclassical Mo and might reflect organ recruitment phenomenon of Mo cells in more severe forms of LN (proliferative Classes III and IV).

Linage cells from Mo/macrophages system constitute one of the most important cells involved in the inflammatory process of several renal diseases. Several studies have shown that the amounts of macrophages found in damaged tissues not only are bystanders of the inflammatory process but also play a role as active cells as occurs in some other in vitro studies [16]. Macrophages are distributed in tissues throughout the body and contribute to both homeostasis and disease. The recent increase in the availability of diverse surface markers for the determination of Mo/macrophages allowed the identification of different subpopulations in the kidney and other tissues. Mo subpopulations are functionally different. Some of these subpopulations have been related with a selective pattern of cytokine production [7, 8].

In vitro studies have demonstrated that macrophages can be polarized by activation with several cytokines. Activated and polarized cells have different functions. Initially, polarized cells were known as "classic" or "alternative" Mo. However, some other authors suggest that Mo should be labeled according to their phenotype (based on surface molecules) or according to their function [17–19]. The difference in the expression of lipopolysaccharide (LPS) receptor (CD14) and of Fcγ receptor III (CD16) has been used to distinguish various Mo subpopulations [4, 20].

We found a greater amount of diffuse infiltrations and aggregates of $CD16^+$ cells in patients with more severe forms of LN. $CD16^+$ are considered as nonclassic or intermediate Mo. It is well known that $CD16^+$ cells produce TNF-α and interferon gamma (IFNγ) and participate in inflammatory process. Additionally, $CD16^+$ express Class II molecules with a more efficient capacity for antigen presentation.

Previously, we observed that patients suffering from SLE had lower levels of $CD16^+$ in peripheral blood, suggesting a differentiation process out of organs and cell recruitment in damaged organs [6]. Mo recruitment in inflammatory tissues could be explained in part by the active participation of Mo during all stages of organ damage process due to autoimmune phenomena. Mo participate during the clearance process of apoptotic bodies and immune complexes. In addition, Mo can induce the production of several cytokines involved in the pathogenesis of LN (for instance, IFNγ). Finally, Mo promote fibrosis and loss of epithelial cells and microvasculature [21, 22]. Given the association between chronicity index score and high degree of $CD16^+$ infiltrates in our study, it is possible that CD16 Mo participate not only during early acute glomerular damage process but also during chronic fibrotic and microvascular processes as we mentioned previously.

Fractalkine (CX3CL1) and its receptor, CX3CR1, are known to mediate both cell adhesion and cell migration. In humans, CX3CR1 is expressed on Mo/macrophages and cytotoxic effector lymphocytes such as natural killer cells and cytotoxic T cells. In mice, its expression in circulating blood cells is restricted to Mo/macrophages and NK cells. Murine and human studies focused on the role of Mo in LN are limited. Using MRL/lpr murine model, Nakatani and colleagues [11] showed that fractalkine expression and $CD16^+$ Mo infiltration increase with progression of the LN. In another study, a fractalkine antagonist was administered to MRL/lpr mice during early stages of LN [23]. MRL/lpr mice that received fractalkine antagonist exhibited significantly reduced glomerular hypercellularity, glomerulosclerosis, crescent formation, and vasculitis when compared with control mice.

Yoshimoto et al. [12] evaluated glomerular expression of fractalkine and $CD16^+$ Mo in patients with LN. The authors found correlation of fractalkine glomerular expression with histopathologic activity index and proliferative forms of LN. Additionally, the amounts of infiltrating $CD16^+$ Mo were higher in proliferative glomerular lesions of patients with SLE.

To the best our knowledge, this is the first study that correlated the levels of Mo in peripheral blood with Mo infiltrates in renal tissues. Our study suggested an inverse correlation among peripheral levels of nonclassic Mo and higher diffuse $CD16^+$ infiltrative cells in glomerular tissue in patients with proliferative forms of LN.

Our study has some limitations. First, we analyzed a relative small number of patients with biopsy proven LN. However, despite this small sample we found significant differences among groups (severe and nonsevere) according to $CD16^+$ infiltrates and subsets of Mo in peripheral blood. Given the nature of the study, we were not able to measure at the same time subsets of Mo in peripheral blood in all patients tested for Mo infiltrates on renal samples. Likewise, as our hospital is a reference center for systemic autoimmune diseases and predominantly received patients with limited access to health care, therefore our patients could be a selected sample of more severe SLE patients with LN. Finally, given that the majority of our patients were Mestizo, our results must be interpreted carefully and must be confirmed in other populations with different racial/ethnic distributions.

In conclusion our results in Mestizo patients with biopsy proven LN suggest that those patients with more severe forms of LN had lower peripheral levels of nonclassical Mo ($CD14^+CD16^{++}$). Reduction of these Mo subsets could be explained in part by a recruitment process in renal tissues. Given the small sample of the current study, our results must be interpreted carefully. Although the information about the role of Mo in LN is limited in clinical studies, animal model studies using fractalkine antagonist open a potential new target for the treatment of patients suffering from severe forms of LN. So far, there are no ongoing clinical trials evaluating the potential benefit of fractalkine antagonist in patients with LN.

Abbreviations

DC: Dendritic cells
IFNγ: Interferon gamma
LN: Lupus nephritis
LPS: Lipopolysaccharide
Mo: Monocytes
SLE: Systemic lupus erythematosus
SLEDAI: Systemic Lupus Erythematosus Disease Activity Index.

Competing Interests

The authors declare that they have no competing interests.

Authors' Contributions

Anabel Barrera García conceived the study, participated in data analysis, and approved the final version of the manuscript. José A. Gómez-Puerta participated in its design and wrote and approved the final version of the manuscript. Luis F. Arias participated in data analysis of kidney biopsies and approved the final version of the manuscript. Catalina Burbano and Mauricio Rojas participated in data analysis of monocytes subsets and reviewed and approved the final version of the manuscript. Mauricio Restrepo, Adriana L. Vanegas, Carlos H. Muñoz, and Luis A. González participated in patient recruitment and reviewed and approved the final version of the manuscript. Gloria Vásquez participated in the design of the study, supported data analysis, and reviewed and approved the final version of the manuscript. All authors read and approved the final manuscript.

Acknowledgments

This work was supported by Colciencias Project no. 11556933532 (Contract no. 575-2013) and by Programa de Sostenibilidad, Universidad de Antioquia. J. A. Gómez-Puerta was supported by Colciencias (no. 656/2014).

References

[1] L. Lisnevskaia, G. Murphy, and D. Isenberg, "Systemic lupus erythematosus," *The Lancet*, vol. 384, no. 9957, pp. 1878–1888, 2014.

[2] M. Adler, S. Chambers, C. Edwards, G. Neild, and D. Isenberg, "An assessment of renal failure in an SLE cohort with special reference to ethnicity, over a 25-year period," *Rheumatology*, vol. 45, no. 9, pp. 1144–1147, 2006.

[3] J. A. Gómez-Puerta, C. H. Feldman, G. S. Alarcón, H. Guan, W. C. Winkelmayer, and K. H. Costenbader, "Racial and ethnic differences in mortality and cardiovascular events among patients with End-stage renal disease due to lupus nephritis," *Arthritis Care & Research*, vol. 67, no. 10, pp. 1453–1462, 2015.

[4] E. Grage-Griebenow, H.-D. Flad, and M. Ernst, "Heterogeneity of human peripheral blood monocyte subsets," *Journal of Leukocyte Biology*, vol. 69, no. 1, pp. 11–20, 2001.

[5] L. Ziegler-Heitbrock, "The CD14+ CD16+ blood monocytes: their role in infection and inflammation," *Journal of Leukocyte Biology*, vol. 81, no. 3, pp. 584–592, 2007.

[6] C. Burbano, G. Vasquez, and M. Rojas, "Modulatory effects of cd14+cd16++ monocytes on cd14++cd16- monocytes: a possible explanation of monocyte alterations in systemic lupus erythematosus," *Arthritis and Rheumatology*, vol. 66, no. 12, pp. 3371–3381, 2014.

[7] K.-U. Belge, F. Dayyani, A. Horelt et al., "The proinflammatory $CD14^+CD16^+DR^{++}$ monocytes are a major source of TNF," *Journal of Immunology*, vol. 168, no. 7, pp. 3536–3542, 2002.

[8] J. Skrzeczyńska-Moncznik, M. Bzowska, S. Loseke, E. Grage-Griebenow, M. Zembala, and J. Pryjma, "Peripheral blood $CD14^{high}$ $CD16^+$ monocytes are main producers of IL-10," *Scandinavian Journal of Immunology*, vol. 67, no. 2, pp. 152–159, 2008.

[9] D. Strauss-Ayali, S. M. Conrad, and D. M. Mosser, "Monocyte subpopulations and their differentiation patterns during

infection," *Journal of Leukocyte Biology*, vol. 82, no. 2, pp. 244–252, 2007.

[10] D. M. Mosser and J. P. Edwards, "Exploring the full spectrum of macrophage activation," *Nature Reviews Immunology*, vol. 8, no. 12, pp. 958–969, 2008.

[11] K. Nakatani, S. Yoshimoto, M. Iwano et al., "Fractalkine expression and CD16+ monocyte accumulation in glomerular lesions: association with their severity and diversity in lupus models," *American Journal of Physiology—Renal Physiology*, vol. 299, no. 1, pp. F207–F216, 2010.

[12] S. Yoshimoto, K. Nakatani, M. Iwano et al., "Elevated levels of fractalkine expression and accumulation of $CD16^+$ monocytes in glomeruli of active lupus nephritis," *American Journal of Kidney Diseases*, vol. 50, no. 1, pp. 47–58, 2007.

[13] Y. Li, P. Y. Lee, E. S. Sobel et al., "Increased expression of FcγRI/CD64 on circulating monocytes parallels ongoing inflammation and nephritis in lupus," *Arthritis Research & Therapy*, vol. 11, no. 1, article R6, 2009.

[14] B. H. Rovin, "The chemokine network in systemic lupus erythematous nephritis," *Frontiers in Bioscience*, vol. 13, no. 3, pp. 904–922, 2008.

[15] I. Heimbeck, T. P. J. Hofer, C. Eder et al., "Standardized single-platform assay for human monocyte subpopulations: lower $CD14^+CD16^{++}$ monocytes in females," *Cytometry Part A*, vol. 77, no. 9, pp. 823–830, 2010.

[16] J. S. Duffield, "Macrophages and immunologic inflammation of the kidney," *Seminars in Nephrology*, vol. 30, no. 3, pp. 234–254, 2010.

[17] S. Goerdt and C. E. Orfanos, "Other functions, other genes: alternative activation of antigen-presenting cells," *Immunity*, vol. 10, no. 2, pp. 137–142, 1999.

[18] V. A. Fadok, D. L. Bratton, A. Konowal, P. W. Freed, J. Y. Westcott, and P. M. Henson, "Macrophages that have ingested apoptotic cells in vitro inhibit proinflammatory cytokine production through autocrine/paracrine mechanisms involving TGF-β, PGE2, and PAF," *Journal of Clinical Investigation*, vol. 101, no. 4, pp. 890–898, 1998.

[19] A. Mantovani, A. Sica, and M. Locati, "Macrophage polarization comes of age," *Immunity*, vol. 23, no. 4, pp. 344–346, 2005.

[20] H. W. L. Ziegler-Heitbrock, "Heterogeneity of human blood monocytes: the $CD14^+CD16^+$ subpopulation," *Immunology Today*, vol. 17, no. 9, pp. 424–428, 1996.

[21] J. S. Duffield, L.-P. Erwig, X.-Q. Wei, F. Y. Liew, A. J. Rees, and J. S. Savill, "Activated macrophages direct apoptosis and suppress mitosis of mesangial cells," *The Journal of Immunology*, vol. 164, no. 4, pp. 2110–2119, 2000.

[22] J. S. Duffield, P. G. Tipping, T. Kipari et al., "Conditional ablation of macrophages halts progression of crescentic glomerulonephritis," *The American Journal of Pathology*, vol. 167, no. 5, pp. 1207–1219, 2005.

[23] A. Inoue, H. Hasegawa, M. Kohno et al., "Antagonist of fractalkine (CX3CL1) delays the initiation and ameliorates the progression of lupus nephritis in MRL/lpr mice," *Arthritis and Rheumatism*, vol. 52, no. 5, pp. 1522–1533, 2005.

34

Relationships among Antibodies against Extractable Nuclear Antigens, Antinuclear Antibodies, and Autoimmune Diseases in a Brazilian Public Hospital

Fernanda Weyand Banhuk,[1] **Bruna Corrêa Pahim**,[2]
Alex Sandro Jorge,[2] **and Rafael Andrade Menolli**[1]

[1] *Laboratory of Applied Immunology, Center of Medical and Pharmaceutical Sciences, Western Parana State University, Cascavel/PR 85819-110, Brazil*
[2] *Laboratory of Clinical Immunology, Western Parana University Hospital, Western Parana State University, Cascavel, PR 85806-470, Brazil*

Correspondence should be addressed to Rafael Andrade Menolli; rafael.menolli@unioeste.br

Academic Editor: Ricard Cervera

One characteristic of autoimmune diseases (ADs) is the production of autoantibodies for extractable nuclear autoantigens, which may aid in the discrimination of the different types of autoimmune diseases and is related to different antinuclear antibody (ANA) patterns. The present study verified the profile of patient samples tested for extractable nuclear antigens (ENA) antibodies in a public hospital and correlated the ENA results with ANA patterns and patient diagnoses. The study reviewed data in the medical records of patients who underwent anti-ENA tests at a public hospital in the West of the State of Paraná from February 2011 to January 2017. Patients were classified according to age, ethnicity, gender, anti-ENA test results, ANA results, and the presence or absence of AD. Thirty-six (20.9%) samples of the 172 anti-ENA tests were positive, seven (4.1%) samples were undetermined, and 129 (75%) exhibited negative results. The ANA reagent was found in 84.3% of the anti-ENA-positive samples. The anti-SSA/Ro autoantibody exhibited the highest frequency in the group, 41.7% (15/36). The most common pattern was nuclear fine speckled, which was found in 24.3% of the samples. The association results indicated a significant relationship between ANA titer and diagnosis in the anti-ENA- and ANA-positive patients. The anti-ENA-negative patients were diagnosed with an AD in 35% (45/129) of the cases, and 75% (27/36) of the anti-ENA-positive patients were diagnosed with an AD. Systemic lupus erythematosus and scleroderma were the most common pathologies in the antigen-positive patients. The anti-ENA test is a good marker to aid in the complex clinical diagnosis of patients with autoimmune diseases.

1. Introduction

Multiple factors cause autoimmune diseases and involve a wide variety of genes and environmental factors, such as stress, age, sex, hormones, and infection exposure [1]. Autoimmune diseases are characterized by autoaggression of the immune system against constitutive antigens of an individual via production of autoantibodies, which exhibit clinical significance when associated with other disease manifestations [2, 3].

The detection of antibodies against cellular antigens (AACA) in HEp-2 cells, also known as antinuclear antibodies (ANA HEp-2), using indirect immunofluorescence (IFI) is the methodology of choice for the screening and identification of various autoantibodies [4, 5]. The ANA assay detects a range of antibodies that react with antigens in the nucleus, nucleolus, cytoplasm, and mitotic cellular apparatus [6]. However, this test should be complemented by the research and identification of autoantibodies and specific autoantigens, many of which exhibit great clinical utility and may play roles as diagnostic markers, as prognostic indicators, or for the monitoring of autoimmune diseases [7–9]. In addition, the presence of positive ANA does not necessarily indicate a disease state, because low levels of ANA are detected in 30% of healthy individuals [10, 11].

The most frequent antigens described in autoimmune diseases exhibit a nuclear localization and are called extractable nuclear antigens because of the purification process; they are most commonly represented by the acronym ENA (*extractable nuclear antigens*) [12].

Anti-ENA research is used to identify a group of specific autoantibodies, including anti-SSA/Ro, anti-SSB/La, anti-RNP, anti-Sm, anti-Scl-70, anti-Jo-1, anti-CENP-B, anti-NUC, and anti-dsDNA. These autoantibodies are detected using several methodologies, such as immunoblot, counter-immunoelectrophoresis, immunodiffusion, enzyme-linked immunosorbent assay (ELISA), and hemagglutination. However, variations in the results can be found because these techniques differ in sensitivity and specificity [13–15]. DNAds as an antigen is not included as ENA by some authors, because the anti-DNA test is commonly performed with another methodology (IIF with Crithidia as antigen), but in this study it was named as ENA, once the sera of patients were tested together with the other ENA antigens by immunoblot method. It is important to note that although the Jo-1 antigen is common in the ENA group, it is a cytoplasmic antigen.

Further analysis of reactivity to ENA may contribute to an improved discrimination among the different types of autoimmune rheumatic diseases (ARD). For example, the presence of anti-ribonucleoprotein (RNP) antibodies is part of the diagnosis of mixed connective tissue disease (MCTD), and positive results for ANA and the presence of anti-dsDNA or anti-Sm constitute three of the six immunological criteria for the diagnosis of systemic lupus erythematosus (SLE) [16, 17]. The presence of antibodies directed against SS-A (Ro) or SS-B (La) ribonucleoproteins is a criterion for the diagnosis of Sjögren's syndrome (SS), and the appearance of antibodies against histidyl-sRNA synthetase (Jo-1) is a major immunological characteristic of polydermatomyositis. The appearance of anti-centromere antibodies (CENP-B) or topoisomerase 1 (Scl-70) aids in the diagnosis of systemic sclerosis [18–20].

The presence of anti-ENA is related to the different patterns of ANA tests, which are associated with manifestations of some autoimmune diseases. Therefore, the present study retrospectively evaluated the correlation between anti-ENA-positive and -negative sera, ANA patterns, and clinical data.

2. Material and Methods

2.1. Casuistry. A cross-sectional, uncontrolled study was performed via a review of the medical records of patients who underwent anti-ENA examination at the Western Paraná University Hospital (HUOP) from February 2011 to January 2017. Patients were selected only on the condition that they had undergone the anti-ENA test, i.e., not considering if preliminary tests were performed, such as the ANA test, since it is common to perform the anti-ENA test as a complementary test to the ANA test.

Patients were classified according to age, ethnicity, gender, anti-ENA, and ANA test results, diagnosis, and specialty that requested the tests. These factors were collected from records in the Tasy® electronic hospital management system, which allowed for verification of laboratory tests issued and stored and the test results in the support, diagnostic, and therapeutic service (SDTS), and patient's archive/history department. The averages and percentages were obtained from the data of each patient.

The ethics committee in research involving human beings of the Western Paraná State University approved the study under number 861.960.

2.2. ANA and Anti-ENA. The ANAs were determined semi-quantitatively in HEp-2 cells using immunofluorescence (Viro-Immun Diagnostics GmbH), according to the manufacturer's protocol. The slides were read on an Olympus epifluorescence microscope, with a mercury vapor lamp of 100 watts power, by two observers, at 400X magnification. Samples were classified into reactives or non-reactives by comparing the fluorescence intensity observed for the sample and the fluorescence intensity observed in the control slide (FITC-QC slide Immuno Concepts N.A. Ltd.) at the second reactivity threshold level (1+). According to the staining of the nucleus and cytoplasm of the cells, different patterns were described, following the Brazilian consensus of ANA-HEp2.

Anti-ENA research was performed using a membrane-based immunoblot assay (Nucleo-9-Line, ORGENTEC Diagnostika GmbH) for the semiquantitative determination of IgG autoantibodies against dsDNA, nucleosome (NUC), SS-A (Ro), SS-B (La), Sm, RNP/Sm, Scl-70, Jo-1, and CENP-B antigens in serum or plasma.

2.3. Statistical Analysis. An association between the diagnosis of AD and ANA patterns, ANA titer, and diagnosis were tested for positive and negative anti-ENA patients using the nonparametric chi-square test with 95% reliability [21]. Patients with indeterminate anti-ENA results lacked sufficient data for conclusive statistical tests, and these data were excluded. The tests were run in software R version 3.4.1 [22] using FunChisq [21] and the ggplot2 graphic package [23].

3. Results

Thirty-six (20.9%) of the 172 anti-ENA tests performed between 2011 and 2017 were positive, seven (4.1%) samples were undetermined, and 129 (75%) exhibited a negative result. These patients showed an age range from 4 to 80 years, averaging 38.01 years, with a prevalence of females and white ethnicity (77.3% and 78%, respectively).

Table S1 (Supplementary Material) presents the behavior of patients with anti-ENA-positive sera with respect to ANA patterns and titers, diagnosis for autoimmune diseases, and sociodemographic data.

The anti-ENA-positive patients aged from 13 to 71 years, averaging 41.8 years, and a prevalence of females and white ethnicity was observed (86.1% and 77.7%, respectively).

ANA positivity in anti-ENA-positive patients was found in 84.3% (27/32) of the samples analyzed that underwent the ANA test. Five of the 36 anti-ENA-positive patients exhibited negative ANA, and the ANA test was not performed in four patients.

The anti-SSA/Ro autoantibody exhibited the highest frequency in the group (41.7%; 15/36). Eleven sera were

Table 1: Titers of ANA tests and clinical diagnosis of autoimmune diseases in anti-ENA-positive patients.

ANA Titles	Diagnosis AD	
	N	Y*
1:80 – 1:160	0	1
1:160- 1:320	3	2
1:640 - >1:640	1	19

Y = presence of autoimmune disease; N = no diagnosis of autoimmune disease; * = positive association between AD presence and ANA titers.

Table 2: Titers of ANA tests and clinical diagnosis of autoimmune diseases in anti-ENA-negative patients.

ANA Titles	AD Diagnosis	
	N	Y
1:80 – 1:160	3	3
1:160- 1:320	10	24
1:640 - >1:640	2	10

Y = presence of autoimmune disease; N = no diagnosis of autoimmune disease.

exclusive for anti-SSA/Ro, and four sera were associated with other autoantibodies. The other most frequently isolated autoantibodies were anti-NUC (13.9%), followed by anti-Scl-70 (11.1%), anti-CENP-B and anti-RNP/Sm (both 8.33%), and SS-B (La) (5.6%). Four of the five patients who were anti-ENA-positive and ANA-negative were anti-SS-A/Ro-positive patients.

The seven patients with undetermined results for anti-ENA included 42.8% who were indeterminate for SS-A (Ro), and four ANA-positive and three ANA-negative patients.

The following ANA patterns occurred in patients with positive anti-ENA (patients in whom it was possible to obtain such data): nuclear fine speckled (28.1%); nuclear large/coarse speckled (12.5%); nuclear dense fine speckled (9.4%); centromere (8.3%); nuclear homogeneous (6.3%); and nucleolar pattern (5.6%). The presence of more than one ANA pattern was verified in three samples, which were identified as a mixed pattern (8.3%).

Some anti-ENA-positive patients (27.8%) did not exhibit ANA patterns or titers because the test was negative or unsolicited.

The association results indicated a significant relationship between ANA titer and diagnosis in anti-ENA- and ANA-positive patients (p *value*=0.0069) (Table 1).

Most anti-ENA-negative patients were women (73.6%), white (79.7%), and aged from four to 80 years (average of 36.3 years). Positive ANA results were observed in 47.3% of the samples (54/112) (no results for the ANA test were found in the medical records of 17 anti-ENA-negative patients). The following immunofluorescence patterns were observed: nuclear fine speckled pattern (37.7%); nuclear dense fine speckled (18.9%); mixed patterns (18.9%); nuclear large/coarse speckled (9.4%); nuclear homogeneous (7.8%); cytoplasmic (7.5%); nucleolar (1.9%); and mitotic apparatus (1.9%).

Complete information about the immunofluorescence pattern was not obtained in some anti-ENA-negative/ANA-positive samples. Only the titer was recorded in these samples.

Table 2 provides that most (65.4%) anti-ENA-negative patients exhibited an intermediate titer range (positive/negative diagnosis). However, Table 1 shows that 76.9% of the samples were obtained from anti-ENA-positive patients in the highest range. We also observed that 84.6% of anti-ENA- and ANA-positive patients had a diagnosis of AD (Table 1), and only 71.1% of the anti-ENA-negative and ANA-positive patients had an AD diagnosis.

Anti-ENA-negative and ANA-positive patients exhibited no association between ANA and AD diagnosis (p *value*= 0.2983). Two patients were not included in Table 2 because no data of titers in their ANA tests was found.

There were no significant associations between the different ANA patterns and AD diagnoses in positive and negative anti-ENA patients, suggesting no specific association of ANA patterns with AD for these samples.

Of the total number of anti-ENA tests performed, 14 (8.1%) were requested by rheumatologists and 158 (91.9%) by physicians from other specialties. At the anti-ENA-positive tests, 16.7% were requested by rheumatologists and the others by other specialties, while in anti-ENA negative tests, rheumatologists were responsible for the request of only 6.2% of the exams.

Twenty-seven (75%) of the 36 anti-ENA-positive patients were diagnosed with an AD. Nine of these patients (33.3%) were diagnosed with SLE, and five patients were diagnosed with SLE associated with another autoimmune disease (Table 3). Anti-ENA-negative patients were diagnosed with an autoimmune disease in 35% of the sample (45/129). Twelve (26.7%) of these patients were diagnosed with SLE, and four (8.9%) patients were diagnosed with SLE associated with another autoimmune disease.

4. Discussion

Numerous studies have demonstrated that a positive ANA test is a strong indicator of an autoimmune disease, and this test is a good methodology to extensively screen for autoimmunity. However, progressive and vigorous improvements in the technology of the various elements composing the assay, including the quality of the HEp-2 cell slides, fluorescent conjugates, and fluorescence microscopes, have revised this concept [24].

These technological improvements greatly increased test sensitivity, and current tests detect antibodies at lower serum levels and less avidity than earlier assays. Therefore, the screening for antibodies against cellular antigens also exhibits a lower specificity [25]. In addition, the prescription of the ANA test started to be made by a broad spectrum of medical specialists, which was once primarily prescribed solely by rheumatologists. Therefore, the pretest probability of autoimmunity was high and favored the diagnostic performance of the test [24, 26].

A wide variety of specialists, who obviously treat different patients in whom the diagnosis of autoimmune rheumatic

TABLE 3: Distribution of autoimmune diseases and autoantibodies against extractable nuclear antigens (anti-ENA).

AD in Anti-ENA-positive patients	Antigens found
SLE (9/27)	SS-A (Ro), SS-B (La), Smith, Scl-70, NUC, dsDNA, RNP/Smith
Scleroderma (4/27)	SS-A (Ro), Scl-70, CENP-B
Sjögren's syndrome (3/27)	SS-A (Ro), SS-B (La)
Polymyositis (2/27)	SS-A (Ro), Smith, Scl-70, RNP/Smith
Behçet's disease (1/27)	SS-A (Ro)
Rheumatoid arthritis (1/27)	SS-A (Ro), SS-B (La), Smith, Scl-70, CENP-B, Jo-1, RNP/Smith
Autoimmune hemolytic anemia (1/27)	NUC
Autoimmune hepatitis and scleroderma (1/27)	CENP-B
SLE and scleroderma (1/27)	Scl-70
SLE and polymyositis (1/27)	RNP/Smith
SLE, MCTD and scleroderma (1/27)	RNP/Smith
SLE and Evans syndrome (1/27)	NUC
SLE and Sjögren's syndrome (1/27)	SS-A (Ro), Smith, RNP/Smith

SLE = systemic lupus erythematosus.
MCTD = mixed connective tissue disease.

disease is less prevalent, are requesting ANA examinations with less discretion. Therefore, the chance for positive results in healthy individuals or individuals with less expressive clinical presentations is greater [27–29]. This increase shows the importance of requesting tests for the identification of specific autoantibodies after receiving a positive ANA test.

Our results demonstrated that 76.9% of the anti-ENA-positive patients were in the highest ANA titer range, and 84.6% of patients who were anti-ENA- and ANA-positive were diagnosed with an AD. This result is very similar to that reported by Jeong [30], who used an anti-ENA test with the same methodology (line immunoassay) and found 83.9% positivity in ANA and anti-ENA tests in a cohort of Asian patients with AD. A study in Bangladesh [31] showed autoimmune diseases in 85.5% of double positivity (ENA and ANA tests), working with dot-blot methodology for ENA detection. This demonstrates that association of these two tests (ANA for screening and anti-ENA to confirm) is essential for diagnosis of AD [10].

Anti-ENA-positive with ANA-negative was found in five (15.2%) sera, which was unexpected because ANA-Hep2 tends to have a higher sensitivity than immunoblot tests. However, the occurrence is not uncommon [12, 27, 32] and some of these ANA-negative results could be patients in immunosuppressive therapy [33]; a revision of their medical records should be necessary to clarify this point. Although five samples showed ANA-negative with anti-ENA-negative, only one patient was diagnosed with AD. The methodology used in this objective is important, as Kidd [34] argued that samples that were previously negative turned out to be positive when subjected to another analysis with a different methodology. Finally, the association of different techniques ensures greater sensitivity and specificity [30].

Anti-SSA/Ro are the antigens that cause the higher number of "false-positive" anti-ENA tests [35]. In this study, this happened in four of five ANA-negative results with anti-ENA-positive. This gives rise to the question that it was highly recommended to use anti-SSA antibody assays in addition to the ANAHEp-2 test in the function of this characteristic [36]. Based on these observations, over three decades ago a transfected HEp-2 cell line overexpressing SS-A/Ro60 was developed and this cell-based IIF assay was marketed as HEp- 2000 cells [37]. According to Bossuyt et al. [38], this characteristic of SSA/Ro happened due to the loss of this antigen in the process of fixing HEp-2 cells to make ANA test kits.

Another point is the sensibility of different methodologies or different antigens used in ENA tests, with authors demonstrating that in some laboratories line immunoassays have also been used as a screening test for disease-specific autoantibodies that are seen in SLE, Sjögren's syndrome, Idiopathic Inflammatory Myopathies, paraneoplastic, and autoimmune liver diseases [35]. Also, the methodology of LIA used here shows good sensitivity, and various studies demonstrate a great correlation between data obtained by LIA and other techniques. Chandratilleke et al. [12] compared LIA with an automatized fluorescent assay (FIDIS) in 529 samples and found a 90.5% concordance. A work conducted in Korea [30], with patients with AD, showed a similar performance among three anti-ENA methods (two automatized immunoenzymatic assays and LIA). Vercammen et al. [39] analyzed 174 ANA-positive samples by immunodiffusion, LIA, and an automatized fluorescent immunodetection methodology, showing no difference between them. However, most studies with comparisons between different techniques of anti-ENA tests are conducted with patients who have been diagnosed with AD.

The highest frequency of the anti-SSA/Ro autoantibody (43.2%) in anti-ENA-positive patients was also reported by Lora et al. [40], with 67.7% predominance, and Sanchez-Guerrero et al. [41], who reported a 40% frequency of antigen-positive samples.

The most prevalent association of autoantibodies in the present study was anti-RNP/Sm (27%), which is similar to the results of Arbuckle et al. [42], who found a prevalence of anti-RNP/Sm in 32% of the samples analyzed. The ANA-HEp2 pattern associated with RNP and Sm autoantigens was nuclear large/coarse speckled [43]. Four of the five patients who exhibited the nuclear large/coarse speckled pattern, although this was associated with mixed patterns of ANA-HEp2, also exhibited anti-RNP/Sm in their sera and a clinical association with SLE.

In general, patients with autoimmune diseases tend to exhibit moderate (1/160 and 1/320) and high (≥ 1/640) ANA titers, and healthy subjects with positive ANA tend to exhibit low titers (1/80) [15, 44]. However, exceptions may exist in both cases [45]. In this study, a significant association was detected between ANA titers and the presence of ADs in patients who were anti-ENA-positive; and these patients exhibited the highest ANA titers (≥1: 640), which is consistent with the literature [15, 25]. Craig [46] showed that, in a large cohort, the number of diagnoses of AD increased with the titer of ANA (13.3% in low levels to 43.4% in high levels), which is consistent with the present data; diagnosis of AD occurred in 55 (71.14%) patients with high titers of ANA (>1:160). Thus, the chance of finding anti-ENA increases with increasing ANA titers [28, 46], as demonstrated in this study, with only one sample with anti-ENA-positive results in the range of lower titers of ANA-positive results.

The ANA patterns for anti-ENA-positive and -negative sera were not significantly associated with ADs. Therefore, it was not possible to establish a relationship between an ANA pattern and a specific disease in this sample.

The homogeneous nuclear fluorescence pattern is primarily associated with systemic autoimmunity [47]. This pattern was observed in two patients who had a clinical condition of SLE: one of these patients exhibited the anti-SSA/Ro antibody; the other patient exhibited anti-Scl-70, anti-Smith, and anti-RNP/Sm; and the last two antibodies listed are markers for SLE [48]. Three of the five patients diagnosed with scleroderma exhibited anti-CENP-B and a centromere pattern (NC) in the ANA test. Göring et al. [49] reported a strong association between scleroderma, anti-CENP-B, and NC pattern.

The NDFS pattern is frequently observed in people without autoimmune diseases and with a positive ANA test [44]. However, the present study observed that two of the three patients who exhibited the nuclear dense fine speckled pattern were diagnosed with rheumatic autoimmune diseases. This is corroborated by some authors [50, 51], who showed that the antigen most related with NDFS pattern is DSF70, but the appearance of others antigens can occur when the sample is from a patient with an autoimmune disease. The frequency of NDFS in other studies varied from 0.3 to 27% [50, 52, 53], showing that differentiation between the NDFS pattern and other patterns can be difficult and it is likely that laboratories in the past have reported NDFS as a mixed pattern. IIF is a subjective test and recognition of this pattern is open to interpretation [54].

A high prevalence of rheumatic autoimmune diseases (75%) was found in anti-ENA-positive patients. The most common diagnosis in these patients was SLE (33.3%), which is consistent with Lora et al. [40], who evaluated the ANA patterns and clinical diagnoses of anti-SS-A/Ro positive patients, and SLE was also the predominant clinical association in these patients with 50.8% frequency.

The diagnostic accuracy of anti-ENA antibodies in AD patients is known to vary with patient selection and detection technique. Previous studies conducted by Albon et al. [55] and Vercammen et al. [39] have compared several methods of ENA testing and shown overall equivalence for most antigens. However, unlike the approach of this study, recruitment in these studies and others [30, 31, 56] was based on patients with known diseases or a positive ANA, which alters the pretest probability of a positive ENA test.

Some associations between extractable nuclear antigens and AD are close and frequently reported in the literature, for example, between Scleroderma and Scl-70 or Sjögren's Syndrome and SS/A or SS/B [2, 3], which were found in this study. Nevertheless, some uncommon associations occurred between anti-ENA and clinical manifestations, as rheumatoid arthritis (RA) and SS/A or autoimmune hemolytic anemia and nucleosome. Association between antibodies against ENA and RA occurred in a minority of patients and was not related to symptoms, and a variety of antigens could occur in RA [57, 58]. Occurrence of anti-ENA in patients with Behçet's disease is uncommon, around 10% [59, 60], but the most frequent antigen is SS/A. An association found in this work, which has not been reported in the literature, was between autoimmune hemolytic anemia and anti-nucleosome. Hemolytic anemia is a pure autoimmune disease and usually does not entail the presence of autoantibodies such as ANA or anti-ENA. In this case, it should be an initial manifestation of some systemic autoimmune diseases, such as SLE [17].

Forty-five of the anti-ENA-negative patients (35%) exhibited manifestations of AD. Twelve of these patients (26.7%) were diagnosed with SLE, and four patients were diagnosed with SLE associated with other autoimmune diseases. These results show the importance of the clinical association of the ANA examination, which is the screening test for autoimmunity [15].

Seven of the 172 antigen tests performed exhibited antibody levels that were very close to the detection limit, and these patients had inconclusive or undetermined anti-ENA results. Two of these patients exhibited clinical signs of AD, and no information on the diagnosis was found for two other patients.

The sensitivity of the tests performed, the experience of the professionals during the execution, interpretation of the results, erroneous requests for anti-ENA tests, and the lack of ANA results when necessary are the primary limitations of the present study. ANA examination should be requested only in the presence of a convincing suspicion of autoimmune disease because a positive result does not necessarily imply autoimmunity. However, when a positive ANA result occurs, it is important to identify the specific autoantibody involved.

5. Conclusions

The anti-ENA test was a good method to aid in the clinical diagnosis of rheumatological autoimmune diseases. In this study, several anti-ENA tests have been solicited without an

ANA test, which should not occur once sensitivity of the first test is lower than the second test.

It is essential to characterize the presence of antibodies that are particular to autoimmune pathologies using specific techniques in ANA-positive patients.

Professionals that directly or indirectly work with anti-ENA and ANA examinations must perform an accurate and constant review of the paradigms that guide the interpretation of the results so that the clinical diagnosis and subsequent treatment of the patients can be successfully achieved.

Conflicts of Interest

The authors declare that there are no conflicts of interest regarding the publication of this paper.

Acknowledgments

The authors are grateful to Rodrigo A. Barcella of Western Parana University Hospital for his technical support and revisions of the text.

References

[1] J. H. Cho and P. K. Gregersen, "Genomics and the multifactorial nature of human autoimmune disease," *The New England Journal of Medicine*, vol. 365, no. 17, pp. 1612–1623, 2011.

[2] J. Suurmond and B. Diamond, "Autoantibodies in systemic autoimmune diseases: Specificity and pathogenicity," *The Journal of Clinical Investigation*, vol. 125, no. 6, pp. 2194–2202, 2015.

[3] C. Campochiaro and E. C. Derrett-Smith, "Autoantibodies in autoimmune rheumatic disease," *Medicine*, vol. 46, no. 2, pp. 78–83, 2018.

[4] American College of Rheumatology Position Statement, "Methodology of Testing for Antinuclear Antibodies," *Am. Coll. Rheumatol*, 2015.

[5] P. L. Meroni and P. H. Schur, "ANA screening: an old test with new recommendations," *Annals of the Rheumatic Diseases*, vol. 69, no. 8, pp. 1420–1422, 2010.

[6] F. d. Brito, S. M. Santos, G. A. Ferreira et al., "Detection of anti-nuclear antibodies by indirect immunofluorescence on HEp-2 cells: setting the appropriate screening dilution for the diagnosis of autoimmune rheumatic diseases," *Revista Brasileira de Reumatologia (English Edition)*, vol. 54, no. 1, pp. 13–20, 2014.

[7] V. P. K. Nell, K. P. Machold, T. A. Stamm et al., "Autoantibody profiling as early diagnostic and prognostic tool for rheumatoid arthritis," *Annals of the Rheumatic Diseases*, vol. 64, no. 12, pp. 1731–1736, 2005.

[8] H. Wu, J. Zeng, J. Yin, Q. Peng, M. Zhao, and Q. Lu, "Organ-specific biomarkers in lupus," *Autoimmunity Reviews*, vol. 16, no. 4, pp. 391–397, 2017.

[9] W.-T. Ma, C. Chang, M. E. Gershwin, and Z.-X. Lian, "Development of autoantibodies precedes clinical manifestations of autoimmune diseases: A comprehensive review," *Journal of Autoimmunity*, vol. 83, pp. 95–112, 2017.

[10] Z. Hu and A. Deng, "Autoantibodies in pre-clinical autoimmune disease," *Clinica Chimica Acta*, vol. 437, pp. 14–18, 2014.

[11] E. P. Nagele, M. Han, N. K. Acharya, C. DeMarshall, M. C. Kosciuk, and R. G. Nagele, "Natural IgG autoantibodies are abundant and ubiquitous in human sera, and their number is influenced by age, gender, and disease," *PLoS ONE*, vol. 8, no. 4, Article ID e60726, 2013.

[12] D. Chandratilleke, R. Silvestrini, S. Culican et al., "Comparison of two extractable nuclear antigen testing algorithms: ALBIA versus ELISA/line immunoassay," *Pathology*, vol. 48, no. 5, pp. 491–497, 2016.

[13] T. G. Phan, R. C. W. Wong, and S. Adelstein, "Autoantibodies to extractable nuclear antigens: Making detection and interpretation more meaningful," *Clinical and Diagnostic Laboratory Immunology*, vol. 9, no. 1, pp. 1–7, 2002.

[14] A. Kavanaugh, R. Tomar, and J. Reveille, "Guidelines for clinical use of the antinuclear antibody test and tests for specific autoantibodies to nuclear antigens," *Arch Pathol Lab Med*, vol. 124, pp. 71–81, 2000.

[15] P. L. Francescantonio, W. d. Cruvinel, A. Dellavance et al., "IV Brazilian Guidelines for autoantibodies on HEp-2 cells," *Revista Brasileira de Reumatologia (English Edition)*, vol. 54, no. 1, pp. 44–50, 2014.

[16] P. Ungprasert, C. S. Crowson, V. R. Chowdhary, F. C. Ernste, K. G. Moder, and E. L. Matteson, "Epidemiology of Mixed Connective Tissue Disease, 1985-2014: A Population-Based Study," *Arthritis Care & Research*, vol. 68, no. 12, pp. 1843–1848, 2016.

[17] M. Petri, A-M. Orbai, and GS. Alarcón, "Derivation and validation of the Systemic Lupus International Collaborating Clinics classification criteria for systemic lupus erythematosus," *Arthritis Rheum*, pp. 2677–2686, 2014.

[18] I. N. Targoff, "Update on myositis-specific and myositis-associated autoantibodies," *Current Opinion in Rheumatology*, vol. 12, no. 6, pp. 475–481, 2000.

[19] P. García de La Peña-Lefebvre, Y. Chanseaud, M. C. Tamby et al., "IgG reactivity with a 100-kDa tissue and endothelial cell antigen identified as topoisomerase 1 distinguishes between limited and diffuse systemic sclerosis patients," *Clinical Immunology*, vol. 111, no. 3, pp. 241–251, 2004.

[20] T. T. Provost, "Anti-Ro(SSA)and Anti-La(SSB)Antibodies in Lupus Erythematosus and Sjoegren's Syndrome.," *The Keio Journal of Medicine*, vol. 40, no. 2, pp. 72–77, 1991.

[21] Y. Zhang and M. Song, "Deciphering interactions in causal networks without parametric assumptions," 2013, https://arxiv.org/abs/1311.2707.

[22] R Foundation for Statistical Computing, *R: A Language and Environment for Statistical Computing*, Austria, Vienna, Austria, 2016.

[23] H. Wickham, *ggplot2: Elegant Graphics for Data Analysis*, Springer, New York, NY, USA, 2009.

[24] L. E. Andrade, "O fator antinúcleo para além do bem e do mal," *Jornal Brasileiro de Patologia e Medicina Laboratorial*, vol. 45, no. 3, pp. 0–0, 2009.

[25] A. Dellavance and L. E. Andrade, "Como interpretar e valorizar adequadamente o teste de anticorpos antinúcleo," *Jornal Brasileiro de Patologia e Medicina Laboratorial*, vol. 43, no. 3, 2007.

[26] V. d. Viana, C. Bueno, and J. F. Carvalho, "Fator antinuclear: do valor diagnóstico ao valor preditivo de doenças autoimunes," *Revista Brasileira de Reumatologia*, vol. 49, no. 2, pp. 85-86, 2009.

[27] I. E. A. Hoffman, I. Peene, E. M. Veys, and F. De Keyser, "Detection of specific antinuclear reactivities in patients with negative anti-nuclear antibody immunofluorescence screening tests," *Clinical Chemistry*, vol. 48, no. 12, pp. 2171–2176, 2002.

[28] X. Bossuyt, A. Hendrickx, and J. Frans, "Antinuclear antibody titer and antibodies to extractable nuclear antigens," *Arthritis & Rheumatism*, vol. 53, no. 6, pp. 987-988, 2005.

[29] R. Hira-Kazal, P. Shea-Simonds, J. L. Peacock, and J. Maher, "How should a district general hospital immunology service screen for anti-nuclear antibodies? An 'in-the-field' audit," *Clinical & Experimental Immunology*, vol. 180, no. 1, pp. 52–57, 2015.

[30] S. Jeong, H. Hwang, J. Roh et al., "Evaluation of an automated screening assay, compared to indirect immunofluorescence, an extractable nuclear antigen assay, and a line immunoassay in a large cohort of Asian patients with antinuclear antibody-associated rheumatoid diseases: A multicenter," *Journal of Immunology Research*, vol. 2018, Article ID 9094217, 12 pages, 2018.

[31] S. Sharmin, S. Ahmed, A. A. Saleh, F. Rahman, M. Choudhury, and M. Hassan, "Association of Immunofluorescence pattern of Antinuclear Antibody with Specific Autoantibodies in the Bangladeshi Population," *Bangladesh Medical Research Council Bulletin*, vol. 40, no. 2, p. 74, 2015.

[32] J. M. Kim, C. H. Ihm, D. H. Sin, M. K. Ihm, and S. C. Sim, "Detection of Anti-ENA and anti-dsDNA antibodies using line immunoassay in systemic autoimmune diseases," *Korean Journal of Laboratory Medicine*, vol. 28, no. 5, pp. 353–361, 2008.

[33] K. F. Thomson, A. Murphy, M. J. D. Goodfield, and S. A. Misbah, "Is it useful to test for antibodies to extractable nuclear antigens in the presence of a negative antinuclear antibody on Hep-2 cells? [4]," *Journal of Clinical Pathology*, vol. 54, no. 5, p. 413, 2001.

[34] K. Kidd, K. Cusi, and R. Mueller, "Detection and identification of significant ANAs in previously determined ANA negative samples," *Clin Lab*, vol. 51, pp. 517–521, 2005.

[35] S. A. Lee, J. Kahng, Y. Kim et al., "Comparative Study of Immunofluorescent Antinuclear Antibody Test and Line Immunoassay Detecting 15 Specific Autoantibodies in Patients With Systemic Rheumatic Disease," *Journal of Clinical Laboratory Analysis*, vol. 26, no. 4, pp. 307–314, 2012.

[36] C. Dahle, T. Skogh, A. K. Åberg, A. Jalal, and P. Olcén, "Methods of choice for diagnostic antinuclear antibody (ANA) screening: Benefit of adding antigen-specific assays to immunofluorescence microscopy," *Journal of Autoimmunity*, vol. 22, no. 3, pp. 241–248, 2004.

[37] I. Peene, W. Van Ael, M. Vandenbossche, T. Vervaet, E. Veys, and F. De Keyser, "Sensitivity of the HEp-2000 Substrate for the Detection of Anti-SSA/Ro60 Antibodies," *Clinical Rheumatology*, vol. 19, no. 4, p. 291.

[38] X. Bossuyt, J. Frans, A. Hendrickx, G. Godefridis, R. Westhovens, and G. Mariën, "Detection of anti-SSA antibodies by indirect immunofluorescence," *Clinical Chemistry*, vol. 50, no. 12, pp. 2361–2369, 2004.

[39] M. Vercammen, P. Meirlaen, J. Sennesael et al., "Diagnostic accuracy of the FIDIS multiplex fluorescent microsphere immunodetection system for anti-extractable nuclear antigen (ENA) antibodies in connective tissue diseases," *Clinical Chemistry and Laboratory Medicine*, vol. 45, no. 4, pp. 505–512, 2007.

[40] P. S. Lora, C. C. Laurino, A. E. Freitas, J. C. Brenol, O. Montecielo, and R. M. Xavier, "Padrões de imunofluorescência do fator antinuclear (FAN) em células HEp-2 de soros reagentes para anti-SSA/Ro," *Revista Brasileira de Reumatologia*, vol. 47, no. 1, pp. 4–9, 2007.

[41] J. Sánchez-Guerrero, R. A. Lew, A. H. Fossel, and P. H. Schur, "Utility of anti-Sm, anti-RNP, anti-Ro/SS-A, and anti-La/SS-B (extractable nuclear antigens) detected by enzyme-linked immunosorbent assay for the diagnosis of systemic lupus erythematosus," *Arthritis & Rheumatology*, vol. 39, no. 6, pp. 1055–1061, 1996.

[42] M. R. Arbuckle, M. T. McClain, M. V. Rubertone et al., "Development of autoantibodies before the clinical onset of systemic lupus erythematosus," *The New England Journal of Medicine*, vol. 349, no. 16, pp. 1526–1533, 2003.

[43] A. Dellavance, P. G. Leser, and L. E. Andrade, "Análise crítica do teste de anticorpos antinúcleo (FAn) na prática clínica," *Revista Brasileira de Reumatologia*, vol. 47, no. 4, pp. 265–275, 2007.

[44] E. M. Tan, T. E. Feltkamp, J. S. Smolen et al., "Range of antinuclear antibodies in "healthy" individuals," *Arthritis & Rheumatism*, vol. 40, no. 9, pp. 1601–1611, 1997.

[45] K. Conrad, M. P. Bachmann, E. Matsuura, and Y. Shoenfeld, "From animal models to human genetics: Research on the induction and pathogenicity of autoantibodies," *Autoimmunity Reviews*, vol. 4, no. 3, pp. 178–187, 2005.

[46] W. Y. Craig and T. B. Ledue, "The relationship between antinuclear antibody data and antibodies against extractable nuclear antigens in a large laboratory cohort," *Clinical Chemistry and Laboratory Medicine*, vol. 50, no. 3, pp. 497–502, 2012.

[47] D. Almeida González, A. Cabrera de León, M. D. C. Rodríguez Pérez et al., "Efficiency of different strategies to detect autoantibodies to extractable nuclear antigens," *Journal of Immunological Methods*, vol. 360, no. 1-2, pp. 89–95, 2010.

[48] C. R. Marçon, M. R. Moraes, S. M. Lanzelotti, D. R. Simis, and G. S. Novaes, "Marcadores de envolvimento sistêmico no lúpus eritematoso crônico discóide," *Revista Brasileira de Reumatologia*, vol. 44, no. 5, pp. 333–338, 2004.

[49] M. Panzner and K. Dessau, "Association of scleroderma and primary biliary cirrhosis results of a systematic study on a dermatological clientele," *Hautarzt*, vol. 49, pp. 361–366, 1998.

[50] J. B. Carter, S. Carter, S. Saschenbrecker, and B. E. Goeckeritz, "Recognition and Relevance of Anti-DFS70 Autoantibodies in Routine Antinuclear Autoantibodies Testing at a Community Hospital," *Frontiers in Medicine*, vol. 5, 2018.

[51] A. Broadfoot, T. Sivertsen, and K. Baumgart, "Dense fine speckled indirect immunofluorescence pattern in an Australian population," *Pathology*, vol. 48, no. 3, pp. 247–250, 2016.

[52] K. Conrad, N. Röber, L. E. Andrade, and M. Mahler, "The Clinical Relevance of Anti-DFS70 Autoantibodies," *Clinical Reviews in Allergy & Immunology*, vol. 52, no. 2, pp. 202–216, 2017.

[53] M. Mahler, T. Parker, C. L. Peebles et al., "Anti-DFS70/LEDGF antibodies are more prevalent in healthy individuals compared

to patients with systemic autoimmune rheumatic diseases," *The Journal of Rheumatology*, vol. 39, no. 11, pp. 2104–2110, 2012.

[54] C. Bentow, M. J. Fritzler, E. Mummert, and M. Mahler, "Recognition of the dense fine speckled (DFS) pattern remains challenging: results from an international internet-based survey," *Autoimmunity Highlights*, vol. 7, no. 1, 2016.

[55] S. Albon, C. Bunn, G. Swana, and Y. Karim, "Performance of a multiplex assay compared to enzyme and precipitation methods for anti-ENA testing in systemic lupus and systemic sclerosis," *Journal of Immunological Methods*, vol. 365, no. 1-2, pp. 126–131, 2011.

[56] H. Nawaz Tipu and M. Mukarram Bashir, "Determination Of Specificity And Pattern Of Antinuclear Antibodies (ana) In Systemic Rheumatic Disease Patients Positive For Ana Testing," *Journal of College of Physicians and Surgeons Pakistan*, vol. 28, no. 1, pp. 40–43, 2018.

[57] D. P. Molden, H. Suzuki, and R. M. Nakamura, "Assays for Sm and RNP antibodies: Pitfalls and technical considerations," *Diagn Immunol*, pp. 24–28, 1985.

[58] P. J. Venables, C. C. Erhardt, and R. N. Maini, "Antibodies to extractable nuclear antigens in rheumatoid arthritis: Relationship to vasculitis and circulating immune complexes," *Clin Exp Immunol*, vol. 39, pp. 146–153, 1980.

[59] A. Al Ghafri and H. Al Wahshi, "Demographic features and clinical aspects of Behçet's disease in Omani patients," *Rheumatology Practice and Research*, vol. 3, 2018.

[60] Y. Shang, S. Han, J. Li, Q. Ren, F. Song, and H. Chen, "The Clinical Feature of Behçet's Disease in Northeastern China," *Yonsei Medical Journal*, vol. 50, no. 5, p. 630, 2009.

35

[^{18}F]-Fluoro-Deoxy-Glucose Positron Emission Tomography Scan Should Be Obtained Early in Cases of Autoimmune Encephalitis

C. R. Newey,[1] A. Sarwal,[2] and S. Hantus[3,4]

[1] *Department of Neurology, University of Missouri, 5 Hospital Drive, CE 540, Columbia, MO 65211, USA*
[2] *Neurology and Critical Care, Wake Forest University School of Medicine, Reynolds M, Medical Center Boulevard, Winston-Salem, NC 27157, USA*
[3] *Department of Adult Neurology, Cleveland Clinic, 9500 Euclid Avenue, Cleveland, OH 44195-5245, USA*
[4] *Epilepsy Center, Neurologic Institute, Cleveland Clinic, 9500 Euclid Avenue, Cleveland, OH 44195-5245, USA*

Correspondence should be addressed to C. R. Newey; neweyc@health.missouri.edu

Academic Editor: Corrado Betterle

Introduction. Autoimmune encephalitis (AE) is a clinically challenging diagnosis with nonspecific neurological symptoms. Prompt diagnosis is important and often relies on neuroimaging. We present a case series of AE highlighting the importance of an early [^{18}F]-fluoro-deoxy-glucose positron emission tomography (FDG-PET) scan. *Methods.* Retrospective review of seven consecutive cases of autoimmune encephalitis. *Results.* All patients had both magnetic resonance imaging (MRI) and FDG-PET scans. Initial clinical presentations included altered mental status and/or new onset seizures. Six cases had serum voltage-gated potassium channel (VGKC) antibody and one had serum N-methyl-D-aspartate (NMDA) antibody. MRI of brain showed mesial temporal lobe hyperintensity in five cases of VGKC. The other two patients with VGKC or NMDA AE had restiform body hyperintensity on MRI brain or a normal MRI, respectively. Mesial temporal lobe hypermetabolism was noted in three cases on FDG-PET, despite initial unremarkable MRI. Malignancy workup was negative in all patients. *Conclusion.* A high index of suspicion for AE should be maintained in patients presenting with cognitive symptoms, seizures, and limbic changes on neuroimaging. In cases with normal initial brain MRI, FDG-PET can be positive. Additionally, extralimbic hyperintensity on MRI may also be observed.

1. Introduction

Autoimmune encephalitis (AE) is a clinically challenging diagnosis usually suspected in cases of altered mental status or seizures after excluding other more common diagnoses. (Anderson 2008) Common presenting signs are nonspecific-memory impairment, hallucinations, anxiety, irritability, depression, seizures, or sleep alterations [1, 2]. These symptoms may develop over a course of weeks to months. AE may be of infectious, paraneoplastic, or immune-mediated etiology. Differential diagnoses, diagnostic approaches, and clinical criteria for diagnosis of paraneoplastic AE have been proposed previously [3–5]. Most recently, consensus on diagnostic criteria for autoimmune encephalitis has been published [6]. Positive serology with specific antibodies and negative workup for malignancy are important in the diagnosis [6]. With emerging evidence of reversibility of AE with immunotherapy, early diagnosis is important and should not be delayed while awaiting for serological data [6]. Thus, early neuroimaging, along with the initial neurological assessment, plays an important role [6, 7].

Voltage-gated potassium channel (VGKC) and N-methyl-D-aspartate (NMDA) antibodies are increasingly being recognized as associations of AE due to easy availability of serological testing. Since the presenting symptoms are nonspecific, establishing neuroimaging correlates to guide diagnostic workup may allow for timely therapeutic interventions. We present seven patients (six positive for VGKC and one positive for NMDA antibodies) with AE highlighting the importance of early neuroimaging with brain magnetic resonance imaging (MRI) and [^{18}F]-fluoro-deoxy-glucose positron emission tomography (FDG-PET).

2. Methods

We screened medical records of patients evaluated at a tertiary academic medical center between 2004 and 2010 billed under ICD-9 codes 276.1 and 323.9. A retrospective review of 848 case records with clinical diagnosis of AE and/or limbic encephalitis upon presentation was done. Of these, 102 patients had paraneoplastic panel results available with 7 being positive (6 positive for VGK and 1 positive for NMDA antibodies). All panels were processed by Mayo Medical Laboratories (Rochester, MN). The cases were further reviewed for historical information, diagnostic workup, medications administered, and neuroimaging findings. The Institutional Review Board approved the study protocol.

3. Results

Patient characteristics are described in Table 1. Mean age was 56.7 years (range: 22 to 91 years of age; 4 males and 3 females). All presented with the chief complaint of altered mental status and/or seizure. One patient had elevated microsomal antibodies (138.6 IU/mL; normal < 5 IU/mL) and thyroglobulin antibodies (1209 IU/mL; normal < 10 IU/mL) with a normal thyroid stimulating hormone (TSH) (4.63 μU/mL) and free T4 (1.4 μU/mL) in addition to VGKC antibody. None of the patients had diabetes. Computed tomography (CT) of chest, abdomen, and pelvis was negative in all patients. CSF was significant in three patients with elevation of white cell count in two patients and mild elevation of protein in a third patient.

The mean time of symptom onset to positive antibody serology was 102.1 days (range: 8 to 185 days; Table 1). The average VGKC titer on initial presentation was 1.44 nmol/L (normal < 0.03) [8]. NMDA titer was not resulted. All but one patient received intravenous methylprednisolone, intravenous immunoglobulin, and plasmapheresis in various combinations. Four of the six treated patients improved with treatment with minimal residual cognitive deficits. One patient did not receive treatment and improved remarkably prior to discharge and returned to her baseline health five months after presentation. One patient expired from an unrelated medical cause. One patient progressed to persistent vegetative state. At least three patients had serial serology titers for the antibodies. Only one case made significant improvement in titer level following treatment. Six of the seven patients required prolonged antiepileptic agents for seizure control.

The average time between symptom onset and first neuroimaging modality was 48.6 days (range: 4 to 184 days). MRI of the brain was the first modality in four cases (Table 2). CT of head was performed first in the other cases. The average time from onset of symptoms to first positive finding on neuroimaging (i.e., T2/fluid attenuated inversion recovery (FLAIR) hyperintensity on MRI or FDG-PET hypermetabolism) was 80.0 days (range: 16 to 184 days). Four patients had mesial temporal lobe hyperintensity on T2/FLAIR weighted MRI. One patient with VGKC AE had T2/FLAIR weighted hyperintensity of the restiform bodies. The other patient with VGKC AE had global atrophy. The patient with positive NMDA AE had serial MRIs that were all unremarkable except development of generalized atrophy (Table 3).

FDG-PET scans were available in six of the patients. All six patients had hypermetabolism of mesial temporal structures (Table 3). In three of these cases, the FDG-PET was positive (i.e., mesial temporal lobe hypermetabolism) before any changes were visualized on brain MRI. Serial MRI scans in two of the patients subsequently became positive for mesial temporal lobe hyperintensity 1 and 72 days following the FDG-PET scans. These patients were positive for VGKC. The brain MRI for the patient positive for NMDA AE only showed generalized atrophy on subsequent imaging. Figure 1 is an illustrative example of FDG-PET findings prior to MRI findings. CT of head was unremarkable for any acute process in all the presented cases.

4. Discussion

This case series of VGKC and NMDA autoimmune encephalitis illustrates the importance of neuroimaging with emphasis of early FDG-PET particularly in cases of initial nondiagnostic MRIs. It also demonstrates the extralimbic nature that may occur with VGKC antibody positive AE.

It is accepted that paraneoplastic and nonparaneoplastic antibodies can present at distant sites from the limbic system, but they usually do so in addition to limbic involvement [9]. The importance of the solitary finding in this case is not clear. VGKC receptors are known to be found in the peripheral nervous and autonomic nervous systems in addition to the central nervous system. Recent studies have illustrated that antibodies directed to proteins (e.g., contactin-associated protein-like 2 (CASPR2) and leucine-rich glioma-inactivated protein 1 (LGI1)) within the VGKC complex or to Kv1 channels may explain why patients present with such varied clinical and radiological presentations [8, 10, 11]. The diversity in neurologic phenotypes seems to be independent of the VGKC antibody titer level [8]. Even at low levels of positive VGKC, the finding of LGI1 and/or CASPR2 antibodies can result in a diverse spectrum of neurologic phenotypes [8]. Nevertheless, LGI1 antibodies typically result in higher titers of VKGC antibody titers, and LGI1 antibodies will typically have cortical (e.g., seizures and/or altered mental status) presentations [8]. These subtypes of VGKC antibody can be found in patients with extralimbic presentations [8]. This suggests a critical evaluation of extralimbic regions of the brain for MRI changes in patients with suspicion for AE. Importantly, VGKC positivity in the absence of antibodies to either LGI1 or CASPR2 does not seem to be clinically relevant as a marker of autoimmune inflammation [11]. Unfortunately, our seropositive-VGKC patients had serum samples tested prior to the accepted reporting of the subtypes of the VGKC macromolecule complex.

Why VGKC antibodies caused mostly limbic hyperintensity on MRI and the NMDA antibodies did not is not entirely

Table 1: Patient characteristics.

Patient	Sex	Age (years)	Clinical features	Cancer	Antibody monitoring (days)	VGKC titers (nmol/L)	NMDA serology	Symptom onset to diagnosis (days)	CSF WBC (cells/mm^3)	CSF protein (mg/dL)	Treatment	Max number of AEDs
1	F	91	Altered mental status	No	Initial	0.13	NA	8	3	57	None	None
2	M	59	Autonomic seizure	No	Initial 54 161 273	1.58 4.22 15.8 1.94	NA	94	1	40	IVMP × 5 days, PLEX × 5 days	3
3	F	52	Altered mental status, depression	No	Initial	0.13	NA	178	NA	69	IVMP × 5 days, IVIG × 5 days	2
4	F	35	Flu-like symptoms, complex partial seizure, hyponatremia, elevated microsomal and thyroglobulin antibodies	No	Initial 24	2.8 0.77	NA	54	2	34	IVIG × 3 days, IVMP × 3 days, PLEX × 5 days	5
5	M	54	Altered mental status, hyponatremia, gelastic seizure	No	Initial	3.89	NA	185	12	47	IVMP × 5 days, PLEX ×5 days	4
6	M	84	Altered mental status, hyponatremia, tonic seizure	No	Initial	0.13	NA	177	2	48	IVMP × 5 days, PLEX × 3 days/week for 2 weeks	2
7	M	22	Psychosis	No	Initial 56	NA	Positive Positive	19	64	23	IVMP × 5, PLEX × 10 d, IVIG × 5, cyclophos-phamide, prednisone 5 qd	5
Average:		*56.7*			*51.6*	*3.5*		*102.1*	*12.0*	*45.4*		

VGKC, voltage-gated potassium channel antibody; CSF, cerebrospinal fluid; IVMP, 1 gram of intravenous methylprednisolone; IVIG = 0.4 g/kg/d of intravenous immunoglobulin; PLEX, plasma exchange; F, female; M, male; NA, not applicable.

Table 2: Structural and physiological workup.

Patient	Days from onset to first image	First image modality	Days from onset to first positive image finding	First positive image modality	Days from onset to first EEG	Days from onset to first positive EEG findings	EEG finding
1	4	CT	NA	NA	159	NA	Normal
2	46	MRI	109	PET	46	81	Vertex seizure
3	73	MRI	120	PET	83	180	Periodic pattern
4	184	MRI	184	MRI	183	183	Nonlocalizable status
5	10	MRI	18	MRI	53	NA	Generalized slowing
6	14	CT	16	MRI	22	22	Right frontotemporal seizure
7	9	CT	33	PET	14	18	Bifrontal seizure
Average	*48.6*		*80.0*		*80.0*	*96.8*	

EEG, electroencephalogram; CT, computed tomography; PET, positron emission tomography; NA, not applicable.

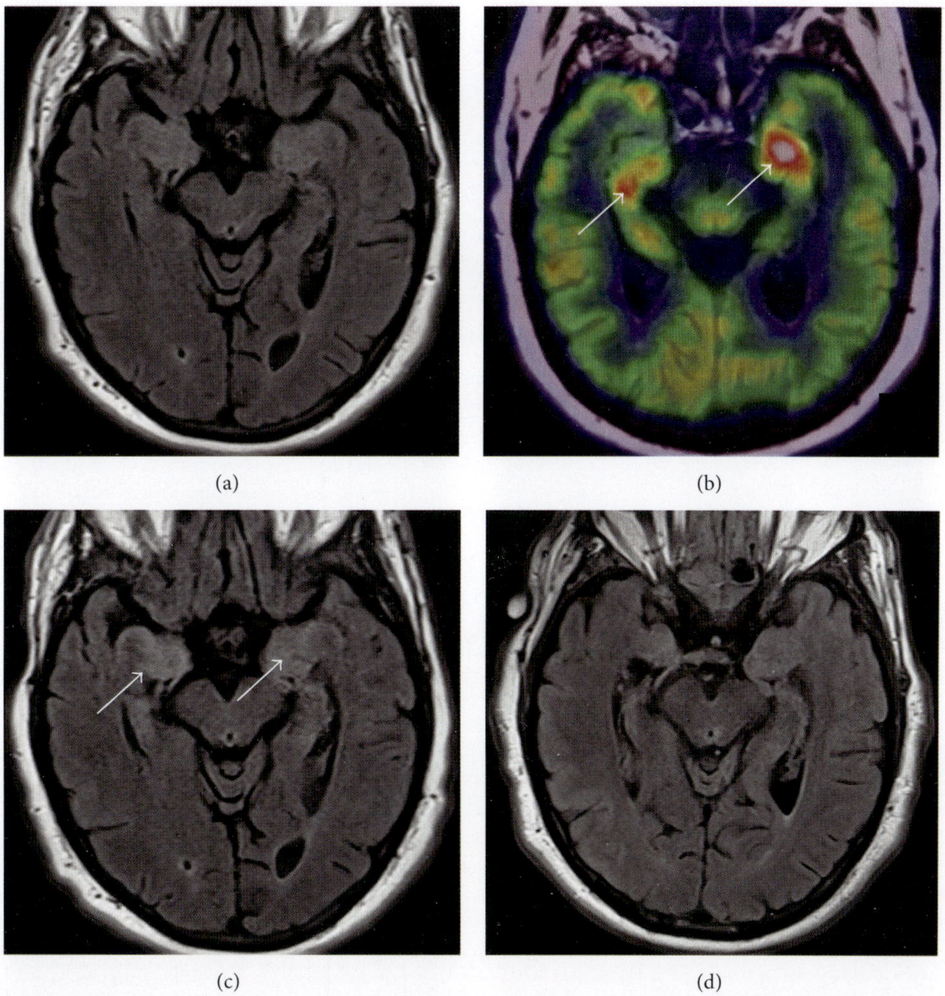

(a) (b) (c) (d)

Figure 1: Neuroimaging of VGKC antibody. The initial, unremarkable axial T2/FLAIR MRI of the brain (a) followed by FDG-PET showing significant asymmetric hypermetabolism of the bilateral mesial temporal lobes (arrows; (b)) with repeat axial T2/FLAIR demonstrating hyperintensity in bilateral mesial temporal lobes (arrows; (c)) that significantly improved by the last T2/FLAIR (d).

TABLE 3: MRI and PET findings.

Patient	MRI brain findings	PET findings
1	Global atrophy out of proportion to patient's age	NA
2	Bilateral mesial temporal lobe hyperintensity on T2/FLAIR without contrast enhancement	Left mesial temporal lobe hypermetabolism
3	Bilateral hyperintensity on T2/FLAIR in the restiform bodies bilaterally without contrast enhancement	Right temporal lobe hypermetabolism
4	Left unilateral mesial temporal lobe hyperintensity on T2/FLAIR without contrast enhancement	Left temporal lobe hypermetabolism
5	Right unilateral mesial temporal lobe hyperintensity on T2/FLAIR without contrast enhancement	Bilateral temporal lobe hypermetabolism
6	Right unilateral mesial temporal lobe hyperintensity on T2/FLAIR without contrast enhancement	Bilateral temporal lobe hypermetabolism
7	Unremarkable brain	Bilateral temporal lobe hypermetabolism

known. It has been suggested that the restricted diffusion seen on the diffusion weighted images (DWI) is due to the presence of abundant number of inflammatory cells along with increased amounts of interstitial water which accounts for the relative normal apparent diffusion coefficient (ADC) images [12]. The hyperintensity is typically asymmetric and rarely enhances with contrast [13]. VGKC are also among the earliest ion channels to appear during brain development. It is not clear whether limbic involvement represents concentration of VGKC in these patients implying a pathogenetic role of the VGKC antibodies or presence of antibodies is an incidental finding. Importantly, the hyperintensity on MRI can persist over months to years and may actually lead to progressive mesial temporal sclerosis [14].

Another important finding in this case series is the lag time in developing noticeable changes on MRI. Two cases showed mesial temporal lobe hypermetabolism on FDG-PET prior to changes on brain MRI. Additionally, the patient with NMDA AE showed mesial temporal lobe hypermetabolism without MRI findings. The utility of FDG-PET in the diagnosis and monitoring of autoimmune encephalitis has been shown to be significant [15–17]. FDG-PET of the brain typically shows hypermetabolism in similar regions as the brain MRI hyperintensity [9]. The described findings on brain MRI have included T2/FLAIR hyperintensities in the mesial temporal lobes (either unilateral or bilateral) that rarely enhance, generalized atrophy, or corpus callosum or basal ganglia hyperintensities [3, 18]. Thus, it is recommended that FDG-PET be obtained early in diagnostic workup of suspected cases of autoimmune encephalitis, especially when the initial MRI of the brain is unremarkable.

In conclusion, FDG-PET is a useful tool in the diagnostic workup of autoimmune encephalitis, such as in patients with VGKC or NMDA receptor antibodies. FDG-PET can be positive despite an unremarkable brain MRI. Additionally, maintaining awareness of extralimbic hyperintensity on MRI is also recommended.

Disclosure

S. Hantus has served as a consultant and on advisory boards for UCB pharma.

Competing Interests

The authors declare that they have no competing interests.

Authors' Contributions

C. R. Newey, A. Sarwal, and S. Hantus contributed equally to the writing of the case and formatting the images. C. R. Newey and A. Sarwal have no financial disclosures to report.

Acknowledgments

The authors would like to thank Welf Saupe of the eResearch Center at the Cleveland Clinic for his assistance in identifying patients for the research project.

References

[1] N. E. Anderson and P. A. Barber, "Limbic encephalitis—a review," *Journal of Clinical Neuroscience*, vol. 15, no. 9, pp. 961–971, 2008.

[2] J. M. Schott, "Another case of voltage-gated potassium channel antibody-related encephalopathy?" *European Neurology*, vol. 55, no. 2, p. 110, 2006.

[3] J. Dalmau and M. R. Rosenfeld, "Paraneoplastic syndromes of the CNS," *The Lancet Neurology*, vol. 7, no. 4, pp. 327–340, 2008.

[4] M. R. Rosenfeld and J. Dalmau, "Update on paraneoplastic and autoimmune disorders of the central nervous system," *Seminars in Neurology*, vol. 30, no. 3, pp. 320–331, 2010.

[5] F. Graus, J. Y. Delattre, J. C. Antoine et al., "Recommended diagnostic criteria for paraneoplastic neurological syndromes," *Journal of Neurology, Neurosurgery and Psychiatry*, vol. 75, no. 8, pp. 1135–1140, 2004.

[6] F. Graus, M. J. Titulaer, R. Balu et al., "A clinical approach to diagnosis of autoimmune encephalitis," *The Lancet Neurology*, vol. 15, no. 4, pp. 391–404, 2016.

[7] H. Gast, K. Schindler, W. J. Z'Graggen, and C. W. Hess, "Improvement of non-paraneoplastic voltage-gated potassium channel antibody-associated limbic encephalitis without immunosuppressive therapy," *Epilepsy and Behavior*, vol. 17, no. 4, pp. 555–557, 2010.

[8] C. J. Klein, V. A. Lennon, P. A. Aston et al., "Insights from LGI1 and CASPR2 potassium channel complex autoantibody subtyping," *JAMA Neurology*, vol. 70, no. 2, pp. 229–234, 2013.

[9] S. Vernino, M. Geschwind, and B. Boeve, "Autoimmune encephalopathies," *Neurologist*, vol. 13, no. 3, pp. 140–147, 2007.

[10] S. R. Irani, C. G. Bien, and B. Lang, "Autoimmune epilepsies," *Current Opinion in Neurology*, vol. 24, no. 2, pp. 146–153, 2011.

[11] A. van Sonderen, M. W. Schreurs, M. A. de Bruijn et al., "The relevance of VGKC positivity in the absence of LGI1 and Caspr2 antibodies," *Neurology*, vol. 86, no. 18, pp. 1692–1699, 2016.

[12] R. N. Sener, "MRI and diffusion MRI in nonparaneoplastic limbic encephalitis," *Computerized Medical Imaging and Graphics*, vol. 26, no. 5, pp. 339–342, 2002.

[13] E. Tüzün and J. Dalmau, "Limbic encephalitis and variants: classification, diagnosis and treatment," *Neurologist*, vol. 13, no. 5, pp. 261–271, 2007.

[14] H. Urbach, B. M. Soeder, M. Jeub, T. Klockgether, B. Meyer, and C. G. Bien, "Serial MRI of limbic encephalitis," *Neuroradiology*, vol. 48, no. 6, pp. 380–386, 2006.

[15] K. M. Tan, V. A. Lennon, C. J. Klein, B. F. Boeve, and S. J. Pittock, "Clinical spectrum of voltage-gated potassium channel autoimmunity," *Neurology*, vol. 70, no. 20, pp. 1883–1890, 2008.

[16] S. Fauser, J. Talazko, K. Wagner et al., "FDG-PET and MRI in potassium channel antibody-associated non-paraneoplastic limbic encephalitis: correlation with clinical course and neuropsychology," *Acta Neurologica Scandinavica*, vol. 111, no. 5, pp. 338–343, 2005.

[17] B. M. Ances, R. Vitaliani, R. A. Taylor et al., "Treatment-responsive limbic encephalitis identified by neuropil antibodies: MRI and PET correlates," *Brain*, vol. 128, no. 8, pp. 1764–1777, 2005.

[18] A. Hiraga, S. Kuwabara, S. Hayakawa et al., "Voltage-gated potassium channel antibody-associated encephalitis with basal ganglia lesions," *Neurology*, vol. 66, no. 11, pp. 1780–1781, 2006.

Permissions

All chapters in this book were first published in AO, by Hindawi Publishing Corporation; hereby published with permission under the Creative Commons Attribution License or equivalent. Every chapter published in this book has been scrutinized by our experts. Their significance has been extensively debated. The topics covered herein carry significant findings which will fuel the growth of the discipline. They may even be implemented as practical applications or may be referred to as a beginning point for another development.

The contributors of this book come from diverse backgrounds, making this book a truly international effort. This book will bring forth new frontiers with its revolutionizing research information and detailed analysis of the nascent developments around the world.

We would like to thank all the contributing authors for lending their expertise to make the book truly unique. They have played a crucial role in the development of this book. Without their invaluable contributions this book wouldn't have been possible. They have made vital efforts to compile up to date information on the varied aspects of this subject to make this book a valuable addition to the collection of many professionals and students.

This book was conceptualized with the vision of imparting up-to-date information and advanced data in this field. To ensure the same, a matchless editorial board was set up. Every individual on the board went through rigorous rounds of assessment to prove their worth. After which they invested a large part of their time researching and compiling the most relevant data for our readers.

The editorial board has been involved in producing this book since its inception. They have spent rigorous hours researching and exploring the diverse topics which have resulted in the successful publishing of this book. They have passed on their knowledge of decades through this book. To expedite this challenging task, the publisher supported the team at every step. A small team of assistant editors was also appointed to further simplify the editing procedure and attain best results for the readers.

Apart from the editorial board, the designing team has also invested a significant amount of their time in understanding the subject and creating the most relevant covers. They scrutinized every image to scout for the most suitable representation of the subject and create an appropriate cover for the book.

The publishing team has been an ardent support to the editorial, designing and production team. Their endless efforts to recruit the best for this project, has resulted in the accomplishment of this book. They are a veteran in the field of academics and their pool of knowledge is as vast as their experience in printing. Their expertise and guidance has proved useful at every step. Their uncompromising quality standards have made this book an exceptional effort. Their encouragement from time to time has been an inspiration for everyone.

The publisher and the editorial board hope that this book will prove to be a valuable piece of knowledge for researchers, students, practitioners and scholars across the globe.

List of Contributors

Andrew W. Campbell
The Wellness Center, 23144 Emerson Way, Land O Lakes, FL 34639, USA

Aristo Vojdani
Immunosciences Lab., Inc., 822 S. Robertson Boulevard, Suite 312, Los Angeles, CA 90035, USA

Gladis Montoya-Ortiz
Center for Autoimmune Diseases Research (CREA), School of Medicine and Health Sciences, Universidad del Rosario, Carrera 24 No. 63C-69, Bogota, Colombia

Emanuele Cozzani, Massimo Drosera, Giulia Gasparini and Aurora Parodi
Di.S.Sal, Section of Dermatology, IRCCS Azienda Ospedaliera, Universitaria San Martino-IST, 16132 Genoa, Italy

Devaraj J. Parasannanavar
Microbiology and Immunology Division, National Institute of Nutrition (ICMR), Jamai-Osmania, Tarnaka, Hyderabad, Andhra Pradesh 500007, India

Anjali Rajadhyaksha
Department of Medicine, King Edward Memorial Hospital, Parel, Mumbai 400 012, India

Kanjaksha Ghosh
National Institute of Immunohaematology (ICMR), King Edward Memorial Hospital, 13th Floor, N.M.S. Building, Parel, Mumbai 400 012, India

Fawzi Abukhalil, Erin Saito and Sejal Mehta
Neurology Department, Los Angeles Biomedical Research Institute, 1124West Carson Street, Building E5, Torrance, CA 90502, USA

Bijal Mehta and Aaron McMurtray
Neurology Department, Los Angeles Biomedical Research Institute, 1124West Carson Street, Building E5, Torrance, CA 90502, USA
Department of Neurology, Harbor-UCLA Medical Center, 1000West Carson Street, Torrance, CA 90509, USA

Christopher B. Toomey
Department of Ophthalmology, Duke University School of Medicine, Albert Eye Research Institute, Durham, NC 27710, USA

David M. Cauvi
Department of Surgery and Center for Investigations of Health and Education Disparities, University of California, San Diego, La Jolla, CA 92037, USA

Kenneth M. Pollard
Department of Molecular and Experimental Medicine, The Scripps Research Institute, La Jolla, CA 92037, USA

Jennifer Ong, Esther Erdei, Curtis Miller, Bernadette Pacheco and Johnnye L. Lewis
College of Pharmacy, Community Environmental Health Program, University of New Mexico Health Sciences Center, 905 Vassar NE, Albuquerque, NM 87106, USA

Robert L. Rubin
School of Medicine, University of New Mexico Health Sciences Center, 1 University of New Mexico, Albuquerque, NM 87131, USA

Carlyle Ducheneaux
Department of Natural Resources, Cheyenne River Sioux Tribe, East Highway 212, Eagle Butte, SD57625, USA

Marcia O'Leary
Missouri Breaks Industries Research, Inc., Hc 64 Timber Lake, SD 57656, USA

Michael Mahler
INOVA Diagnostics, Inc., 9900 Old Grove Road, San Diego, CA 92131, USA

Patricia Nez Henderson
Black Hills Center for American Indian Health, 701 St. Joseph Street, Suite 204, Rapid City, SD 57701, USA

K. Michael Pollard
Scripps Research Institute, 10550 North Torrey Pines Road, La Jolla, CA 92037, USA

Julio C. Sartori-Valinotti and Megha M. Tollefson
The Department of Dermatology, Mayo Clinic College of Medicine, Rochester, MN 55905, USA

Ann M. Reed
The Department of Pediatrics, Mayo Clinic College of Medicine, Rochester, MN 55905, USA

Carolina Muñoz-Grajales
Rheumatology Department, Pablo Tobón Uribe Hospital, Medellín, Colombia

Juan C. Pineda
Internal Medicine Department, Fundación Valle del Lili, ICESI University, Cali, Colombia

Ana Cláudia Guimarães Abreu, Gabriela Guy Duarte and Juliana Yasmin Pains Miranda
Faculdade de Ciências Humanas, Sociais e da Saúde, Universidade Fumec, 30310-190 Belo Horizonte, MG, Brazil

Daniel Gontijo Ramos
Departamento de Dermatologia, Santa Casa de Belo Horizonte, 30150-221 Belo Horizonte, MG, Brazil
Cl´ınica de Dermatologia, Edificio Life Center, 30110-921 Belo Horizonte, MG, Brazil

Camila Gontijo Ramos and Mariana Gontijo Ramos
Faculdade de Ciências Humanas, Sociais e da Saúde, Universidade Fumec, 30310-190 Belo Horizonte, MG, Brazil
Clínica de Dermatologia, Edificio Life Center, 30110-921 Belo Horizonte, MG, Brazil

Licia Maria Henrique da Mota, Leopoldo Luiz dos Santos-Neto and Pedro Luis Tauil
Faculdade de Medicina, Universidade de Brasília, Brasília, DF, Brazil

Ana Cristina Vanderley Oliveira
Faculdade de Medicina, Universidade de Brasília, Brasília, DF, Brazil
CRDF, SHLN Bloco L Centro Cínico Norte II, 70910-900 Brasília, DF, Brazil

Jozélio Freire De Carvalho
Hospital Universitário Professor Edgard Santos da Universidade Federal da Bahia, 70390-700 Salvador, BA, Brazil

Iramaya Rodrigues Caldas
Coordenação de Pesquisa da Fundação Oswaldo Cruz (FIOCRUZ), 41810-080 Brasília, DF, Brazil

Olindo Assis Martins Filho
Laboratório de Biomarcadores de Diagnóstico e Monitoração do Centro de Pesquisas René Rachou, FIOCRUZ, 21040-900 Belo Horizonte, MG, Brazil

Julio E.Molineros, Celi Sun, Prasenjeet Motghare, Xana Kim-Howard and Swapan K. Nath
Arthritis and Clinical Immunology Research Program, Oklahoma Medical Research Foundation, 1025 NE 13th Street, Oklahoma City, OK 73104, USA

Kek Heng Chua
Department of Biomedical Science, Faculty of Medicine, University of Malaya, 50603 Kuala Lumpur, Malaysia

Lay Hoong Lian
Department of Molecular Medicine, Faculty of Medicine, University of Malaya, 50603 Kuala Lumpur, Malaysia

Reidun Stenberg
Department of Pediatrics, Centre for Rehabilitation Research and Department of Clinical Medicine, School of Health and Medical Sciences, Örebro University, 70185 Örebro, Sweden

Marios Hadjivassiliou and Nigel Hoggard
Department of Neurology and Department of Neuroradiology, The Royal Hallamshire Hospital, Sheffield S10 2JF, UK

Pascale Aeschlimann and Daniel Aeschlimann
Matrix Biology and Tissue Repair Research Unit, College of Biomedical and Life Sciences, School of Dentistry, Cardiff University, Cardiff CF14 4XY, UK

Hassan A. N. El-Fawal
Neurotoxicology Laboratory, Albany College of Pharmacy and Health Sciences, 106 New Scotland Avenue, Albany, NY 12208, USA

Farhad Salehzadeh
Pediatric Department, Ardabil University of Medical Sciences (ARUMS), Ardabil 56157, Iran

Ozra Yasrebi, Mahsa Hosseini Khotbesara and Maryam Hosseini Khotbesara
Department of Pediatrics, Ardabil University of Medical Sciences (ARUMS), Bouali Hospital, Iran

Steen Stender and Pal Bela Szecsi
Department of Clinical Biochemistry, Gentofte Hospital, University of Copenhagen, 2900 Hellerup, Denmark

Merete Engelhart, Troels Mørk Hansen and Hanne Slott Jensen
Department of Rheumatology, Gentofte Hospital, University of Copenhagen, 2900 Hellerup, Denmark

Renata Baronaite
Department of Clinical Biochemistry, Gentofte Hospital, University of Copenhagen, 2900 Hellerup, Denmark
Department of Rheumatology, Gentofte Hospital, University of Copenhagen, 2900 Hellerup, Denmark

Gorm Thamsborg
Department of Rheumatology, Glostrup Hospital, University of Copenhagen, 2600 Glostrup, Denmark

Sharada T Rajan, Suganya Ramalingam, Narasimhan Malathi and Harikrishnan Thamizhchelvan
Department of Oral Pathology, Faculty of Dental Sciences, Sri Ramachandra Medical College and Research Institute (Deemed to Be University), Chennai, India

Narasimhan Sangeetha
Oral and Craniofacial Health Sciences, College of Dental Medicine, University of Sharjah, Sharjah, UAE

Benjamin Bienia and Roumen Balabanov
Department of Neurological Sciences, Multiple Sclerosis Center, Rush University Medical Center, 1725W Harrison Street, Suite 309, Chicago, IL 60612, USA

Pankaj S. Kothavade, Vipin D. Bulani, Dnyaneshwar M. Nagmoti, Padmini S. Deshpande, Nitin B. Gawali and Archana R. Juvekar
Department of Pharmaceutical Science and Technology, Institute of Chemical Technology, N. P. Marg, Matunga, Mumbai, Maharashtra 400 019, India

Mei Meng, Jian Liu, Jia-rong Gao, Yue Sun and Chuan-bing Huang
Department of Pharmacy, The First Affiliated Hospital of Anhui University of Chinese Medicine, 117 Meishan Road, Hefei 230031, China

Hui Jiang
Department of Pharmacy, The First Affiliated Hospital of Anhui University of Chinese Medicine, 117 Meishan Road, Hefei 230031, China
College of Basic Medicine, Anhui Medical University, 81 Meishan Road, Hefei 230022, China

Ting Wang and Xiu-juan Qin
College of Pharmacy, Anhui University of Chinese Medicine, 103Meishan Road, Hefei 230038, China

Evagelia Trigoni, Alexandra Tsirogianni, and Chryssa Papasteriades
Department of Immunology-Histocompatibility, "Evangelismos" General Hospital, 10676 Athens, Greece

Elena Pipi
Department of Dermatology, University of Lübeck, 23562 Lübeck, Germany

Gerassimos Mantzaris
Department of Gastroenterology, "Evangelismos" General Hospital, 10676 Athens, Greece

Emilio Besada
Bone and Joint Research Group, Institute of Clinical Medicine, UiT The Arctic University of Norway, 9037 Tromsø, Norway

Ondrej Dolezal
NHS Scotland, Dumfries and Galloway Royal Infirmary, Bankend Road, Dumfries DG14AP, UK

Leila Tahernia
Growth and Development Research Center, Tehran University of Medical Sciences, Tehran, Iran
Children's Medical Center, Pediatrics Center of Excellence, Tehran, Iran

Hosein Alimadadi
Department of Pediatrics, Tehran University of Medical Sciences, Tehran, Iran
Pediatric Gastroenterology and Hepatology Research Center, Tehran University of Medical Sciences, Tehran, Iran

Fatemeh Tahghighi
Children's Medical Center, Pediatrics Center of Excellence, Tehran, Iran
Department of Pediatrics, Tehran University of Medical Sciences, Tehran, Iran

Zahra Amini
Children's Medical Center, Pediatrics Center of Excellence, Tehran, Iran

Vahid Ziaee
Children's Medical Center, Pediatrics Center of Excellence, Tehran, Iran
Department of Pediatrics, Tehran University of Medical Sciences, Tehran, Iran
Pediatric Rheumatology Research Group, Rheumatology Research Center, Tehran University of Medical Sciences, Tehran, Iran

J. B. Winer
Queen Elizabeth Hospital, B15 2TH Birmingham, UK

Somayeh Khezri, Hamid-Reza Mahmoudi, Seyedeh Nina Masoom, Maryam Daneshpazhooh, Kamran Balighi and Cheyda Chams-Davatchi
Autoimmune Bullous Diseases Research Center, Department of Dermatology, Tehran University of Medical Sciences, Razi Hospital, Vahdate-Eslami Square, Tehran 11996, Iran

S. Hamed Hosseini
Knowledge Utilization Research Center, School of Public Health, Tehran University of Medical Sciences, Tehran 1417613151, Iran

Nancy J. Olsen, Carl McAloose and Jamie Carter
Division of Rheumatology, Department of Medicine, Penn State MS Hershey Medical Center, Hershey, PA, USA

Bobby Kwanghoon Han
Division of Rheumatology, Department of Medicine, University of Washington, Seattle, WA, USA

Indu Raman and Quan-Zhen Li
Department of Immunology, University of Texas Southwestern Medical Center, Dallas, TX, USA

Duanping Liao
Department of Public Health Sciences, Penn State University, College of Medicine, Hershey, PA, USA

Alejandro Caro Pérez, M. Consuelo Alonso Cañizal and Lorena Alonso Díez
Gennova Research, Gennova Scientific S.L. Seville, Spain

Sarita Kumble and Krishnanand D. Kumble
Pictor Limited, Auckland, New Zealand

Luis M. Jiménez Jiménez and Pilar Durán Parejo
Department of Metabolopathy, Hospital Virgen del Rocio, Seville, Spain

Tyler T Wright, Rachel V. Jimenez and Alexander J. Szalai
Department of Medicine, The University of Alabama Birmingham, Birmingham, AL 35294, USA

Todd E. Morgan, Namrata Bali, Xiaogang Hou and Caleb E. Finch
Davis School of Gerontology and Department of Biological Sciences, The University of Southern California, Los Angeles, CA 90089, USA

Mark A. McCrory
Department of Pathology, The University of Alabama Birmingham, Birmingham, AL 35294, USA

Zeinab Fagheei Aghmiyuni and Ahmad Khorshidi
Department of Microbiology and Immunology, Faculty of Medicine, Kashan University of Medical Sciences, Kashan, Iran

Rezvan Moniri
Department of Microbiology and Immunology, Faculty of Medicine, Kashan University of Medical Sciences, Kashan, Iran
Anatomical Sciences Research Center, Kashan University of Medical Sciences, Kashan, Iran

Tahereh Soori
Razi Hospital, Tehran University of Medical Sciences, Tehran 11996 63911, Iran

Seyed Gholam Abbas Musavi
Department of Statistics, Health Faculty, Kashan University of Medical Sciences, Kashan, Iran

Fabio Bonilla-Abadía, Carlos A. Cañas, Gabriel J. Tobón and Andrés F. Echeverri
Rheumatology Unit, Fundación Valle del Lili, ICESI University, Carrera 98 18-49, Cali, Colombia

Nicolás Coronel Restrepo
Internal Medicine Unit, Fundación Valle del Lili, CES University, Cali, Colombia

Evelyn Muñoz-Buitrón and Andres Mauricio Castro
Clinical Research Unit, Fundación Valle del Lili, Cali, Colombia

Mercedes Andrade Bejarano
School of Statistics, Universidad del Valle, Cali, Colombia

Anabel Barrera García, Catalina Burbano and Mauricio Rojas
Grupo de Inmunología Celular e Inmunogenética, GICIG, Universidad de Antioquía, Medellín, Colombia

Mauricio Restrepo, Adriana L. Vanegas, Carlos H. Muñoz and Luis A. González
2Grupo de Reumatología, Universidad de Antioquía, Medellín, Colombia

José A. Gómez-Puerta and Gloria Vásquez
Grupo de Inmunología Celular e Inmunogenética, GICIG, Universidad de Antioquía, Medell´ın, Colombia
Grupo de Reumatología, Universidad de Antioquía, Medellín, Colombia

Luis F. Arias
Grupo de Patología Renal y Trasplante, Universidad de Antioquía, Medellín, Colombia

Fernanda Weyand Banhuk and Rafael Andrade Menolli
Laboratory of Applied Immunology, Center of Medical and Pharmaceutical Sciences, Western Parana State University, Cascavel /PR 85819-110, Brazil

Bruna Corrêa Pahim and Alex Sandro Jorge
Laboratory of Clinical Immunology, Western Parana University Hospital, Western Parana State University, Cascavel, PR 85806-470, Brazil

C. R. Newey
Department of Neurology, University of Missouri, 5 Hospital Drive, CE 540, Columbia, MO 65211, USA

A. Sarwal
Neurology and Critical Care, Wake Forest University School of Medicine, Reynolds M, Medical Center Boulevard, Winston-Salem, NC 27157, USA

S. Hantus
Department of Adult Neurology, Cleveland Clinic, 9500 Euclid Avenue, Cleveland, OH 44195-5245, USA
Epilepsy Center, Neurologic Institute, Cleveland Clinic, 9500 Euclid Avenue, Cleveland, OH 44195-5245, USA

Index